Here are your

1997 WORLD BOOK HEALTH & MEDICAL ANNUAL Cross-Reference Tabs

For insertion in your WORLD BOOK set

The Cross-Reference Tab System is designed to help link THE WORLD BOOK HEALTH & MEDICAL ANNUAL'S major articles to related WORLD BOOK articles. When you later look up a topic in your WORLD BOOK and find a Tab by the article, you will know that one of your HEALTH & MEDICAL ANNUALS has newer or more detailed information.

How to use these Tabs

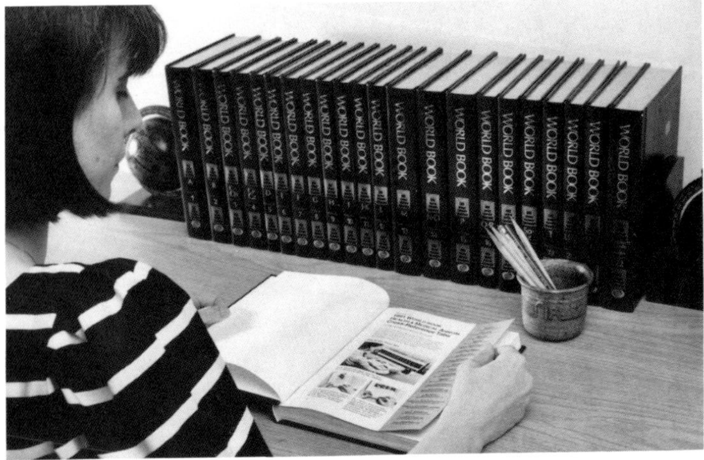

First, remove this page from THE HEALTH & MEDICAL ANNUAL.

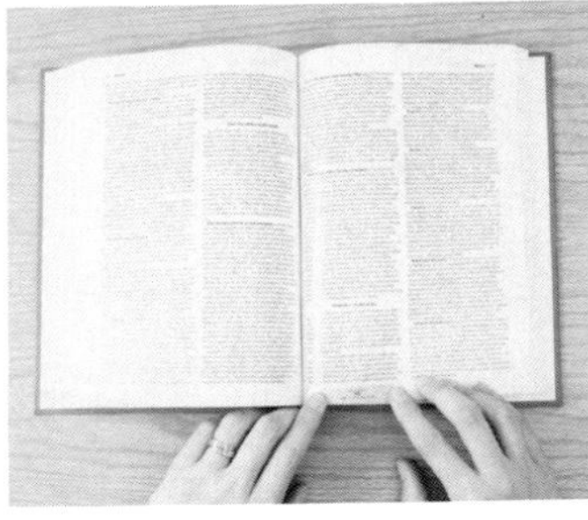

Begin with the first Tab, **AIDS.** Take the *A* volume of your WORLD BOOK set and find the **AIDS** article. Moisten the **AIDS** tab and affix it to that page by the article.

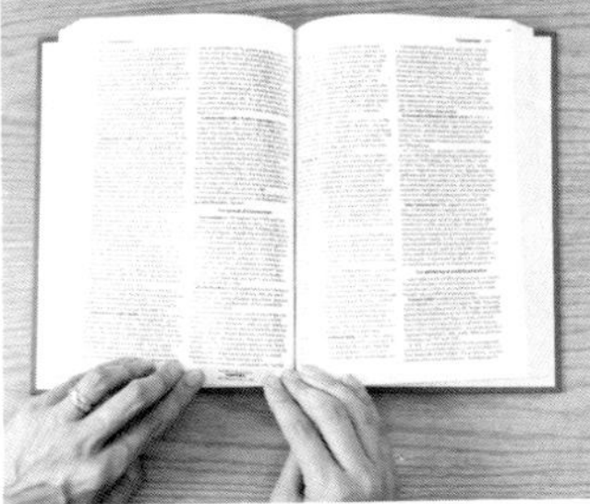

Glue all the other Tabs in the appropriate volumes. Your *H* volume does not have an article on **HEALTH RISKS.** Put that tab in its correct alphabetical location in the *H* volume—near the **HEALTH MAINTENANCE ORGANIZATION** listing.

On the Medical Frontier
AIDS
1997 Health & Medical Annual, p. 194

Medical and Safety Alerts
ALLERGY
1997 Health & Medical Annual, p. 140

A Healthy Family
ESTROGEN
1997 Health & Medical Annual, p. 70

Medical and Safety Alerts
EYE
1997 Health & Medical Annual, p. 154

A Healthy Family
FOOT
1997 Health & Medical Annual, p. 42

Medical and Safety Alerts
GLAUCOMA
1997 Health & Medical Annual, p. 154

A Healthy Family
HEALTH RISKS
1997 Health & Medical Annual, p. 116

A Healthy Family
HEARTBURN
1997 Health & Medical Annual, p. 98

A Healthy Family
HORMONE
1997 Health & Medical Annual, p. 70

On the Medical Frontier
JOINT
1997 Health & Medical Annual, p. 208

On the Medical Frontier
LASER
1997 Health & Medical Annual, p. 180

A Healthy Family
MEMORY
1997 Health & Medical Annual, p. 56

Medical and Safety Alerts
OFFICE HEALTH HAZARDS
1997 Health & Medical Annual, p. 124

A Healthy Family
OLD AGE
1997 Health & Medical Annual, p. 82

A Healthy Family
STOMACH
1997 Health & Medical Annual, p. 98

Spotlight on Stress
STRESS
1997 Health & Medical Annual, p. 10

On the Medical Frontier
SURGERY
1997 Health & Medical Annual, p. 180

A Healthy Family
TEETH
1997 Health & Medical Annual, p. 106

On the Medical Frontier
VIRUS
1997 Health & Medical Annual, p. 194

On the Medical Frontier
WEIGHT CONTROL
1997 Health & Medical Annual, p. 166

THE WORLD BOOK

HEALTH & MEDICAL ANNUAL

1997

World Book, Inc.
a Scott Fetzer company
Chicago London Sydney Toronto

THE YEAR'S MAJOR HEALTH STORIES

From early reports of success in combating the AIDS virus with a combination drug therapy to the promise of new weapons against obesity, it was an eventful year in medicine. On these two pages are stories that *Health & Medical Annual* editors selected as among the year's most important, memorable, or promising, along with information about where to find them in the book. The Editors

AIDS drug therapies

"Cocktails" made from several drugs show promise in early tests of stopping the AIDS virus from reproducing and wreaking its havoc. In the section On the Medical Frontier, see SCIENCE VERSUS THE AIDS VIRUS.

Clot-buster clouts strokes

The clot-busting drug TPA, used to treat heart attacks, wins approval for treating strokes in June 1996 after studies show it prevents damage to the brain if administered promptly. In the Health Updates and Resources section, see STROKE.

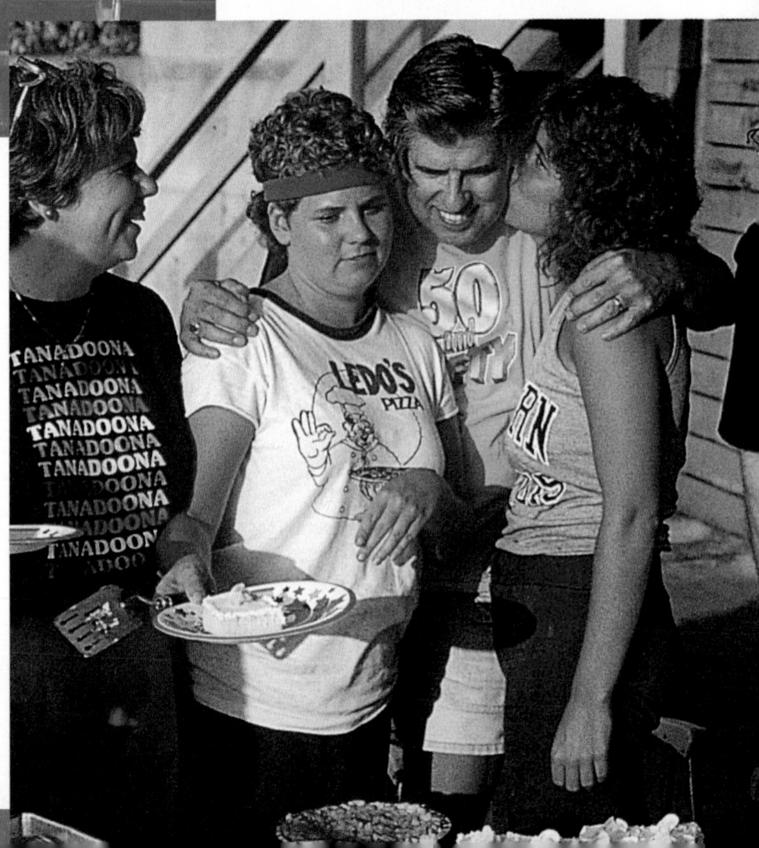

The graying of America

The first baby boomers hit 50 in 1996, and 10,000 Americans on average will turn 50 every day for the next decade. In the Health Updates and Resources section, see AGING.

World Book, Inc.
525 W. Monroe
Chicago, IL 60661

ISBN 0-7166-1197-X
ISSN 0890-4480
Library of Congress Catalog Card Number: 87-648075
Printed in the United States of America

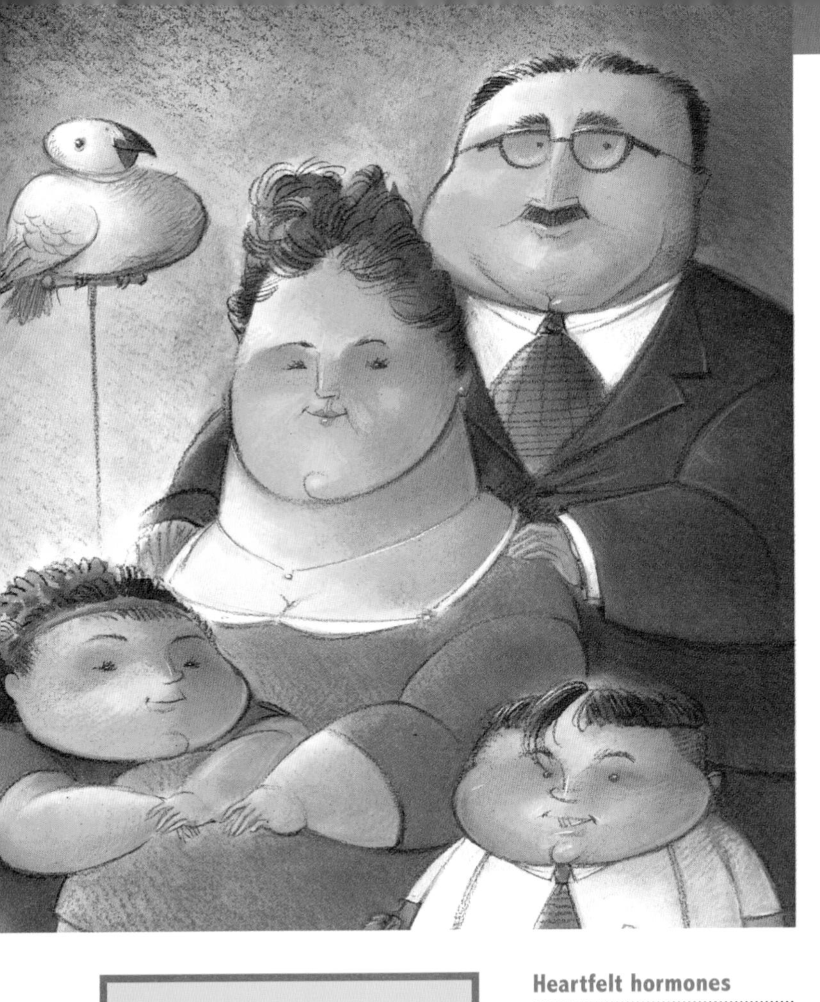

Waist disposal

A weight-loss drug based on the hormone leptin goes into human testing in 1996 after animal studies find that leptin turns obese mice thin. In the section On the Medical Frontier, see NEW WEAPONS IN THE WAR AGAINST WEIGHT.

Hair-raising heredity

Novelty-seeking behavior is tied to a gene in January 1996, marking the first known (though unconfirmed) link between a gene and a specific normal personality trait. In the Health Updates and Resources section, see GENETIC MEDICINE.

Heartfelt hormones

Evidence mounts in 1996 on the benefits of hormone replacement therapy for women's health—the heart in particular. In the section A Healthy Family, see HORMONE REPLACEMENT THERAPY.

Mad cow disease

A scientific report by British scientists in March 1996 links a human brain disorder with beef from infected cattle. In the Health Updates and Resources section, see INFECTIOUS DISEASES.

See page 28.

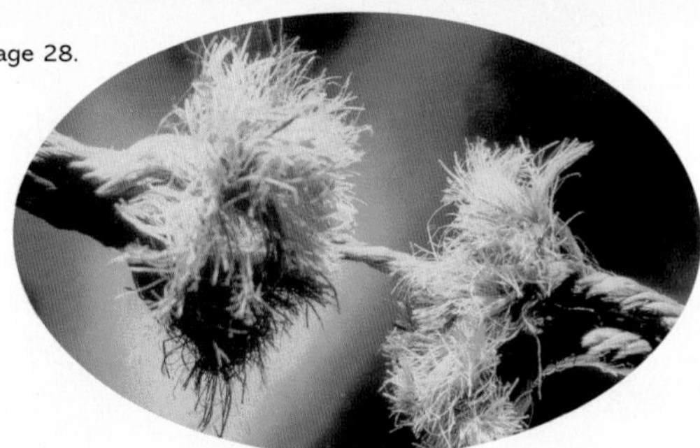

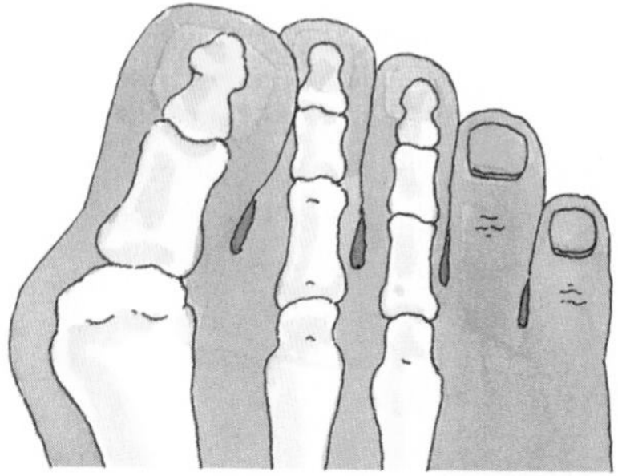

See page 44.

CONTENTS

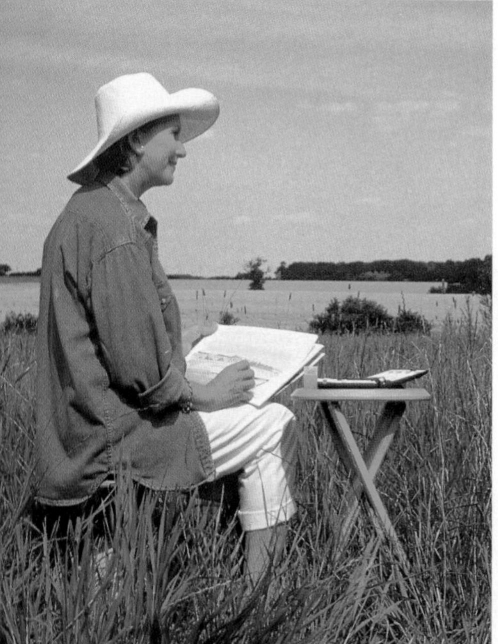

See page 82.

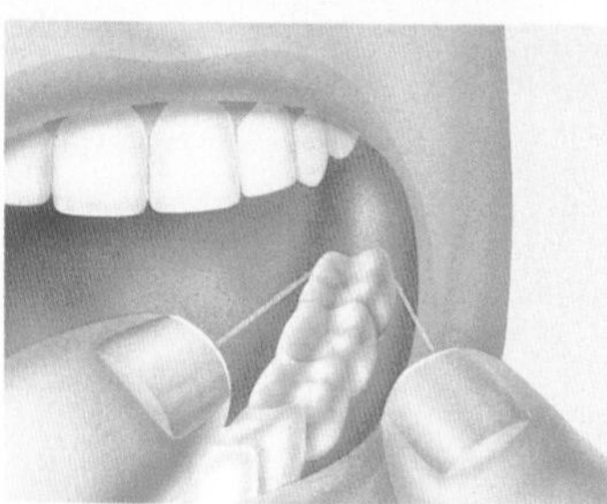

See page 112.

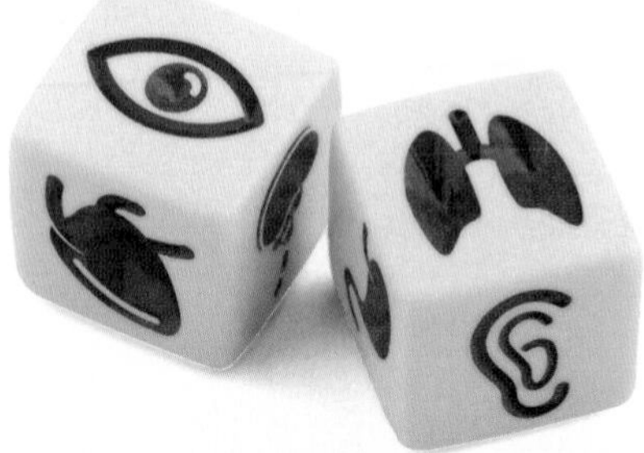

See page 116.

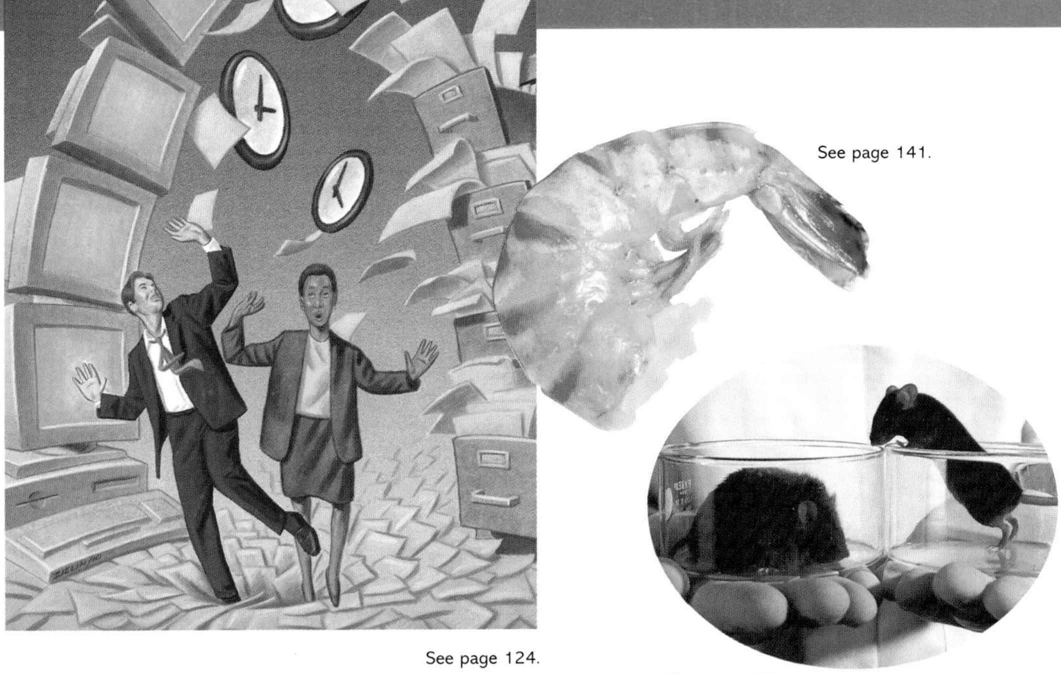

See page 141.

See page 124.

See page 171.

122 Medical and Safety Alerts

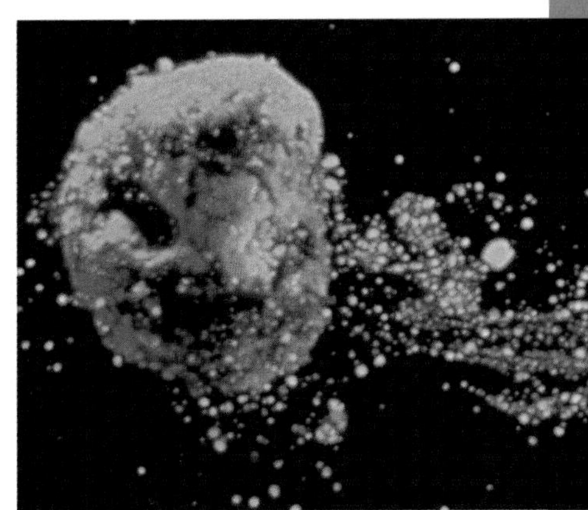

See page 191.

164 On the Medical Frontier

222 Health Updates and Resources

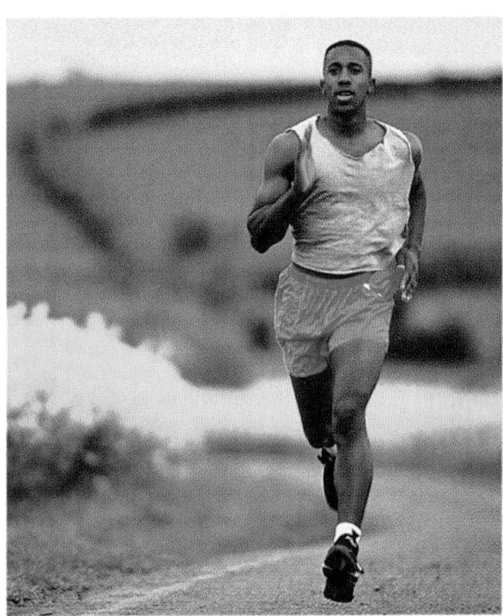

See page 270.

Staff

IMPORTANT NOTE: The information contained in *The World Book Health & Medical Annual* is not intended to take the place of the care and attention of a physician or other medical or health care professional. The information contained in *The World Book Health & Medical Annual* is believed to be accurate but cannot be warranted. On any matters related to health, always consult a physician or other appropriate health care professional.

EDITORIAL ADVISORY

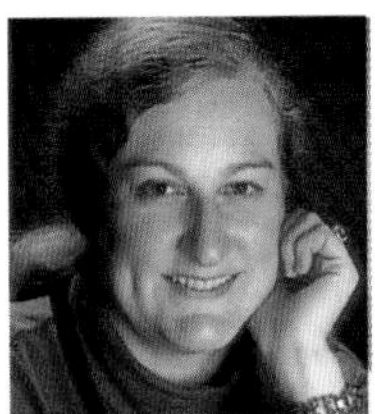

Nadine Bruce, M.D., is Chief of the Division of General Internal Medicine and Program Director of the Internal Medicine Residency at Mt. Sinai Medical Center in Cleveland, Associate Professor of Medicine at Case Western Reserve University School of Medicine, and Medical Director of the Margaret Wagner House in Cleveland Heights. She received the B.S. degree in 1964 from the College of St. Francis and the M.D. degree in 1970 from the University of Illinois at Chicago. She is board-certified in both Internal Medicine and Geriatrics. Dr. Bruce is a Master of the American College of Physicians and former Governor of the College.

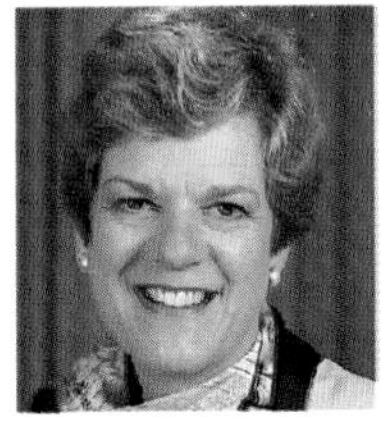

Linda Hawes Clever, M.D., is Chairman of the Department of Occupational Health at California Pacific Medical Center and Clinical Professor of Medicine at the University of California at San Francisco. She received the A.B. degree in 1962 and the M.D. degree in 1965, both from Stanford University. Dr. Clever served on both the Board of Governors of the American College of Physicians and its Board of Regents. Since 1990, she has been Editor of the *Western Journal of Medicine*. She is a member of the Institute of Medicine of the National Academy of Sciences and the Board of Scientific Counselors of the National Institute of Occupational Safety and Health.

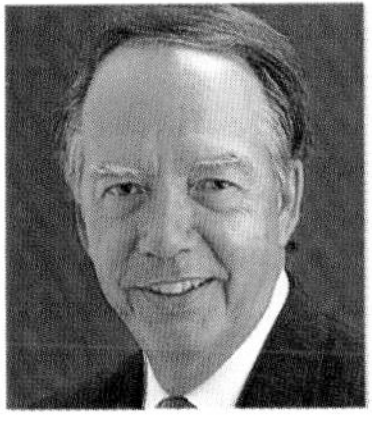

Robert B. McCall, Ph.D., is Professor of Psychology at the University of Pittsburgh and Co-Director of the University's Office of Child Development. He received the B.A. degree from DePauw University in 1962 and the Ph.D. degree from the University of Illinois in 1965. Professor McCall was a contributing editor of *Parents* magazine from 1980 to 1990 and is currently an Associate Editor of the journal *Child Development*. He is a fellow of the American Psychological Association, the American Psychological Society, and the American Association of Applied and Preventive Psychology.

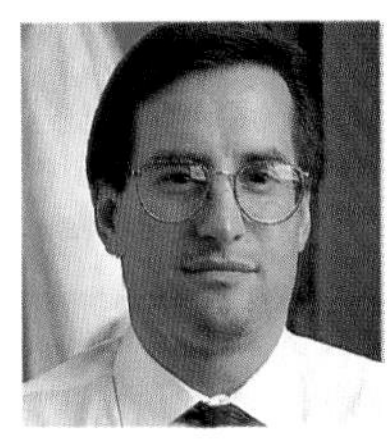

Mark W. Stolar, M.D., is on the faculties of Northwestern University Medical School and Rush University Medical School, where he is Associate Professor of Clinical Medicine. He is also Associate Chief of the Section of General Internal Medicine at the Northwestern Medical Faculty Foundation. Dr. Stolar received the B.A. degree from Northwestern University in 1975 and the M.D. degree from the University of Illinois in 1979. He is on the board of the Endocrine Fellows Foundation and is a member of the American College of Physicians, the Endocrine Society, and the American Society of Clinical Endocrinologists.

CONTRIBUTORS

Balk, Robert A., M.D.
Director of Pulmonary Medicine,
Rush-Presbyterian-St. Luke's
Medical Center.
[Health Updates and Resources:
Respiratory System]

Barone, Jeanine, M.S.
Nutritionist and Contributing
Editor,
*University of California at Berkeley
Wellness Letter.*
[Health Updates and Resources:
Nutrition and Food]

Ben-Gad, Meira, B.A.
Free-Lance Writer and Editor.
[A Healthy Family: *Evaluating
Health Risks*]

Benowitz, Steven I., B.S., M.A.
Free-Lance Science Writer.
[On the Medical Frontier: *Active
Lives with Artificial Joints*]

Birnbaum, Gary, M.D.
Professor of Neurology,
University of Minnesota.
[Health Updates and Resources:
Brain and Nervous System]

Bowers, Kathryn E., M.D.
Associate Dermatologist,
Beth Israel Hospital.
[Health Updates and Resources:
Skin]

Clarke, Peggy, M.P.H.
President, American Social Health
Association.
[Health Updates and Resources:
Sexually Transmitted Diseases]

Cohen, Donna, Ph.D.
Professor and Chair,
Department of Aging and Mental
Health,
University of South Florida.
[A Healthy Family: *Planning Your
Happily Ever After*]

Cohen, Sanford I., M.D.
Senior Vice Chair and Professor,
Department of Psychiatry and
Behavioral Sciences,
University of Miami.
[Spotlight on Stress, *Stress and
Mental Health*]

Crawford, Michael H., M.D.
Robert S. Flinn Professor and
Chief of Cardiology,
University of New Mexico
Health Sciences Center.
[Health Updates and Resources:
Heart and Blood Vessels]

Davis, James N., M.D.
Professor and Chairman,
Department of Neurology,
State University of New York at
Stony Brook School of Medicine.
[Health Updates and Resources:
Stroke]

Eisdorfer, Carl, Ph.D, M.D.
Professor and Chairman,
Department of Psychiatry and
Behavioral Sciences,
University of Miami.
[Spotlight on Stress: *Stress and
Physical Health*]

Franklin, James L., M.D.
Associate Professor,
Rush-Presbyterian-St. Luke's
Medical Center.
[A Healthy Family: *Heartburn:
Taking Aim at Fire;* Health
Updates and Resources:
Digestive System]

Friedman, Emily, B.A.
Health Policy and Ethics Analyst,
Health Policy Section Editor,
*Journal of the American Medical
Association.*
[Health Updates and Resources:
Health-Care Issues]

Gartland, John J., A.B., M.D.
James Edwards Professor
Emeritus of Orthopedic Surgery,
Thomas Jefferson University.
[Health Updates and Resources:
Bone Disorders]

Gerber, Glenn S., M.D.
Assistant Professor,
Department of Surgery,
University of Chicago.
[Health Updates and Resources:
Urology]

Harris, Jules E., M.D.
Samuel G. Taylor III Professor of
Medicine,
Rush University.
[Health Updates and Resources:
Cancer]

Hecht, Jeff, B.S.E.E., M.E.
Contributing Editor,
Laser Focus World magazine.
[On the Medical Frontier: *Laser
Surgery Comes into Focus*]

Hermann, Richard C., M.D.
Staff Psychiatrist, McLean Hospital,
and Research Fellow, Department
of Psychiatry,
Harvard Medical School.
[Health Updates and Resources:
Mental Health]

Hussar, Daniel A., B.S., M.S., Ph.D.
Remington Professor of Pharmacy,
Philadelphia College of Pharmacy
and Science.
[Health Updates and Resources:
Drugs]

Kass, Philip H., D.V.M., Ph.D.
Associate Professor of
Epidemiology,
University of California at Davis.
[Health Updates and Resources:
Veterinary Medicine]

Lapp, Danielle C.
Cognitive Rehabilitation
Specialist,
Department of Psychiatry,
Stanford University Medical
School.
[A Healthy Family: *Remembering
Not to Forget*]

LaRosa, Judith H., R.N., Ph.D.
Clinical Professor of Public Health,
Tulane University.
[A Healthy Family: *Hormone
Replacement Therapy*]

Levine, Carol, M.A.
Executive Director,
The Orphan Project,
Fund for the City of New York.
[Health Updates and Resources:
Medical Ethics]

Lewis, David, C., M.D.
Professor of Medicine and Community Health,
Brown University.
[Health Updates and Resources: *Alcohol and Drug Abuse; Smoking*]

Lewis, Ricki, B.S., M.A., Ph.D.
Adjunct Assistant Professor of Biology,
State University of New York at Albany and University of Miami.
[Health Updates and Resources: *Weight Control*]

Maugh, Thomas H., II, Ph.D.
Science Writer,
Los Angeles Times.
[Health Updates and Resources: *Environmental Health*]

McInerney, Joseph D., B.S., M.A., M.S.
Director, Biological Sciences Curriculum Study.
[Health Updates and Resources: *Genetic Medicine*]

Minotti, Dominick, A., M.D., M.P.H.
Staff Physician,
Northwest Asthma and Allergy Center.
[Health Updates and Resources: *Allergies and Asthma*]

Moore, Margaret E., A.M.L.S., M.P.H.
Head, Education Services,
Health Sciences Library,
University of North Carolina at Chapel Hill.
[Health Updates and Resources: *Books of Health and Medicine*]

Osborn, June E., M.D.
Professor of Epidemiology and Pediatrics,
University of Michigan School of Public Health.
[On the Medical Frontier: *Science Versus the AIDS Virus*]

Pisetsky, David S., M.D., Ph.D.
Chief, Division of Rheumatology, Allergy and Clinical Immunology,
Duke University Medical Center.
[Health Updates and Resources: *Arthritis and Connective Tissue Disorders*]

Prinz, Richard A., M.D.
Helen Shedd Keith Professor and Chairman,
Rush-Presbyterian-St. Luke's Medical Center.
[Health Updates and Resources: *Surgery*]

Reese, Jennifer M.
Free-Lance Writer.
[Medical and Safety Alerts: *Health Hazards at the Office*]

Rinehart, Rebecca D.
Associate Director, Publications,
American College of Obstetricians and Gynecologists.
[Health Updates and Resources: *Pregnancy and Childbirth*]

Roodman, G. David, M.D., Ph.D.
Chief of Hematology Section,
Audie Murphy Veterans Administration Medical Center.
[Health Updates and Resources: *Blood*]

Siscovick, David S., M.D., M.P.H.
Professor of Medicine and Epidemiology,
University of Washington.
[Health Updates and Resources: *Exercise and Fitness*]

Stephenson, Joan, B.S., Ph.D.
Associate Editor, *Journal of the American Medical Association*.
[Medical and Safety Alerts: *Food Allergies: When Common Foods Cause Uncommon Reactions*]

Thompson, Jeffrey R., M.D.
President,
Dallas Kidney Specialists.
[Health Updates and Resources: *Kidney*]

Tideiksaar, Rein, Ph.D.
Director, Department of Geriatric Care Coordination,
Sierra Health Services, Inc.
[Health Updates and Resources: *Aging*]

Tremaine, M. David, M.D.
Orthopedic Surgeon and Director,
Foot and Ankle Center,
Anderson Clinic.
[A Healthy Family: *Feet: A User's Manual*]

Trubo, Richard, B.A., M.A.
Free-Lance Medical Writer.
[On the Medical Frontier: *New Weapons in the War Against Weight;* Health Updates and Resources: *AIDS; Child Development; Diabetes; Ear and Hearing*]

Van Herle, Andre J., M.D.
Professor of Medicine,
UCLA School of Medicine.
[Health Updates and Resources: *Glands and Hormones*]

Weiss, Sharlene M., R.N., Ph.D.
Associate Professor and Director,
the Cortelis Center,
University of Miami.
[Spotlight on Stress: *Managing Stress*]

Weiss, Stephen M., M.P.H., PH.D.
Professor of Psychiatry and Behavioral Sciences,
University of Miami.
[Spotlight on Stress: *The Nature of Stress; The Stress Response*]

Wilensky, Jacob T., M.D.
Professor of Ophthalmology,
University of Illinois at Chicago College of Medicine.
[Medical and Safety Alerts: *Glaucoma Watch*]

Woods, Michael, B.S.
Science Editor, *The Toledo Blade*.
[A Healthy Family: *Healthy Gums;* Health Updates and Resources: *Dentistry; Eye and Vision, Infectious Diseases; Safety*]

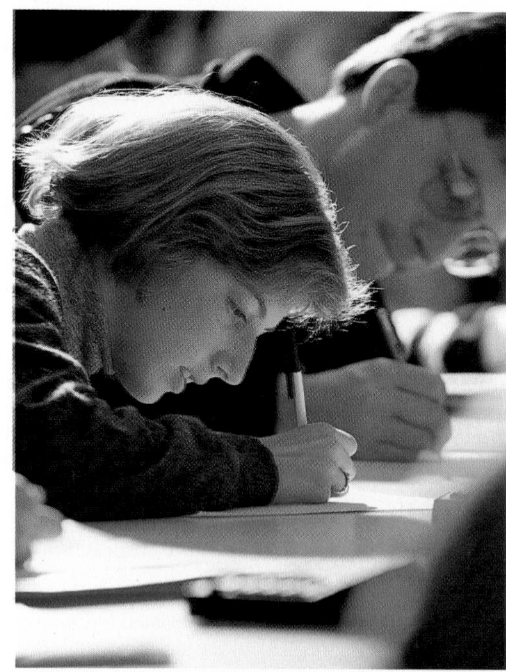

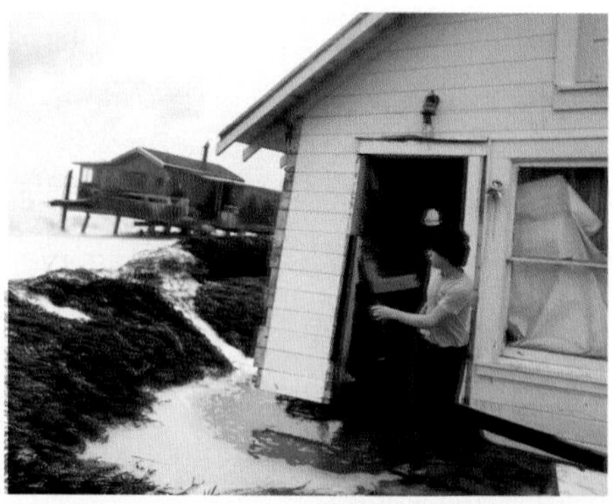

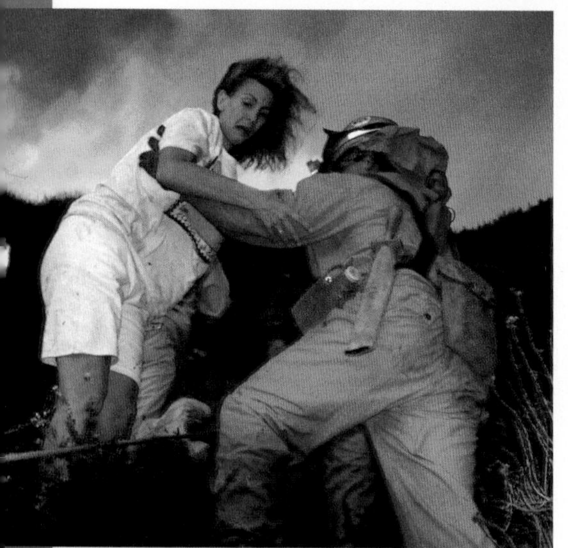

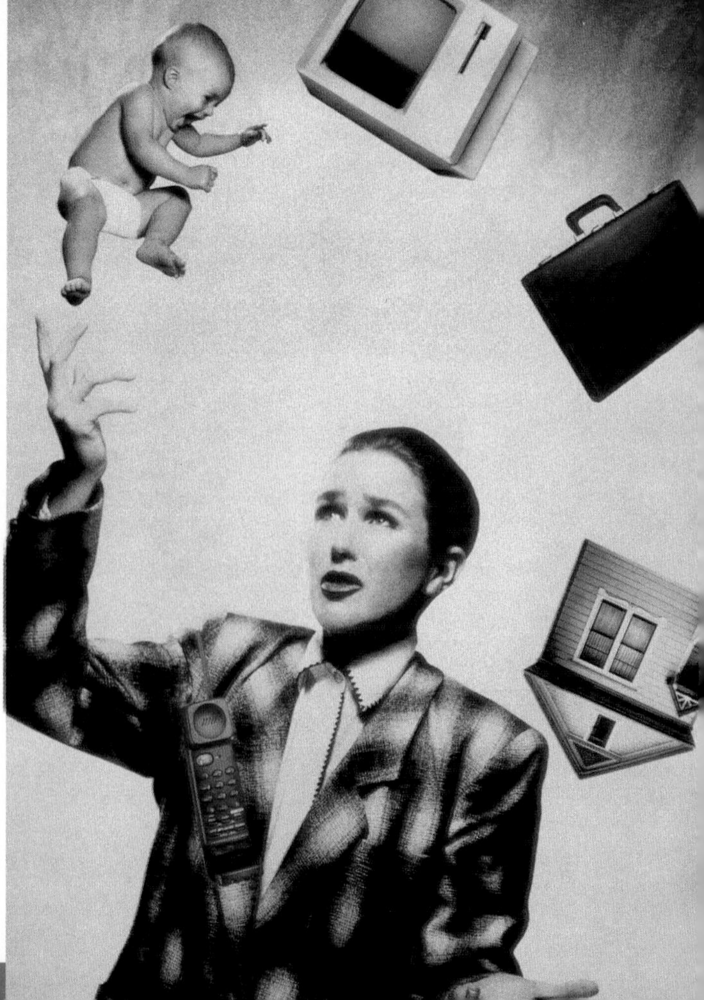

Spotlight on Stress

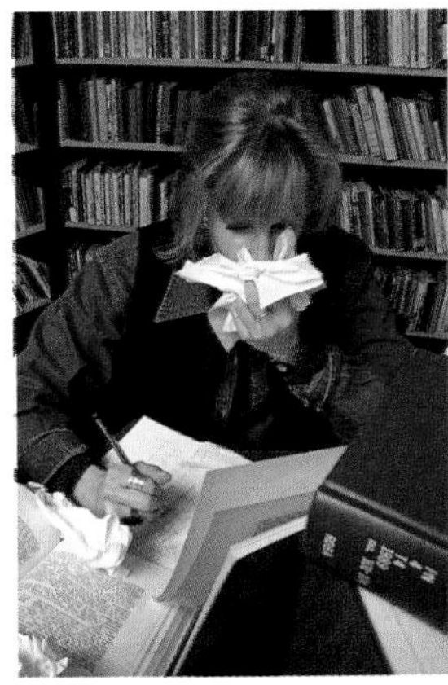

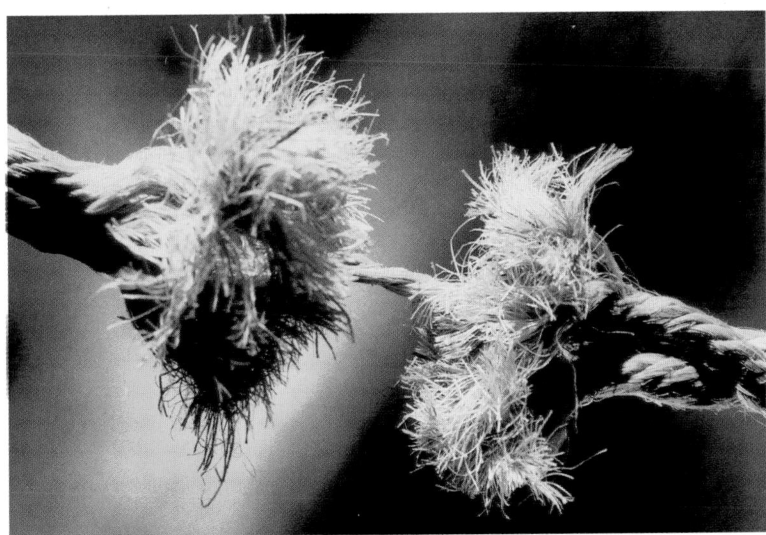

Understanding stress and its influence on health is one of the more complex tasks facing scientists today.

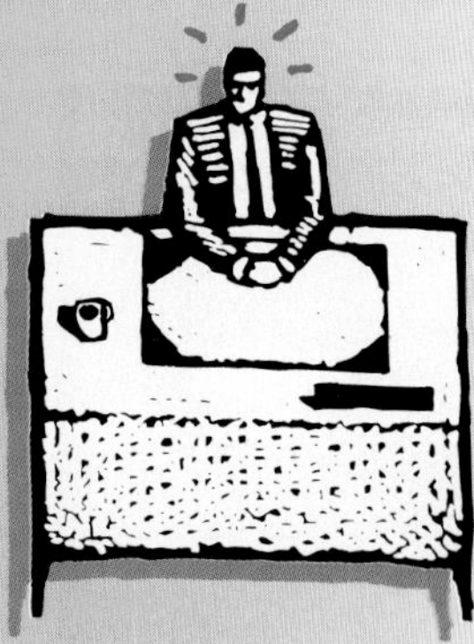

The Nature of STRESS

By Stephen M. Weiss

STRESS IS PROBABLY ONE OF THE MOST MISUNDERSTOOD WORDS in the English language. Thousands of books, scientific papers, and popular articles have attempted to explain the concept, defining stress in dozens of ways.

The term stress was borrowed from physics and first used in connection with health issues in 1936 by Hans Selye, a Canadian physician-researcher who became one of the most prolific writers on the subject. Selye defined stress as the body's response to any real or imagined demand placed upon it.

In everyday speech, when people talk about stress, they are usually referring to a situation or experience that puts them under a strain—for example, "stress at work." Selye, however, applied the term *stressor* to such demands upon an individual. He reserved the word stress for the body's physiological and biochemical response to those demands. The body's response to stressors, Selye believed, could be positive—a condition he called *eustress*—or negative, which he termed *distress*.

A certain amount of stress in life helps people be productive and feel challenged and energized. In the early 1900's, two American psychologists, Robert Yerkes and John Dodson, charted a relationship between stress and performance. Up to a point, they found, stress improves performance. But at some point, stress becomes overwhelming and counterproductive, and then it can lead to health problems.

The author:

Stephen M. Weiss is Director of the Division of Behavioral Medicine at the University of Miami School of Medicine.

Two main types of stressors

Scientists divide *stressors* (factors that produce stress) into two groups: external and internal. Stressors can work individually or in combination to trigger a stress response.

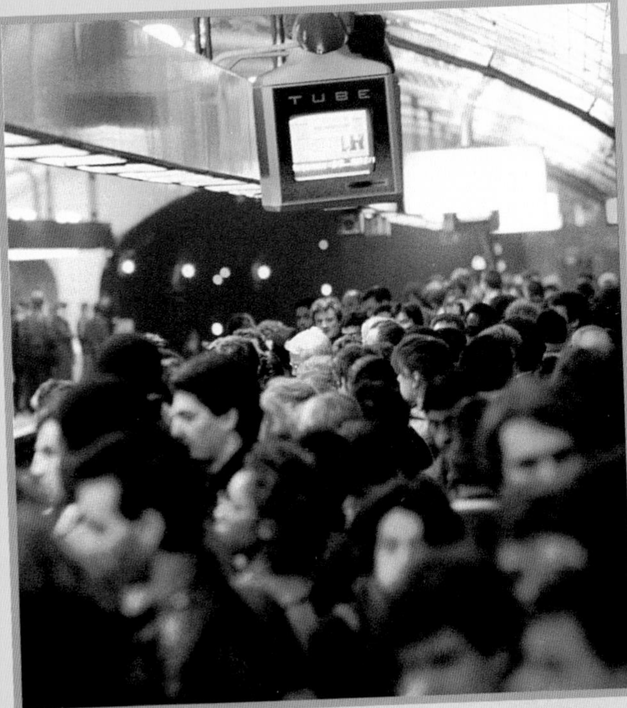

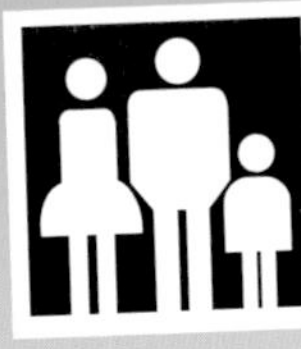

External stressors

External stressors are found in the physical environment in which people live and work and in social, cultural, and political circumstances.

- Environmental stressors include noise, crowding, and extreme temperatures.
- Social stressors include conflict with family members, unrewarding social interactions, and difficulties at work.
- Cultural and political stressors include racial tensions and national upheaval.

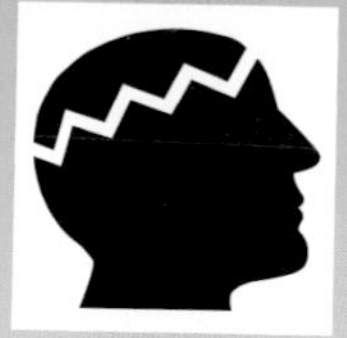

Internal stressors

Internal stressors, also referred to as emotional or psychological stressors, involve thoughts, memories, and feelings. Internal stressors are usually harder to pin down than external stressors, and their effect on health is less direct. Examples include:

- Worrying about money, one's job, or performing well on a test.
- Remembering an angry confrontation.
- Feeling sad after the loss of a loved one.

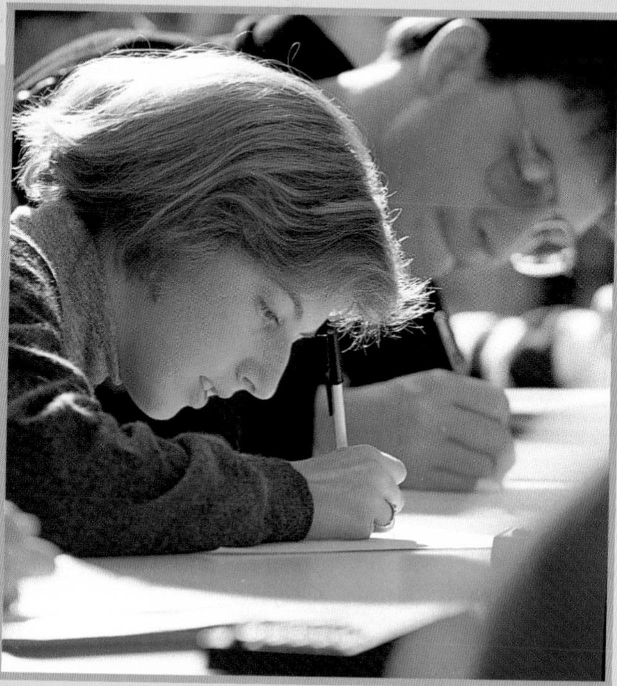

Scientists divide the demands that produce stress into two main groups: external and internal. External stressors can be found outside us, in the physical environment in which we live and work and in our social, cultural, and political circumstances. Examples of stressors in the environment include crowding, noise, and extreme temperatures. Social stressors might be unfulfilling family relationships, unsatisfying work, and unrewarding social interactions. Cultural and political stressors include racial tensions, national upheaval, and government repression.

Internal stressors, also described as psychological and emotional stressors, come from within—from thoughts, memories, and feelings. Recalling an angry confrontation, for example, can reawaken the stressful emotions it initially provoked. Anticipatory anxiety that a performance won't be good enough can be more stressful than the performance itself. Internal stressors are typically more difficult to pin down than external stressors, and their effect on health is less direct.

All types of stressors can affect health, both individually and in combination. If people lived in controlled laboratory conditions, scientists could probably determine exactly which stressors provoke what kind of stress response in any given individual. But real life is far too complex, making it next to impossible for researchers to isolate particular stressors and observe people's responses to them. What scientists have learned is that similar stressors can provoke greatly different stress responses. An individual's response to stressful situations is governed by genetics, experience, personality, and perception.

Shaping the stress response

The genes that we inherit from our parents provide predispositions to particular resistances or vulnerabilities. For example, some people are more resistant to pain-induced stress than others or more vulnerable to stress-provoked allergies. These built-in sensitivities and resistances influence the way that people's bodies react to their environment.

Experience means our personal history. People cannot change what has happened to them, but how they remember the past colors their reactions to future events. Thus, a person who experienced a disruptive move as a child may find changing homes stressful as an adult. Personality also affects reactions to events. Someone who is cautious by nature may experience severe stress in response to a change in routine that another person barely notices.

All these factors influence perceptions—whether someone perceives a particular situation as challenging, threatening, or joyful, for example. The imminent prospect of jumping out of an airplane at 10,000 feet would be likely to evoke very different stress responses in a 26-year-old experienced sky diver and a 55-year-old surgeon who was trying the sport for the first time. But their individual perceptions would be quite different in a situation in which they were both called on to save the life of a severely injured accident victim.

As the example indicates, people's responses to various situations depend on their perceptions of those situations. Such perceptions, which are shaped by one's personality and experience, are what give personal meaning to a situation and determine the individual stress response.

Perceptions also determine the way people remember past events. Many circumstances, particularly age, influence these perceptions. Going back to visit a childhood home often brings the awareness that a house remembered as huge is actually rather small. In a similar way, stressful, emotionally charged memories from early years may become "enlarged" over time, increasing a person's vulnerability to similar experiences later in life. For example, a child who is often bullied may become an adult who is timid and afraid of confrontation.

How important is control?

The amount of control people feel that they have over the events affecting their lives also influences a person's stress response. This sense of control affects decisions people make on the job, their willingness to take risks, their ability to take charge of their health, and other personal qualities. But even a sense of control does not shield people from the stress response.

Since the 1960's, scientists have studied the relationship between stress and control through experiments with rats, mice, and monkeys. In the studies, the animals are exposed to a stressor, such as a mild electric shock. One group of animals is able to control the stressor in some way—for example, by pressing a lever to stop the shock. The other group has no control over the stressor.

The studies have found that animals lacking control demonstrate a greater stress response at first. However, as the stressor gradually increases in magnitude, the situation is reversed: The animals that are allowed to control the situation show a larger stress response than the other animals, whose responses remain about the same regardless of the magnitude of the stressor.

The animals lacking control seem to accept their situation; the animals accustomed to having control struggle to manage the extreme stressor. These experiments show that in dealing with extremely stressful situations, a sense of control does not necessarily lessen the stress response. At times, power may be more stressful than powerlessness.

Understanding stress and its effects on health is one of the more complicated tasks facing scientists who study human behavior and its biological basis. Although researchers have begun to unravel the workings of the stress response, much remains to be learned about countering the negative effects of stress. •••

The stress response helps people meet the challenges of daily life, but it can also become a danger to health.

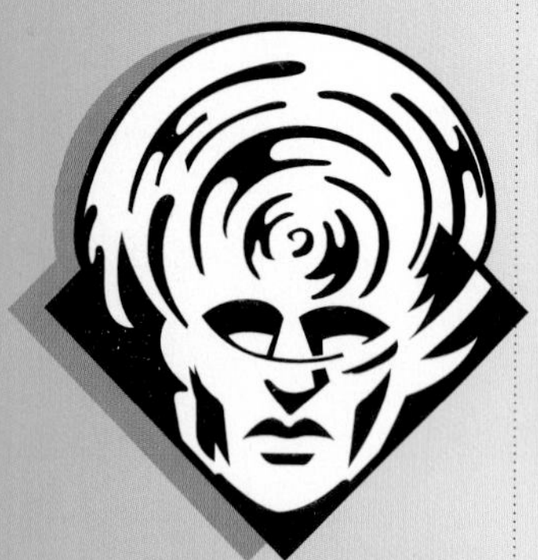

The Stress Response

By Stephen M. Weiss

STRESS IS THE REACTION OF OUR BODIES to the challenges and complexities of daily life. In response to stressful situations, physical, chemical, and emotional changes that serve an important purpose occur in our bodies. But the stress response can become dangerous when triggered in the wrong situations or when it is too intense or continues too long.

Scientists have just begun to unravel the intricate, multilayered interaction of biology, behavior, and environment involved in stress. Their discoveries are part of a new field called behavioral medicine. This specialty enlists the modern technology of medicine to clarify the stress response and to determine the effects of stress on health and human performance.

We have essentially the same biological equipment as our earliest ancestors, who often faced such immediate physical dangers as the possibility of being eaten by saber-toothed tigers or stepped on by woolly mammoths. Early human beings needed instant energy and lots of it to help them deal with these emergencies. In the 1930's, physiologist Walter Cannon described the "fight-or-flight response," a fundamental surge of physical resources to provide peak efficiency during emergency situations. With the body revving in high gear,

The author:

Stephen M. Weiss is Director of the Division of Behavioral Medicine at the University of Miami School of Medicine.

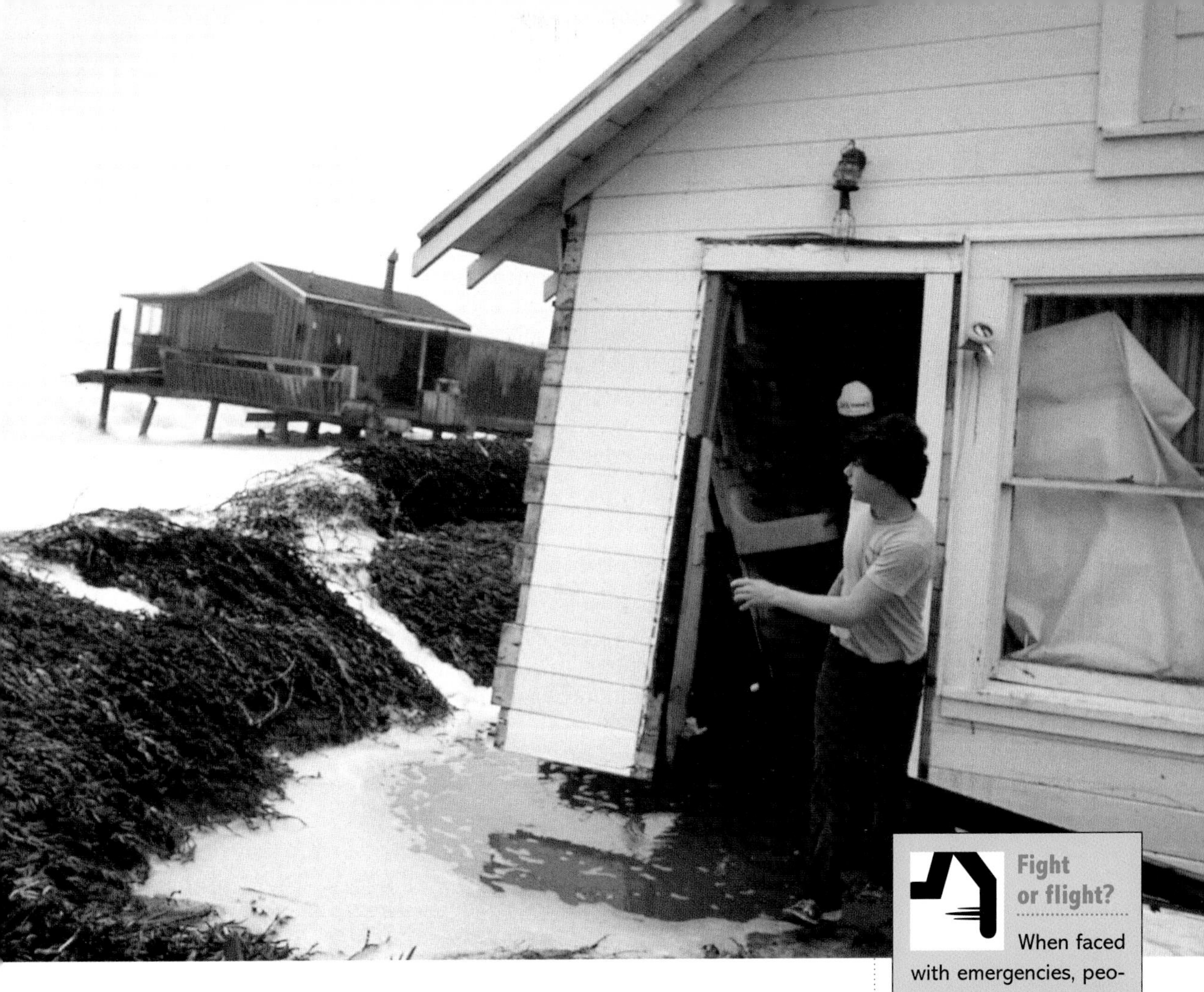

we are primed to confront the challenge or to escape from it. To balance this outlay of resources, bodily functions that are not needed in the crisis, such as digestion or salivation, are slowed down or stopped.

In an emergency, a part of the brain called the hypothalamus commands the release of *hormones* (chemical messengers that control various body activities) from different places in the body. The main stress hormones are epinephrine and norepinephrine. Epinephrine is produced by the adrenal glands, located just above the kidneys; norepinephrine is produced in many places. Together, they stimulate a range of physical responses in the body's organs. The heart rate speeds up, blood pressure rises, breathing grows deeper and faster, blood flow is rerouted from digestion to muscles, and blood clots faster. Simultaneously, hormones release stored fats and sugars to provide a surge of energy. All of these changes ready the body for fight or flight.

The Canadian physiologist Hans Selye, a pioneer stress researcher, called this stress response the General Adaptation Syndrome, dividing the body's response to *stressors* (real or imagined external demands) into three stages: alarm, resistance, and exhaustion.

Fight or flight?

When faced with emergencies, people need instant energy to help them either fight or flee. In the 1930's, physiologist Walter Cannon described the "fight-or-flight response," a surge of physical resources that allows the body to operate at peak efficiency during high-stress situations. To balance this outlay of energy, bodily functions not needed during the crisis, such as digestion or salivation, are slowed down or stopped.

In the alarm stage, defenses are mobilized through the release of stress hormones, which prepare the body for fight or flight. In the resistance stage, the body deals with the stressor but continues to release stress hormones in reduced amounts. Although it appears that the body has returned to a normal state, physiological responses continue to occur. In the exhaustion stage, physiological responses consume the body's resources and energy fails.

The fight-or-flight response was well-suited to the stressors faced by early human beings. The typical stressful situation in prehistoric times resolved itself quickly: You won and ate—or you lost and were eaten. The urgent nature of such situations was matched by the instant nature of the stress response.

A prehistoric response to modern challenges

Today's life stressors are different from those faced by our ancestors. Modern society exposes us to such stressors as gridlocked traffic, long working hours, money worries, thwarted career ambitions, and complex emotional and social desires and demands. Yet our biological equipment has not changed with the times. Adapted for reaction to life-threatening physical danger, our stress response now kicks in while we wait in traffic or when we anticipate giving an important presentation at work. This discrepancy in cause and effect becomes a problem when the stress response is triggered too often, is too intense, or lasts too long. Wear and tear on the body increases, and the eventual result is a stress-related disease or disorder.

Selye's theory of the stress response has been criticized by other researchers. One of his contemporaries, Yale University psychiatrist John Mason, argued that Selye had ignored the emotional component of stress, which he viewed as central to the stress response. Mason held that external stressors are not sufficient to cause disease. When exposed to the same stressors, some people become susceptible to disease and others remain healthy. Mason argued that individual differences must be considered in order to understand stress.

In the 1980's, psychologist Richard Lazarus and his colleagues at the University of California at Berkeley formulated a comprehensive theory of how *chronic* (persistent) stress affects health. Lazarus emphasized the importance of *cognitive factors* (thoughts) and the personal meaning given to events in determining whether someone experiences stress-related disorders and in what manner. He singled out *vulnerability* and *coping* as fundamental concepts critical for understanding stress. Vulnerability is a lack of social or physical resources necessary to meet a particular challenge. Coping is the process of changing one's thoughts and behavior to deal with stressors that threaten to exceed one's resources.

People who cope successfully are people who believe in their ability to bring about desired results. In addition, successful copers tend to be healthy, high-energy individuals with good problem-solving skills, social support, and financial resources.

For Lazarus, the key to the stress response was neither an external event nor the emotional response to the event, but rather a person's perception of the situation. Success or failure in a stressful encounter shapes the expectation of success in future encounters. According to Lazarus, individual differences in assessing and coping with stressful situations determine the magnitude of the stress response and the likelihood of developing stress-related disorders.

Measuring stress

Laboratory researchers have taken several approaches to measuring stress. The Yerkes-Dodson Curve, for example, charts a relationship between stress and performance. Performance tests typically measure the effects of exposure to a stressor, such as crowding or noise. A difference between an individual's performance of a given task before and after exposure suggests to researchers that the change was caused by the stressor. Performance tests are very useful in measuring the effects of short-term stressors.

Questionnaires and surveys since the late 1950's have attempted to document and quantify stressors in daily life. Perhaps the best known of these tests, which are called self-report scales, is the Social Readjustment Rating Scale (SRRS), developed by American psychiatrists Thomas Holmes and Richard Rahe in 1967. Using the results of stress questionnaires given to people of various ages, ethnic groups, and backgrounds, Holmes and Rahe ranked 43 "life events" according to their severity as stressors. They ranked the death of a spouse and divorce as the two most stressful life events, and minor violations of the law, Christmas, and vacations as the least stressful.

Holmes and Rahe maintained that any change in life patterns had an associated "stressor value," regardless of whether the change was perceived as positive or negative. For example, marriage and outstanding personal achievement were both assigned moderate to high stressor values in the SRRS.

Lazarus and his colleagues developed another

The stress response

In an emergency, changes occur throughout the body. This is the stress response, which prepares a person for the intense effort of attack, defense, or escape.

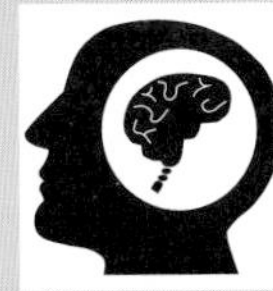

- **Epinephrine is secreted**
  The brain signals the adrenal glands, located just above the kidneys, to secrete the hormone epinephrine. Together with other stress hormones, epinephrine stimulates physical responses throughout the body.

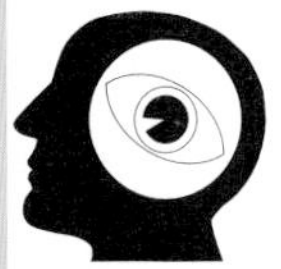

- **Pupils dilate**
  The pupils of the eyes *dilate* (widen) to enhance vision.

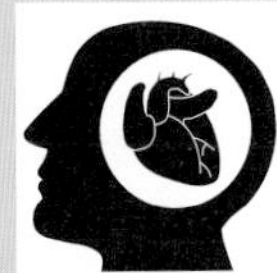

- **Heartbeat accelerates**
  The heart beats faster in order to speed blood, containing oxygen and energy, to where it is needed.

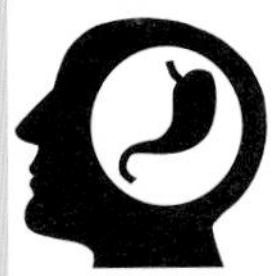

- **Digestion is inhibited**
  The digestive system, not needed during the emergency, shuts down.

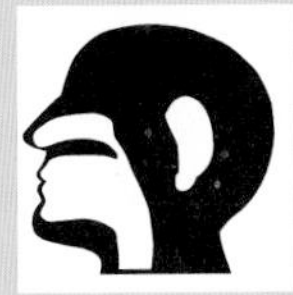

- **Salivation is inhibited**
  Production of saliva, which helps break down food for digestion, is decreased.

Measuring stress: hassles and uplifts

Psychologist Richard Lazarus and his colleagues at the University of California at Berkeley developed a useful method for measuring stress. They devised scales that list events often perceived as stressful (hassles) and those often perceived as positive (uplifts). Individuals indicate the hassles and uplifts they have experienced in a given time period—for example, one month. Below are the hassles and uplifts most frequently cited in a study of 100 white, middle-class adults aged 45 to 64.

Daily hassles scale: Ten most frequent hassles

Item	% Mentioning*
1. Concerns about weight	52.4
2. Health of a family member	48.1
3. Rising prices of common goods	43.7
4. Home maintenance (inside)	42.8
5. Too many things to do	38.6
6. Misplacing or losing things	38.1
7. Yardwork or outside-home maintenance	38.1
8. Property, investment, or taxes	37.6
9. Crime	37.1
10. Physical appearance	35.9

*Percentage of people checking item each month averaged over nine months.
Source: Hassles and Uplifts Scales by Richard S. Lazarus and Susan Folkman.

Uplifts scale: Ten most frequent uplifts

Item	% Mentioning*
1. Relating well with spouse or lover	76.3
2. Relating well with friends	74.4
3. Completing a task	73.3
4. Feeling healthy	72.7
5. Getting enough sleep	69.7
6. Eating out	68.4
7. Meeting responsibilities	68.1
8. Visiting, phoning, or writing someone	67.7
9. Spending time with family	66.7
10. Being pleased with home (inside)	65.6

*Percentage of people checking item each month averaged over nine months.
Source: Hassles and Uplifts Scales by Richard S. Lazarus and Susan Folkman.

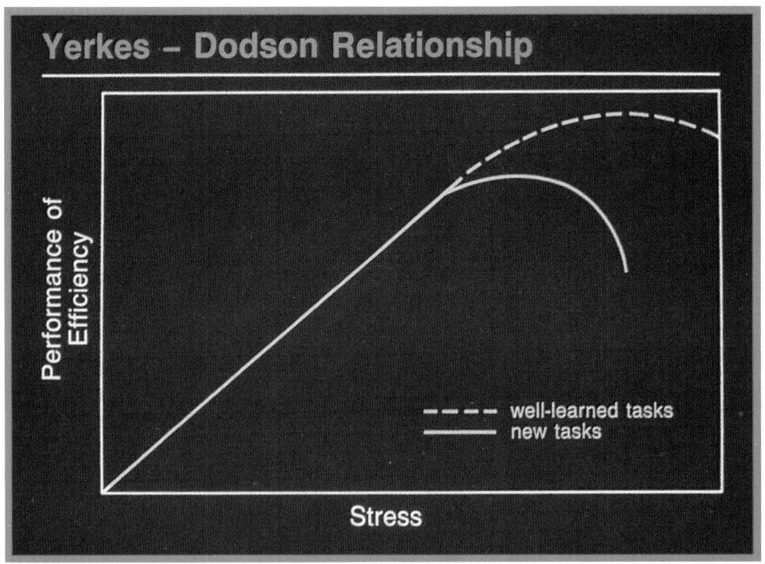

Based on Yerkes and Dodson, 1908.

How stress affects performance

American psychologists Robert Yerkes and John Dodson charted a relationship between stress and performance. Up to a point, stress improves performance, especially on well-learned tasks. But when stress levels are too high, performance declines.

way to measure stress. Rather than focus on major life events, they devised two scales to measure daily "hassles" and "uplifts." Their scoring system strongly weighs how a hassle or uplift is perceived by the person experiencing it.

Scores on the daily hassles scale are stronger predictors of mental and physical illnesses than either the SRRS or the uplifts scale. This agrees with current thinking that one's health status is more closely related to chronic stressors than to major life events, which are generally briefer in nature. Whether uplifts may protect health is still unclear, but they do not seem to have a negative impact.

Devices created for the continuous monitoring of astronauts' physiological status have enormously expanded researchers' ability to measure the effects of stress on the body. Modern technology allows researchers to monitor the brain, heart, blood pressure, and many other stressor-sensitive systems. Changes in sweat gland activity, muscle tension, and breathing can also be detected.

Experiments that measure patterns of stress-related fluctuation in a person's blood pressure may help predict future *hypertension* (high blood pressure) and coronary heart disease. For example, a person's response to stressors in the laboratory, such as being asked to complete a complex task in a limited amount of time, indicates how that individual's cardiovascular system probably responds to the hassles of daily life, such as waiting in lines or having car trouble.

Physiological measures appear to provide the best predictions of stress-related health problems. This area of behavioral medicine holds great potential to reveal in detail the body's extraordinarily complex reaction to real and perceived demands. With this knowledge, modern medicine can seek remedies for disorders arising from our ancestors' successful survival mechanisms. •••

Stress has been linked to many physical ills, but scientists are just beginning to understand how it acts on the body.

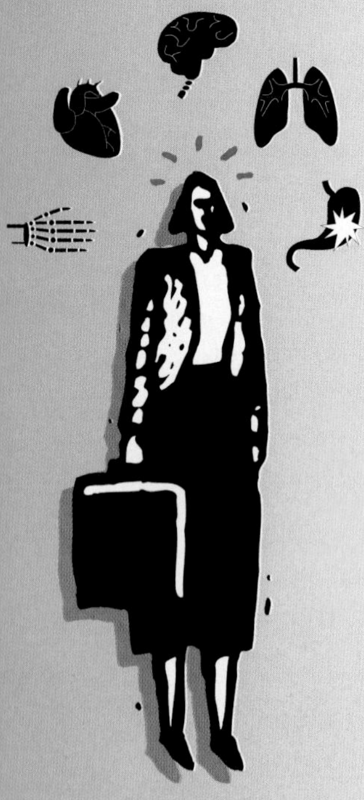

Stress and PHYSICAL HEALTH

By Carl Eisdorfer

ON JAN. 17, 1994, THE DAY A MAJOR EARTHQUAKE ROCKED LOS ANGELES, the number of fatal heart attacks recorded in the region was five times the expected number—24 compared with a daily average of 4.6 for the preceding week. The heart attack rate also soared when Iraqi missiles hit Israeli cities during the Persian Gulf War of 1991. The first day that missiles struck, deaths from heart attacks and strokes in Israel rose to 147, from the usual average of 92.9.

These dramatic events underscored the threat that severe stress poses to the heart. But events need not be so dramatic to endanger the heart. Robert Eliot, a cardiologist who heads the Institute of Stress Medicine in Scottsdale, Arizona, estimates that stress-related heart conditions claim the lives of as many as half a million Americans each year.

Nor are heart attacks the only physical damage to the body inflicted by stress. Researchers in various fields have linked stress to a suppressed immune system and other physical ills, including *hypertension* (high blood pressure), migraine headaches, sleep disorders, eating problems, asthma, and allergies. And physicians report that stress-based complaints such as fatigue, headache, and insomnia account for a large number of office visits. But scientists are just beginning to understand how stress affects the body.

What we call stress is actually the body's response to demanding

The author:

Carl Eisdorfer is Chairman of the Department of Psychiatry and Behavioral Sciences at the University of Miami School of Medicine.

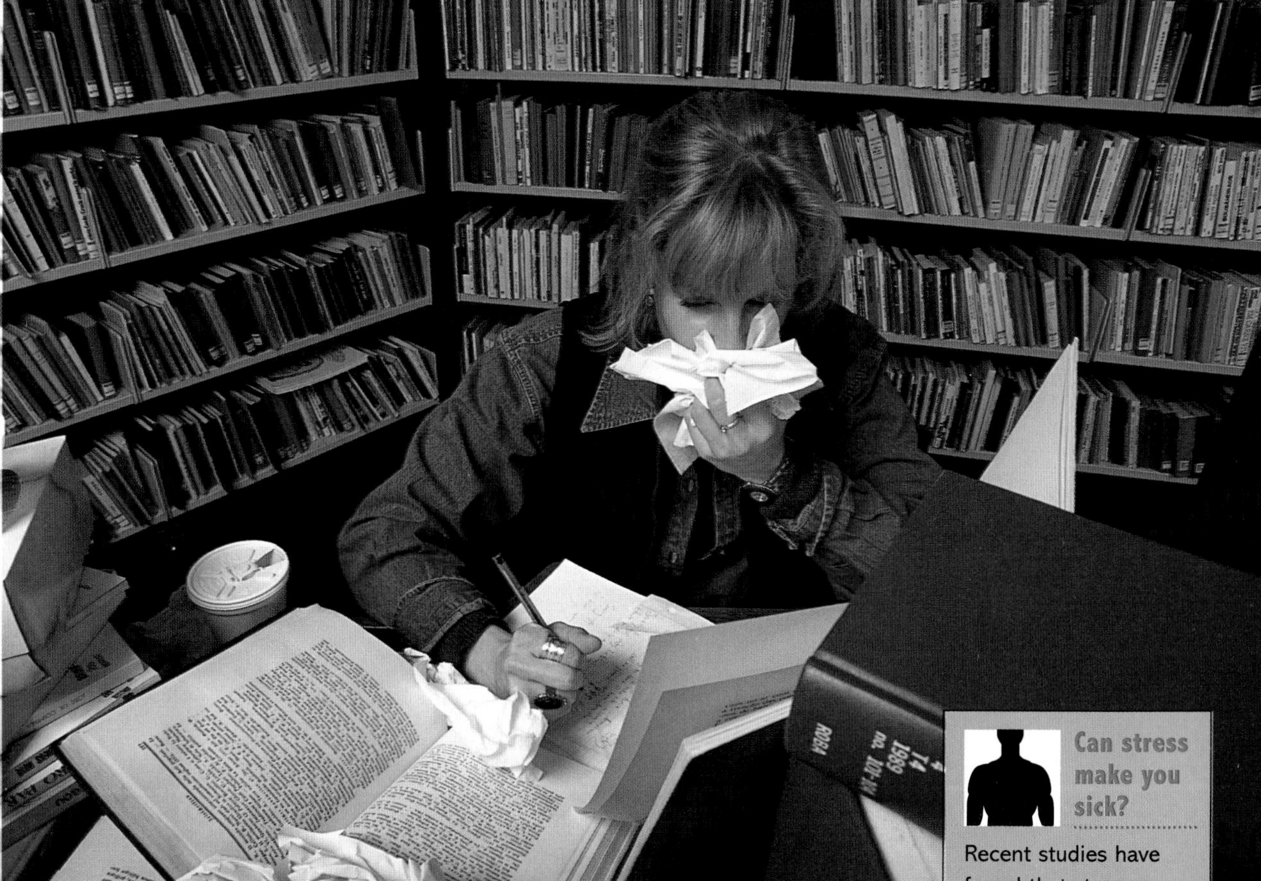

Can stress make you sick?

Recent studies have found that stress can affect the immune system. Researchers at Carnegie Mellon University in Pittsburgh, Pennsylvania, had students complete surveys to determine their stress levels, and then gave them nose drops containing cold viruses. The students who had scored high on the stress test had a 90-percent chance of catching cold; those who scored lower had only a 74-percent chance. The researchers found that stress increases levels of cortisol, a hormone that has been shown to suppress the immune system.

situations or events known as stressors. Stressors can be external—an earthquake, for example—or internal, such as anxiety over an upcoming exam. Stressors can also be positive events, such as marriage, or a promotion at work. In response to stressors, the eyes, ears, skin, and other sense organs send signals to a part of the brain called the hypothalamus. On the basis of these signals and of past experience with stressors, the hypothalamus activates the stress response. It signals the nearby pituitary gland, which releases a *hormone* (chemical messenger) called adrenocorticotropin-releasing hormone (ACTH).

ACTH makes its way through the bloodstream to the adrenal glands, which sit atop the kidneys and release a number of hormones critical to the stress response. These include glucocorticoids, which supply the body with instant energy and suppress the immune response, and epinephrine (also called adrenaline) and norepinephrine (also called noradrenaline), which step up heart rate and blood pressure. This sequence is referred to as the hypothalamic, pituitary, adrenal axis, and the hormones the adrenal glands release are known collectively as stress hormones.

The stress hormones bring about changes throughout the body, not only elevating heart rate and blood pressure and providing energy, but also speeding up breathing, reducing hunger, stimulating thirst, and even widening the pupils of the eye to enhance vision.

Through the body's feedback system, we experience these physical changes as tension, fear, excitement, and other emotions.

This stress response is useful for reacting to an urgent, life-threatening situation, but when prolonged it can harm the body. In the short term, blood flow increases to the parts of the body that require energy, such as the arms and legs, thus improving the body's ability to respond by "fight or flight." Systems not needed in the emergency, such as the digestive system, are put on hold by directing blood flow away from them. But when the stress response remains activated for an extended period, the redirection of blood flow may lead to hypertension, digestive system upsets, and other health problems.

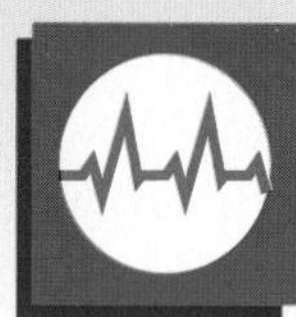

Diseases and disorders linked to stress

Researchers in various fields have linked stress to a number of physical ills, including heart disease, hypertension, and suppression of the immune system. But scientists are just beginning to understand the connections between stress and physical health.

Stress and the heart

Because heart disease is such a major health risk, much early research on stress-related illness concentrated on the heart. The so-called Type A personality—aggressive, controlling, driven—quickly became associated with an increased risk for heart disease. Although this association was accepted for many years, long-term studies eventually determined that most Type A traits were unrelated to heart disease. However, one personality trait did appear to be consistently associated with heart disease: anger and general hostility.

This effect of stress on the *cardiovascular system* (heart and blood vessels) can crop up years after the initial exposure to a stressor. A recent study of 556 World War II veterans, conducted at Yale University, found that the rate of stroke among men who had been prisoners of war was eight times higher than that of men who had not been captured. (Stroke occurs when a rupture or blockage of a blood

Heart attack

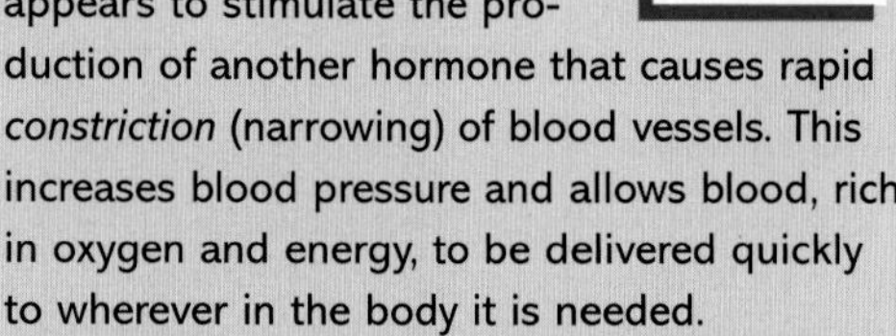

The stress hormone epinephrine appears to stimulate the production of another hormone that causes rapid *constriction* (narrowing) of blood vessels. This increases blood pressure and allows blood, rich in oxygen and energy, to be delivered quickly to wherever in the body it is needed.

If a person has heart disease—clogged coronary arteries, for example—blood flow to the heart muscle is deficient. The constriction caused by the hormone limits blood flow even further and can lead to a heart attack. Thus, the activity of epinephrine could account for the increased number of heart attacks recorded after major disasters such as earthquakes.

Peptic ulcers

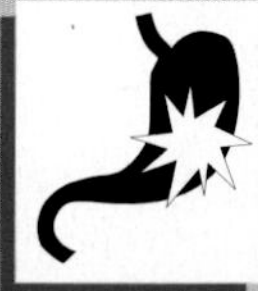

For years, people believed stress caused ulcers. The theory was that stress increased the production of stomach acid, which ate holes in the lining of the stomach or the *duodenum* (the top of the small intestine). But in the early 1980's, Australian researchers found that *helicobacter pylori,* a common form of bacteria, could promote ulcer formation by irritating the stomach lining.

In some parts of the world, 90 percent of the population carries the *H. pylori* bacterium in their stomachs—yet few of them develop ulcers. Thus, another factor—perhaps stress—acting in combination with *H. pylori* appears to be involved in ulcer formation. Researchers are investigating the role that stress may play in this process.

vessel causes injury to the brain.) The researcher who conducted the study concluded that the impact of severe stress on the body may be long-lasting, raising the body's sensitivity to future stressors.

Animal studies support the theory that stress early in life can have lasting consequences. In a study of monkeys, young monkeys separated from their mothers for 15 minutes a day showed only a slight change in their stress response. But monkeys separated from their mothers for three hours a day during the first months of life had a greatly heightened stress response thereafter. Once sensitized to stress, they were likely to race around their cage or cower in a corner when exposed to even a mild stressor.

Chronic stress can also set in motion a slow but prolonged attack on the cardiovascular system by elevating blood pressure. The role stress plays in hypertension and the extent of its effect are still being investigated. But studies have found that the strain of a high-pressure job can lead to a chronic elevation of blood pressure, a condition that increases the risk of heart disease. Studies have repeatedly shown that people working at high-strain jobs over which they have little control, such as waitresses, assembly-line workers, and people in middle-management positions, are at greater risk for hypertension.

Researchers at Duke University in Durham, North Carolina, reported in June 1996 that the amount of stress people are experiencing may provide a more accurate indication of heart disease risk than the standard physical test of heart function, running on a treadmill while heart rate is monitored. The researchers administered mental stress testing, such as complex math problems that had to be solved in a limited amount of time, to 126 people. They used sophisticated

Stroke

The effect of stress on the *cardiovascular system* (heart and blood vessels) may not appear until years after a person is exposed to a stressor. Researchers have found a link between stress and stroke, which occurs when a rupture or blockage of a blood vessel causes injury to the brain.

A recent study of 556 World War II veterans, conducted at Yale University in New Haven, Connecticut, found that men who had been prisoners of war suffered strokes at a rate about eight times higher than that of men who had not been captured. Researchers concluded that the impact of severe stressors on the body may be long-lasting, raising its sensitivity to future stressors.

Autoimmune disorders

Studies have shown that stress may play a role in *autoimmune disorders*—diseases that occur when the immune system attacks the body's own tissues. One such disease is rheumatoid arthritis, which involves swelling and pain in the joints. Some people who have arthritis claim that stress makes the condition worse.

Researchers at Arizona State University conducted a study of 100 rheumatoid arthritis patients. They found that those who reported high levels of stress in their relationships with others had twice the level of the hormone prolactin in their blood as those who said they were not under such stress. Research has shown that prolactin sets in motion a series of reactions that results in swollen joints.

imaging techniques to detect changes in blood flow to the heart while the participants underwent testing. During a five-year follow-up, the investigators found that 27 percent of the people who responded poorly to the testing, as indicated by a greater reduction in blood flow, had suffered a heart attack, were experiencing *angina* (chest pain), or had severely clogged coronary arteries. By contrast, only 12 percent of the participants who did not have trouble with the tests had experienced serious heart problems.

While the role of stress in cardiovascular disease has been studied for decades, recent study of chronic stress's impact on health has focused on its relationship with the immune system. The workings of the immune system are extremely complex and the ways in which stress interacts with this system are exceedingly difficult to unravel.

But scientists are beginning to identify these links. Although it had been demonstrated that injury to certain parts of the brain altered the immune response, the prevailing view among scientists had long been that the brain did not communicate with the immune system and that psychological factors such as stress did not influence immunity. Recent discoveries, however, have brought that view into question.

Stress and the immune system

In the 1980's, scientists at Ohio State University measured the ways that anxiety reduces the body's ability to produce interferon, a protein that is crucial to fighting disease. The researchers found that during college examination weeks, students had less interferon in their bodies and were far more likely to contract colds or the flu than at other times of the year.

This finding mirrors results obtained by researchers at Carnegie Mellon University in Pittsburgh. Study participants first answered a questionnaire aimed at determining their levels of stress. They then received nose drops containing cold viruses. Participants with high scores on the stress scale had a 90-percent chance of catching cold, compared with a 74-percent chance among participants with lower scores. The researchers found that stress boosted levels of a hormone called cortisol, which has been shown to suppress the immune system.

Studies conducted at Ohio State University in the 1990's have shown that hostile feelings may disturb the immune response. The investigators asked 90 newlywed couples to resolve difficult issues, such as feelings about their mothers-in-law. While the couples tried to iron out their differences, instruments to which they were connected drew small blood samples at regular intervals. The blood was tested for levels of stress hormones. The researchers found that when couples became more hostile, blood levels of hormones that boosted immune response fell and levels of hormones that weakened the response rose.

Other scientists have explored the role that stress might play in *autoimmune* disorders—diseases that result from an attack by the immune system on the body's own tissues. What causes the immune system to tag a body tissue as foreign and mount an attack remains a mystery, but some findings implicate stress as a factor.

One of the most common autoimmune diseases is rheumatoid arthritis, a disorder that involves swelling, pain, and tenderness in the joints. Some people with this disease report that stress makes their arthritis worse. Researchers at Arizona State University studied 100 rheumatoid arthritis patients and found that those who said they were experiencing high levels of stress in their relationships with other people had twice the level of the hormone prolactin in their blood as those who did not report such stress. Other studies have shown that prolactin travels to the joints, where it sets in motion a series of reactions that results in swollen joints.

There is also good reason to suspect a role for stress hormones in disturbances of the large intestine—spastic colon, for example, which may produce chronic diarrhea, constipation, and cramping. Some cases of colitis—chronic inflammation of the colon—are also suspected of resulting from sustained stress, where no other clear cause can be found.

Can emotional strain cause illness?

As researchers work to link stress with disorders of specific organs and systems, some more general vulnerabilities to stress have become clear. For example, studies have established that people who are widowed are at risk of dying within a year or so of their spouse. Anniversaries—of deaths, for example—and major events, such as a wedding or the loss of a job, also arouse emotions strong enough to constitute stressors.

Research reported in 1995 suggested that stress levels can alter the immune response in patients with AIDS, especially when major stressors such as the death of a loved one occur. An ongoing study, conducted by researchers at the University of Florida and the University of North Carolina, followed 93 HIV-infected men for 6 months to 3½ years. The more stressors the men encountered, the study found, the more likely that their condition worsened. Other research has found that cynical, hostile HIV-infected men had poorer immune function than those with a more positive attitude.

Chronic stress takes a toll on the body. Where it strikes and how we respond depends to a great extent on genetic predisposition, our past experience with stress, and other physiological factors not yet discovered. As a growing number of scientists examine the effects of stress on health, a new field known as psychoneuroimmunology has emerged. This discipline investigates the complex interactions of the nervous system, immune system, and hormonal system and the effects that human behavior—including stress—has on these systems and on health. Future findings may help us to avoid many illnesses caused by stress. •••

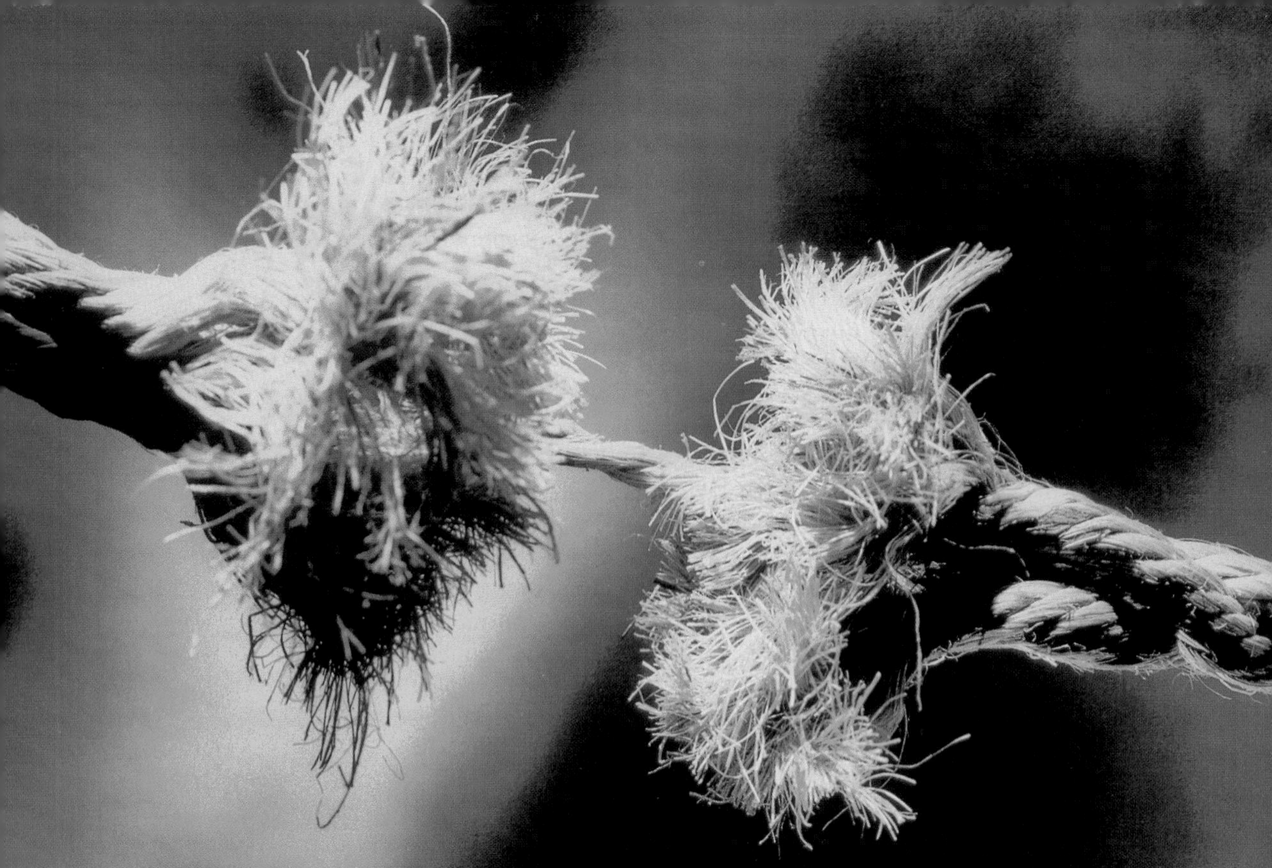

When people feel unable to cope with stress, their mental well-being may be at risk.

Stress and Mental Health

By Sanford I. Cohen

The author:

Sanford I. Cohen is Senior Vice Chairman of the Department of Psychiatry and Behavioral Sciences at the University of Miami School of Medicine.

LIFE IS FULL OF EXPERIENCES THAT PEOPLE FIND STRESSFUL—driving in traffic, waiting in line, working against a deadline, arguing, or performing demanding tasks. However, it is not these stress-ors themselves, but rather people's perceptions of them, that cause stress. The level of stress that people experience is related to their sense of how adequately they can control or cope with stressful situations. When people feel that they do not have the resources to handle stressors, their level of stress increases sharply.

The emotions set off by stressful situations vary considerably. The same stressor might excite one person and fill another person with fear. A confrontation with an angry lion, for example, would produce a much different reaction in an experienced big-game hunter carrying a large rifle than it would in a tourist armed with nothing but a camera. Emotional reactions are specific to each person and depend on the significance or meaning the individual attaches to a particular stressor. In the example just cited, the hunter sees a trophy, while the tourist sees a terrifying predator.

Individuals who feel threatened by a situation typically experience fear. Fear can arise from the threat of immediate physical harm or from the more subtle threat that people may feel when starting a new job or meeting a group of strangers. A feeling of fear is normal and appropriate. It acts as a danger signal that informs us of the need to deal with a threat.

People deal with perceived threats and other stressors in various ways. The process of managing the discrepancy between demands and personal resources is referred to as coping.

Learning to cope

Problem-focused coping is a behavioral effort to reduce the demands of a stressful situation or to expand one's resources. Everyday life provides many examples of problem-focused coping, such as quitting a difficult job, devising a new work schedule, seeking medical or psychological treatment, or learning new job skills.

Emotion-focused coping, on the other hand, aims at controlling emotional responses to a stressful situation. People often use emotion-focused coping when they feel helpless to change a stressor and so seek to reduce its impact. This kind of coping may involve activities that distract attention from the stressor, such as participating in sports, watching television, or finding support from friends or relatives.

When people feel overwhelmed by life and unable to cope, stress becomes a serious problem. People experiencing sustained stress may grow socially isolated, uncaring, or angry. Anger may lead to aggressive behavior. For example, a man who is angry and frustrated over the loss of a job may respond by abusing his children.

High levels of stress can damage one's mental health in a variety of ways. If stressors are prolonged or intense, or if a person lacks the resources to handle them, a stress-related illness

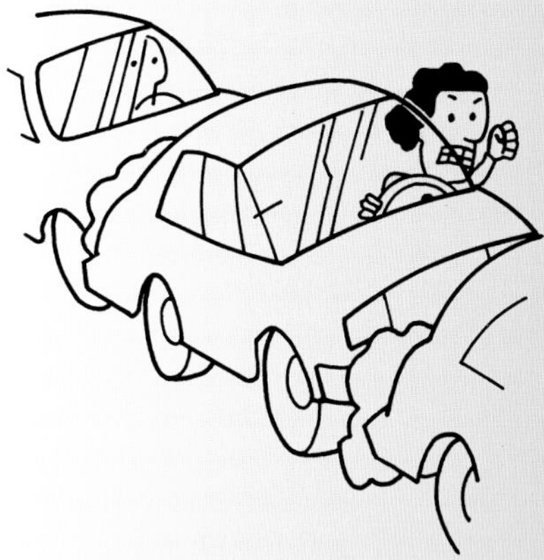

Common emotional responses to stress

People's emotional responses to stress depend on how they perceive stress. These perceptions, in turn, are colored by their previous experiences with situations they found stressful. Some common emotional responses to stress include:

- **Anger**
  Some people perceive stress as an attack and respond with anger.
- **Depression**
  People who experience stress in response to a loss or who feel overwhelmed by demands placed on them become vulnerable to depression.
- **Excitement**
  Not all responses to stress are negative. Stress can generate a sense of excitement and challenge.
- **Fear and anxiety**
  Threatening experiences, such as having an accident while driving on a wet road, can produce fear at the time and evoke anxiety later, whenever the person encounters the situation again.

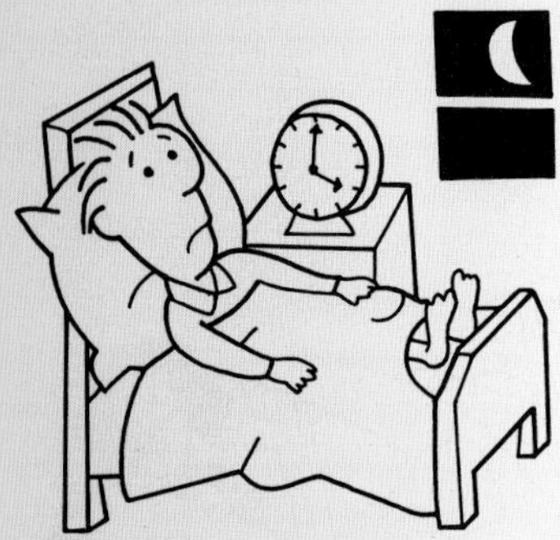

Common behavioral responses to stress

The cumulative effects of stress may bring about a number of changes in behavior. Some common behavioral responses to stress include:

- **Aggressive behavior**
  People who become angry when under stress may exhibit aggressive behavior toward those around them.
- **Alcohol and drug use**
  People sometimes increase their consumption of alcohol or dependence on drugs—including cigarettes, caffeine, tranquilizers, and illicit drugs—as a way of dealing with stress.
- **Fatigue**
  The experience of stress can be exhausting.
- **Irritability**
  People may lose their temper easily and often when they are under stress. Or they may explode over minor incidents.
- **Minor accidents**
  Stress can make people accident-prone. In some cases, this is the result of other stress-related behavior, such as increased alcohol use.
- **Overeating**
  Seeking comfort from food is a fairly common response to stress.
- **Sleep disturbances**
  People under stress may experience changes in their sleep habits—for example, an inability to fall asleep, waking early, or sleeping too much.

may develop. When stressors are extreme and overwhelming, a condition known as post-traumatic stress disorder (PTSD) may result. Other mental illnesses can also be triggered by stress.

Early warning signals that stress is affecting the mind may be emotional or intellectual. Emotional reactions include feeling burned-out or sad for long periods of time or feeling devoid of all emotions except anger and irritation. Familiar signs of intellectual strain are an inability to concentrate, forgetfulness, and difficulty in making decisions.

Unhealthy behaviors may also be indications that a person is overcome by stress. Society is full of props that people use to distract their attention from stressors. These props include alcohol, caffeine, tobacco, tranquilizers, and illicit drugs. People may come to rely heavily on these substances and lose their ability to manage stress without them. In the short run, it may be easier to pop a pill or have a stiff drink than to make an appropriate change in one's life.

People also use food to distract themselves from the stressors in their lives. If work isn't going well, a bar of chocolate may provide immediate comfort. Such stopgap behaviors can become dangerous if they are perceived as a necessary part of life.

Alcohol use and carelessness, two common behavioral responses to stress, probably play a role in the relatively high accident rates of people in stressful circumstances. Studies have found that individuals experiencing high levels of stress are more likely than other people to suffer accidental injuries at home, in sporting activities, on the job, or while driving a car.

Post-traumatic stress disorder

Some people are exposed to extreme, devastating stressors that are outside the range of normal human experience. These stressors include fires, floods, and other disasters; military combat or other violent situations; and train and aircraft accidents. Such extreme stressors can produce severe mental health problems.

The most common disorders occurring in the aftermath of devastating personal experiences are

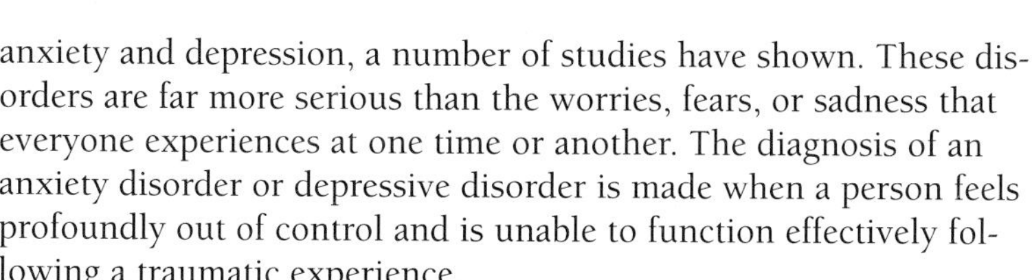

anxiety and depression, a number of studies have shown. These disorders are far more serious than the worries, fears, or sadness that everyone experiences at one time or another. The diagnosis of an anxiety disorder or depressive disorder is made when a person feels profoundly out of control and is unable to function effectively following a traumatic experience.

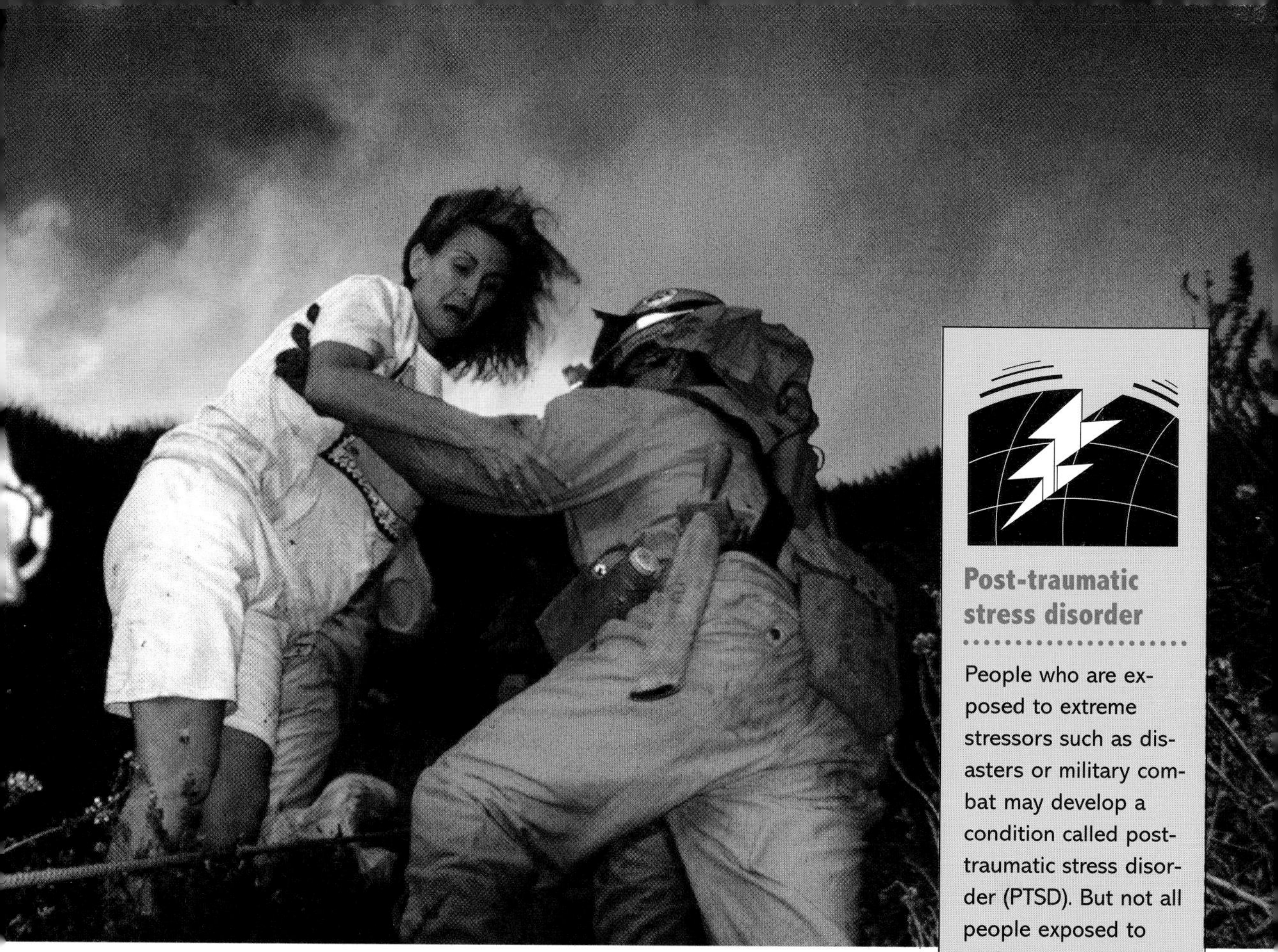

A substantial number of people exposed to severe stressors of a life-threatening nature develop PTSD or related syndromes. The symptoms of PTSD vary considerably, but researchers have found that they can be classified into three groups.

Recognizing the signs

One group of symptoms is known as *reexperiencing*. People with this form of PTSD become preoccupied with a trauma they have lived through, and thoughts and memories related to the event continually intrude upon their daily lives. Reexperiencing also takes the form of recurrent nightmares. Unlike normal dreams, these nightmares feature a relatively realistic replaying of the traumatic event. Even more literal reexperiencing can take the form of flashbacks, episodes in which a person feels as if he or she is once again in the midst of the trauma.

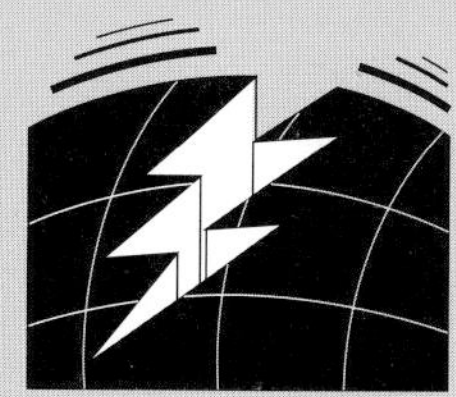

Post-traumatic stress disorder

People who are exposed to extreme stressors such as disasters or military combat may develop a condition called post-traumatic stress disorder (PTSD). But not all people exposed to such stressors develop the disorder, suggesting that traumatic experiences in themselves do not cause PTSD. A variety of factors, including personality, education, and family history, may be involved.

What are some of the symptoms?

- Nightmares and flashbacks related to the trauma
- Feelings of detachment from others
- Difficulty sleeping
- Feeling constantly "on the alert"
- Panic attacks

Another group of PTSD symptoms includes *emotional numbing*, in which people lose interest in activities, experience feelings of detachment from others, exhibit a restricted range of emotion, and have a pessimistic outlook on the future. People with this form of PTSD may also try to avoid thoughts, feelings, and situations that remind them of the traumatic event.

Heightened arousal is another major symptom group. People with these symptoms of PTSD may have difficulty sleeping. They may be constantly "on the alert" and easily startled. For example, war veterans who have not recovered from the trauma of their wartime experience may respond to a car's backfiring by taking cover. People with heightened-arousal PTSD may also suffer panic attacks, during which they experience breathing difficulties, an increased heart rate, dizziness, and nausea.

Who is most vulnerable?

Research has found that certain character traits may make a person more vulnerable to PTSD. Shyness, irritability, impulsiveness, and pessimism may increase a person's risk of developing PTSD, according to findings reported in May 1996 by psychologist Paula Schnurr of the National Center for Post-Traumatic Stress Disorder at the Veterans Affairs Medical Center in White River Junction, Vermont. Schnurr based this conclusion on psychological tests given to college students who later fought in the Vietnam War during the 1960's and 1970's.

Other studies suggest that a family history of depression may put people at higher risk of PTSD, which indicates that heredity is sometimes involved. Education and intelligence seem to protect against PTSD, however. Studies of people in the war-torn country of Bosnia have found that those who did not finish high school had a 50 percent greater risk of developing PTSD than those who got their diplomas. All of this research suggests that traumatic experiences do not in themselves cause PTSD. A variety of factors seem to determine how a person responds to an extreme stressor.

A number of studies suggest that major psychiatric disorders, such as clinical depression, may be brought on by stress in people who are vulnerable to such disorders. Most people do not become mentally ill, even if they are confronted by major life stressors. But for those who are susceptible to depression, the disorder may be triggered by deaths and other stressful events. Further, people are more likely to develop depression if they confront a number of major life stressors simultaneously than if they meet them one at a time.

Stress alone does not threaten mental health. To the contrary, good mental health can help us cope with stress. But everyone has a breaking point, and prolonged, severe, or overwhelming stress can push the mind to its limits. It is vital that we get the stress in our lives under control before that limit is reached. •••

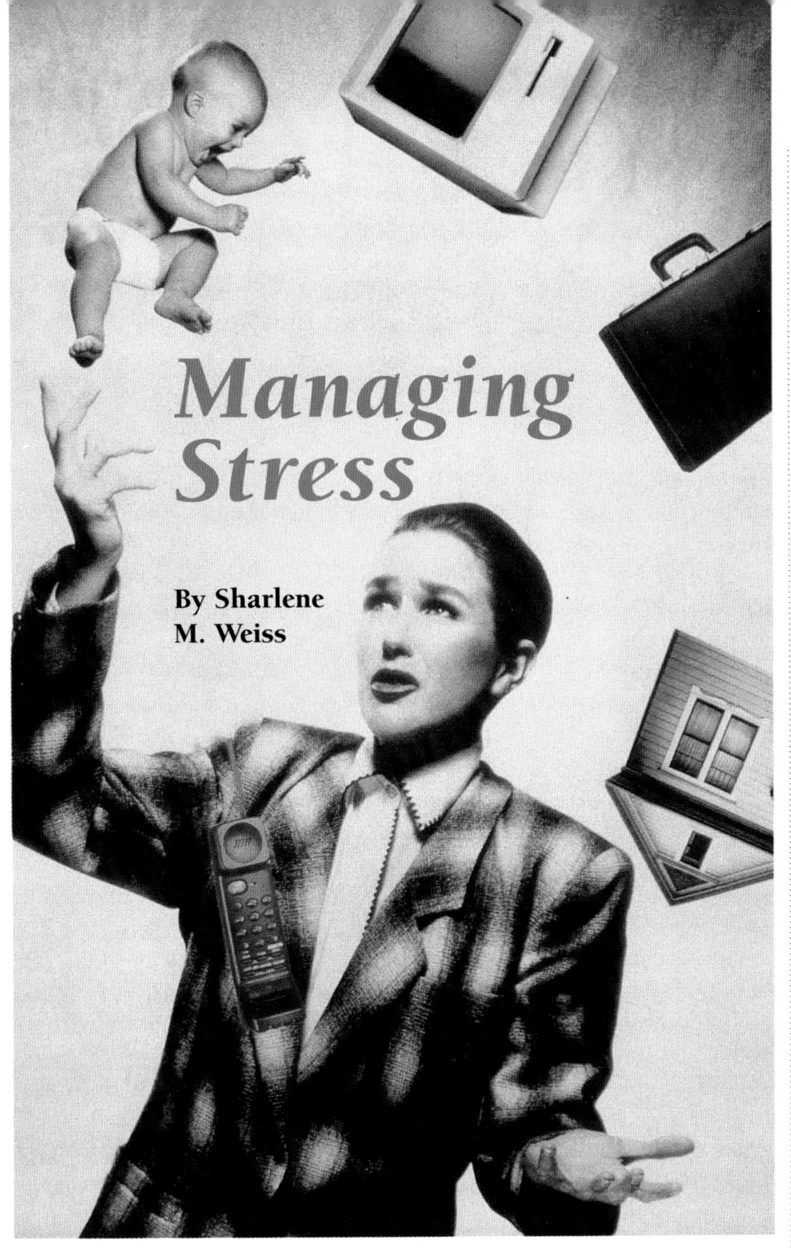

Managing Stress

By Sharlene M. Weiss

Counteracting the negative effects of stress is important to our physical and mental health.

AN IMPORTANT FIRST STEP TOWARD MANAGING STRESS is learning to recognize its warning signs. Although our bodies "talk" to us all the time, many people have not learned to heed the physical, emotional, and behavioral signals the body sends. For some people, the reaction to stress is physical: a headache, a backache, a stomachache, gas or diarrhea, muscle tension in the neck or shoulders, a racing heartbeat, or cold hands. Sometimes, the reaction is emotional: irritability, depression, anxiety, or anger. A change in behavior can also be a warning flag. People may eat or sleep more or less than usual, drink or smoke heavily, or turn to drugs. The stress response can also be a combination of physical, emotional, and behavioral signals.

The author:

Sharlene M. Weiss is Director of the Courtelis Center for Research and Treatment in Psychosocial Oncology at the University of Miami.

If such signals occur with increasing frequency or intensity and last longer than usual, professional help may be needed. Unfortunately, many people decide to do nothing about the stress they are experiencing until they have been diagnosed with a stress-related disease or disorder, such as heart disease. But it's possible to recognize the negative effects of stress and do something about them before illness develops.

Gaining control over personal stressors

To manage stress, people need first to recognize their own personal stressors—the sorts of demanding situations or circumstances that they have trouble dealing with. Some people have a strong negative reaction to environmental stressors, such as noise, crowding, poor ventilation, or extremes of heat or cold. Others respond more strongly to interpersonal or social stressors, such as conflict with angry or aggressive people, communication difficulties, or giving or receiving criticism. And some react most strongly to stressors at work or at home, such as schedules they can't keep up with, family arguments, or boredom.

Some of the most common stressors come from within—for example, when our performance on a certain task does not match our expectations. Just thinking about a stressful situation can evoke a stress response in the body. For example, a situation many people find stressful is making a presentation at a meeting. A moderate amount of stress can be helpful, enabling the person to speak in a stronger, fuller voice; gesture and stand more confidently; and think in a clear, organized way. But as a result of excessive worry, perhaps about how the boss will evaluate the presentation, the stress response can become intense. In that case, performance may decline—the person may speak too quickly, tremble, and lose concentration while speaking to the audience.

Once people learn to recognize their own stressors, they can formulate a plan for dealing with them. Avoiding the situation that evokes stress, or minimizing its effects, is one solution. For example, a person who finds traffic congestion stressful could take a different route, carpool, use public transportation, or listen to books on tape for distraction while stuck in traffic.

Gaining control over stressors by learning new skills is another effective way to manage stress. Training programs can sometimes help people change their response to a stressor. Through such programs, a person might improve communication skills or practice techniques for dealing with difficult people.

Some people engage in negative "self talk" when confronted with a stressor, telling themselves "I can't do this" or "I'm not smart enough." Others grow anxious and think irrationally. If people learn to recognize when they are sending themselves negative messages, they can gain control over stressors by replacing those messages with positive ones.

Some stressors, however, are impossible to avoid or control. But people can learn to counteract the negative effects of the stress response. Exercise and relaxation techniques are two effective ways of managing unavoidable stress.

Counteracting the effects of stress

Exercise helps counteract the negative effects of the stress response by speeding up the process by which the body breaks down stress hormones. These hormones are released when the stress response is activated, and they trigger physiological changes throughout the body. Blood pressure and pulse rate rise, breathing becomes faster and deeper, and muscles tense, as the body prepares itself for action. Once the stressful event is over, however, it is important that the body rid itself of the stress hormones before they cause damage. So after a long, hectic day, it's a good idea to get some exercise rather than just flopping down in front of the television.

Another way to counteract the stress response is by evoking the *relaxation response*—the body's natural calming system. Relaxation techniques can be used to shut off the stress response or to lessen the strength of the response. Once a stressful event has passed, these techniques can also speed the body's recovery.

The stress response and the relaxation response are both important in maintaining the body's balance. The stress response can be compared to the accelerator of a car; the relaxation response, to the brakes. When stimulated appropriately, the stress response can help people meet deadlines, work effectively, and maintain a high level of energy. But when it occurs too frequently or remains active too long, the stress response can harm the body.

Many studies have shown that the relaxation response decreases pulse and breathing rates, lowers blood pressure and levels of stress hormones, and eases muscle tension and anxiety. Studies have also demonstrated that people who practice and use relaxation techniques tend to increase their work efficiency, mental clarity, self-esteem, concentration, creativity, and ability to cope with stress.

By trying a variety of relaxation techniques, you can choose the technique or techniques you find most effective. All relaxation techniques share certain characteristics. Most importantly, they require daily practice in a quiet setting free of distractions and sensory stimulation. Rather than trying to force relaxation, assume a comfortable position and a mental attitude that allows relaxation to occur. Practicing with an audiotape can be helpful while learning a relaxation routine. After practicing different relaxation exercises, you can construct your own routine, incorporating portions of several exercises.

One of the simplest relaxation techniques to learn is diaphragmatic *(dye uh fruh MAT ic)* breathing, also called belly breathing. Diaphragmatic breathing is a particularly good technique because it can be used throughout the day, in a variety of situations. It empha-

EFFECTIVE WAYS OF REDUCING STRESS

Learning to relax

People can learn to counteract the negative effects of the stress response through exercise and the practice of relaxation techniques. Relaxation techniques require daily practice in a quiet setting free of distractions. By experimenting with a variety of relaxation methods, people can choose the ones that work best for them.

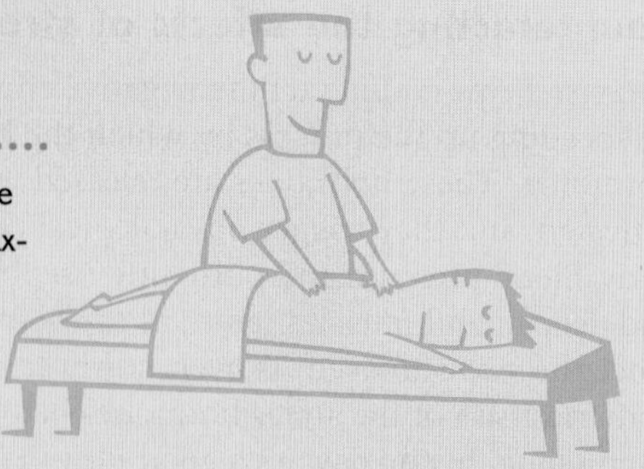

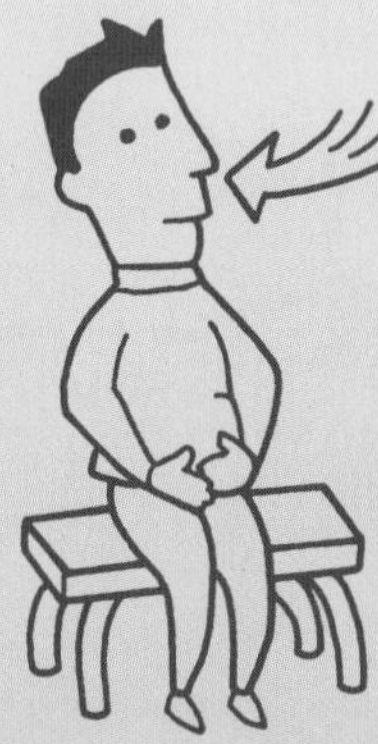

Diaphragmatic breathing

A simple relaxation technique is diaphragmatic (*dye uh fruh MAT ic*) breathing. This slow, deep breathing helps restore the body's state of balance after a stressful event.

- **INHALE:** Many people tighten their abdomens when breathing in. In diaphragmatic breathing, the abdomen protrudes when one inhales. Placing the hands on the abdomen while inhaling can help people ensure that they are breathing correctly.
- **EXHALE:** As one exhales, the abdomen flattens.

If combined with the repetition of a word or phrase, such as *re* on the in breath and *lax* on the out breath, diaphragmatic breathing is even more effective.

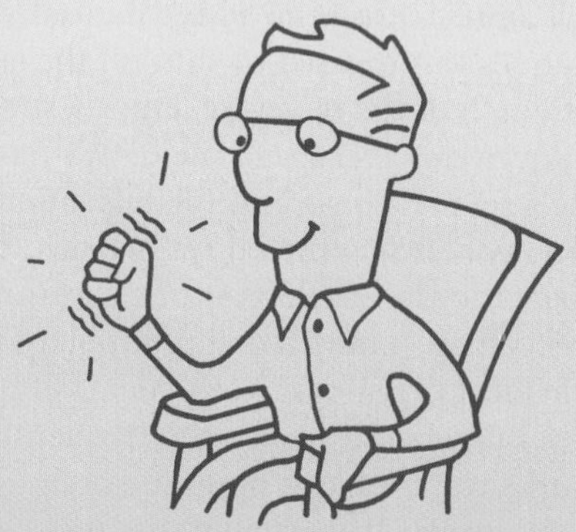

Progressive muscle relaxation

Progressive muscle relaxation involves tensing muscles to the utmost and then relaxing them, thus learning to "let go" of tension. This tensing and relaxing process progresses from the feet to the head, working through all of the major muscle groups.

Developed by a physician in the 1930's, progressive muscle relaxation can help reduce anxiety and lessen muscle tension. The technique is particularly effective for people who tighten their muscles in response to stress and for those who prefer structured exercise.

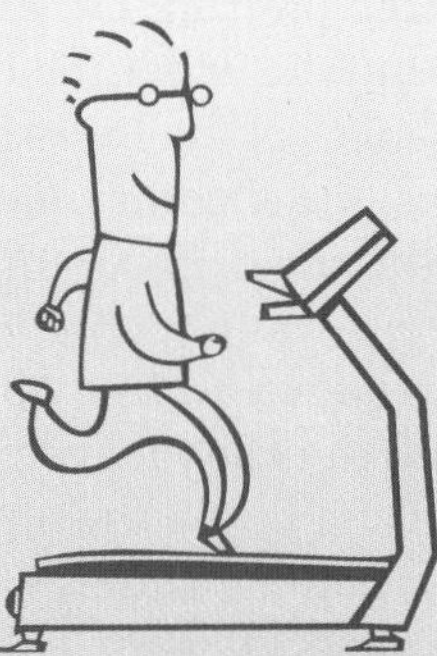

Exercise

Exercise is an effective way to counteract the negative effects of stress. When the stress response is activated, stress hormones are released into the bloodstream. If the body doesn't rid itself of these hormones after the stressful situation is over, the hormones can cause damage. Exercise helps speed up the process by which the body breaks down stress hormones.

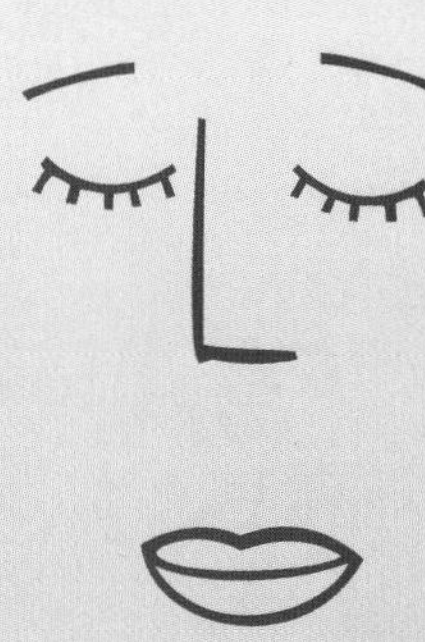

Meditation

Meditation is an effective relaxation technique. The goal is to focus on a word, sound, or object, or simply on one's breathing, blocking out all other thoughts. People attempting to use this technique should remember that learning to stay focused and avoid distracting thoughts takes practice and may be difficult at first.

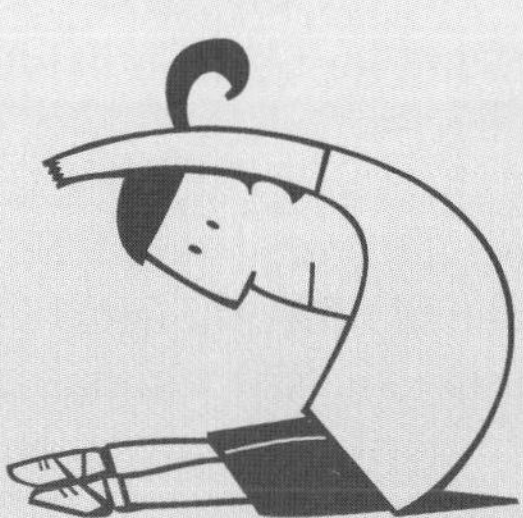

Yoga

Yoga is a series of postures and breathing exercises, performed slowly and with concentration. Many people enjoy yoga because it is a gentle form of exercise that requires no special equipment. The goal of yoga is to achieve a unity of body, mind, and spirit.

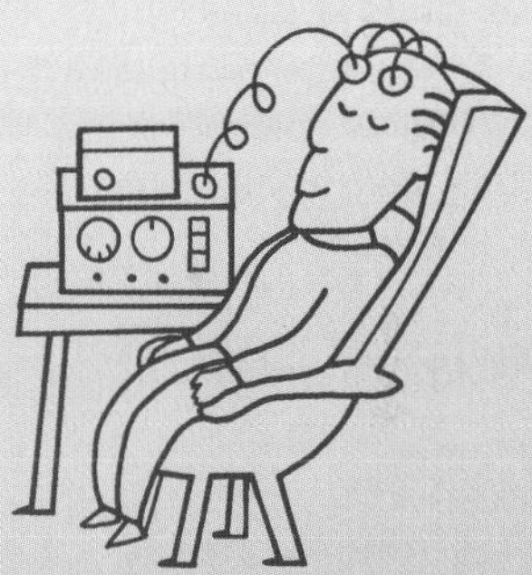

Biofeedback

Biofeedback can help teach people to control various body functions that are affected by stress. Sensors attached to the body record information about such activities as muscle tension, pulse rate, and sweat gland activity. This feedback is converted into a tone or pulse that is displayed on a monitor. The goal is to change the display by consciously altering a body function.

sizes slow, deep breathing and helps counteract the tendency to breathe rapidly when under stress.

Many people tighten their abdominal muscles when breathing in. In diaphragmatic breathing, the abdomen protrudes when the person inhales. The *diaphragm* (the large muscle under the lungs) drops down and the lower lobes of the lungs fill with air. As the person exhales, the abdomen flattens.

Diaphragmatic breathing helps restore the body's state of balance after a stressful event. This breathing technique is even more effective when combined with the repetition of a word or phrase, such as *re* on the in breath and *lax* on the out breath. Simply by changing breathing patterns, people can begin to manage the stress response.

Other relaxation techniques can also help alleviate stress. Among them are progressive muscle relaxation, meditation, yoga, biofeedback, talk therapy, and behavioral therapy.

Progressive muscle relaxation was developed by American physician Edmund Jacobson in the 1930's as a way for his patients to reduce anxiety and lessen muscle tension. Jacobson instructed people to tense their muscles to their utmost and then release them to "let go" of tension. The tensing and relaxing process progresses through all of the major muscle groups, from the feet to the head. Progressive muscle relaxation is particularly effective for people who respond to stress by tightening their muscles and for those individuals who prefer structured exercise.

Meditation is an effective means of relaxation. The goal is to focus on a word, sound, breath, or object, and block out all other thoughts or worries. It takes practice to stay focused without letting the mind wander and to learn not to dwell on or be distracted by other thoughts.

Yoga is a discipline aimed at uniting the body, mind, and spirit. It includes a series of postures and breathing exercises, all performed slowly and with concentration. Many people use yoga as their form of relaxation because it is gentle, requires no special equipment, and can be done almost anywhere.

Biofeedback is a tool that can give people moment-by-moment information on what is happening in their bodies as they practice relaxation techniques. Sensors attached to different places on a person's body record information on body functions such as muscle tension, pulse rate, sweat gland activity, and even brain wave patterns. This biological feedback is converted into a

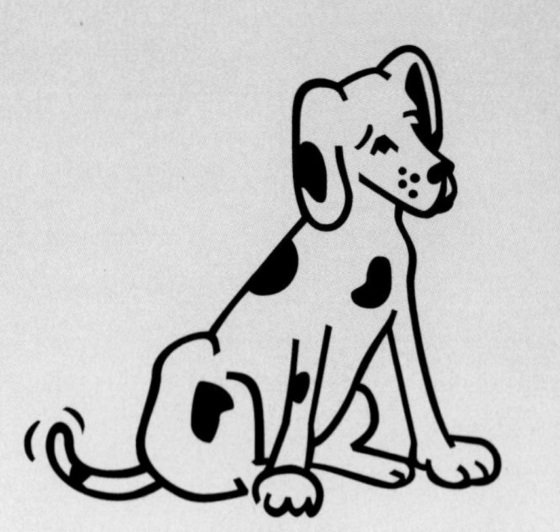

Can pets help relieve stress?

Research reported in March 1996 suggested that pets can lower people's stress levels. Married couples were asked to complete stressful tests under different conditions. Physical indicators of stress levels—blood pressure and heart rate—were lowest when only a dog was present during the tests. They were highest when just a spouse was present.

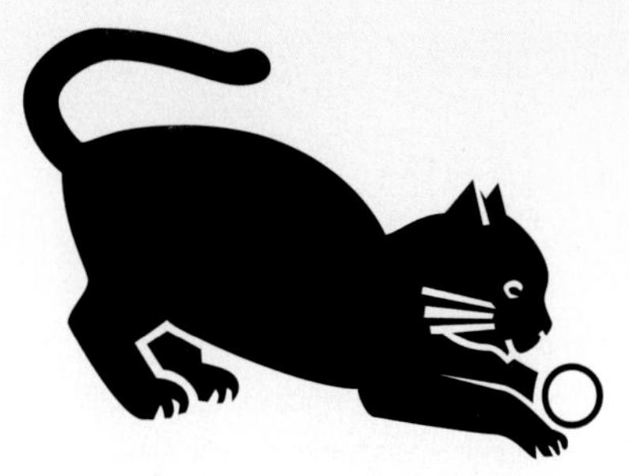

tone or pulse that is displayed on a monitor. The goal is to change the display by consciously altering a body function. People who feel frustrated because they don't know which relaxation techniques work best for them can turn to biofeedback. It can help speed up the learning process and also demonstrate the ability to control many body functions once considered to be automatic.

Talk therapy and behavioral therapy are methods of helping people become aware of their personal stressors and stress signals. These techniques, provided by professional therapists, teach people how to deal with stress through strategies that change their patterns of response to stressors. Such strategies can include avoiding stressors, minimizing or modifying exposure to them, and developing skills for reducing excessive reactions to stressors. Through such therapeutic approaches, people can learn to maintain a healthy stress response that enhances performance, though use of these techniques alone may not be effective for people with serious disorders.

Most therapists agree that short-term drug therapy can also be effective in helping to manage stress, particularly in relieving such symptoms as anxiety or depression that interfere with other forms of therapy. The goal of prescribing medications, such as antianxiety or antidepressant drugs, is usually to reduce symptoms in order to permit other, more lasting forms of treatment to take effect.

Many people do not concern themselves with managing stress until they have developed a stress-related disease or disorder. But they should listen to what their bodies are telling them and act sooner. With effective stress management, many of the health problems caused by excessive stress can be prevented.

Slowing the progress of disease

For people who have already developed a serious illness, stress management may be just as important. Studies have found that by managing stress, people with illnesses such as cancer and AIDS may be able to assist the healing process, reduce disease symptoms, and extend their lives. One often-cited study showed that women with advanced breast cancer who belonged to a support group lived on average twice as long as those who lacked this form of assistance. The women in support groups also reported less pain and discomfort.

Another study showed that patients with melanoma—a potentially deadly form of skin cancer—had a stronger immune response to the disease if they were able to openly express their feelings of anger. When researchers measured the growth rate of the patients' tumors, they found a lower rate of cell growth and more immune system cells among patients who expressed their anger than among those who responded to their condition with stoicism or helplessness.

Research in this area is still at an early stage. But preliminary investigations suggest that in addition to helping prevent disease, stress management may be an effective weapon for fighting serious illness when it develops. •••

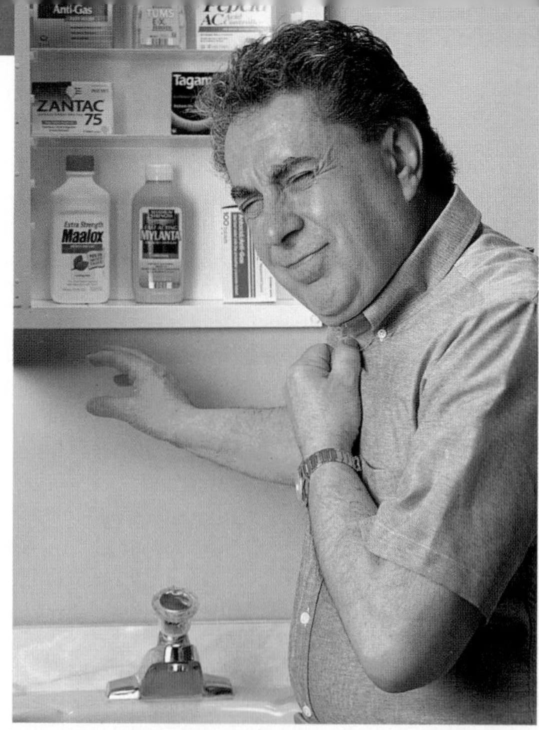
Anti-Gas
TUMS
ZANTAC
75
Extra Strength
Maalox
MYLANTA

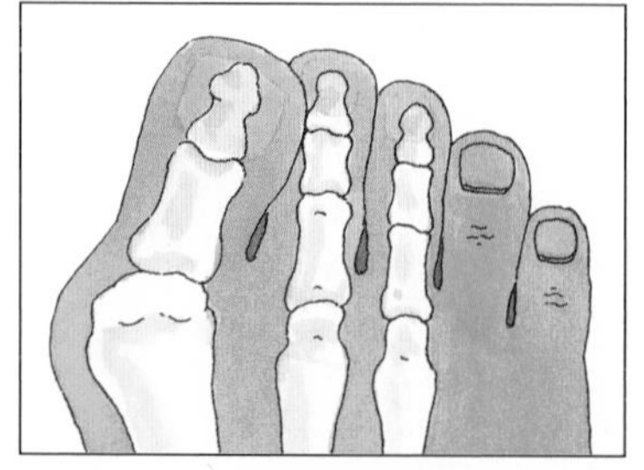

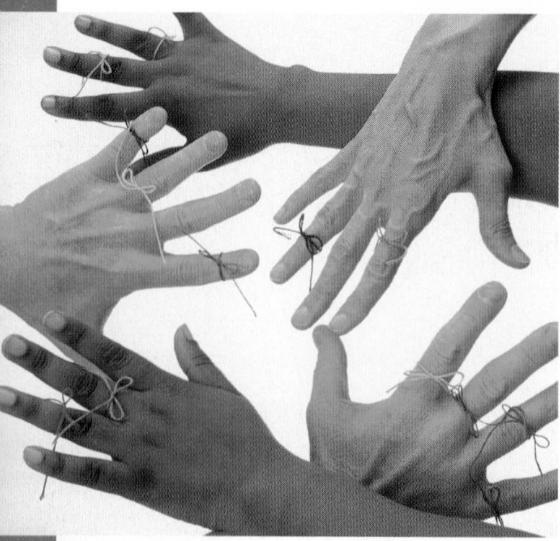

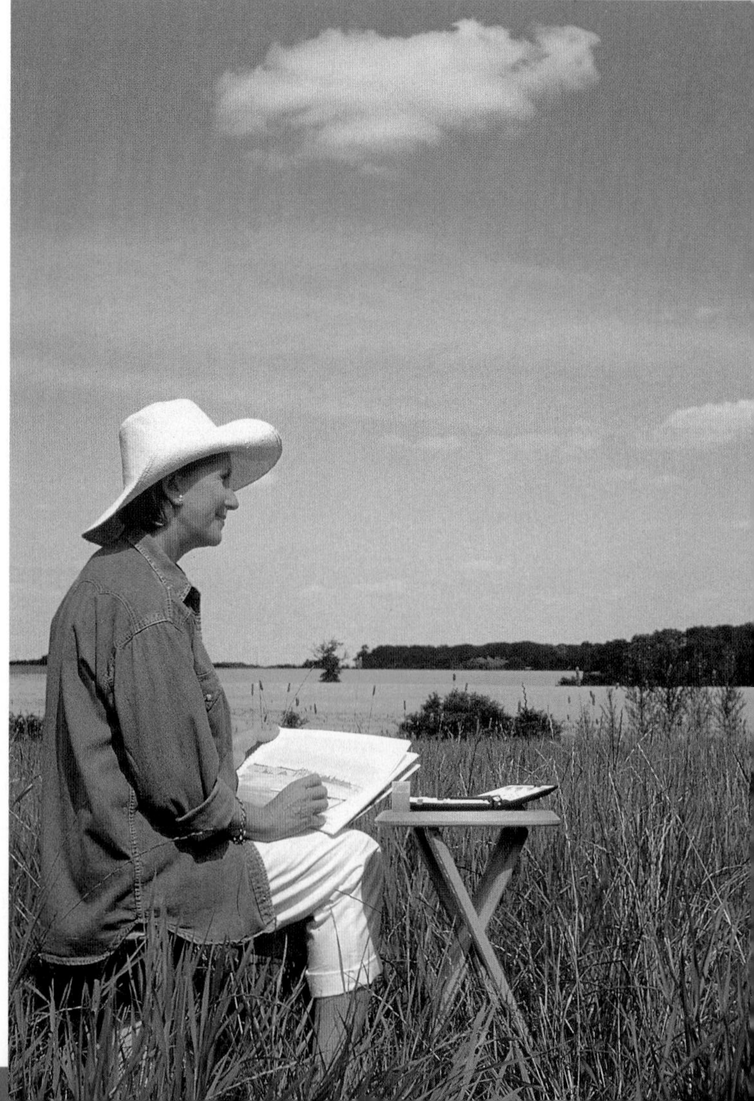

A Healthy Family

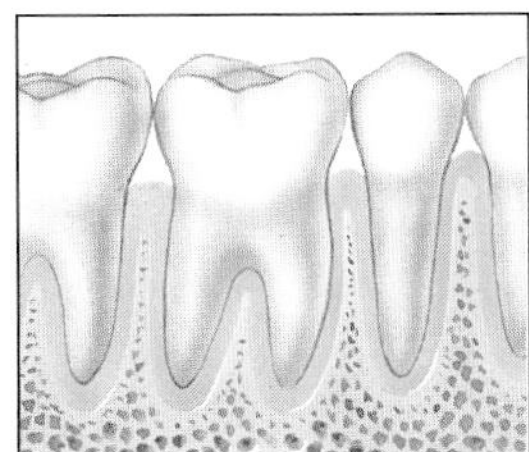

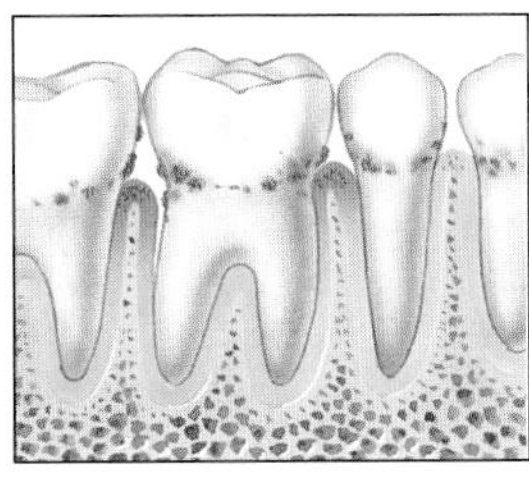

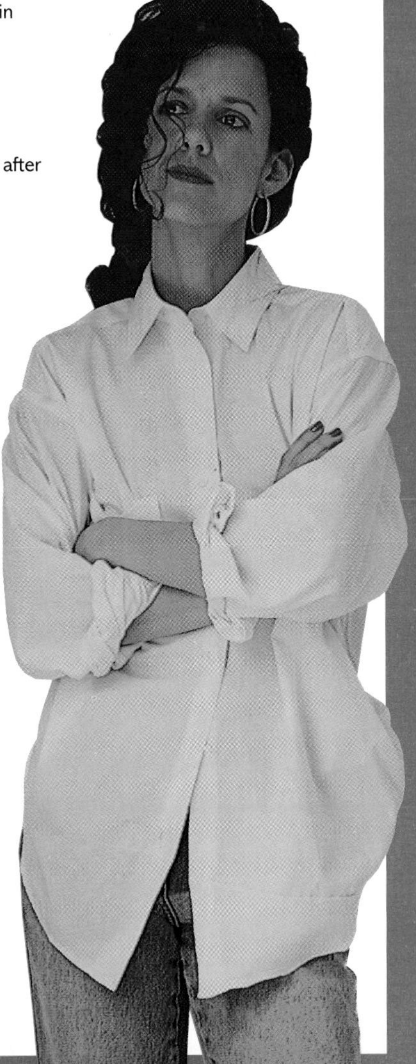

Feet are among the hardest-working parts of the body, so it's important to take care of them. Here's how.

Feet:
A User's Manual

By M. David Tremaine

WE TOO OFTEN UNDERESTIMATE THE IMPORTANCE OF OUR FEET—until they start to hurt! Then we learn that even a seemingly minor problem like a blister or a callus can impair one of our most valued abilities: the ability to move around. Feet are among the hardest-working parts of the body, and they account for a substantial number of our health problems.

With every walking step, the foot carries the full force of the body's weight. This force is multiplied two or three times when a person jogs. Running transmits tons of force to the feet. Sports physicians estimate that people weighing 150 pounds (68 kilograms) place a total of 6 million pounds (2.7 million kilograms) of force on their feet during a marathon run.

The foot is a complex structure. When we stand or walk, 33 small joints and 26 bones keep the foot flexible and help it adapt to a variety of surfaces. Ligaments, elastic tissues that hold bones in position, provide stability at the joints. Several muscle groups start and control the many movements the foot is capable of.

In addition to the daily pounding that feet get, they develop some of the ills that often plague the rest of the body with age: a general weakening of the muscles and bones, the added stress of weight gain, and various disorders that limit movement, impair blood circulation, and inflame joints. But we can increase our comfort if we understand the foot and its care.

The author:

M. David Tremaine, M.D., is an orthopedic surgeon in Arlington, Virginia, and author of *The Foot & Ankle Sourcebook*.

The amazing foot

The intricate, powerful structure of the foot makes it possible for us to perform such movements as dancing, leaping, running, climbing, and pedaling. Each foot has 26 bones and 33 joints that provide stability and flexibility. As we walk, the big toe maintains balance while the little toes act as a springboard. The metatarsal bones on the outside of the foot adjust to uneven walking surfaces, while the three inner metatarsals remain rigid to provide support.

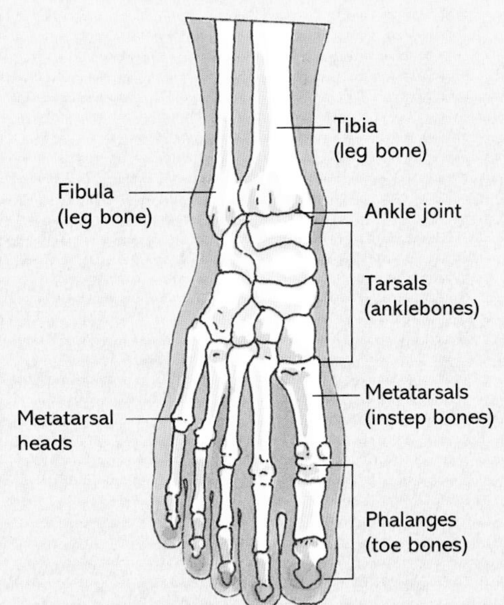

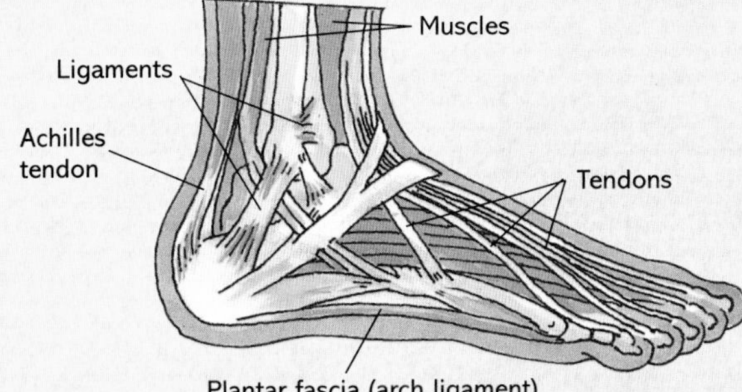

Muscles control the movement of the foot, and tendons attach the muscles to bones. The Achilles tendon, one of the strongest tendons, links the heel bone with the calf muscles. More than 100 elastic tissues called ligaments hold the ends of bones together. The plantar fascia, one of the strongest ligaments, forms the arch.

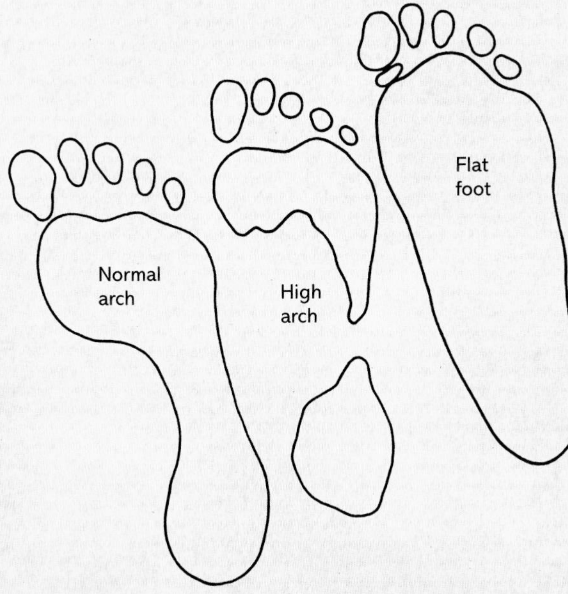

Our footprints show the type of arch we have. In a normal foot, the bones form an arch, supported by muscles and ligaments, that lifts the instep, *far left*. In someone with a high arch, *middle,* the instep is lifted excessively, causing the foot to rotate outward when the heel hits the ground. In someone with a flat foot, *near left,* the instep rests on the ground, usually because weak muscles, tendons, and ligaments do not support the arch.

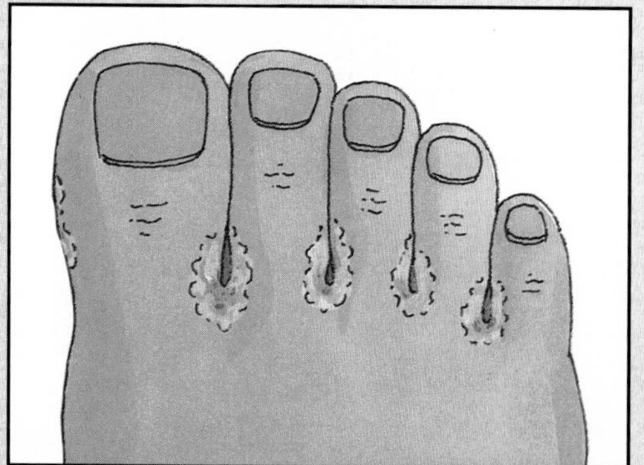

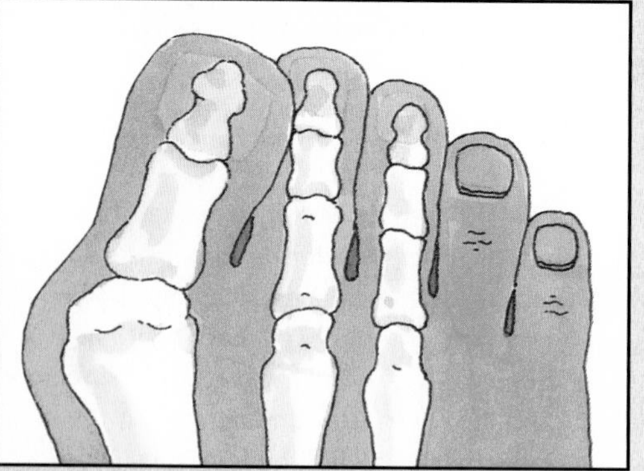

Athlete's foot

Athlete's foot is a skin infection caused by a fungus. It usually occurs between the toes, making the skin whitish and scaly. In severe cases, the skin may develop cracks or open sores. The presence of itching, a smelly discharge, and redness indicate that a bacterial infection has developed as well.

Cause: Sweat or other moisture on the skin serves as an excellent breeding ground for the fungus and for bacteria as well. The chances of developing athlete's foot increase in hot, humid climates and from contact with floor surfaces in public showers and swimming pools, which may harbor the fungus. The disease affects many athletes whose feet regularly become hot and sweaty.

Prevention: Feet should be kept dry. Dry them especially carefully after bathing and swimming. Wear cotton socks, which absorb sweat and let air in, and avoid shoes made of synthetic materials that do not "breathe." Change your socks and shoes daily. Wear shower shoes in public facilities to avoid picking up the fungus.

Treatment: If the infection has not yet caused the skin to crack, an over-the-counter antifungal cream marketed for athlete's foot should help. Apply it on the affected area twice a day for at least 30 days. If the treated skin shows no signs of improvement within 7 to 10 days, it's a good idea to consult a physician. Any crusting, oozing, pus, or redness suggests a bacterial infection and requires medical attention.

Bunions

A bunion is an enlargement of the joint at the base of the big toe, where the toe meets the rest of the foot. It results from a bone misalignment in which the metatarsal bone projects inward at the joint and the toe bone points outward.

A bump on the side of the foot just below the big toe is the first noticeable sign of a bunion. As the misalignment progresses over time, the size of the bump increases and pressure on it causes pain, making it increasingly difficult to find comfortable shoes. The skin over the bump may turn red and become thick.

Other problems can accompany a bunion. Among the most common is a second toe that rides over or under the big toe—a condition known as a hammertoe. As weight is shifted away from the deformed big toe, a painful *callus* (area of thickened skin) may develop on the ball of the foot below the second toe. A callus may also appear on the side of the big toe, where shoes rub against the bunion, and the toenail of the big toe may become ingrown.

Cause: A tendency to develop bunions appears to be hereditary, though this tendency troubles far more women than men. Women's shoes with narrow pointed toes contribute to the problem, as do high-heeled shoes that thrust weight forward onto the front part of the foot.

Prevention: For those with an inherited tendency toward bunions, wearing shoes that fit properly is the best means of prevention. Avoid shoes with pointed toes that contort the foot, and wear high heels only occasionally.

Treatment: After a bunion develops, finding shoes that fit properly becomes especially important. Because the enlarged joint makes the foot wider, shoes with square or rounded toes and extra length are recommended. Low heels also are advisable. When buying shoes, watch for seams that might irritate the bunion.

Other self-treatments for bunions include wearing arch supports or shoes that support the arch. This reduces spreading of the front of the foot, relieving pressure on the bunion. Foam rubber or lambswool "spacers" can be placed between the toes to ease pressure on the bunion. These measures help relieve pain, but they do not halt the progression of the bunion.

Surgery can help correct large bunions. In almost all cases, the procedure requires cutting away the bony protrusion and a part of the metatarsal bone. The surgeon then realigns the ligaments that connect these bones at the joint.

After a bunion develops, stress on the big toe from normal activity leaves the toe susceptible to *arthritis* (joint inflammation). When arthritis has developed in the toe joint, the standard bunion-removal procedures cannot relieve pain and the surgeon may fuse the bones at the joint. The toe loses flexibility as a result.

Bunion surgery rarely requires an overnight hospital stay or general anesthesia. Numbing the foot and ankle usually suffices. The surgeon may insert pins, wires, or other surgical devices to hold the toe in position during and after surgery.

For several days after bunion surgery, patients must limit their activity. Elevating the foot and applying an ice pack are recommended to reduce swelling. Patients need to use crutches for three to six weeks after surgery and wear a strap-on surgical shoe. After six to eight weeks, they can usually return to regular shoes that have extra length, open toes, or a cut-out toe. Most patients can resume their normal activities in comfort from three to six months after the surgery. In approximately 15 to 20 percent of cases, however, the bunion recurs after a few years.

As with any surgery, complications may occur in a few cases. The most common complications are numbness around the big toe and stiffness. Swelling of the foot is common and may persist for months. In such cases, the patient may need to continue wearing a surgical shoe and keep the foot elevated during periods of inactivity.

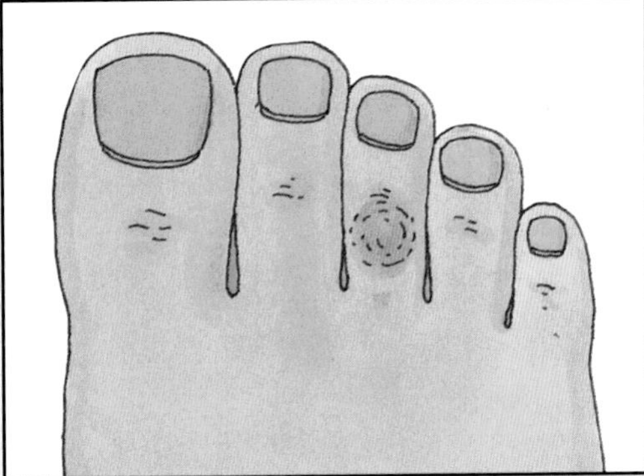

Calluses and corns

A callus is a thickening of the skin that is the body's protective response to recurring friction or pressure. Calluses typically form on the bottom of the feet, though they can form on the fingers and other parts of the body. A corn is a callus that develops between the toes or on top of them.

Cause: The pressure responsible for calluses and corns can stem from foot abnormalities and from ill-fitting shoes. For example, calluses commonly form on bunions that press against the inside of shoes. High arches, which cause the instep bones to push downward, can lead to calluses on the ball of the foot. High heels thrust the bones of the instep forward, thus putting added pressure on the ball of the foot.

Prevention: Calluses and corns can best be prevented by avoiding high heels and shoes that pinch the toes.

Treatment: The first step in treating a corn or callus is to remedy the problem causing it: Don't wear shoes that are too narrow or too short, and consider buying a larger size. A cushioned corn pad with an opening over the corn can reduce friction. Special metatarsal pads can reduce pressure on calluses that form on the balls of the feet. Padded sole inserts and soft-soled shoes also help. Over-the-counter remedies for corns that work by burning the skin should be avoided.

The larger the callus, the more pain it causes. To reduce the callus's size, soak it in warm water to soften it, and then file it down with a pumice stone. People who have poor eyesight, limited dexterity, or reduced sensation in their feet as a result of diabetes should not trim their calluses.

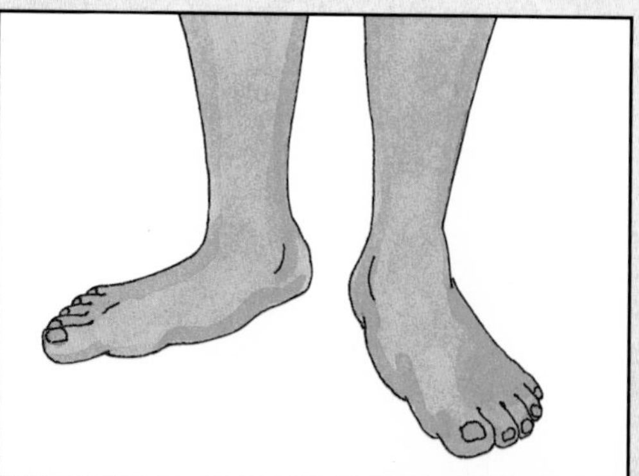

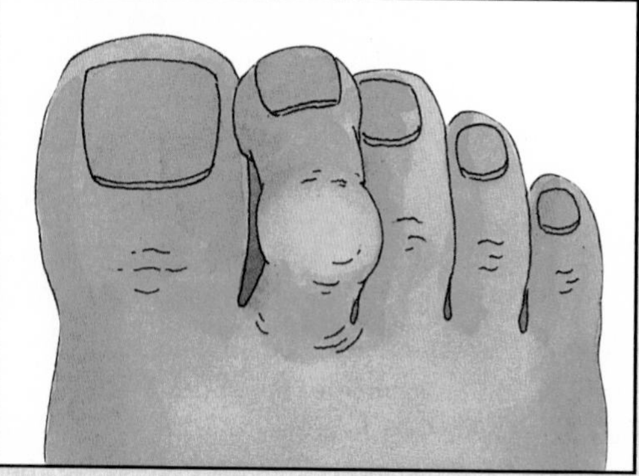

Flat feet and fallen arches

A flat foot is one that has little or no arch. Many flat feet cause no problem. However, when the condition develops in adulthood—a disorder known as fallen arches—it is characterized by pain and swelling in the arch and the inside of the ankle. Fallen arches occur most often in overweight adults in middle age or later. The condition progresses until the rupture of the tendon that attaches to the muscles supporting the arch.

Cause: All children have flat feet until the ligaments and muscles of the foot complete their development at about age 6. Sometimes, for unknown reasons, the muscles that normally support the arch remain weak and no arch develops.

Prevention: Little can be done to prevent flat feet. Seriously overweight adults can lessen their risk of fallen arches by losing weight.

Treatment: Flat feet may require no treatment unless they present problems. Fallen arches are usually treated nonsurgically first, with a cast on the foot or a molded arch support in the shoe.

Because fallen arches tend to worsen over time, surgery is often necessary. The surgical procedure used depends on the extent of the foot's collapse. In less severe cases, the surgeon may support the arch by transplanting a tendon from another part of the foot and by realigning some of the bones in the midfoot.

In more severe cases, the surgeon may fuse small joints of the midfoot and hind foot to prevent further collapse. This leaves the foot less flexible and less able to adapt to uneven surfaces. The foot remains in a cast for three months after surgery, and crutches must be used for six weeks. The foot can then gradually begin to bear weight.

Hammertoes

A hammertoe is a deformed toe in which the two end joints bend downward in a clawlike position and the joint nearest the rest of the foot bends upward. A mallet toe is similar but involves only the joint nearest the tip of the toe. When the deformity first becomes apparent, the toe is still flexible and capable of being straightened. Over time, the toe becomes inflexible, and so early treatment is important.

The affected toe is usually the second one, though the curling can occur on one or more toes and on one or both feet. Many people who have a hammertoe first developed a bunion on the big toe. A painful callus frequently develops over the uplifted joint or under the tip of the toe. Pain also may arise from a callus that forms on the ball of the foot. This condition—pain in the ball of the foot—is known as metatarsalgia.

Cause: Although some people develop a hammertoe following an injury, many cases have no known cause. However, the problem stems in part from an imbalance in pulling power between the muscles and tendons on the top of the toe and those on the bottom.

Bunions, which can cause toes to overlap, can contribute to the formation of a hammertoe. High heels and shoes with pointed toes can aggravate the condition.

Prevention: The basic measure for preventing hammertoes and metatarsalgia is wearing shoes with low heels and a roomy toe. High heels aggravate metatarsalgia by angling the rounded ends of the metatarsal bones downward against the ball of the foot. Shoes that are too tight or too short can contribute to the formation of a hammertoe or a mallet toe by bending the toes.

Treatment: A hammertoe strap—a cushioned pad placed beneath the ball of the foot with a strap that fits over the toe—can pull down the hammertoe, thereby relieving pressure on both the toe and the ball of the foot. A metatarsal pad placed inside the shoe shifts weight from the ball of the foot to the heel, relieving metatarsalgia. A foam or moleskin cushion can ease pressure on calluses and corns that form where the hooked toe rubs against the shoe. To lessen painful pressure on a callus at the tip of the toe, a pad called a toe crest can be placed under the mallet toe to lift the toe from the sole of the shoe.

When these measures fail to relieve the pain, surgery becomes an option. Surgery can, if necessary, be performed on more than one toe at a time. In the standard procedure, the physician releases tendons and ligaments to bring pulling power back into balance and then fuses the toe joint nearest the rest of the foot. In some cases, the hammertoe must be shortened by cutting away some of the bone. If a bunion is contributing to the hammertoe or mallet toe, that condition requires surgical correction as well. While the toe is healing, a pin holds it in a straight position. The pin is removed in the doctor's office after three or four weeks.

If the main problem is metatarsalgia, the physician may cut and reposition the metatarsal bone to lift the metatarsal head so that it applies less pressure to the ball of the foot. Unfortunately, this procedure carries the risk of transferring pressure to one of the other metatarsals, and further surgery may later be needed as a result.

After surgery, the patient usually wears a surgical shoe or an elastic bandage. The recovery period is similar to that following bunion surgery, except that patients spend less time on crutches after hammertoe surgery.

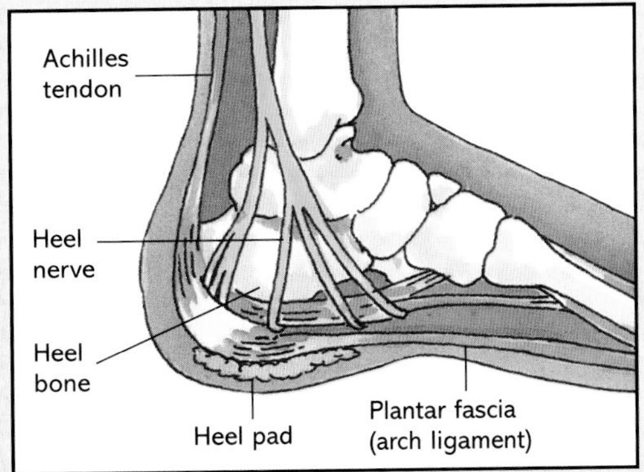

Heel pain

Heel pain is a fairly common condition that occurs primarily in middle age or later as the result of cumulative stresses on the heel. The day-to-day pounding the heel takes is enormous and becomes six to nine times greater when we run or jump than when we walk. The fatty pad that covers the heel bone acts as a shock absorber when we move about and our heels strike the ground. But over time, these heel pads wear down.

Pain in the heel results primarily from inflammation of the soft tissues covering the heel bone—particularly the arch ligament, known as the plantar fascia, which extends along the arch and connects the heel to the toes. Heel pain ranges from a mild ache upon waking to severe pain that lasts all day. The pain may occur in one heel or in both.

Tightness of the Achilles tendon, which extends from the heel along the ankle to the calf, is often associated with heel pain. When this is the case, the pain is usually worst upon rising and subsides over the course of the day as the tendon stretches out. The pain can recur at the end of the day, however, especially after standing on the feet all day.

Cause: Heel pain has many causes, but the primary instigator is inflammation of the plantar fascia. The function of this ligament is to hold the foot steady as we move about and our weight shifts onto the balls of our feet.

Many things can overstress the plantar fascia and lead to inflammation. The chief culprit is a tight Achilles tendon, especially in people who have flat feet or a high arch. When the Achilles tendon is tight and inflexible, the foot compensates by rolling inward when it hits the ground. This motion, known as pronation, puts extra stress on the plantar fascia and is more pronounced in people with flat feet. In people with high arches, the tightness of the arch ligament and Achilles tendon leave the foot susceptible to plantar fasciitis.

Inflammation of the plantar fascia was once thought to result from a heel spur—a tiny projection of the heel bone at the point where the arch ligament joins the bone. Although a heel spur is present in many people who have heel pain, most foot surgeons now believe that the spur has little or nothing to do with the pain.

In rare cases, heel pain appears to be associated with another disease that involves inflammation, including certain forms of arthritis and colitis, an inflammatory disease of the bowel. Irritation of the nerve that passes over the heel bone also can produce heel pain. Obesity, which increases the pressure on the feet, can contribute to heel pain. So can taking up running or jogging after a long period of inactivity.

Prevention: Exercises that stretch the Achilles tendon can help prevent heel pain. Prolonged standing and obesity, which place extra stress on the heel area, should be avoided, especially by people with high arches or flat feet. People who take up running or jogging should start gradually and wear sports shoes with well padded soles.

Treatment: Stretching the ligaments and tendons that attach to the heel is the most effective self-treatment for heel pain. Before getting out of bed in the morning, point your feet toward your nose. Hold the stretch for 15 seconds without wiggling the toes, and then repeat the stretch three times. Taking a warm shower or soaking in a warm tub followed by more stretching can reduce heel pain dramatically. People who sit for long periods should repeat the stretches before standing up, extending their legs parallel to the floor and pointing their feet toward their nose.

Other helpful steps include placing a heel cushion or sole insert in the shoe and wearing soft-soled rather than leather-soled shoes. Taking aspirin or a nonsteroidal anti-inflammatory drug such as ibuprofen can help reduce inflammation, though prolonged use of these drugs should be monitored by a physician. Massaging the heel with ice for a few minutes several times a day also may help reduce pain and inflammation.

Medical attention is called for if heel pain persists or worsens. The physician may inject the drug cortisone into the heel to reduce inflammation or suggest the use of molded foot supports to control pronation.

The physician may perform surgery in the rare cases that fail to respond after six to nine months of nonsurgical treatment. The usual procedure involves partially cutting the arch ligament to relieve the tension on it. If the nerve to the heel is irritated, the nerve may be severed as well. Recuperation from surgery takes from six weeks to three months. Although the surgery is successful in 75 to 80 percent of cases, some patients continue to experience pain after the procedure.

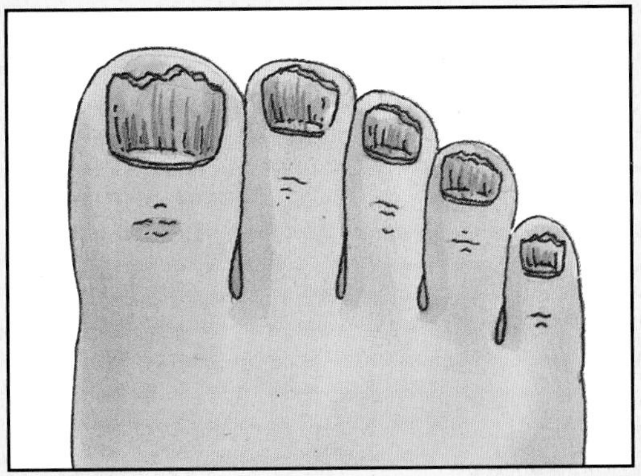

Nail problems

Toenails are a common site for fungus infections. Various symptoms can indicate the presence of an infection. The infection may produce white or yellow dots or streaks on the nail, or the entire nail may become discolored. The nail may thicken and loosen or even separate entirely from the nail bed. It can also crumble. In some cases, the entire nail becomes green and painful. This suggests a more serious infection that requires professional medical treatment.

Cause: Warm, moist environments serve as excellent breeding grounds for fungi, and moisture or dirt that accumulates under the toenails can foster their growth.

Prevention: Keep the toenails clean and dry. Avoid shoes made of synthetic materials that make the feet sweat and hold moisture in. Follow the steps for preventing athlete's foot.

Treatment: Once established, toenail fungus infections are difficult to get rid of. Treatment is successful in only about half the cases, and over-the-counter remedies are rarely effective. For these reasons, fungus infections that cause no pain are probably best left untreated. For more serious cases, doctors can prescribe creams or oral medications. When the nail is severely damaged, the physician may recommend surgical removal of the nail. People who have diabetes should seek medical treatment at the first sign of a nail infection.

An ingrown toenail is a painful condition in which one or both corners of the nail press into the soft tissue alongside the nail, producing inflammation and, in many cases, infection. In the most severe cases, a red streak runs up the foot and along the leg. This complication indicates blood poisoning, which requires emergency medical treatment.

Cause: Ingrown toenails are most often caused by wearing tight shoes or by trimming the nails down the sides rather than straight across, thus exposing delicate tissue. This tissue easily becomes infected when punctured by the toenail itself or by any other object. People with other foot abnormalities, including bunions and hammertoes, are especially vulnerable to ingrown toenails. In addition, injury can cause the nail to grow at an abnormal angle, increasing the likelihood of irritation to tissue.

Prevention: Ingrown toenails can usually be prevented by trimming the nails properly and by wearing shoes with sufficient room in the toe. When trimming the nails, cut them straight across. Avoid cutting the corners of the nails at an angle.

Treatment: Soaking the foot in warm water can relieve pain while the nail is growing out. If infection occurs, medical treatment is needed, and an antibiotic ointment or an oral antibiotic may be prescribed. It's also important to determine the cause of the ingrown toenail to prevent its recurrence. If the condition persists, the physician may recommend surgery to remove part of the nail.

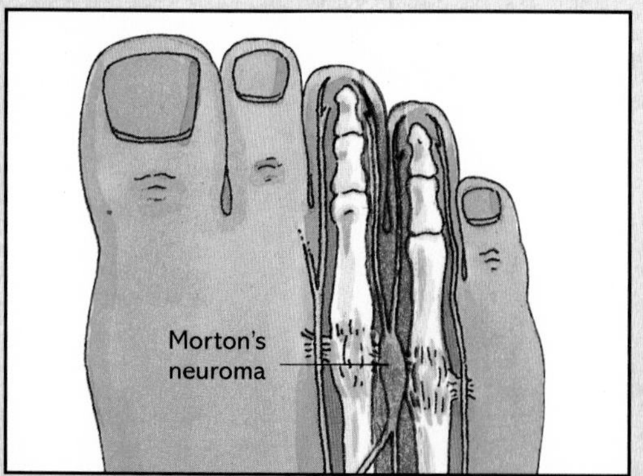

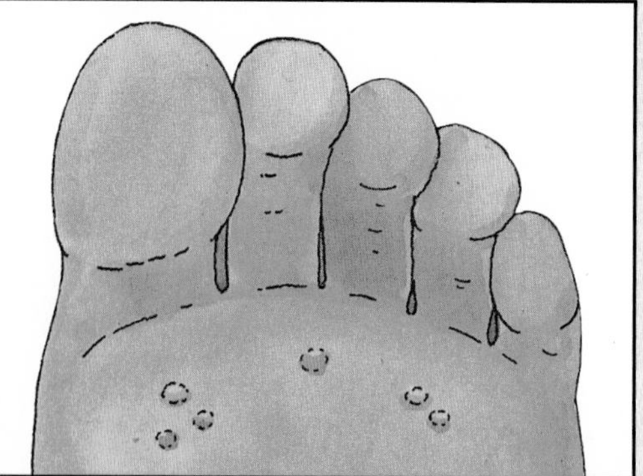

Neuromas

A neuroma is an inflammation of a nerve or of the tissue around the nerve. The symptoms can include numbness, burning, or tingling radiating from the area. In some cases, pain that occurs in the ball of the foot can be disabling.

Cause: Any injury to a nerve can lead to a neuroma. The most common foot neuroma, called Morton's neuroma, usually results from pinching of the nerve that extends between the metatarsal bones into the toes. It typically produces numbness and tingling between the third and fourth toes or the second and third toes. Neuromas are seven to eight times more common among women than men. Shoes with pointed toes that pinch and high heels, which thrust body weight onto the ball of the foot, can aggravate a neuroma.

Prevention: Avoiding high heels and shoes that pinch helps prevent irritation of the nerve.

Treatment: The first response to a neuroma in the foot should be to wear shoes with low heels. A small metatarsal pad beneath the ball of the foot can relieve pressure on the nerve.

Anyone with the symptoms of a neuroma should consult a physician. An injection of the drug cortisone and an anesthetic can reduce inflammation and produce quick pain relief, but the benefit is often only temporary. In such cases, surgery may be recommended. The standard procedure involves cutting out the inflamed nerve and releasing the ligaments putting pressure on the nerve. This leaves the area between the toes permanently numb but does not affect the functioning of the foot. Patients use crutches for two or three weeks after surgery. A new neuroma sometimes forms where the old one was cut.

Warts

A wart is a skin growth caused by a virus. Warts known as plantar's warts occur singly or in clusters on the soles of the feet, where minor cuts provide an entry for the virus. These warts are often mistaken for calluses. Both are thickened, raised areas of skin. But unlike calluses, warts have tiny, dark dots in their center formed by blood vessels. Warts also are painful when squeezed from the sides, whereas calluses hurt only when pressure is applied directly on them.

Cause: The virus that causes plantar's warts most commonly enters the skin through minor cuts on the soles of the feet. Walking barefoot, especially on dirty or littered ground, increases the likelihood of developing warts.

Prevention: The best means of preventing plantar's warts is to keep the feet clean and dry. Wash cuts on the soles of the feet immediately, and apply an antiseptic lotion.

Treatment: Warts may disappear in time without treatment. To remove isolated warts or several small warts, an over-the-counter solution of salicylic acid or trichloricedic acid can be applied each evening. The surrounding skin should be protected by a moleskin doughnut to prevent irritation. In the morning, soak the foot in warm water and gently rub the area of the warts with a pumice stone or stiff cloth. The treatment should continue until the skin is clear, but it should not be used to treat large clusters of warts.

If warts persist, stronger medications or surgical removal are possibilities. Physicians remove warts by several methods, including cutting them off, heating them with a laser or electric needle, or freezing them with a chemical.

Diabetes and feet

Foot care is especially important to people with diabetes—some 14 million Americans and about 120 million people worldwide. Many of them are unaware that they have the disease. If diabetes is not properly controlled, it can cause damage to nerves, resulting in a loss of sensation, especially in the legs and feet. As a result, cuts and infections may go unnoticed and untreated. By the time the problem is detected, amputation may be necessary to save the patient's life. Even a seemingly minor infection can lead to serious complications. Doctors emphasize that no foot infection is trivial in someone who has diabetes.

Loss of sensation is not the only complication of diabetes associated with the feet. Poor blood circulation can cause pain while walking. Open sores on the feet also can result from circulation problems—and from ill-fitting shoes. Such sores require immediate and aggressive treatment to control infection. Sudden swelling of the feet also calls for emergency treatment.

Only proper foot care by medical professionals and by the patient and the patient's family can prevent serious problems. Basic guidelines on foot care for people with diabetes include the following:

- Maintain a proper weight to ease the burden on the feet, and follow a low-fat, high-fiber diet to aid blood circulation by keeping arteries healthy.
- Exercise regularly, and include exercises that pump the feet up and down and improve blood circulation.
- Inspect the feet daily; more often if there is a loss of sensation. Look for such signs of problems as redness, swelling, blisters, ulcers, or increased warmth. Any of these signs require immediate medical attention.
- Avoid tobacco and caffeine, which *constrict* (narrow) the blood vessels and reduce the blood supply to the legs and feet.
- Wash the feet daily and dry them carefully between the toes to reduce the chances of infection from fungi and other microbes.
- Avoid walking barefoot, which increases the chances of injury and infection.
- Inspect the insides of shoes every day for signs of wear and anything that might rub against the feet. Always shake shoes out before putting them on.
- Avoid wearing shoes without socks, and wear socks that are not constrictive or mended. Cotton socks, which absorb moisture, are best.
- Do not use chemicals or over-the-counter skin products on your feet. To alleviate dry skin, apply baby oil or mineral oil and then wipe away any excess oil.
- Don't trim calluses. Get professional care.
- Don't use elastic bandages or tape on the feet or ankles. They can reduce circulation.
- Avoid hot surfaces and hot water. Lack of sensation can prevent people from feeling the heat and lead to a burn.
- Elevate the feet whenever possible to keep swelling under control.
- Be sure shoes fit properly, and have feet measured each time before buying shoes.

Buying shoes that fit

For years, fashion demanded that women jam their feet into shoes with narrow, pointed toes, and women developed foot problems as a result. Today, it's easier to find shoes that fit properly, especially if you know what to look for.

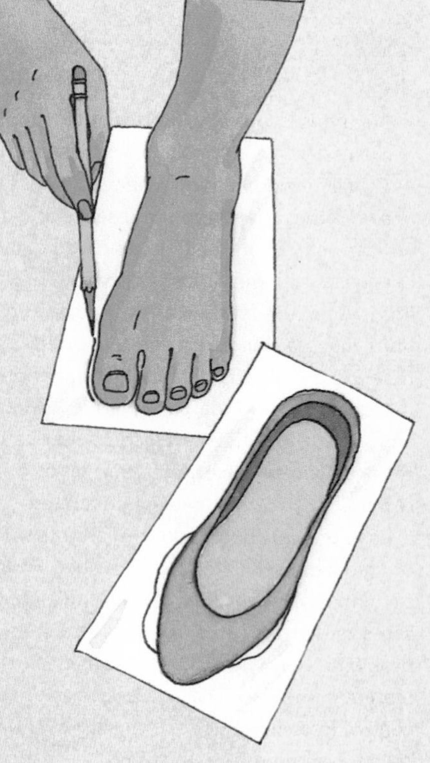

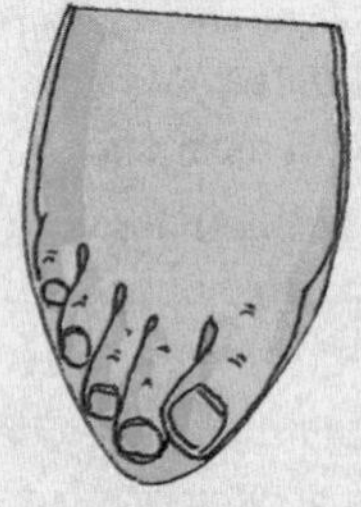

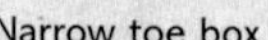

Narrow toe box

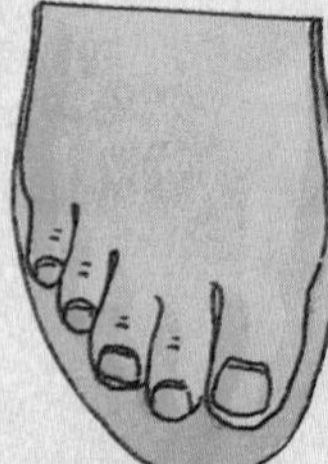

Wide toe box

The toe box of a shoe that fits should be roomy. The toes should be able to wiggle, the shoe shouldn't pinch, and there should be space between the tip of the longest toe and the end of the shoe. It's possible to test the fit of shoes by tracing the outline of the foot while standing on a piece of paper, *top right.* Then place the shoe over the outline. If the outline of the foot extends beyond the outline of the shoe, the shoes are too narrow.

Tips for a good fit

- If shoes don't feel comfortable, don't buy them.
- Don't expect your feet to stretch tight shoes.
- Have your feet measured each time you buy shoes; feet stretch with age.
- Have both feet measured, as feet may differ in size. Buy shoes that fit the larger foot.
- Try on shoes late in the day, when feet have swollen to their largest size.
- If you cannot find shoes that fit, ask your doctor for advice.

What a well-fitting shoe should have

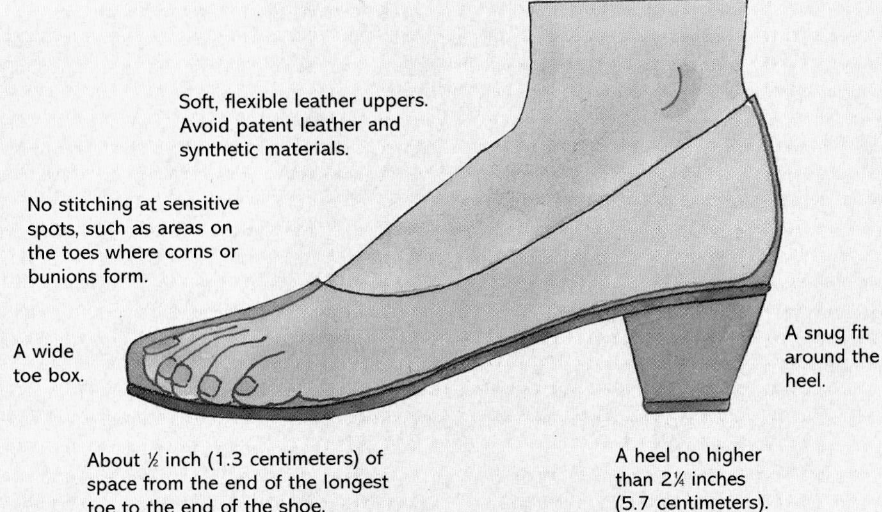

Buying children's shoes

It is important that children's shoes fit properly because their feet are still developing. An ill-fitting shoe can deform a child's pliable foot.

In addition to general guidelines for choosing shoes that fit, some additional guidelines apply to children:

- Children do not need to wear shoes until they begin to walk. The main purpose of shoes for toddlers is to protect their feet from injury.
- Toddlers do not need high-topped shoes to support their ankles. Tennis shoes or oxfords work just as well for them.
- Parents should check a child's shoes often to see if they still fit. Children's feet are very flexible and can be stuffed into shoes that are too small. Parents cannot count on the child to complain about ill-fitting shoes.
- Children should not wear hand-me-down shoes because shoes mold themselves to an owner's foot. A hand-me-down shoe will have the shape of its original owner's foot.

The shoe should fit the sport

All sports shoes are designed to enhance athletic performance. But there are many types, each made to protect feet from the stresses of a particular sport. Two features that all sports shoes should offer are support and shock absorption. Foot specialists suggest that you wear a sport-specific shoe for any sport you engage in more than three times a week. Cross-training shoes are good for people who participate in different sports.

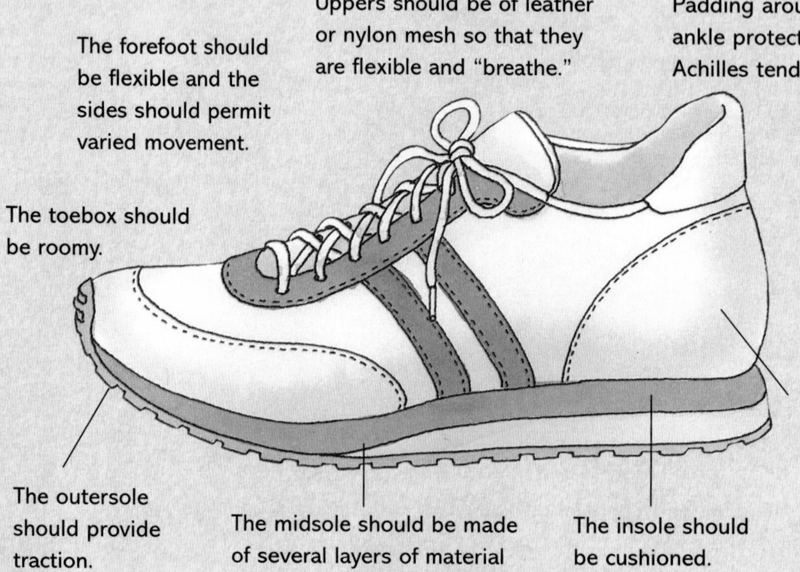

The sole should be flexible to allow rapid movement.

Who treats feet?

Primary care physicians can treat many foot ailments. But feet, like other parts of the body, sometimes require specialized care. The following specialists are trained to provide foot care.

An orthopedist is a physician who specializes in the treatment of problems of the body's musculo-skeletal system—that is, the bones, joints, muscles, tendons, and ligaments. Orthopedists, also called orthopedic surgeons, can diagnose and treat various foot and ankle deformities, injuries, and disorders.

An orthopedist receives four years of training at a medical school, leading to the degree of Doctor of Medicine (M.D.). This is followed by a five-year postgraduate residency in orthopedic surgery, which includes training in foot and ankle problems. Some orthopedists complete additional training in foot and ankle problems and are said to have a subspecialty in the foot and ankle.

Physicians who pass written and oral qualifying examinations are certified to practice orthopedic surgery by the American Board of Orthopedic Surgeons. The American College of Orthopedic Surgeons is the professional organization for board-certified orthopedists.

A podiatrist is a doctor of podiatric medicine. Podiatrists diagnose and treat a variety of diseases, malfunctions, and injuries involving the foot, ankle, and related structures. Podiatrists may perform surgery, prescribe medication, and prescribe and fit corrective shoes and other corrective devices.

A podiatrist receives four years of training at a college of podiatric medicine, which leads to the degree of Doctor of Podiatric Medicine (D.P.M.). Most podiatrists also complete a postgraduate residency of at least one year. Podiatrists who pass written and oral qualifying examinations are certified to practice podiatry. The American College of Foot and Ankle Surgeons is the professional organization for podiatric surgeons.

A pedorthist is a specialist in the design, fitting, and modification of footwear and in *orthotics* (molded inserts to place in the shoe) for relieving foot pain. Pedorthists are usually associated with a shoe store or foot clinic.

People who pass qualifying examinations are certified to prescribe footwear and assist in the design of orthotics by the Board of Certification in Pedorthics.

For more information:

American Academy of Orthopedic Surgeons.
6300 North River Road
Rosemont, Illinois 60018-4226
(800) 346-AAOS.

American Orthopedic Foot and Ankle Society
701 16th Avenue
Seattle, Washington 98122
(800) 235-4855

American College of Foot and Ankle Surgeons
444 North Northwest Highway
Park Ridge, Illinois 60068
(708) 292-2237

Pedorthic Footwear Association
9861 Broken Land Parkway
Columbia, Maryland 21046-1151
(800) 673-8447

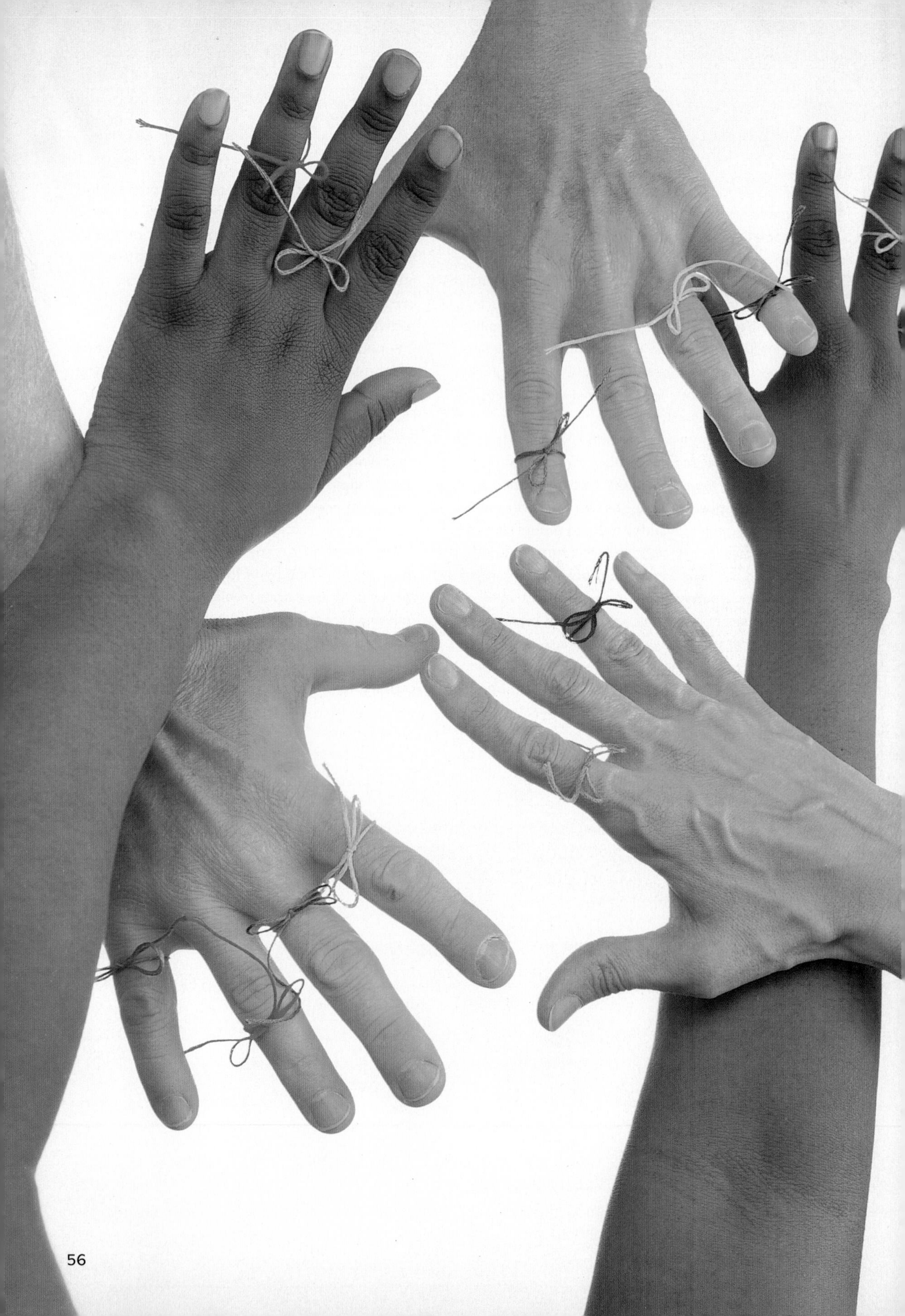

Remembering Not to Forget

By Danielle C. Lapp

WHEN PEOPLE FIRST NOTICE that their memory is failing, they may fear that Alzheimer's disease is just around the corner. People who are in their 20's or 30's don't find it especially worrisome to walk into a room and not remember why they're there. But by the time they reach their 50's, such lapses can seem ominous.

Some degree of forgetfulness is normal at any age. But if you can remember later what it was you forgot to do—pick up the cleaning or call your mother—your memory is still working, even if not to your satisfaction. Before jumping to the conclusion that you have a serious memory problem, ask yourself two questions: "Do I remember what I *need* or *want* to remember?" and "How good was my memory in the first place?"

Forgetting is part of memory's normal operation. If you could remember everything you thought, read, heard, saw, and felt, life would be impossible. Imagine how awful it would be to remember every hurt feeling or the dialogue of every movie you have seen. In fact, the only way to pay attention to what's happening at the moment is to put aside most other thoughts. Overall, people are better off if they have a sense of what's worth remembering and what's not.

Forgetfulness increases with normal aging, but there are techniques to improve memory at any age.

Memory researchers like myself have found that people can regain control over their memories if they understand something about the processes of remembering and forgetting. This understanding helps them actively participate in the encoding, storage, and recall of information they want to retain. Memory failures typically trigger anxiety, and anxiety is one of memory's worst enemies. People become far less anxious about memory problems once they realize that these are a normal part of aging and that there are strategies they can employ to improve recall.

For example, when you can't remember a familiar word, such as the name of a street you pass every day, the best strategy is to relax and let memory's mental "scanner" take over. Most words come back within 30 seconds. The inability to recall a name or a particular word—the tip-of-the-tongue phenomenon—is one of the most common memory lapses.

The links in memory's chain

People are rarely aware of memory's workings until they experience a memory lapse. They typically expect memory to operate automatically, storing information until they are ready to retrieve it. A major reason for forgetfulness is, in fact, this reliance on spontaneous processes. But by making conscious use of mental strategies to form a strong impression, or memory trace, it's possible to greatly improve the likelihood of recall.

Imagine memory as a chain with the following links:

Need or Interest—>Motivation—>
Attention—>Concentration—>Organization

A need to remember something or a keen interest in something provides the motivation for paying attention. Only then does a person apply the concentration and organization needed to store the information properly. When memory problems arise, something has happened to break this chain and interfere with the storage of the information, thereby preventing recall.

Consider a student who wishes to do well in a course. This desire provides the motivation to pay attention in class. With sustained attention, the student concentrates more fully on what the instructor is saying. Concentration enables the student to organize the instructor's lecture in a meaningful way. Organization works as an index, enabling the mind to locate the desired information in its storage site in the brain—during the final examination, for example.

Sustained attention is the key to storing information. If you are not paying attention while something is happening, you are unlikely to remember it afterward. Among the chief reasons for inattention is lack of motivation. If you don't need to recall something or you are not interested in it, you have little motivation to pay attention to it. So before saying "I forgot," stop and think. Perhaps a more accurate assessment would be "I couldn't pay attention" or "I didn't listen."

Many situations can make it difficult to sustain attention. When

The author:

Danielle C. Lapp is a cognitive rehabilitation specialist at Stanford University and the author of articles and books on improving memory.

you're rushed, stressed, depressed, or anxious, for example, your worries monopolize your attention and make it difficult to concentrate. Attention can fade if you're tired or drowsy; some medications also contribute to drowsiness. Digressions and interruptions can sabotage attention. But what probably subverts attention most of all is the automatic gesture. Anything done automatically or by habit, such as parking the car, may mean trouble later on—when you go to find the car and can't remember where you parked it.

Paying greater attention means intensifying awareness of sense perceptions. All information enters the brain through one or more of the five senses—hearing, sight, smell, taste, and touch. But these sense perceptions stay in the mind less than a second and fade quickly unless transferred to short-term memory. Short-term memory is also called working memory because it holds information in active use—for example, a phone number while you are dialing it. Information remains in short-term memory only about 20 seconds after you stop thinking about it. Then, it either enters long-term memory or is forgotten. The more sense perceptions—such as images, sounds, and tastes—that people attach to information, the "deeper" the processing of the memory trace and the easier it is to recall later.

Sometimes sensations cue memories to surface spontaneously. The classic example comes from *Remembrance of Things Past* by French author Marcel Proust. Proust's narrator tells of dipping a small cake called a madeleine into a cup of tea. As he tastes the cake, happy memories of his childhood flood over him. Most of us have experienced such spontaneous recall, perhaps while smelling

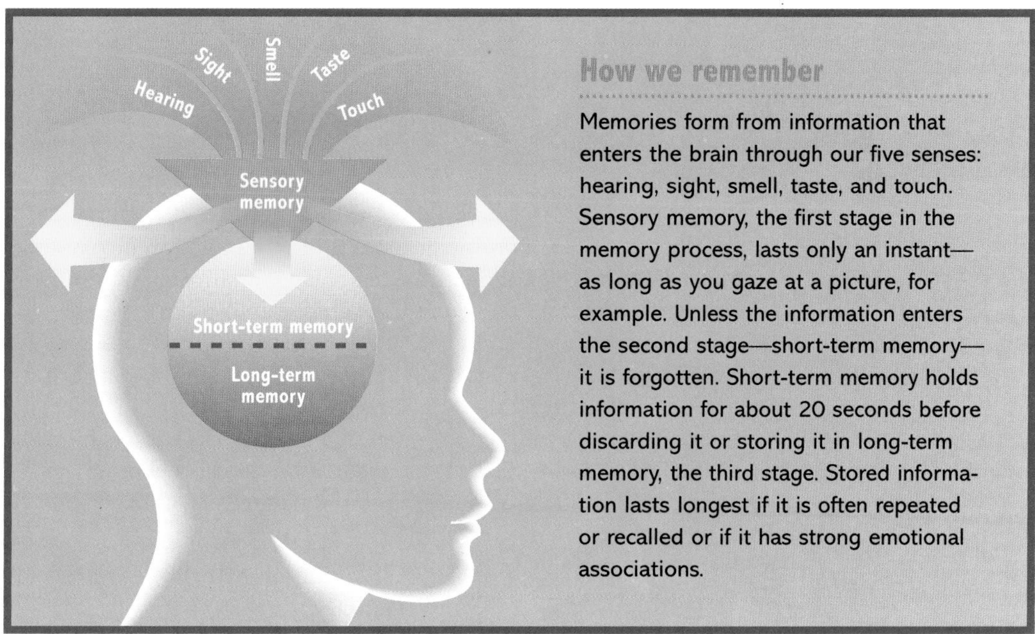

How we remember

Memories form from information that enters the brain through our five senses: hearing, sight, smell, taste, and touch. Sensory memory, the first stage in the memory process, lasts only an instant—as long as you gaze at a picture, for example. Unless the information enters the second stage—short-term memory—it is forgotten. Short-term memory holds information for about 20 seconds before discarding it or storing it in long-term memory, the third stage. Stored information lasts longest if it is often repeated or recalled or if it has strong emotional associations.

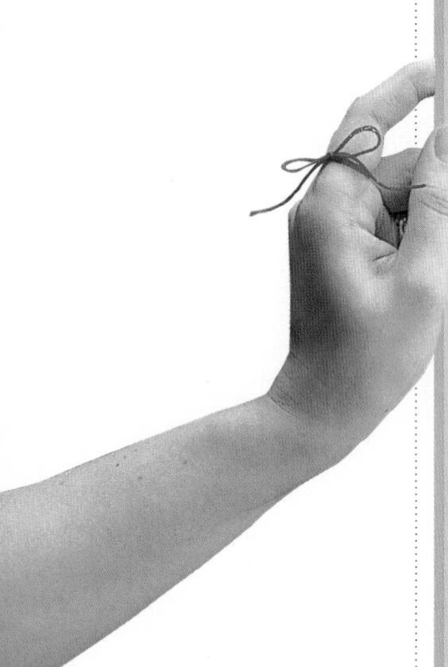

How aging affects memory

Various changes that accompany aging can alter our ability to store and retrieve information: the two keys to memory. Aging can interfere with storage and retrieval in the following ways, but there are ways of managing these limitations.

- **Impaired vision and hearing.** Have them tested regularly because you can't remember what you don't hear or see.
- **Shortened attention span.** If you find you tire or your attention wanders more easily than before, take frequent breaks.
- **Slowed response time.** Take your time and try not to be impatient. The missing word or thought will resurface.
- **Reduced memory capacity.** Accept the fact that memory function declines with age and try not to worry about lapses.
- **Greater difficulty organizing thought.** With age, it takes conscious effort to organize thinking, a process that occurred automatically when we were young.
- **Greater difficulty doing several things at once.** Focus on one task at a time and you'll have less trouble finishing it.
- **More sensitivity to distraction.** When undertaking a task, try to minimize interruptions and distractions that can make you forget what you were doing.
- **Reduced activity and need to remember.** After retirement, there's less incentive to stay active and alert, so find activities you enjoy and set specific goals.
- **Greater vulnerability to depression** as a result of losses—of career, health, or loved ones. Seek professional help if the blues don't lift. Depression is treatable.

Source: Danielle C. Lapp.

a particularly pungent aroma or looking at a photograph or painting.

Repetition provides another means of tagging information for long-term storage. When you repeat something such as a phone number for longer than about 20 seconds, the information enters long-term memory. The more often you repeat the number or call it to mind, the more durable the memory becomes.

Information also enters long-term memory through association with intense emotion. The anxious anticipation before a prom, sorrow over a pet's death, or other emotion-charged situations create lasting memories that often are retrievable for a lifetime.

Memory experts make a distinction between remembering how to do something—performance memory—and the more intellectual skill of remembering facts and other verbal and visual information,

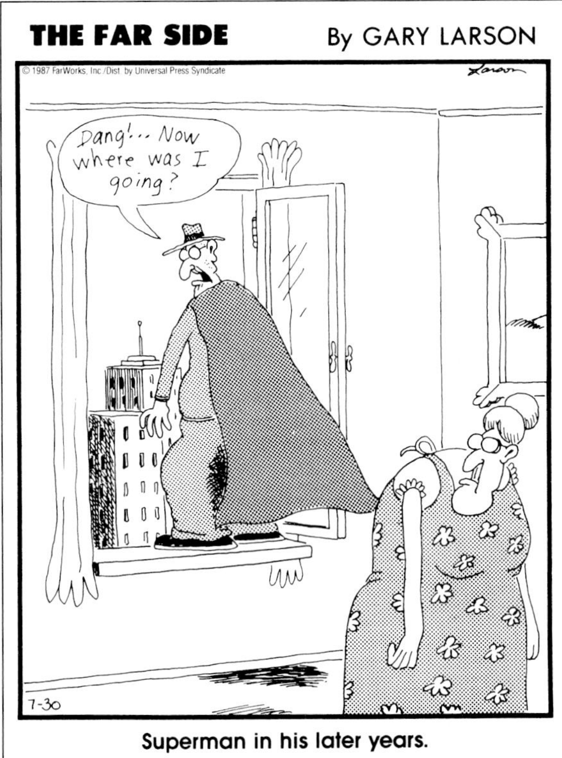

Superman in his later years.

Common—and normal—memory lapses

Memory lapses occur at all ages, though they become more frequent with age. Some things we commonly forget include:

- Faces and names.
- Specific words—the tip-of-the-tongue phenomenon.
- Directions.
- Where we've left objects in regular use, such as keys and eye glasses.
- What we've just heard.
- What we've just read.

Source: Danielle C. Lapp.

known as declarative memory. Learning to ride a bicycle, for example, conditions muscles and reflexes, and this physical information is stored in performance memory. Learning how the parts of a bicycle work calls for analytic skills, and this information is stored in declarative memory.

Skills stored in performance memory are especially long lasting. But how well people retrieve information from declarative memory depends upon their current analytic ability. In general, retrieval from declarative memory becomes more difficult with age, reflecting a decline in analytic ability.

How memories become altered

Time alters memories, both through disuse and through use. An incident that is never recalled may disappear from memory. Repetition, though key to memory storage, can also transform memories. In recalling an incident, a person may unconsciously tamper with the memory—leaving some things out, for example, or adding a detail that seems relevant at the moment.

These alterations occur because the context in which people recall a memory differs from the original experience, and the new circumstances may prompt them to call up different details. In recalling an important conversation, someone might omit what now seem to be embarrassing moments, while adding remarks that should have been made, which then become part of the remembered conversation. Moreover, the recollections and comments of other people involved may enter in, so that the next time the conversation is recalled, these are included as the person's own.

Other circumstances also can interfere with memory in various ways. Sometimes, expectations override sense perceptions, and so we remember what we had expected to hear or see. Or the imagination may fill in details to complete a memory.

Signs of abnormal memory loss

Some types of memory loss are not a part of normal aging and may reflect a more serious disorder, such as Alzheimer's disease. Forgetfulness that interferes with daily life is not a normal part of aging. Other signs of abnormal memory loss include:

- Difficulty remembering how to perform familiar tasks, such as getting dressed or making dinner.
- Difficulties with language, such as substituting inappropriate words, finishing thoughts, or following instructions.
- Difficulties with abstract thinking, such as adding up a column of numbers.
- Disorientation, such as forgetting the way home.
- Poor judgment.
- Loss of interest in appearance and in everyday activities.

Source: The Alzheimer's Disease Association.

Aging and memory

For many years, memory researchers concentrated on retrieval difficulties as the primary source of long-term memory problems in older adults. In tests of recall, older people experience much more difficulty than younger people in recalling numbers shown to them an hour or so earlier. But in prompted recall, when they are shown a list of numbers, older people recognize which numbers they saw earlier as well as younger people do. This finding indicates that the information was stored in memory but that older people had lost the ability to recall it unless prompted.

Researchers now believe, however, that most of these retrieval problems stem from poor storage of the information in the first place. Many older adults remark that they have no problem remembering what happened 60 years ago, but they just can't remember what happened last week. In other words, they still have access to the deep memory traces created when they were young. Their present problem lies in encoding new information for long-term storage.

Subtle changes in memory begin at about age 20, though people do not usually notice memory problems until much later, perhaps when they enter middle age or after they retire. The extent of these problems varies a great deal. Memory powers show much more variation among people over age 55 than among younger people.

The first noticeable sign of flagging memory powers usually is slower recall. In tests of mental functioning, older people's brain waves exhibit less activity than those of younger people. This inevitable decline means that older people must expect to give more time and effort to processing and retrieving information.

Faulty vision or hearing loss can play havoc with awareness as people age, causing them to overlook what is around them or to mishear what is said, so that accurate memory is impossible. In such cases, eyeglasses or a hearing aid may not only correct the impaired faculty but improve the recording of information in memory as well.

Aging also reduces attention span. Tasks such as reading that require concentration become difficult to sustain over long periods, and people may notice that they have repeatedly read the same passage without remembering its contents. When this happens, it's a good idea to take a break and resume reading later.

Reduced attention leaves people vulnerable to distractions. When interrupted, older people may have difficulty remembering what they were engaged in prior to the interruption. Whereas teen-agers may have no trouble doing homework while listening to the radio, older people are more likely to find their train of thought interrupted by the sound of a radio when they are writing or reading.

In fact, doing more than one thing at a time becomes increasingly difficult with age. Someone may make a mistake when writing a check while listening to the clerk behind the counter, or may drive a car past the turn while carrying on a conversation. Researchers have found that people with "type A" personalities, who are accustomed to taking on many tasks at once and doing everything themselves, are especially frustrated by the need to slow down and concentrate on doing one thing at a time.

Older people also do not seem to form mental pictures as easily as they did when younger. A young woman who is asked where she bought her shoes is likely to answer the question by first calling up a mental image of the shoes in the store, while an older person may not visualize the store so readily. Recall becomes more difficult when fewer visual cues are available to aid the brain in its search for the appropriate response.

As people age, thinking in an organized manner becomes less automatic. This decline becomes apparent in tests that involve matching faces with names: Younger test subjects automatically devise some mental strategy to connect the two, whereas older subjects often do not and simply give up.

Improving memory

People of any age can learn strategies to improve memory. These strategies increase our concentration and help us form strong memory traces. They also improve our recall.

- Take some time to think about what's important for you to remember and focus your attention on that.
- Use visual and verbal cues to form clear impressions. For example, visualize an object or task you wish to remember, and repeat or comment upon it aloud.
- Form associations to reinforce memories and set up cues for retrieval.
- Analyze the information you wish to store. What is its essential function or message? What are the key details?
- Recall the information often.

Source: Danielle C. Lapp.

Abnormal memory loss

Some types of memory loss go beyond normal aging and involve damage to the brain. The brain disorder most often linked with memory loss is Alzheimer's disease, which affects an estimated 3 to 5 percent of Americans in their 60's, according to the National Institute on Aging, and about 20 percent of people over age 80. The fact that the "oldest-old"—people over age 85—constitute the fastest-growing age group in the U.S. population means that more and more people are living long enough to develop the disease.

The memory loss that characterizes Alzheimer's disease interferes with everyday functioning. People with the disease may forget how to perform once-familiar tasks, such as balancing a checkbook, getting dressed, or finding the way home. Other signs of Alzheimer's disease include the inability to complete a thought or follow instructions and the incorrect or inappropriate use of words when speaking. When prompted with the correct word, a person with Alzheimer's will still not use the word, whereas a person experiencing a momentary lapse will incorporate it.

Although the memory loss caused by Alzheimer's disease is irreversible, many other disorders that contribute to memory loss are treatable. Imbalances of thyroid hormone, which may leave people mentally sluggish, can be corrected with thyroid supplements. Dehydration and malnutrition—especially an inadequate intake of B vitamins—also may interfere with mental functioning. *Anemia* (a reduction in the number of red blood cells) and poor blood circulation impair mental functioning by depriving the brain of an adequate supply of oxygen. Surgery patients may experience memory failures temporarily, until the effect of the anesthesia wears off, usually within a few days. Strokes and certain head injuries also can produce memory loss. In some cases, training can "rewire" nerve connections in the injured brain and improve memory.

Learning the art of remembering

Training can also help overcome the memory lapses that result from aging. The art of remembering might be described as the art of planting cues to facilitate recall. The keys are image-association, organization, and selective attention.

Image-association means developing a clear picture in the mind's eye, and it underlies strategies to remember all kinds of information. For example, one way to avoid mislaying objects in everyday use is to visualize where they are placed, by looking at a pocket while dropping keys into it, or by taking a mental snapshot of the desk while laying eyeglasses next to the telephone there. These conscious associations between object and location deepen the memory trace, easing the task of locating items when they are again needed.

For most people, learning to plant sensory cues requires sharpening their powers of observation. Consider the problem of locating a car parked in the crowded lot of a shopping mall. By paying careful attention to where the car is parked in relation to nearby buildings and the closest mall entrance, it's possible to plant visual cues that later help locate the car among the hundreds in the lot. Including other sensory cues—the smells from a nearby restaurant, the sound

Techniques to remember faces and names

Spend about one minute looking at each face. Decide on a dominant feature: hair, nose, mouth, facial shape. Read the name below the picture, and look for a meaning in the name, some visual cue that will trigger recall. Then, arbitrarily place the image onto the dominant feature and visualize the composite image until you know it well. Say the image aloud. As an example, suppose a man named Dennis Sterling has glossy gray hair, which suggests silver. The composite image could be a silver tray balanced on his hair. Turn the page after forming composite images for all the faces.

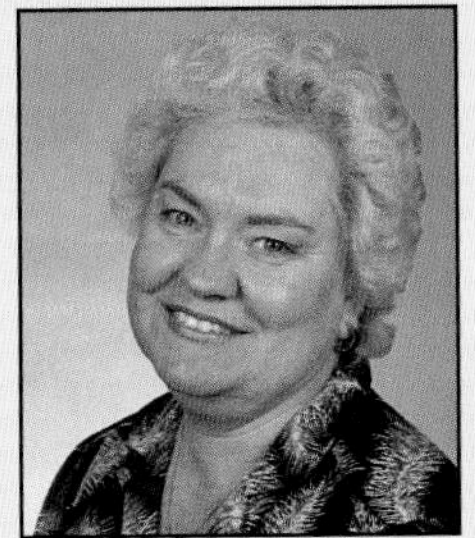
Elizabeth Laski

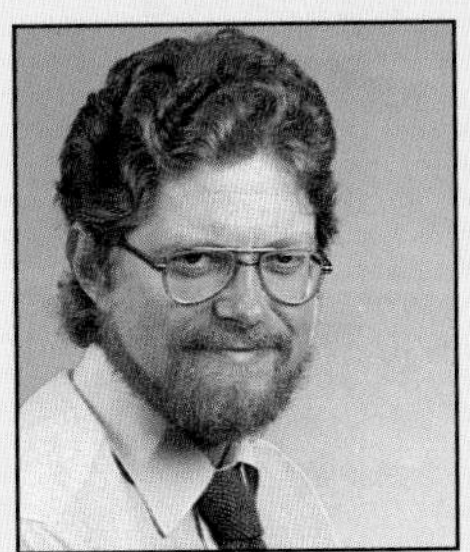
George Andersen

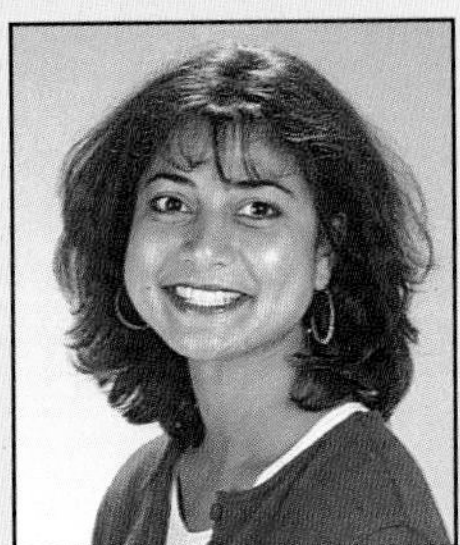
Tia Menendez

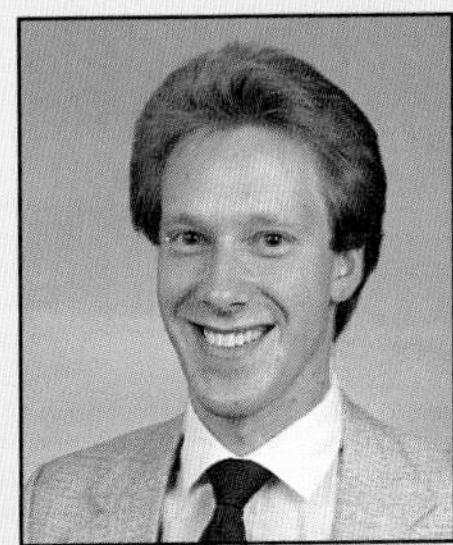
Jonathan Willis

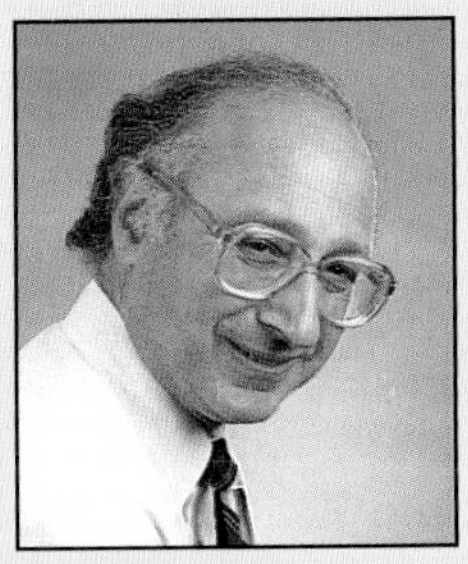
Victor Raffia

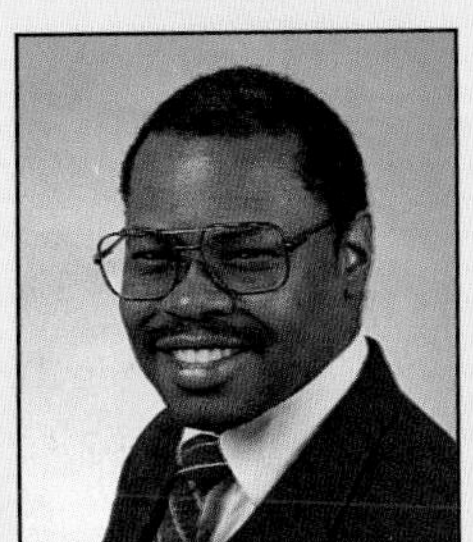
Steven Carleton

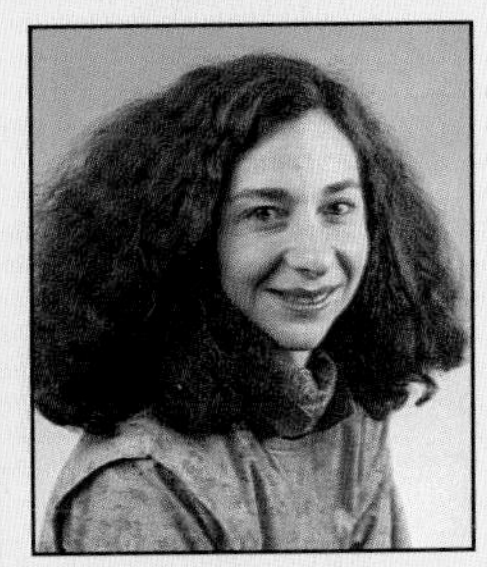
Allison Kouros

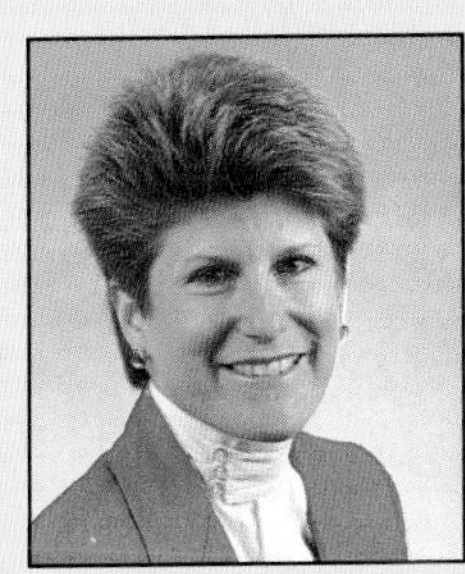
Paula Van Dyke

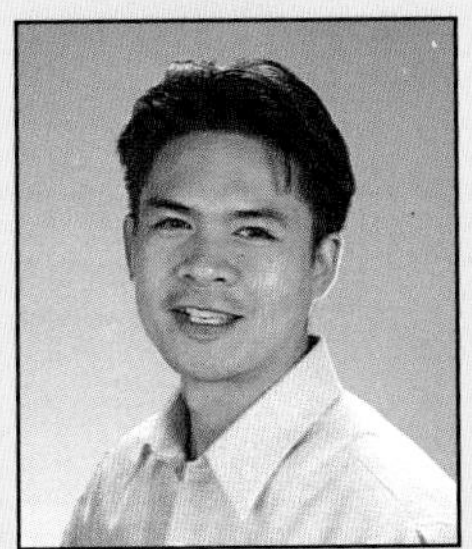
Joseph Cardozzo

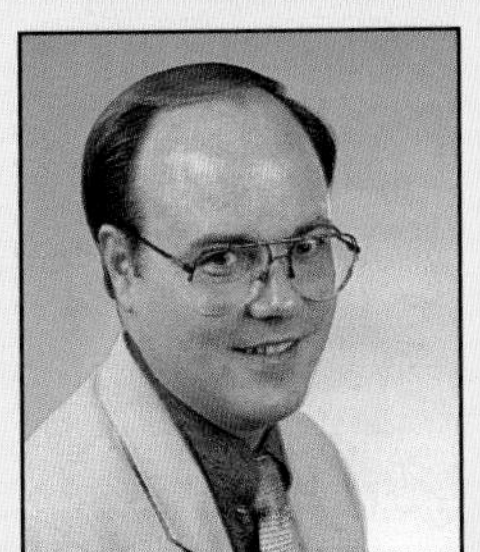
Allen Ackerman

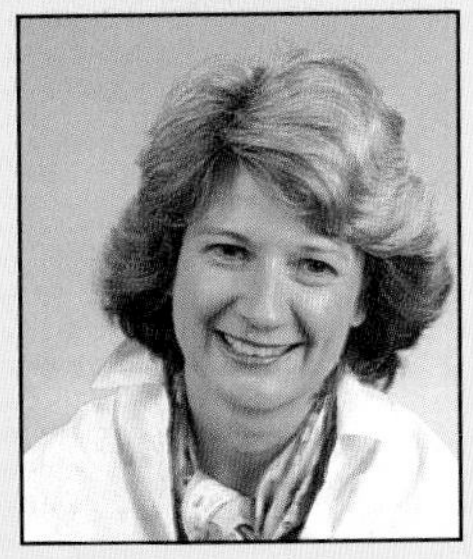
Monica O'Brien

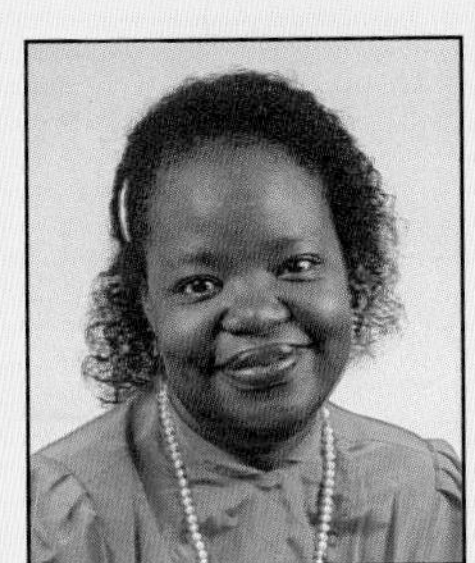
Anna Jaye

Techniques to remember faces and names

Now look at the faces again. The composite images that you created should help call to mind some of the names. Below the photographs write the names of as many faces as you can recognize. The average for people who have not had memory training is six correct identifications, and seven or eight is good. More than eight correct identifications is excellent.

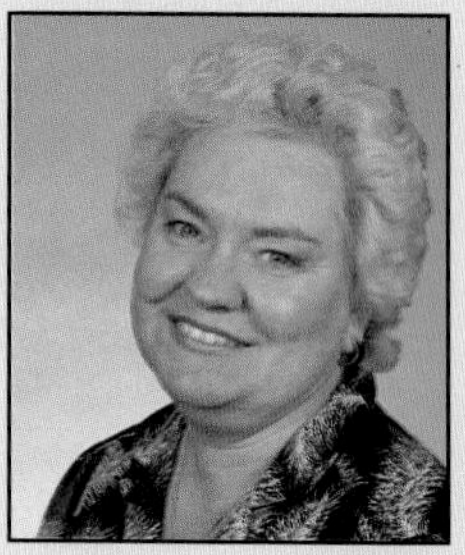
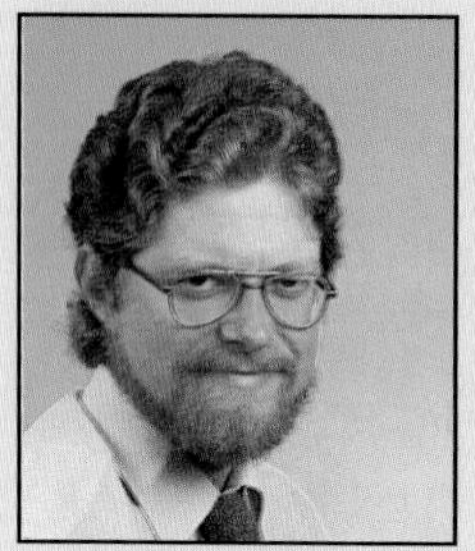
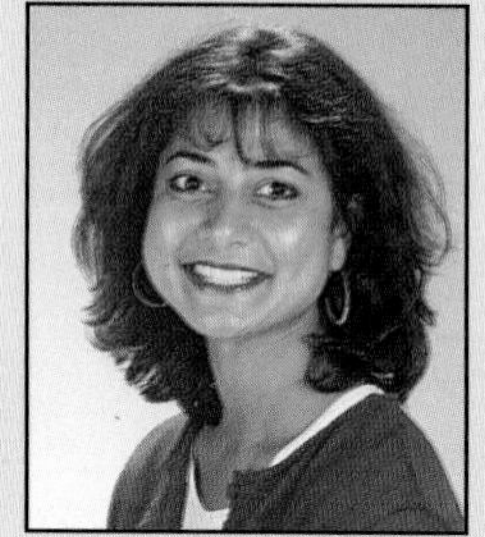
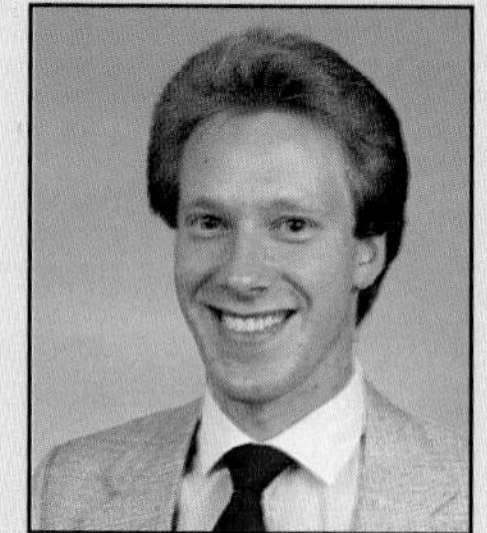

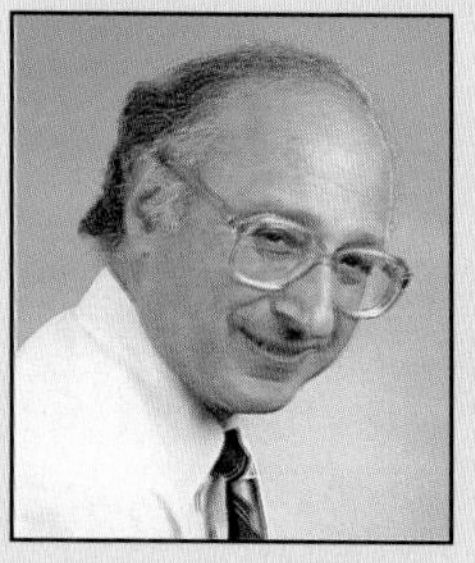
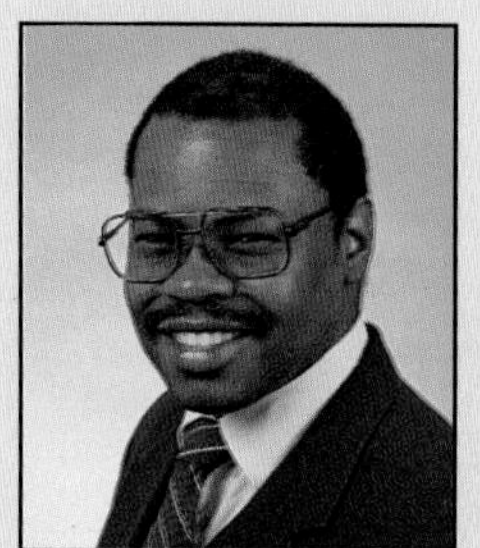
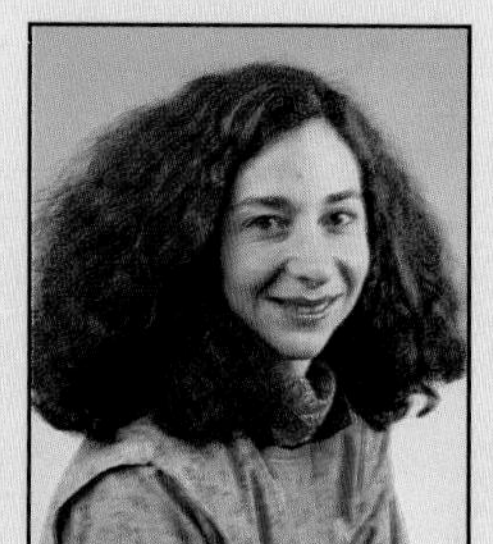
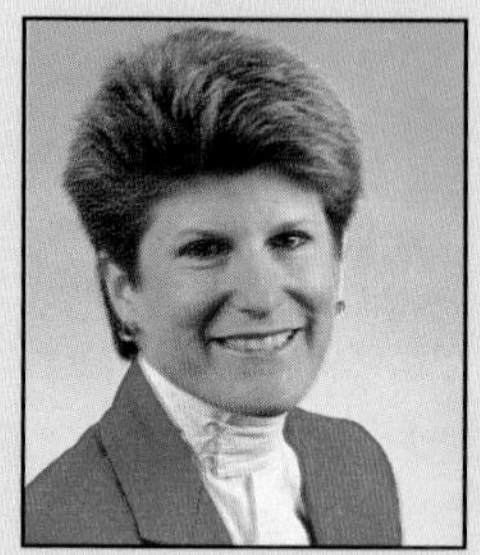

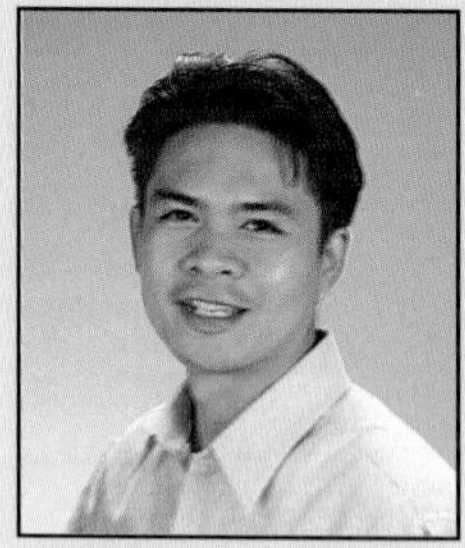
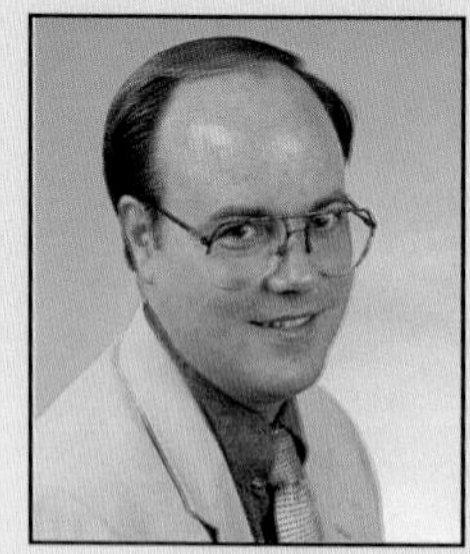
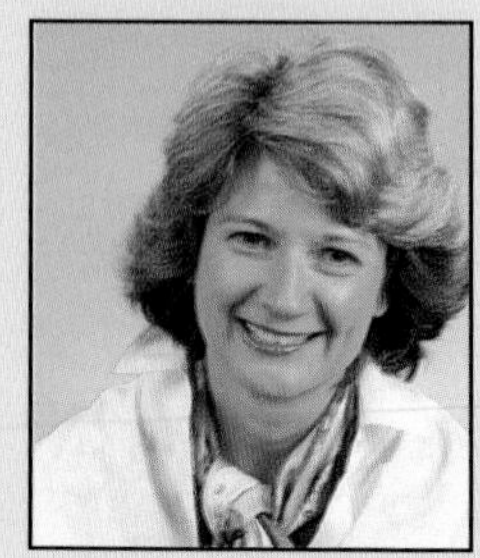
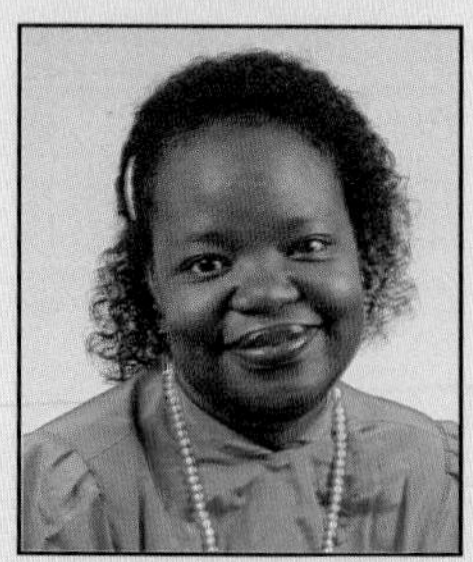

of traffic just beyond the lot—also deepens the memory impression.

Verbal cues can reinforce visual cues and leave a still stronger memory trace. In parking the car at the mall, for example, the shopper might say aloud, "As I face the driver's side, I see a white building. Directly in front of the car, I see the entrance to the mall."

Association plays a major role in organization. These associations can be intellectual, sensory, or emotional. It is helpful to analyze information by asking such questions as: "What are its most important features? Why do I want to recall it? What does it resemble? How do I feel about it? Asking and answering such questions creates associations that aid recall.

Becoming better organized in daily life helps control anxiety and helps avoid the last-minute rushing that heightens anxiety and thus adds to memory problems. Even small changes, such as always putting objects back in the same place and using a calendar to keep track of things to do, reduce anxiety and aid memory. Other techniques that reduce anxiety include deep breathing (inhaling and exhaling slowly through the nose) and visualization exercises (closing the eyes and picturing waves slowly breaking, for example).

Selective attention is the personal "filter" we apply in deciding how important it is to remember something. No one can hope to remember everything. People with what we term a photographic memory are exceptional. Most of us have far more limited memories. Rather than worry about what we forget, it's more productive to focus on what we want to remember.

Setting priorities for daily or weekly tasks is one application of selective attention. If you have four errands to run, organize them by importance and by efficient use of your time, deciding first to fill the tank with gas, then pick up the bread, and last of all take the clothes

Testing visual memory using abstract figures

Look at these four figures for 30 seconds. Wait two minutes before turning the page. Then, look at the eight figures on that page and mark the ones you recognize from this page. People who have not had memory training correctly identify three figures on average.

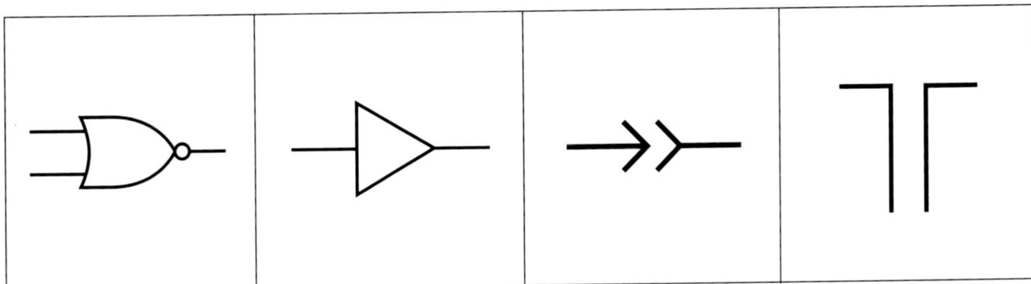

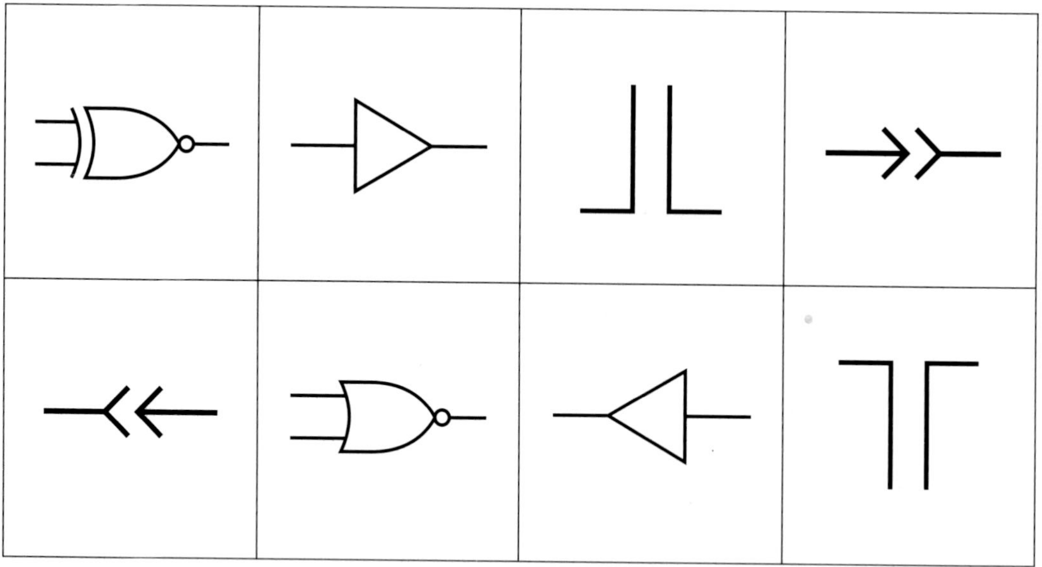

Testing memory using numbers

Read these lines of numbers one at a time, spending about a second on each while hiding the others with your hand. After each line, stop, look up, say the numbers aloud in reverse order, and then write them down in that order. If you see 493, for example, you would write down 394 without looking. Writing five lines correctly is the average for people who have not had memory training. Writing six correct lines is very good.

1 9 8

3 2 8 4

5 6 1 9

1 9 3 6 7

8 2 5 7 4

9 7 6 2 3 8

5 1 8 3 9 4

to the cleaner's. If an errand is urgent, try using visual cues as well—for example, putting the clothes for the cleaners in front of the door, where they cannot be overlooked. Or stick a note on the dashboard as a reminder to pick up the cleaning.

Doing it now is a useful tool for freeing up memory. If you undertake tasks as you think of them, then you don't need to keep them in mind. When you telephone someone, for example, start the conversation by stating the reason for the call. Then you can turn to chitchat. That way you won't hang up having forgotten to say why you called. A related way of freeing memory is to make notes as you think of things, using one list, which is easier to find than several.

No matter what your age, it's a good idea to recognize situations when attention is difficult to sustain. Irritation, triumph, and other emotions can distract people from what they are doing, so it's wise in such situations to pause and take stock. For example, when you are angry with a clerk for overcharging you, check to make sure that the clerk has returned your credit card.

While the emotions of the moment can get in the way of efficient recall, over the long term, emotional associations make memory traces more durable. To illustrate this point, I ask people to think of the teachers they had in grade school. The teachers they remember usually struck an emotional chord, positive or negative. A teacher remembered fondly may have singled the person out for praise. Or people may still bristle at the recollection of a teacher who humiliated them before the class. Because age does not diminish the effect of emotion on memory, coating today's memories in emotion can preserve them for a lifetime.

Memory training also relies on *mnemonic devices*—strategies for prompting memory. Most people are familiar with the use of acronyms, which consist of the first letter or syllables of the words to be remembered. For example, HOMES is an acronym to remember the Great Lakes—Huron, Ontario, Michigan, Erie, and Superior.

Another mnemonic device, based on image association, is useful for remembering the name of someone you have just met. The first step is to identify one prominent feature—a man's silver hair, for example. The next step is to attach a meaning to the person's name. Say the name over to yourself. Does it suggest any other words? It's important to choose a meaning that you can visualize. The name Sterling, for example, might suggest silverware. Visualize the meaning to reinforce the image. Finally, superimpose one image on the other, silver hair on sterling silver, and then take a mental snapshot of the composite image. At the next meeting, this image will help recall his name.

Practice makes perfect

Memory is a complex process that relies on a network of connections and associations. Through practice, it's possible to maintain that network and keep memory reasonably sharp. In the same way that active exercise contributes to physical vigor, regular exercise of memory skills can enhance and prolong the speed and strength of mental recall. •••

For further reading:

Baddeley, Alan. *Your Memory: A User's Guide.* Avery, 1994.

Lapp, Danielle C. *Don't Forget! Easy Exercises for a Better Memory.* Addison Wesley, 1995.

Lapp, Danielle C. *(Nearly) Total Recall. A Guide to a Better Memory at Any Age.* Stanford Alumni Association, 1992.

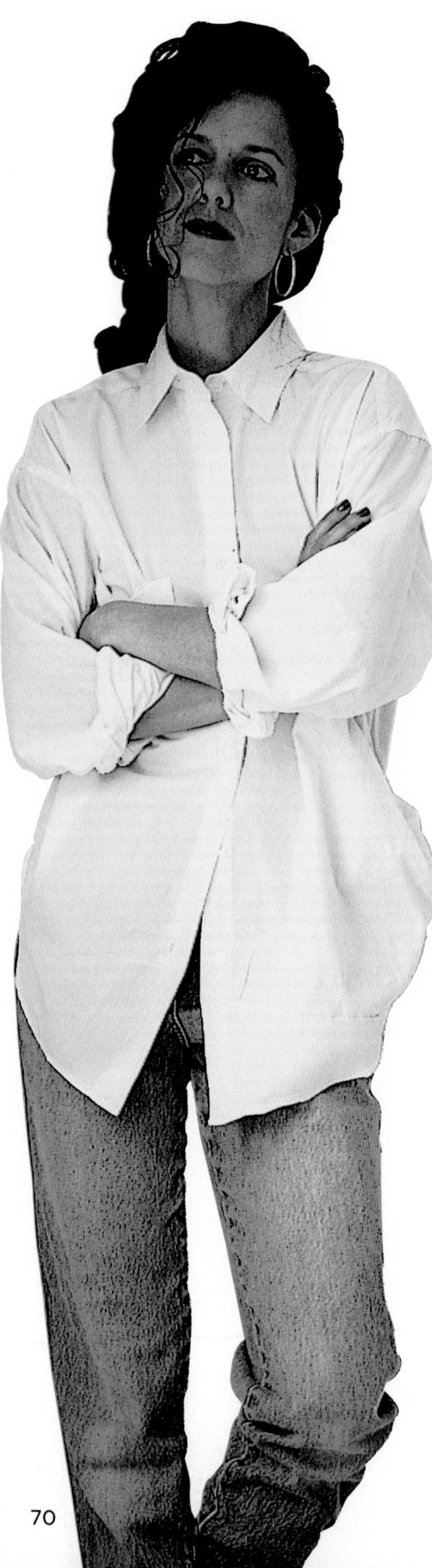

Female sex hormones offer relief from menopausal symptoms and certain effects of aging but pose some risks.

Hormone Replacement Therapy

By Judith H. LaRosa

EACH YEAR, THE MORE THAN 1 MILLION AMERICAN WOMEN who reach menopause face a complicated decision for which there is no right answer—only the best answer for each woman. This decision is whether to take hormone replacement therapy (HRT), a treatment of female sex hormones that can relieve the unpleasant symptoms which may accompany the end of menstruation. HRT also may have a profound effect on the skeletal and cardiovascular systems. But arriving at this decision is very much a balancing act.

On one hand, a woman, with the aid of her physician, must examine the enormous benefits of the treatment, including relief from hot flashes and other hormonally induced symptoms of menopause. (Menopause is defined as a woman's final menstrual period.) Over the longer term, HRT helps forestall some potentially life-threatening effects of aging. Medical researchers have found that it very likely reduces the risk of heart disease—the leading killer of American women—

and that it prevents or nearly halts a sometimes crippling loss of bone known as osteoporosis.

On the other hand, each woman must also consider the treatment's risks. These include a possible increase in her chances of developing breast cancer. Further complicating the process are uncertainties about the long-term benefits and risks of HRT and the sometimes conflicting conclusions of medical studies evaluating it. Mix in some women's reservations about the long-term use of drugs that may themselves cause unpleasant side effects—when the women otherwise feel fine—and this health decision can become one of the most thoughtful a woman will ever have to make.

Preserving vitality after menopause

In the mid-1990's, from 15 to 25 percent of American women in their menopausal years were taking HRT, according to the North American Menopause Society, an organization for health-care professionals. And interest in the treatment soared as the oldest of the 40 million female baby boomers approached menopause. Not until 1910 did average life-expectancy for women born in America reach the average age of menopause: 51. Today, the majority of American women can expect to live more than one-third of their lives after menopause. And as life expectancy has risen, so too have expectations about preserving vitality into middle age and beyond. Many advocates view HRT as a valuable means of protecting health and well-being while pushing back the disabilities of old age.

Menopause, like menstruation, is triggered by changes in blood levels of certain *hormones* (chemical messengers that control body functions), particularly estrogen and progesterone. Estrogen is actually a group of chemically similar hormones produced mainly by the ovaries that orchestrates every event in a woman's reproductive life. Estrogen also helps maintain tissues of the genitals, the urinary tract, and some of the muscles that support these organs. Beyond that, estrogen influences the health and functioning of more

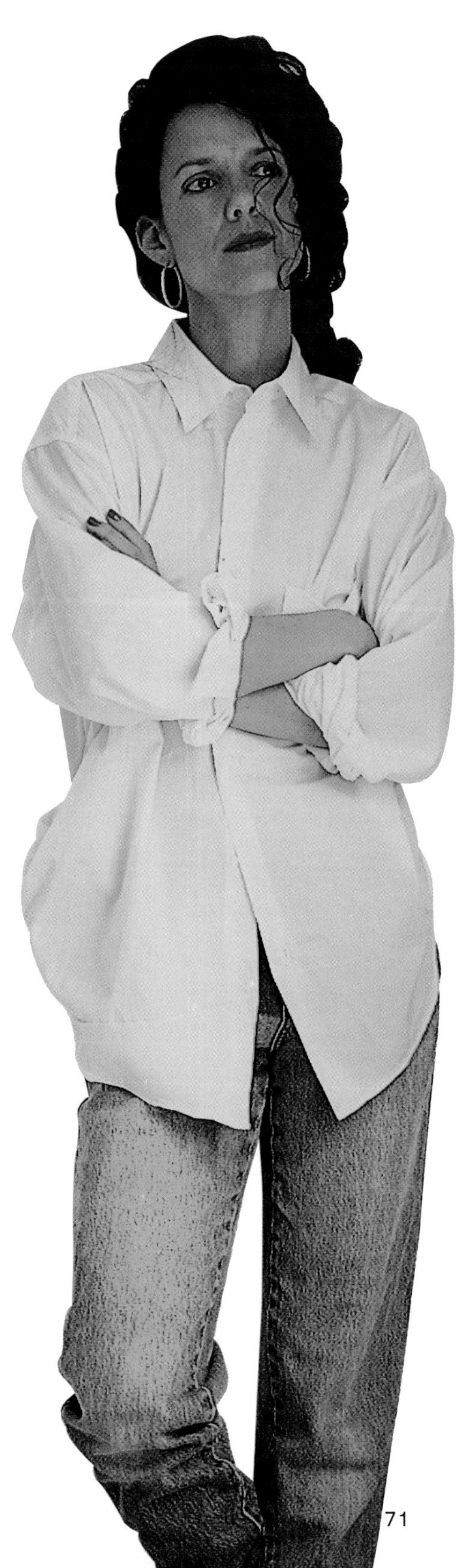

than 300 types of body tissue, including the brain, liver, skin, and blood vessels. Progesterone also is produced mainly by the ovaries and works with estrogen in preparing the uterus for pregnancy. If pregnancy does not occur, progesterone levels decline, and the uterine lining is shed in menstruation.

While a woman is in her 30's, her estrogen and progesterone levels begin a gradual decline that accelerates when she reaches her 40's. For another 10 years or so, hormone levels continue to drop, until they become so low that menstruation ceases. For most women, menopause occurs between the ages of 45 and 55.

Easing the symptoms of menopause

HRT consists of either estrogen alone, which is often referred to as ERT, or estrogen in combination with progesterone or progestin, a synthetic version of progesterone. ERT was introduced in the 1950's in the form of supplementary estrogen to relieve the unwelcome symptoms of menopause that about 85 percent of women experience in varying degrees. In that respect, it is extremely successful. In 95 percent of women, estrogen relieves hot flashes, also called hot flushes—sudden feelings of heat in the face and upper body that are often followed by sweating—and night sweats (hot flashes that occur during sleep). Estrogen also reduces menopause-related sleep problems and reverses the uncomfortable drying and thinning of the linings of the vagina and urinary tract that occurs as estrogen levels fall. Moreover, estrogen often eases the irritability, mood swings, fatigue, and feelings of depression that affect some women during the menopausal years.

In the late 1970's, however, medical studies began warning that women who took supplementary estrogen were five times more likely than nonusers to develop cancer of the *endometrium* (lining of the uterus). To reduce this risk, doctors began prescribing progesterone in combination with estrogen. They theorized that the higher incidence of endometrial cancer was linked to a chronic overgrowth of the uterine lining, caused by estrogen, that created conditions favorable to the growth of cancerous tumors. Since then, numerous studies have confirmed that progesterone reduces the risk of endometrial cancer to that of a woman not taking HRT. Unless a woman has had a *hysterectomy* (surgical removal of the uterus), both estrogen and progesterone should be prescribed if she undertakes HRT.

The estrogen component of HRT may be administered by means of pills, patches, creams, or vaginal suppositories, all of which are absorbed into the bloodstream to varying degrees. Many women on oral HRT take one estrogen pill daily for 20 to 25 days, though taking a pill daily is becoming more common, according to the American College of Obstetricians and Gynecologists (ACOG). Taking estrogen continuously is often less confusing, the ACOG notes, and it prevents a reappearance of menopausal symptoms. Patches also deliver a continuous dose of estrogen, though they probably don't pro-

Glossary

Estrogen: A group of chemically similar hormones produced mainly by the ovaries that orchestrates every event in a woman's reproductive life and affects the health and functioning of more than 300 types of body tissue.

Estrogen replacement therapy: A treatment of estrogen that relieves the symptoms of menopause and may forestall some life-threatening effects of aging.

Hormone replacement therapy: A treatment of estrogen and progestin that relieves the symptoms of menopause and may forestall some life-threatening effects of aging.

Hormones: Chemical messengers that control body functions.

Progesterone: A female sex hormone that prepares the uterine lining for pregnancy.

Progestin A synthetic version of progesterone.

The author:

Judith H. LaRosa is Professor and Chair of the Department of Applied Health Sciences at Tulane University.

What is hormone replacement therapy (HRT)?

HRT consists of the hormone estrogen alone or estrogen in combination with progestin, a synthetic version of the hormone progesterone. Progestin is generally prescribed with estrogen to reduce the risk of cancer of the *endometrium* (uterine lining) for women with a uterus. Women who have had a hysterectomy can probably take estrogen alone safely.

How is HRT taken?

The estrogen in HRT may be administered by means of pills, skin patches, creams or vaginal suppositories. Estrogen pills may be taken daily or cyclically, for 20 to 25 days in the month. Estrogen creams and suppositories can be used directly on vaginal tissue to alleviate dryness. Progestin pills may be taken daily or cyclically, for about 12 days in the month. Women on the daily progestin regimen usually will not have a menstrual period, while those on the cyclic regimen may have withdrawal bleeding for a few days.

vide the same protection against heart disease that oral HRT does.

Estrogen creams and suppositories are prescribed for women interested chiefly in reversing the drying and thinning of the tissues of the genitals and the urinary tract. These forms, which contain a lower dose of estrogen than do pills or patches, stimulate cell growth in the walls of the vagina, keep the vaginal lining moist and reduce the risk of vaginal infections and discomfort with intercourse. But unless a woman uses creams or suppositories infrequently and in small amounts (or has had a hysterectomy), she also will need to take progesterone for protection against endometrial cancer.

Progesterone is taken in pill form, usually for 12 days each month. Many women find that its side effects temper the boost estrogen gives to energy levels and disposition. Progesterone may bring on bloating, breast tenderness, irritability, and other premenstrual symptoms. Also, a woman on progesterone usually experiences a menstrual period beginning a day or two before she takes her 12th pill, though these periods are usually shorter and lighter than those occurring before menopause. These side effects may be temporary or they may last as long as a woman takes the hormone.

In the 1990's, some physicians began prescribing progesterone in a smaller dose taken daily, in an effort to reduce side effects. Daily pills also may eliminate monthly bleeding. Switching to pills with a different formulation of estrogen and progesterone or changing the method of delivery also may lessen side effects.

In the absence of official guidelines, opinions differ on when HRT should begin. Some doctors recommend starting only at menopause. Others believe treatment should begin before menstruation ceases if a woman experiences bothersome menopausal symptoms or is at high risk for osteoporosis or heart disease.

About half of women who begin taking HRT halt treatment on their own within six months, according to the North American Menopause Society. Some women stop because of side effects. Many women stop after their body adjusts to lower estrogen levels and hot flashes and other menopausal symptoms diminish or vanish. Questions about the long-term effects of HRT also have made some women wary. And some women simply do not like taking pills.

Some health experts, however, believe that women should continue taking HRT even after their menopausal symptoms disappear, perhaps for the rest of their life. These advocates focus on HRT's beneficial effect on two health risks that increase greatly after menopause: heart disease and osteoporosis. Health experts also point to a 1995 study by the American Cancer Society suggesting that women who take HRT have half the risk of developing cancer of the colon as do nonusers. And they say that the estrogen in HRT helps women maintain a more youthful appearance and preserve an enjoyable sex life. Furthermore, several small studies suggest that HRT enhances memory, may counter depression, and may even help shield women against the mental deterioration of Alzheimer's disease.

Protection against heart disease

HRT's most profound long-term benefit may be a reduction in the risk of *cardiovascular* (heart and blood vessels) disease, which kills nearly one in every two American women who die after age 50, according to the National Center for Health Statistics. Before menopause, a woman's risk of a fatal heart attack is only about one-fifth that of a man of similar age. But by age 54, the American Heart Association reports, that risk has risen dramatically to about one-half that of men. And by the time a woman reaches her mid- to late-60's, her chances of dying of a heart attack nearly equal those of a man of the same age.

Health experts link the rising incidence of cardiovascular disease after menopause to falling estrogen levels. Estrogen appears to protect against heart disease by keeping arteries healthy. In animal studies, estrogen raised levels of artery-clearing HDL-cholesterol while lowering levels of artery-clogging LDL-cholesterol. As estrogen levels drop, cholesterol is more likely to stick to artery walls, forming

What are the benefits of HRT?

Demonstrated benefits	Probable benefits
• Relieves bothersome menopausal symptoms—such as hot flashes, night sweats and insomnia—which many women experience as a result of fluctuating hormone levels. • Halts or slows the rate of bone loss, which accelerates after menopause and can result in porous, brittle bones—a condition known as osteoporosis. Women are at above-average risk for developing osteoporosis if they are thin or small-boned, have fair skin and blonde hair, drink or smoke heavily, get little exercise, or have a low-calcium diet. • Relieves vaginal dryness and a thinning of vaginal tissue that can accompany menopause and make intercourse painful.	• Appears to reduce the risk of heart disease, which rises dramatically for women following menopause. Women are at higher-than-average risk for heart disease if they have high cholesterol levels or a family history of heart disease. • May reduce the risk of colon cancer, which is the second most common cancer killer for women, following lung cancer. • Appears to ease the irritability, mood swings, fatigue and mental fogginess that can accompany menopause. • May keep the skin thicker, moister, and more youthful. Many women experience dry skin as their estrogen levels drop.

What are the risks of HRT?

Demonstrated risks	Potential risks
• Increases the risk of cancer of the uterine lining if estrogen is taken alone. The addition of progestin to HRT lowers this risk. • Can produce premenstrual symptoms, such as fluid retention and irritability.	• May raise the risk of breast cancer, though studies on this subject are not conclusive. • May lead to weight gain. • May increase the risk of developing gallstones in some women. • May lead to headaches.

plaques that narrow the artery and reduce blood flow. Estrogen also slows abnormal contractions of the artery that can cause a blockage of the artery. In addition, estrogen appears to keep down blood levels of fibrinogen, a protein that promotes clotting.

The evidence for supplementary estrogen's benefit to the heart is considerable. More than 30 medical studies have reported that postmenopausal women who take estrogen substantially lower key risk factors linked to cardiovascular disease. These factors include high blood pressure and high blood levels of cholesterol,which can result in high levels of fatty plaques.

One of the most extensive studies used data from the Nurses Health Study, an ongoing long-term study of 122,000 women nurses

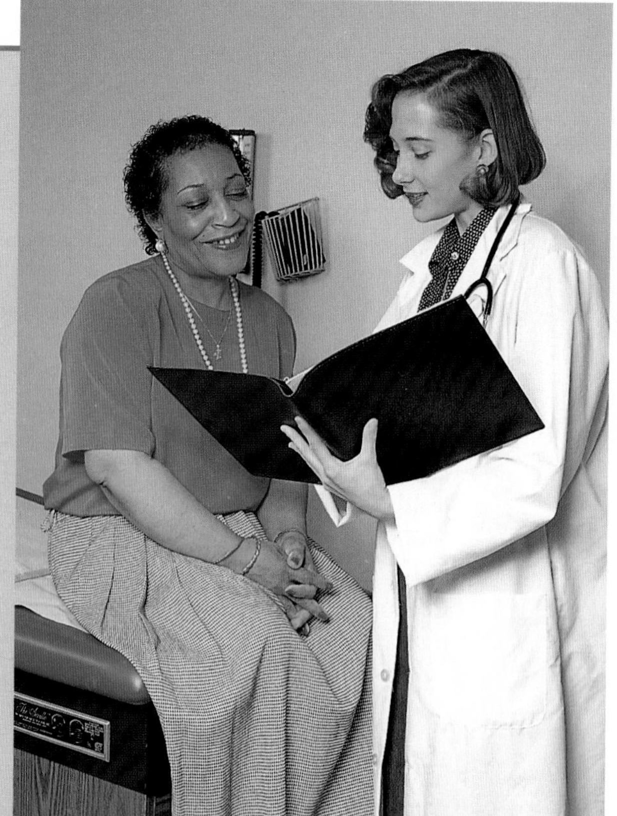

Weighing the risks and benefits of HRT: What should women consider ?

Menopausal women at above-average risk for heart disease or osteoporosis and with no increased risk for breast cancer may want to consider taking HRT. For these women, the benefits of HRT in protecting against heart disease and osteoporosis greatly outweigh the much smaller risk of developing breast cancer. HRT is generally not recommended for women who have had breast cancer, because estrogen is associated with an increased risk for the disease. Women at above-average risk for breast cancer face a difficult decision and should carefully weigh their individual risks in consultation with their physician.

How long is HRT usually taken?

To quell menopausal symptoms, women usually take HRT for less than five years. To preserve HRT's long-term benefits—for the heart and bones— a postmenopausal woman may need to continue HRT for the rest of her life. When estrogen is discontinued, bone loss accelerates rapidly. However, HRT's long-term effects have not been fully studied.

by researchers at Harvard Medical School in Boston. Among the 48,470 nurses in the study who passed through menopause from 1976 to 1986, those taking estrogen had a 44 percent lower risk of developing major heart disease than those not taking HRT.

A January 1995 study by the National Institutes of Health (NIH) provided additional evidence of HRT's cardiovascular benefits. This study, known as the Postmenopausal Estrogen/Progestin Interventions (PEPI) Trial, examined the health histories of 875 women aged 45 to 64, over a three-year period. Some of the women had not taken hormones. Others had taken estrogen alone or a combination of estrogen and progestin. While the women taking estrogen alone had the lowest risk of heart disease, the researchers found the combination therapies to be only slightly less beneficial. This finding alleviated persistent concerns that the addition of progesterone or progestin to HRT might significantly weaken estrogen's beneficial effect on the heart and blood vessels.

Despite such findings, some questions remain about HRT's long-term effects on the heart. The most significant question, raised by the PEPI researchers themselves, is whether HRT's cardiovascular benefits will actually prevent heart attacks and strokes.

New evidence, reported in January 1996, strongly suggests that HRT reduces the death rate from heart attack and stroke. Researchers at the University of California studied the health histories of 454 women who were born from 1900 to 1915 and had used estrogen for at least one year, beginning in 1969. They found that the estrogen users—about half the women in the study—were 60 percent less likely to have suffered a fatal heart attack and 73 percent less likely to have suffered a stroke. They noted that the death rate from all causes was 46 percent lower among the estrogen users than among the nonusers.

Health experts stress that women should not rely solely on HRT to maintain a healthy heart. Even women taking HRT should eat a low-fat diet, maintain an appropriate weight, avoid smoking, and exercise regularly.

Getting a jump on osteoporosis

As a result of the drop in estrogen levels that occur before menopause, women lose on average an estimated 15 to 20 percent of their bone mass within five years of menopause, according to the National Osteoporosis Foundation. Thereafter, the rate slows to about 1 percent per year. This erosion of bone can leave the bones porous and fragile and prone to fracture. The bones of the hips and wrists and the vertebrae of the spine are especially susceptible to deterioration. Both men and women lose bone mass as they age, but women are four times more likely to develop osteoporosis because they typically start with smaller bones and hence less bone mass. While bone loss occurs in women of all racial and ethnic groups, it is most pronounced in Caucasian and Asian women, thin women, and women who smoke or who drink heavily.

About half of all American women suffer an osteoporosis-related fracture after age 50, according to the National Osteoporosis Foundation. Hip fractures are the most prevalent and the deadliest. From 5 to 20 percent of hip-fracture patients die within one year from complications related to the fracture, according to the National Osteoporosis Foundation. More than 50 percent of those over age 65 who fracture a hip remain incapacitated for the rest of their life.

Although several drugs have proved useful in treating osteoporosis, estrogen is the only drug approved for both preventing it and halting its progress. During the past 20 years, numerous studies have demonstrated that estrogen significantly slows bone loss. Overall, studies have found, estrogen users are at least 25 percent less likely to suffer a fracture than are nonusers.

A study reported in January 1995 suggests an even larger reduction in risk. This six-year study, led by researchers at the University of Pittsburgh Graduate School of Public Health in Pennsylvania, found that women who began taking estrogen within five years of menopause and continued to take it reduced their risk of all nonspinal fractures by 50 percent and their risk of wrist and hip fractures by 71 percent. Women in the Pittsburgh study who began HRT more than five years after menopause showed a 25 percent drop in the risk of all nonspinal fractures. But the study also found that women who stopped taking the hormone, even after 10 years, were just as likely to experience a fracture as women who had never taken the hormone.

In October 1995, the first of a new class of drugs for treating osteoporosis won approval from the U.S. Food and Drug Administration. That drug, named Fosamax, appears to build tissue in patients with the disease by slowing the biochemical processes that cause bone to break down. As a result, the drug helps the body's bone-building cells restore bone tissue lost to osteoporosis. Drugs like Fosamax may provide an alternative to estrogen.

Health experts stress that estrogen is only one weapon against osteoporosis. Even women taking estrogen should follow a diet rich in calcium or boost their intake with calcium supplements. Postmenopausal women should also engage in regular weight-bearing exercises for the legs, such as walking, dancing, or weight lifting, which aid in strengthening bones. Not smoking also lessens the risk of osteoporosis, as does maintaining an appropriate weight. After menopause, the body's remaining estrogen is stored in fat cells, and very thin women enter their later years at a disadvantage.

The question of breast cancer

Like any powerful drug, HRT is not without risk. HRT may stimulate the growth of *benign* (noncancerous) uterine tumors and may increase the risk of gallstones. A 1995 study by the American Cancer Society suggested that women who took estrogen for at least 6 to 11 years increased their risk of fatal ovarian cancer by 40 to 70 percent. That is, during the seven years of the study, 436 of the 240,073 postmenopausal women followed developed fatal ovarian cancer. But experts point out that more studies are needed before conclusions can be drawn about a possible relationship between estrogen and ovarian cancer. At present, the primary risk from estrogen, in addition to endometrial cancer, appears to be a slightly elevated risk of breast cancer.

For many women, breast cancer is the most worrisome question about HRT. Estrogen's ability to stimulate the growth of existing cancer cells in the breast is well established. Much less certain, however, is whether estrogen itself causes cancer. Some studies suggest that women on HRT are no more likely than nonusers to develop breast cancer, whereas other studies report a slightly increased risk for those who take hormones.

Two contradictory studies reported in summer 1995 underscored

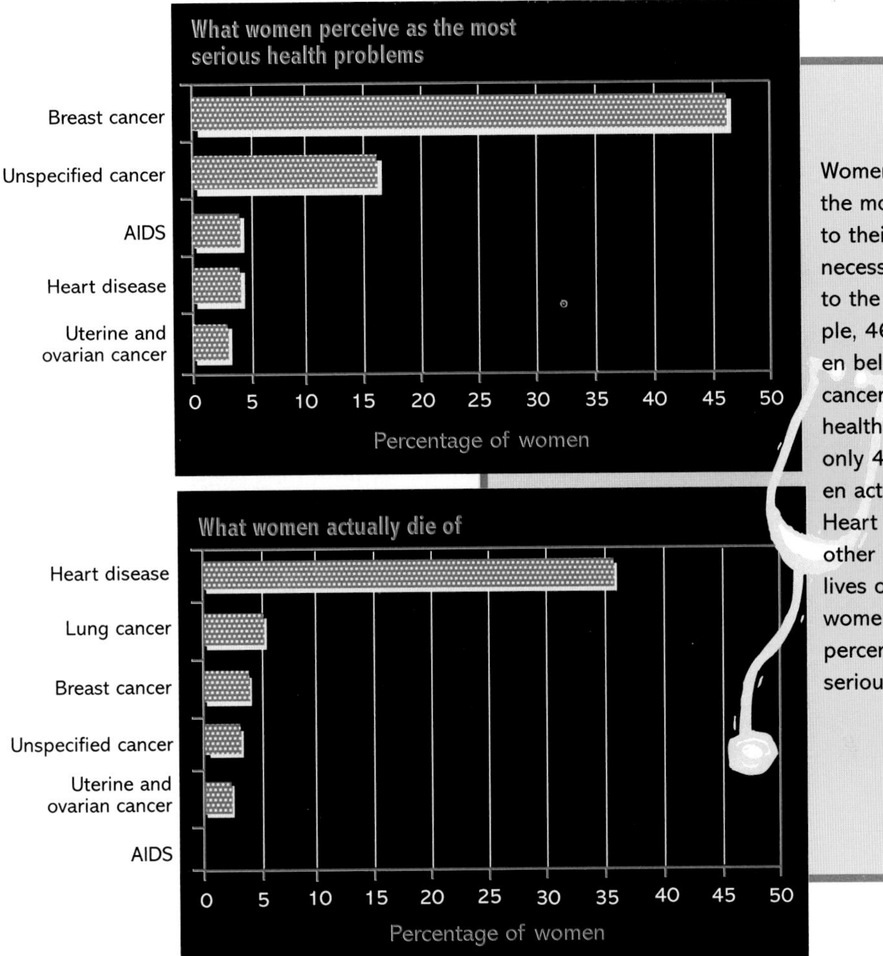

Source: Gallup Poll; National Center for Health Statistics.

Women's perceptions of the most serious threats to their health do not necessarily correspond to the reality. For example, 46 percent of women believe that breast cancer is their greatest health threat, though only 4 percent of women actually die of it. Heart disease, on the other hand, claims the lives of 36 percent of women, though only 4 percent perceive it as a serious threat.

the need for additional research on this question. The first study, reported in June 1995, was an extension of the Nurses Health Study and examined the incidence of breast cancer among 69,000 nurses who reached menopause from 1978 to 1992. The Harvard researchers reported that the women who had used HRT for at least five years after menopause were from 32 to 71 percent more likely to develop breast cancer than were women who had never used HRT. The highest risk occurred among hormone users age 60 to 64. Although older women normally have a higher rate of breast cancer than younger women, researchers were unable to explain the sharp increase in rates.

The second breast cancer study, reported in July 1995, found no connection between breast cancer and HRT. In this study, reported by researchers at the University of Washington in Seattle, 537 women age 50 to 64 with recently diagnosed breast cancer were compared with a control group of healthy women. The study found that 58 percent of the women with breast cancer had used HRT, compared with 61 percent of women in the control group.

Although both studies looked at the overall relationship between HRT and breast cancer, they were the first major U.S. studies specifically designed to investigate the link between breast cancer and progesterone. The Harvard researchers wanted to learn whether progesterone protects against breast cancer as it does against uterine cancer. The answer was a disappointing no. The Washington researchers sought to determine if adding progesterone to estrogen therapy increased the risk of breast cancer. Their answer was a reassuring no. After the publication of the Nurses Study, the NIH commented, "When all the studies are combined, it appears that there is very little or no overall risk of breast cancer associated with hormone replacement therapy," though, the agency pointed out, some studies suggest a risk associated with prolonged use—10 to 15 years.

Physicians who favor HRT point out that a woman's risk of dying of heart disease is nearly 10 times greater than her risk of dying of breast cancer. Experts say more studies are needed on HRT and breast cancer risk, especially studies that follow participants for more than five years (the maximum length of all major HRT studies so far) and controlled studies in which participants are assigned randomly to one form of therapy or another.

Health experts hope to gain some answers from the Women's Health Initiative, a 15-year study sponsored by the NIH. The study focuses on the causes and prevention of heart disease, osteoporosis, and cancer, particularly breast and colon cancer. The HRT portion of the study will involve 27,500 women, half of whom receive HRT and half, a placebo. Researchers hope to learn how much hormone a woman should take and for how long to obtain maximum benefit while minimizing risks. But preliminary results from this study will not be available until at least 2001.

Cautions for HRT users

Most doctors will not prescribe ERT or HRT for women who have breast cancer or have had a cancerous breast or breast tumor removed. Other women who should not consider hormone therapy, according to the ACOG, are women who have undiagnosed vaginal bleeding, cancer of the endometrium, chronic liver disease, or a recent history of blood clots.

Women at above-average risk for breast cancer should be especially cautious, though they are not necessarily ruled out as HRT candidates. Factors that raise this risk include a family history of breast cancer or of breast cysts or other benign breast diseases; never having been pregnant; giving birth for the first time later in life (after one's 20's); early onset of menstruation (before age 11); and late menopause (after age 55).

Others who may be advised against HRT include women with

seizure disorders, high blood pressure, or benign uterine tumors. Other conditions that may preclude HRT, according to the ACOG, include migraine headaches, *endometriosis* (a disorder in which endometrial cells migrate to other areas of the body), and gallbladder disease.

A woman who decides to take HRT also should take steps to minimize her risks. The ACOG advises women on HRT to have an annual physical examination that includes a breast and pelvic exam, Pap smear, a blood pressure check, and a cholesterol test. In addition, all women over age 50 should have a yearly mammogram, according to the ACOG. A woman on hormone therapy who still has a uterus should be taking progesterone along with estrogen. If for some reason she is not, she should have a yearly endometrial biopsy, a test in which a scraping of tissue from the uterus is examined for precancerous or cancerous cells. The ACOG also recommends that women on HRT have a yearly discussion with their doctor about the treatment's effects and reevaluate their decision to take the medication.

Many doctors believe that for most women, the benefits of HRT outweigh its potential risks. Ultimately, however, each woman must educate herself about HRT, balance its certainties and uncertainties in consultation with her physician, and decide whether HRT is for her. •••

For further reading:

Cherry, Sheldon H., M.D., and Runowicz, Carolyn D. *The Menopause Book: A Guide to Health and Well-Being for Women After 40*. Macmillan, 1994.

Schiff, Isaac, M.D., with Parson, Ann B. *Menopause: The Massachusetts General Hospital Guide*. Times Books, 1995.

Sheehy, Gail. *The Silent Passage*. Pocket Books, 1992.

The Menopause, Hormone Therapy, and Women's Health. U.S. Congress, Office of Technology Assessment, Washington, D.C., 1992.

For more information:

The North American Menopause Society
c/o University Hospitals Department of OB/GYN
11100 Euclid Ave.
Cleveland, OH 44106
216-844-8748

The American College of Obstetricians and Gynecologists
409 12th St., SW
Washington, D.C. 20024-2188
202-638-5577

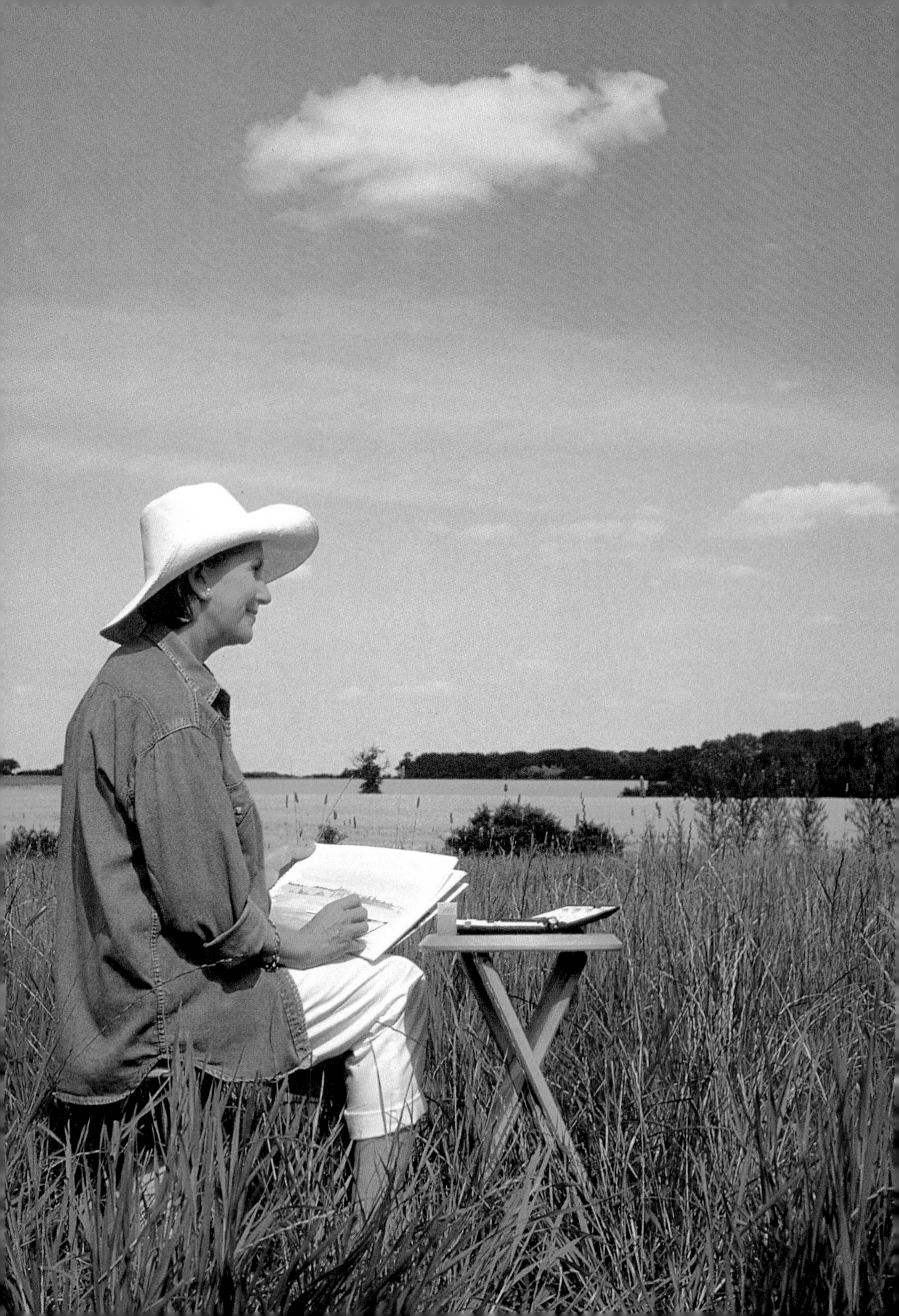

Baby Boomers should start planning now for a healthy and fulfilling life after retirement.

Planning Your Happily Ever After

By Donna Cohen

"Cheshire Puss". . . Alice went on, "Would you tell me, please, which way I ought to walk from here?"

"That depends a great deal on where you want to get to," said the Cat.

"I don't much care where—" said Alice.

"Then it doesn't matter which way you walk," said the Cat.

—Lewis Carroll, *Alice's Adventures in Wonderland*

WHEN IT COMES TO PLANNING FOR OLD AGE, the majority of Americans are as directionless as Alice in Wonderland. Few have even a vague notion of how they want to live out their later years. In the United States, a typical worker logs a lifetime average of 90,000 hours on the job but devotes only about 10 hours to planning what he or she will do after retirement.

Why do so few Americans give thought to the future? After all, as the Cheshire Cat implies, it's hard to know what steps to take if you don't know what goal you're working toward.

But for young adults, the need to build a personal life and career leaves little time and energy to consider the challenges of old age. Many middle-aged people fail to plan for retirement because they mistakenly believe that the federal government, their employer, or family members will adequately care for their needs. Women who devote themselves to homemaking and raising children may consider retirement planning essential only for people with salaried jobs. Finally, every American lives in a culture that considers growing old and retiring to be negative life events. Planning for the future thus requires facing the prospect of losing status in our work-oriented society.

The act of envisioning oneself as a happy and fulfilled retired person may take much of the fear out of aging, however. People who expect to find pleasure and meaning out of life in their 60's, 70's, and 80's may find it easier to set aside money for those years, to develop the skills they will need as an older person, and to keep their body in shape for the long haul.

Studies of people who report being happy and fulfilled into their 80's indicate that most of them traveled, took college courses, read books, or in some other way actively participated in stimulating activities. Research also shows that older people who have fulfilling relationships with family and friends feel better about themselves than those who lack significant social and emotional contacts. The people with strong relationships are more likely to be self-confident, to enjoy sexual activity, and to have lower levels of certain stress-induced hormones associated with disease.

The American way of retiring

Retirement is a fairly new phenomenon. Only in the last 40 years or so have education, employment, and retirement become the standard stages of life for Americans. In 1900, the average life expectancy was 46.3 years, and the relatively few people who made it to age 65 could expect to live only another year or so. But life expectancy has risen dramatically over the course of the century, as has the number of years spent in retirement.

The average lifespan of the first wave of Americans born during the baby boom between 1946 and 1964 is projected to be about 77 years for men and 82 years for women. This means that men who choose to retire at age 62 are likely to live at least 15 years after retirement. Women are likely to have 20 years. On average, as much as one-quarter of an American worker's life will be spent in retirement. Because women in the United States live an average of five years longer than men, the ratio of men to women decreases significantly in later life. American women are quite likely to outlive their husbands, especially if the husband is older than the wife. Although there's no easy way to prepare for widowhood or divorce, it's important for women to develop their own interests and pay attention to their personal needs and wishes during their adult life.

For this and a number of other reasons, the years after 65 do not always bring a cessation of work. For example, many people who earn low wages and have inadequate savings, pensions, and health insurance cannot afford to quit working. In contrast, some highly paid workers find great satisfaction in their careers and are reluctant to leave them, despite financial security. Others continue to work

The author:

Donna Cohen is Professor and Chairman of the Department of Aging and Mental Health at the University of South Florida in Tampa.

because they enjoy the social interaction and mental stimulation of a job as well as the income.

The desire to be near friends and family explains why most people retiring in the 1990's prefer to stay in the area they lived in during their working years. Among today's retirees, the people who are most likely to move away are those who do not feel connected to their community or want to change their lifestyle in retirement, and who have the resources to finance the move.

The coming senior boom

As a result of the baby boom, a large number of Americans will be reaching their 60's, 70's, and 80's in the first several decades after the year 2000. The demographic bulge may force society to make accommodations for older people that other generations never enjoyed. People who want to use their later years in nontraditional ways—by starting a new business, going to law school, or joining the Peace Corps, for example—may find few social barriers and plenty of company.

A 1996 survey of the first group of baby boomers to turn 50 found that most plan to quit their present job by age 58 but to keep working, full-time or part-time, until age 70 or beyond. Baby boomers also appear less likely to stay put than their parents. About 40 percent said they planned to relocate after retirement.

Baby boomers will find their retirement shaped by the corporate restructuring of the 1980's and 1990's. Budget cuts, downsizing, the closing of facilities, and mergers mean that members of this generation of workers are likely to change careers at least once and to adjust to several different employer-employee relationships. They may need to think in terms of multiple retirements, rather than a one-time exit from the workforce.

A 1996 *New York Times* poll indicated just how widespread job insecurity has become. The poll showed that three-fourths of all U.S. households have had a close call with a layoff. A family member had lost a job in one-third of all households. And 1 in 10 adults reported that losing a job had precipitated a major life crisis.

Thus, when thinking about retirement, it's good to bear in mind that it may include an early and unscheduled departure from a job. Although an

Booming population of older Americans

People planning for retirement can expect to have lots of company in their later years. Life expectancies have been extended, *below*, and the number of people over 65 in the United States has grown dramatically, *bottom*.

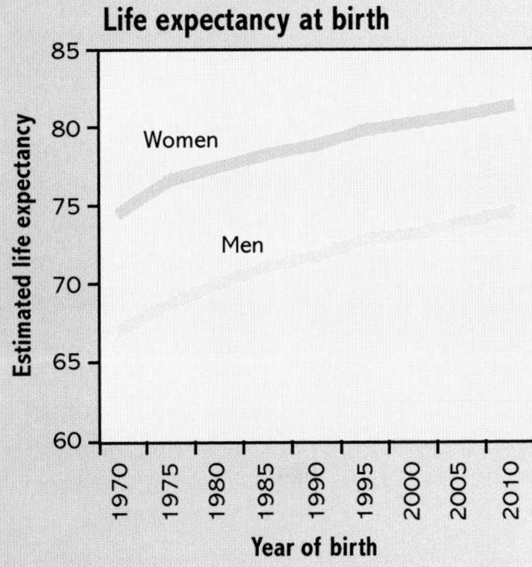

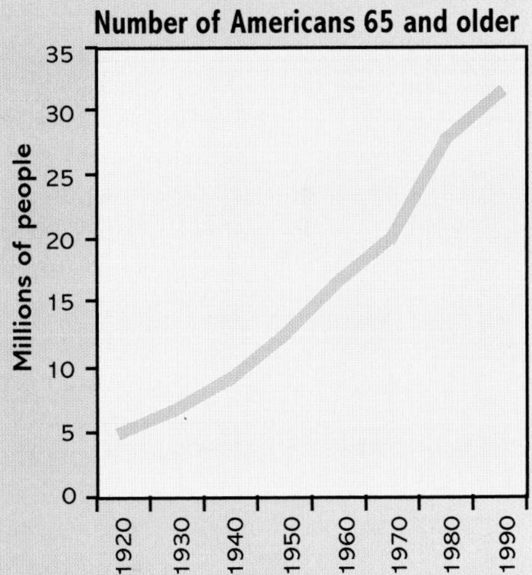

Source: U.S. Bureau of the Census.

insecure present makes planning for a secure future all the more difficult, the absence of job security has served to drive home an important message: There is life beyond work. Other areas in life can also bring satisfaction and fulfillment.

Starting the planning process

For many people, retirement planning means financial planning. But experts agree that when preparing for retirement, it is important to consider more than just finances. Plans should include thinking about where one will live, what one will do for fun and fulfillment, how one will maintain meaningful relationships and social contacts, and what one will do to take care of physical and mental health.

It's a good idea to start setting aside money for retirement early in life—in one's 20's if possible. Planning one's retirement activities, on the other hand, can begin at any age, though some experts suggest that people should start by their early 40's. Others say that 10 years before one hopes to retire is early enough to begin making preparations. Because situations and goals change, retirement goals should be reassessed at regular intervals, perhaps on the same date each year.

At that time, people can review key spheres in life—physical health, emotional well-being, financial health, and intellectual, spiritual, and personal fulfillment. Thinking about the areas that need attention can help in setting tangible goals for retirement and also for the year ahead. Writing down the past year's achievements in each sphere often brings a pleasant surprise at how much has been accomplished.

The planning process is affected not only by one's own attitudes and expectations but also by those of the rest of the family. Couples should make plans together in order to work out differing expectations ahead of time. It is not necessary, however, that both partners quit work at the same time, though it can ease the transition if they go through it together.

Retirement planning courses are offered at many locations—one's place of employment, community centers, local colleges, churches, and other organizations. A more informal option is to create a retirement planning group consisting of four to six people. Members of the group need not be of the same age or occupation. Planning together creates a good environment for brainstorming and learning from each other. The team also provides a mechanism for members to challenge each other to clarify their ideas.

The most important step in retirement planning is deciding how to spend the hours previously devoted to work. A 1995 Canadian study of retired people indicated that those who planned post-retirement activities were more likely to be happy in old age than those who focused only on financial planning. One shouldn't simply make vague plans to "keep busy," however. It's better to come up with specific activities to pursue.

Resources for retirement planning

Several organizations, books, and computer software programs can provide assistance for planning various aspects of retirement.

Organizations. *American Association of Homes for the Aging* provides a list of nonprofit homes for the elderly. Write to: American Association of Homes for the Aging; 1050 Seventeenth Street, NW; Washington, D.C. 20036.

American Association of Retired Persons has information on economic, health, and work issues of retired people. Write to: American Association of Retired Persons, Membership Communications; 601 E Street, NW; Washington, D.C. 20049. Or call toll-free: 1-800-424-3410.

American Institute of Certified Public Accountants provides references for personal financial specialists. Call toll-free: 1-800-862-4272.

Association of Part-Time Professionals assists people who work part-time or wish to do so. Write to: Association of Part-Time Professionals; Flow General Building; 7655 Old Springfield Road; McLean, VA 22102.

The Certified Financial Board of Standards gives consumers information about certified financial planners and disciplinary actions against them. Call 1-303-830-7543.

Money Minds provides accountants and financial experts to answer questions over the telephone for a per-minute fee. Call toll-free: 1-800-ASK-A-CPA.

National Academy of Elder Law Attorneys has information about lawyers specializing in the legal matters of concern to older Americans. Call 1-602-881-4005.

The National Association of Personal Financial Advisors provides references for financial planners who charge on a fee-only (no commission) basis. Call toll-free: 1-800-366-2732.

The Older Women's League offers education material about issues of concern to midlife and older women. Write to: The Older Women's League; 666 11th Street, NW, Suite 700; Washington, D.C. 20001.

Social Security Administration provides information about social security benefits. Write to: Social Security Administration; 64401 Security Boulevard; Baltimore, MD 21235. Or call: 1-800-772-1213.

T. Rowe Price provides a free retirement planning kit upon request. Write to: T. Rowe Price; 100 East Pratt Street, Baltimore, MD 21290.

General books on retirement. *The Adventure of Retirement: It's about More than Just Money,* by Guild A. Fetidge. Prometheus Books, 1994.

How to Plan for a Secure Retirement, by Barry Dickman, Trudy Lieberman, and the editors of Consumer Report Books. Consumer Report Books, 1992.

Over Fifty: The Resource Book for the Better Half of Your Life, by Tom and Nancy Biracree. Harper Collins, 1991.

The 50+ Wellness Plan: A Complete Program for Maintaining Nutritional, Financial, and Emotional Meaning for Mature Adults, by Cori Harris McIlwain, Debra Fulgham, Bruce Steinmeyer, R. E. Fulghum, and Robert Bruce. John Wiley, 1990.

Transitions: A Woman's Guide to Successful Retirement, by Diana Cort-Van Arsdale and Phyllis Newman. Harper Collins, 1991.

Books on physical and emotional health. *Caring for Your Aging Parents,* by Donna Cohen and Carl Eisdorfer. Tracher/Putnam, 1995.

A Second Helping of Chicken Soup for the Soul, by Jack Canfield and Mark Victor Hansen. Health Communications, 1995.

Healthwise for Life: Medical Self Care for Healthy Aging. Healthwise, Inc., 1992.

Seven Habits of Highly Effective People: Restoring the Character Ethic, by Steven R. Covey. Simon and Schuster, 1989.

Stress and Health, by Philip Rice. Brooks/Cole Publishing, 1992.

Books about financial preparations. *The Price Waterhouse Retirement Planning Advisor.* Simon & Schuster, 1990.

You Can Afford to Retire! by William Parrott and John L. Parrott. Simon & Schuster, 1992.

Books about relocating: *Places Rated Almanac: Your Guide to Finding the Best Places to Live in North America,* by David Savageau and Rick Boyer. Prentice Hall, 1993.

Retirement Places Rated: All You Need to Plan Your Retirement or Select Your Second Home, by David Savageau and Rick Boyer. Prentice Hall, 1990.

Computer software about retirement. *Discover for Retirement Planning.* American College Testing Service.

Fred: The Friendly Retirement Education Database. Employee Benefit Systems, Inc.

Relocation Options. Martlet, Inc.

Planning one's retirement lifestyle

One of the first steps in retirement planning is to decide where and how to live and what to do during the time previously spent working. A checklist, *below*, and information about the lives of other seniors, *right and opposite page,* may help the decision-making process.

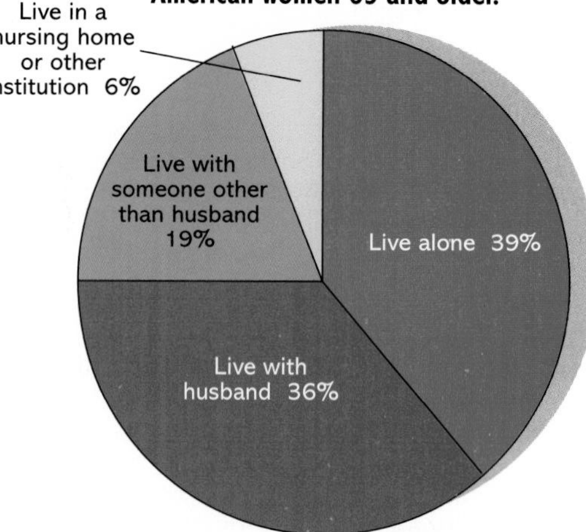

Source: U.S. Bureau of the Census.

Things to do

- If you are not sure how you will fill your days after retirement, write out a list of all the activities you would like to do now but lack the time. Talk to retired friends and relatives about the activities that make them feel satisfied and involved with life.
- To focus your thinking, make out a schedule for your first month of retirement. List the things you will do for fun, but also what you will do to feel you are contributing to society and connected to family and friends.
- Take up a sport or hobby, join a social club, or do volunteer work to develop interests outside work.
- Consider working part-time for a year or two before retirement to ease the transition.
- If you would like to change careers at retirement, plan ahead by taking courses and talking to experts in the new field.
- Brainstorm with your spouse and other family members about travel plans or other activities you can do together after retirement.
- If you plan to relocate, spend considerable time in the new area before making the move. Visit the area often, talk to other retired residents, and subscribe to the local newspaper. Consider a year-long trial period in the new area. Instead of selling your existing home and buying a new one, rent out your home and lease one in the new area to make sure the move is right for you.
- If you are building or renovating a retirement home, incorporate principles of "universal design" that make the dwelling user-friendly for people who have disabilities.

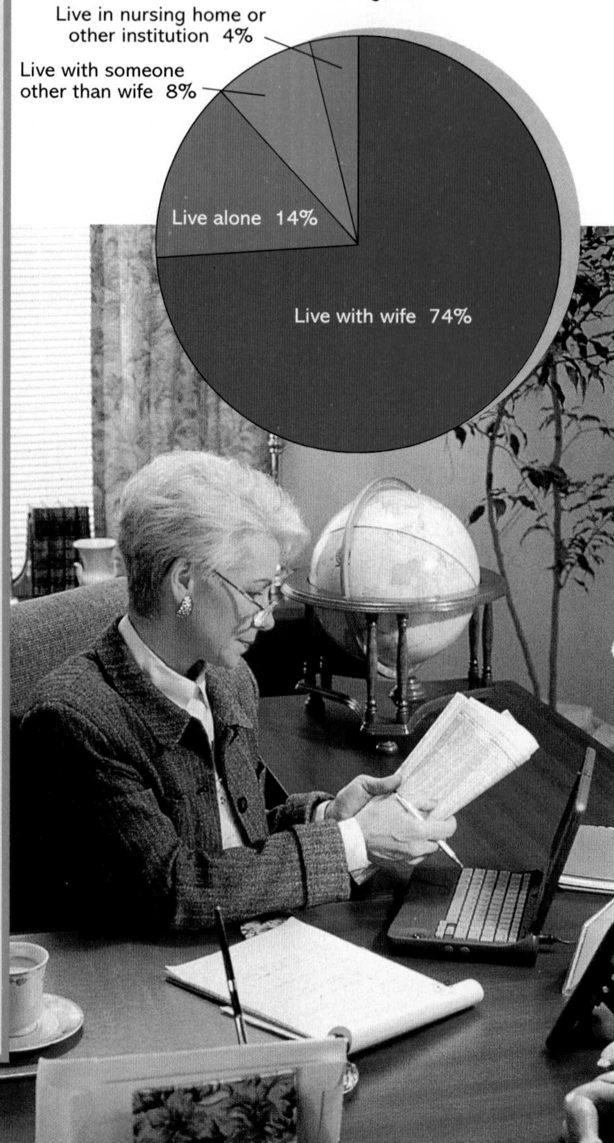

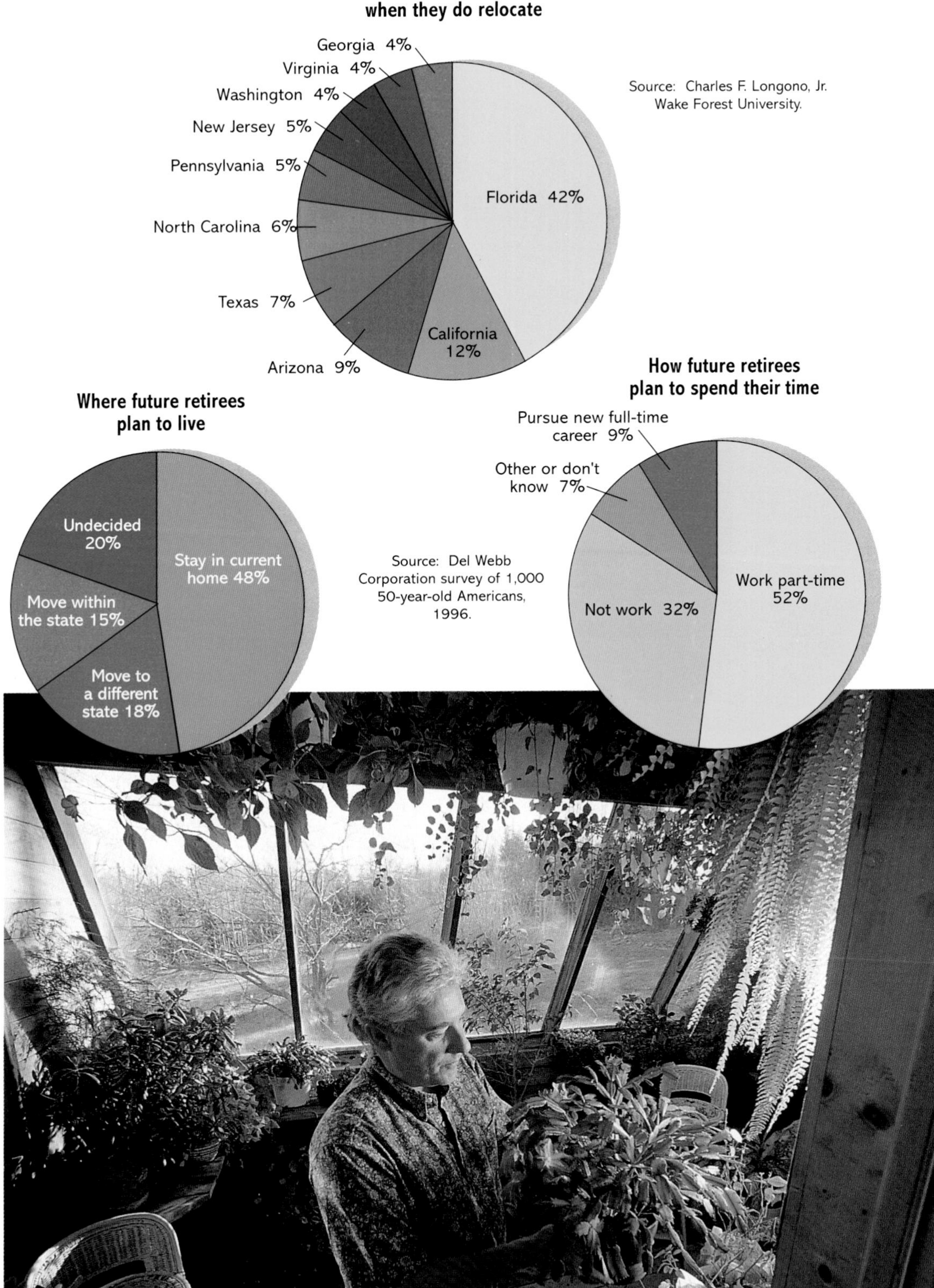
Where retirees move when they do relocate
Georgia 4%
Virginia 4%
Washington 4%
New Jersey 5%
Pennsylvania 5%
North Carolina 6%
Texas 7%
Arizona 9%
California 12%
Florida 42%
Source: Charles F. Longono, Jr. Wake Forest University.
Where future retirees plan to live
Undecided 20%
Stay in current home 48%
Move within the state 15%
Move to a different state 18%
Source: Del Webb Corporation survey of 1,000 50-year-old Americans, 1996.
How future retirees plan to spend their time
Pursue new full-time career 9%
Other or don't know 7%
Not work 32%
Work part-time 52%

Fulfilling activities to fill the time

The easiest way to begin the planning process is by making a list of interesting activities—college courses; artistic, musical, or literary pursuits; sports and hobbies; travel destinations; government and community service activities; and part-time work and consulting opportunities. As retirement approaches, people are likely to become more focused about what they want to do, and they can begin to prepare for those activities by reading books, making contacts in a specific field, or taking appropriate lessons or courses. Doing these things before leaving the job can also help ease the transition to retirement.

While planning this area of life, one should consider the need for scheduled or structured activities. People who find themselves idling away their weekends and weeknights by watching TV may need the discipline of regular classes, meetings, golf dates, or a part-time job to stay involved in life after retirement. On the other hand, "self-starters" who jump out of bed on Saturday morning to write a To Do list may not need such a structured life to keep active.

In any case, most retirees may want to give some thought to the possibility of continuing to work after retirement. Part-time employment after one's official retirement can provide needed income, structure to the days, and a chance to interact with people.

Some people find it extremely difficult to imagine life after retirement, and they may need exercises to "loosen up" their thinking. One way is simply to meet with people who are retired and talk with them about their lifestyle, goals, ambitions, and activities. Another technique is to try to imagine a typical week after retirement and write out a day-by-day schedule for filling the hours.

A more creative strategy involves imagining one's own funeral. In this exercise, the person writes down what words of remembrance a close friend, a family member, and a co-worker might speak at his or her funeral service. The objective of this thought exercise is not to focus on death but to think about what kind of person one is, how one has lived life so far, and what aspects of life may have been neglected. Workaholics may find this a particularly useful strategy for discovering what they would like to focus on other than work.

Options for housing

Once a person knows what he or she would like to do after retirement, it becomes easier to plan living arrangements appropriate to that lifestyle. The ideal home can be anyplace that maximizes the retiree's feelings of comfort, safety, independence, and overall well-being.

People interested in moving to a new city, state, or country after retirement can start by visiting a library or bookstore to find reference works describing the pros and cons of various locations in the United States and abroad. Chambers of commerce and real estate associations also provide information—admittedly somewhat biased—

Planning for a healthy retirement

Old age can bring a variety of health problems, *bottom right*. While planning other aspects of retirement, people can also take steps to protect their health now and into the future, *below*.

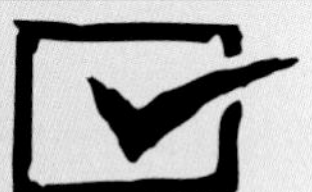

Things to do

- Learn all you can about your family medical history. If certain cancers or other diseases run in your family, find out whether the disease can be prevented or detected early, and take the necessary precautions or screening tests.
- Assemble a trusted health care team, including a primary care physician, dentist, and, if necessary, specialists for chronic medical conditions.
- Break poor health habits and start good ones. If you smoke, quit now while you have the distraction of working at a job. Learn how to prepare nutritious meals, incorporate exercise into your life, and reduce stress.
- Keep abreast of changing regulations regarding Medicare and other types of medical insurance for the elderly.
- Safeguard your mental health by striving to develop emotional characteristics that predict happiness in older people—including the ability to think positively, to be flexible, and to think well of oneself despite changing circumstances.

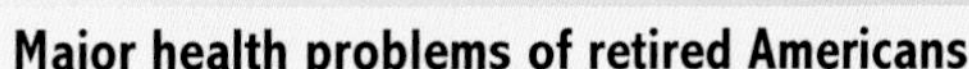

Major health problems of retired Americans

Mobility problems. Difficulty getting around because of osteoporosis, arthritis, cardiovascular disease, or other health conditions.

Loss of function. Impaired ability to see and hear, as well as the loss of control of bladder or bowels.

Mental and emotional problems. Difficulties such as depression, and much less commonly, dementia related to Alzheimer's disease, stroke, or other illnesses that affect the brain.

about their own communities. Some of the factors to consider include the area's climate, cost of living, tax burden, crime rate, medical services, cultural amenities, public transportation, accessibility for visitors, and shopping and restaurants.

Experts suggest that people considering relocation spend as much time as possible in the new area before retirement and try to develop friends and connections there. Many people sell their home, buy a new one elsewhere, and then discover that the new area does not suit them. People can avoid this expensive mistake by renting a home for a year after relocating rather than buying immediately.

Living arrangements often change as the years go by and unforeseen events occur. The birth of a grandchild, the death of a spouse, or the retiree's own health problems may prompt relocation to a new city or a move to a new dwelling.

Some people choose to move to retirement communities, where they can live independently but have easy access to social support and recreational activities. Age and infirmity may eventually necessitate moving to a facility for assisted living. These facilities enable residents to maintain their own apartment while receiving certain services, such as meals, transportation, and in-home care. It's difficult to predict when such services might become necessary, but it is important to explore options before the need for them arises. Some of the most desirable facilities have waiting lists three to four years long.

Many retirees would prefer to remain in their own home after developing a significant health problem. If that is the case, they should look into the availability and cost of in-home assistance before there is an emergency.

Good health in old age

In many people's minds, growing older is primarily associated with health problems and physical decline. However, advancing years do not automatically mean debilitating losses in physical and mental functioning. In fact, only about 5 percent of Americans over 65 live in nursing homes or other institutions. Of those over 85, about 22 percent live in nursing homes.

Although some health problems cannot be prevented, taking care of one's body is an important part of planning for old age. People with chronic conditions such as diabetes or high blood pressure should make sure those conditions are under control to help avoid complications in the future.

It is advisable for people to find out all they can about the diseases that run in their family. This information is particularly helpful if the family has a history of cardiovascular disease, diabetes, or cancers of the prostate, breast, or other organs. Many of these diseases can be prevented or treated in early stages by taking appropriate action in middle age.

Retirement planning is also a natural time to give up poor health habits such as smoking and to begin good ones. People of any age will benefit from starting a program of regular aerobic exercise, eating a low-fat diet with plenty of fruits and vegetables, and learning how to reduce stress.

For those whose health insurance plan allows them to choose their physicians, another good way of preparing for the needs of retirement is by assembling a trusted health-care team. Such a team should include a primary-care physician, dentist, and appropriate specialists.

The most common health problems of older Americans fall into three categories. First, mobility problems affect many older people who can't get around easily because of arthritis, cardiovascular disease, osteoporosis, or other conditions. A second common problem of aging is the loss of function. That refers to diminishing senses such as vision and hearing as well as the loss of bladder or bowel control. The third category consists of mental or emotional problems. Depression is the most common such problem for seniors. Less common is dementia related to Alzheimer's disease, stroke, or other illnesses that affect the brain.

Many of these conditions can be prevented or treated. Physical exercise, for example, combats cardiovascular disease, improves memory and thinking, and increases flexibility and strength. Regular medical checkups can detect glaucoma, cataracts, hearing problems, and other conditions that may lead to a loss of function. Depression can be treated with drugs or psychotherapy at any age. Urinary incontinence is now treatable with medication and surgery.

Another fact of life is that at least 40 percent of middle-aged Americans are now responsible for the care of aging parents and other relatives. The average 50-year-old couple in the United States already spends more time caring for their aging parents than rearing their children. The financial, health, and personal needs of aging parents thus place a big demand on many people nearing retirement. Women in particular tend to shoulder this burden. A middle-aged woman is more likely than her brother to shorten her work hours or quit work entirely to care for their aging parents or other relatives. Her own retirement plans may have to be put on hold because of her early exit from the work force.

People approaching retirement should also stay apprised of legal changes affecting health insurance for older Americans. Changes in the availability of Medicare, for example, may cause retirees to pay more for health care than they had originally budgeted. As of 1996, Medicare covered less than 40 percent of health-care costs for eligible participants.

Preparing for the emotional challenges of old age

Mental health is an important component of overall well-being at any age, and even more so at retirement. People who are prone to depression, for example, may be at risk for a worsening of the condi-

Planning legal and financial details

Retirement planning is also an appropriate time to make legal arrangements, *below*, as well as to assess one's financial resources and future needs, *opposite page*.

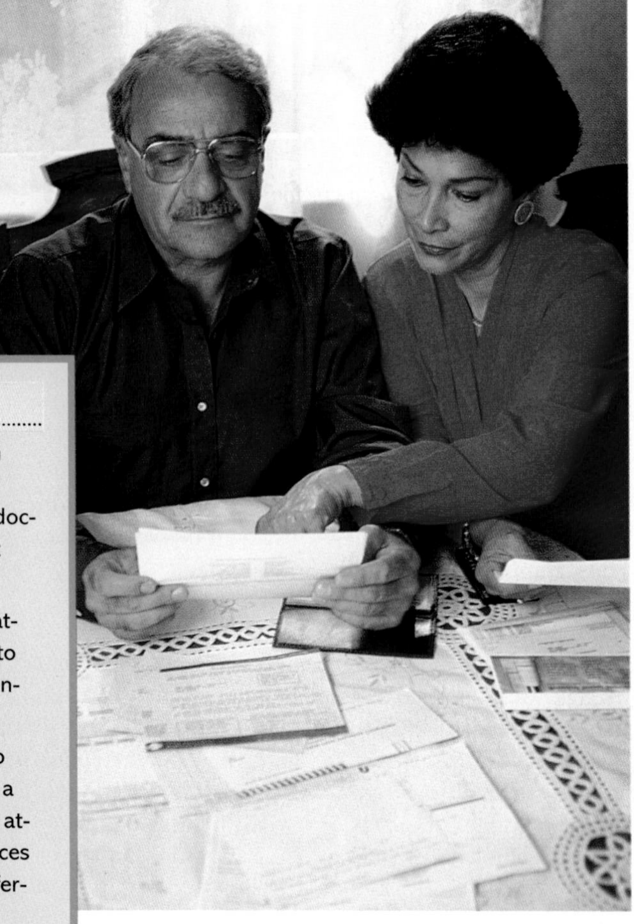

Things to do

- Draw up your will and decide whom you will name as the will's executor. Have a lawyer create or review the document to avoid technical errors that could invalidate the will.
- Have a lawyer draw up a power of attorney to name someone you trust to act on your behalf in case you are unable to do so.
- Consult a lawyer if you would like to create an advance directive such as a living will or a health care power of attorney that spells out your preferences for medical treatment if you are suffering from a terminal illness or injury. Nearly all states recognize the legality of the documents, though requirements vary from state to state.
- Discuss estate planning with a financial adviser or lawyer if you would like to set up trusts, establish joint ownership of some assets, or make gifts to reduce estate taxes.

tion in retirement, particularly when they experience health problems or the death of close friends or a spouse. Giving up work can also cut people off from daily social contact with peers and leave them feeling alone and adrift. It is wise for any older person to be alert for the symptoms of depression, which include changes in sleeping and eating habits, loss of energy, feelings of hopelessness, and thoughts of suicide.

Just as it is possible to improve one's memory by learning certain skills, it is possible to learn skills that will improve psychological health in old age. Research indicates that older people with good mental health are likely to be adept at three psychological skills. The first is sometimes called "reframing"—the ability to see apparently negative events and circumstances in a positive way. A common example of reframing is to think of a glass of water as being half full rather than half empty. People of any age can develop the habit of reframing by actively searching for a more positive perspective when faced with an unpleasant turn of events. For example, someone who

Things to do

- Estimate your needed level of income after retirement. (A rough rule of thumb is 70 to 75 percent of your current income.)
- Contact the Social Security Administration to determine your estimated government benefits.
- Contact your employer's pension administrator to find out what, if any, benefits you will receive on retirement.
- Calculate your income from personal assets such as savings accounts, investments, and rental property.
- Subtract your estimated expenses from your post-retirement income. If there is a shortfall, you may need to find ways to save more before retirement, scale back your living expenses, or remain in the work force longer than you had planned.
- Reassess your financial status at least once a year. For advice on investing, read books or consult a licensed financial planner.

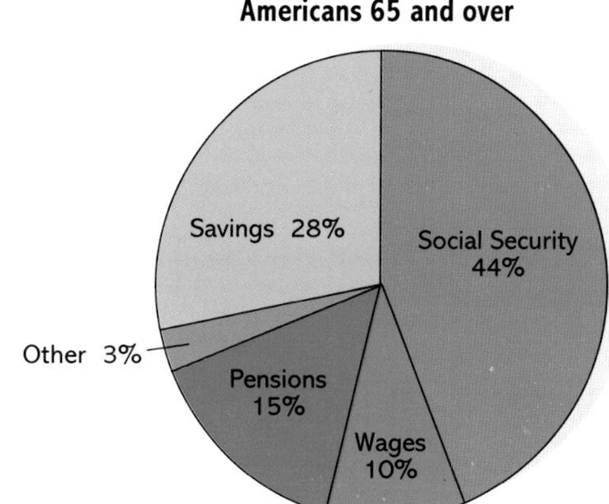

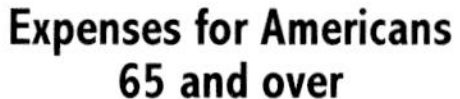

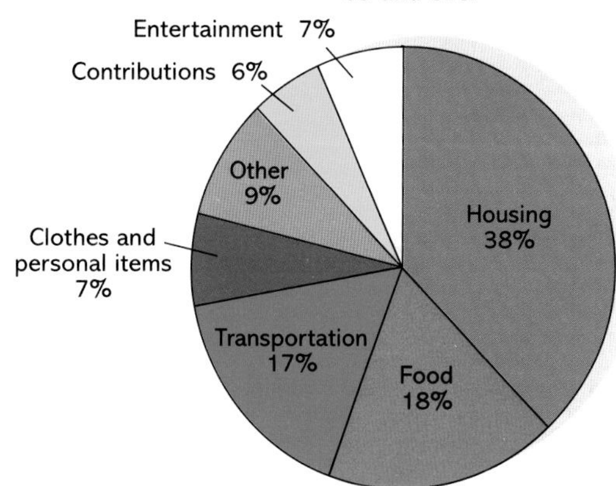

Source: U.S. Bureau of the Census.

The annual inflation rate plays a big role in calculating retirement expenses. To maintain the same standard of living, a person retiring in 5 or more years would need one of the amounts shown at right to replace each $1,000 of current income. Variations in the annual inflation rate produce stunning differences in the amount of income required.

Annual inflation rate	In 5 years	In 10 years	In 15 years	In 20 years	In 25 years
4%	$1,217	$1,480	$1,801	$2,191	$2,666
6%	$1,338	$1,791	$2,397	$3,207	$4,292
8%	$1,469	$2,159	$3,172	$4,661	$6,848
10%	$1,611	$2,594	$4,177	$6,728	$10,835
12%	$1,762	$3,106	$5,474	$9,646	$17,000
14%	$1,925	$3,707	$7,138	$13,743	$26,462

is fired from a job might recognize that the setback is also an opportunity to move in a new direction.

The second skill that is helpful to develop is adaptability, the ability to easily accommodate new situations or "go with the flow." For example, during the ups and downs of a working life, employees are often faced with changing circumstances: a new boss, a relocation, a shift in responsibilities. Some employees will be distressed by these changes, while others will not be terribly bothered. People who can learn to adapt to new situations tend to be less distressed by some of the events that accompany old age—physiological changes, for example, or a decline in status after retirement.

The third psychological skill is developing a sense of self that can evolve and grow over the years. A woman who has long taken pride in being a mother, grandmother, and homemaker, may have difficulty adapting to a move to a small retirement condominium in a state far away from her children. However, if the same woman thinks of herself in broader terms—for example, as a creative and nurturing person—then moving to a new location may not be so difficult. After all, she could continue to express herself and use her talents by taking art courses, organizing a community garden, or starting a day-care center.

Financial preparations

Once details of a person's desired retirement lifestyle have been fleshed out, he or she is in a much better position to make financial plans for supporting that lifestyle. Among the things that should be considered are future expenses—including housing, food, clothing, gifts, travel, entertainment, insurance, and other items. Many retirement planners use 70 to 75 percent of current income as a general rule of thumb for budgeting. A person should also calculate income anticipated from pensions, personal savings, investments, and social security and survivor's benefits. Subtracting the projected need from income shows whether there will be sufficient money for the lifestyle envisioned.

This calculation may well yield an unpleasant shock, according to a Merrill Lynch Investment Company survey of preretirees and managers who administer pension funds. This survey found that most Americans think they are better financially prepared for retirement than they actually are. Nearly 40 percent expected that social security would be their most important source of income. In fact, according to a 1993 U.S. Treasury Department report, only 20 percent of income among retirees living on $20,000 or more a year came from social security. An additional 15 percent came from employee pension plans. Personal savings, investments, and other sources of income made up the remaining 65 percent.

Given an income shortfall, some people may decide to delay retirement for a few years or to begin scaling back their living expenses. Most individuals with pensions, on the other hand, may find that they have a financial incentive to retire after they have reached the required age and years of service.

A financial planner can help workers decide on a timing strategy and get the most out of savings and investments. Some financial planners charge an hourly fee to set up a financial program that the client then carries out. Other planners receive a commission on any financial transactions they make on the client's behalf. In many cases, the former type of professional will be less expensive in the long run than the latter.

Another strategy for handling the financial end of retirement planning is to take a course at a community college or university to learn more about investing. One should exercise caution and common sense before enrolling in expensive seminars in hotels and conference sites, however. Such seminars, particularly those that promise an unusually high yield on investments, may be operated by unscrupulous types rather than legitimate, credentialed financial planners.

In general, the key to success in financial planning is anticipating as many problems as possible. These include one's own financial needs as well as the those of others. Younger as well as older members of the family may require help at some point. Grandparents sometimes assume significant responsibilities for their grandchildren, typically when their adult children suffer economic hardships, become ill, or die. The health problems of spouses and other family members can significantly affect a retiree's finances as well.

Legal details

A final task in preparing for retirement is to contact a lawyer to prepare a will, handle the legal issues of estate planning, prepare a power of attorney, and create an advance directive, or "living will," to spell out one's wishes regarding medical treatment. Books available in a public library offer tips on legal preparations for retirement. In addition, it may be helpful to seek out a lawyer who specializes in elder-law issues. State bar associations can help residents find a lawyer in their area with this specialty.

Clearly, retirement planning involves much more than setting aside a nest egg and investing in life insurance. To successfully plan for retirement means preparing for secure and comfortable housing, good mental and physical health, and involvement in meaningful relationships and activities. But by establishing goals, gathering needed information, and cultivating new skills, it may indeed be possible to live happily ever after. •••

A multitude of remedies promise to keep stomach acid in its place and relieve heartburn woes.

Heartburn: Taking Aim at Fire

By James L. Franklin

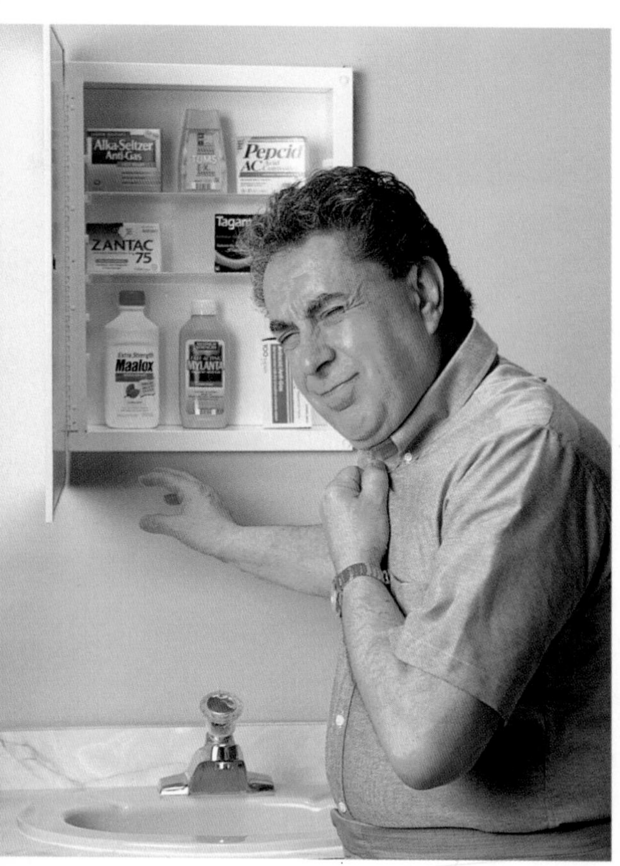

JUDGING FROM THE WAVE OF ADVERTISING that washed over American media in 1995, one might think modern medicine had found a new cure for heartburn. In fact, the advertised drugs had long been prescribed by doctors. What was new was that they were now being sold over-the-counter.

No doubt the ads found an attentive audience. Perhaps 40 percent of American adults know the feeling of a burning pain behind the breastbone that typically occurs after a meal. For some, heartburn is more than occasional. About 1 in 10 adults experiences it daily.

For relief, most heartburn sufferers rely on remedies from the drugstore shelf. Until recently, that usually meant liquid or tablet antacids, which can temporarily neutralize the source of heartburn pain—digestive acids that rise from the stomach into the lower end of the gullet, irritating the tissues there. Then in April 1995, the U.S. Food and Drug Administration approved the prescription medicine famotidine (sold as Pepcid) for over-the-counter distribution as a heartburn remedy. Approvals for two related drugs—cimetidine (Tagamet) and ranitidine (Zantac)—followed within the year.

These drugs offer people a more potent way to stave off heartburn at home, but some doctors worry that their ready availability means people with excessive heartburn may delay seeing a doctor about the problem. Such a delay can be dangerous indeed, because chronic heartburn sometimes signals a more serious condition. Just as important, any of these drugs may be harmful if overused.

What is heartburn?

In most cases, heartburn is the visible sign of a condition called gastroesophageal reflux disease, or GERD, in which stomach acids back up into the *esophagus* (the tube that carries food from the throat to the stomach). Normally, a muscular "pressure zone" called the lower esophageal sphincter tightly controls the connection between the esophagus and the stomach. When a person eats, the sphincter relaxes briefly to allow the food to enter the stomach.

Sometimes, however, the sphincter relaxes for no known reason, enabling the stomach's powerful digestive acids to escape into the esophagus. Studies show that this backflow, called reflux, occurs in many people without causing symptoms. But in some people, the episodes are long enough or frequent enough to irritate the tissues of the lower esophagus, causing pain.

Classic heartburn pain centers in the chest and may radiate to the throat or mouth. It occurs at night and might last for one hour or several. Sufferers may notice an acid or bitter taste or feel fluid rising from the stomach into the throat. Symptoms may worsen if they bend over or lie down.

Heartburn is not always easy to identify. Sometimes the chest discomfort is vague or severe enough to mimic signs of a heart attack. A person may visit the emergency room and undergo batteries of tests, only to receive a diagnosis of heartburn. While a false alarm may be annoying and expensive, the consequences are far worse when someone with a real heart problem assumes it's "only heartburn." Therefore, experts recommend that people with questionable chest pain—particularly pain that occurs with physical exertion—not hesitate to call their doctor or go to an emergency room. Often a brief checkup can ease patients' minds, if not their aching chests.

Causes and contributing factors

Many factors can prompt or aggravate heartburn. High-fat meals can slow the rate at which the stomach empties, leaving acids present for longer periods, and also prompt the sphincter to relax. Some patients report symptoms after consuming acidic foods, such as citrus juices or tomato sauce. Studies also indicate that specific foods can prompt symptoms in some patients regardless of the foods' acid content. Common culprits include coffee (even decaffeinated), alcoholic drinks, onions, garlic, chocolate, and peppermint. Smoking also can make heartburn worse by stimulating acid production and impeding the lower esophageal sphincter's function.

Eating just before bedtime may promote nighttime attacks. When the person lies down to sleep, gravity enables acids to flow more easily from the stomach. People who are overweight are particularly susceptible to heartburn because increased pressure on their internal organs can force acids upward. Pregnant women may also suffer, both because the enlarging womb compresses the stomach and because pregnancy stimulates the release of hormones that may encourage the lower esophageal sphincter to relax.

Some people may simply be naturally prone to heartburn. For example, their systems may be less adept than other people's at clearing acids from the esophagus. Or they may produce less saliva, which helps neutralize acids when swallowed.

Finally, certain medicines can aggravate heartburn—by promoting acid production, relaxing the sphincter, or reducing saliva. Troublesome drugs include such painkillers as aspirin, ibuprofen, and naproxen; the hormone progesterone (used in birth control pills and postmenopausal therapy); anticholinergics (prescribed for irritable bowel syndrome); tricyclic antidepressants (prescribed for depression); calcium-channel blockers (prescribed for high blood pressure); and theophylline (prescribed for asthma).

Until the last 20 years or so, doctors thought that reflux usually stemmed from a condition called hiatal hernia, in which a weakness in the *diaphragm* (the muscle separating the chest and abdomen) allows part of the stomach to bulge upward into the chest, just below the esophagus. Since the 1970's, however, studies have shown that the crucial factor in reflux is not hiatal hernia, but rather the lower esophageal sphincter—in particular, how strong it is and how often it relaxes. Although hiatal hernia is evidently not essential to reflux, doctors believe it may encourage problems by weakening the sphincter's effect and by holding stomach acids close to the esophagus. Hiatal hernia is also commonly present in people with *esophagitis* (inflammation of the esophagus), a complication of reflux.

Glossary

Antacid: A drug that neutralizes stomach acid.

Esophagitis: Inflammation of the esophagus that can develop when reflux is chronic or severe.

Gastroesophageal reflux disease (GERD): A disorder in which stomach acid backs up into the esophagus.

H_2-blocker: A drug that reduces the amount of stomach acid produced.

Hiatal hernia: A condition that can contribute to heartburn by permitting the stomach to bulge upward into the chest.

Lower esophageal sphincter: An area of muscular pressure that normally prevents stomach acid from backing up into the esophagus.

Complications of heartburn

Esophagitis develops when reflux is so severe and frequent that refluxed stomach acids eat away at the tissues lining the esophagus. If the resulting *ulcerations* (open sores) penetrate large blood vessels beneath the surface, the result can be severe bleeding and *anemia* (a shortage of red blood cells). A build-up of scar tissue over the damaged areas may cause a stricture, a narrowing of the esophagus that can make swallowing difficult.

Because so many people with heartburn never seek professional treatment, no one can be sure exactly how many develop esophagitis. Some research suggests that among those whose symptoms are severe enough to drive them to the doctor, about one-third have signs of esophagitis and 10 percent or more have severe cases.

Persistent heartburn also may lead to a rare but serious complication called Barrett's esophagus. Here, the cells that line the esopha-

The author:

James L. Franklin is associate professor of medicine at Rush-Presbyterian-St. Luke's Medical Center.

What is heartburn?

Heartburn—a burning sensation right behind the breastbone—occurs when stomach acid backs up into the lower end of the esophagus. The condition typically occurs after a meal and can last for an hour or more. Heartburn develops when the muscle that normally controls the passage between the esophagus and stomach relaxes, permitting the backflow of stomach acid. It is still unclear what causes this zone of muscular pressure, known as the lower esophageal sphincter, to relax.

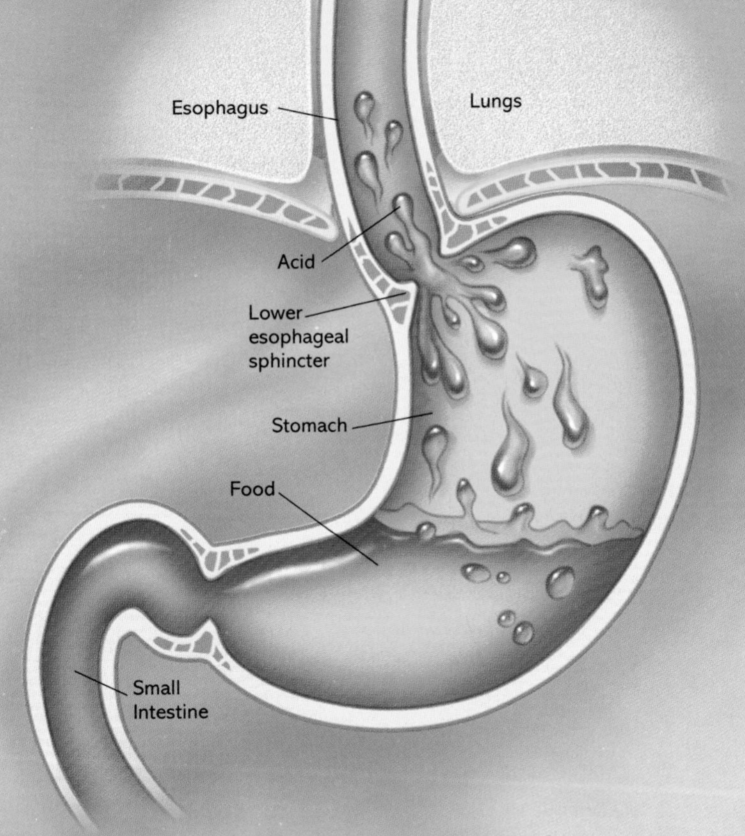

The role of hiatal hernia

Until the early 1970's, physicians thought that most cases of heartburn stemmed from a weakness in the diaphragm—the muscle that separates the chest from the abdomen. As a result of this weakness, part of the stomach bulges upward into the chest, a condition known as hiatal hernia. Although physicians now believe that relaxation of the lower esophageal sphincter is the key factor in heartburn, many people who experience frequent and severe bouts of heartburn also have a hiatal hernia. Hiatal hernia may contribute to heartburn by weakening the sphincter's effect and by keeping stomach acids close to the esophagus.

gus are replaced with another type of cell not normally found in that location. In about 1 in 10 patients with Barrett's esophagus, the abnormal cells develop into cancer of the esophagus, which is frequently fatal. Some experts think that esophagitis alone, even without the detectable changes of Barrett's esophagus, may increase the risk of cancer.

These complications affect the esophagus specifically. But doctors have begun to recognize that reflux may have more far-reaching effects. In particular, research suggests that reflux may contribute to some cases of laryngitis or asthma.

Factors that aggravate heartburn

Many things can prompt or worsen symptoms of heartburn. They include:

- High-fat meals, which can slow the rate at which the stomach empties.
- Acidic foods such as citrus juices or tomato sauce. Certain other foods, including chocolate, peppermint, and onions.
- Coffee, even decaffeinated.
- Alcoholic drinks.
- Smoking.
- Eating just before bedtime.
- Obesity, which puts increased pressure on internal organs and can push stomach acid upward. Pregnancy can do the same.
- Certain medications, including the painkillers aspirin and ibuprofen.

Diagnosing heartburn

Most people with heartburn never see a doctor about it because they get sufficient relief from drugstore remedies. For people with occasional complaints that respond to self-treatment, this may be fine. However, a trip to the doctor is in order if medicines do not curb the pain or if the person experiences unusual symptoms—such as trouble swallowing, chest pain other than burning, persistent abdominal pain, signs of bleeding (coughed-up clots or black stools), hoarseness, wheezing, or frequent coughing or throat-clearing. These may be symptoms of heartburn complications.

When patients do consult their doctors, a careful medical history and description of symptoms may be enough to establish a diagnosis of GERD. Generally, additional tests are necessary only when heartburn doesn't respond to standard medicines or when symptoms are unusual. In these cases, doctors have several ways to determine the cause of the heartburn, the presence of complications, and the best treatment.

An upper gastrointestinal (GI) X ray, taken after the patient drinks a substance that shows up on X rays, can produce an image of the affected organs. This technique can reveal a hiatal hernia or show a stricture, which may be a sign of esophagitis.

Gastrointestinal endoscopy involves inserting a flexible tube down the patient's throat. A miniature videocamera on the end of the tube lets the doctor view the tissues of the esophagus and any abnormalities such as ulcerations, hiatal hernia, stricture, or the abnormal tissues of Barrett's esophagitis. Using a cutting device threaded through the tube, the doctor may take *biopsies* (tissue samples) from suspicious areas to test for cancerous changes. The doctor can also use expandable "balloons" or other devices to *dilate* (widen) an esophagus narrowed by scar tissue.

Neither an X ray nor endoscopy can verify the presence of GERD, which can exist even if there is no hiatal hernia, inflammation, or other visible abnormality. To check for sensitivity to acid, doctors may use a Bernstein test, also known as an acid perfusion study, in which an acid and a neutral solution are in turn deposited in the lower esophagus to see if the acid triggers heartburn symptoms.

The "gold standard" for diagnosing GERD is 24-hour monitoring of acidity in the esophagus. Doctors place into the esophagus a tiny device that measures acidity and transmits this information by means of a wire to a small pack worn by the patient. The resulting record reveals the frequency and intensity of any reflux episodes. Because this test is both uncomfortable and expensive, it is used only when symptoms are unusual and doctors need to verify that GERD is the problem.

Treating heartburn

Heartburn treatment typically follows a set sequence of steps. To begin with, doctors recommend such measures as these to reduce the incidence of reflux:

- Avoid large or high-fat meals and foods that seem to prompt symptoms.
- Don't eat just before lying down to sleep.
- Maintain a healthy weight.
- Don't wear clothes that fit tightly around the waist.
- Avoid drinking alcohol and smoking.
- If nighttime attacks are a problem, elevate the upper body by putting a wedge under the upper part of the mattress or placing blocks under the head of the bed.

When heartburn does occur, the routine response is medication. Whether a patient is following doctor's orders or self-treating, the first choice is usually an antacid. Antacids include ingredients that, when swallowed, neutralize stomach acids on contact. Although relief comes quickly, it may wear off within an hour or less.

The common antacid ingredients vary in their effectiveness and risks. Many antacid preparations combine ingredients to balance their strengths and weaknesses. One preparation (sold as Gaviscon) adds alginic acid to two standard antacid agents. This combination is thought to float on top of the contents of a full stomach, where it can intercept refluxed acids. Calcium-based antacids often remain effective for a short time only, and stomach acidity may increase when their effect wears off.

If antacids do not work, the next step is to try the more potent histamine H_2-receptor antagonists (also known as H_2-blockers), which reduce the amount of acid the stomach produces in the first place. These drugs include not only cimetidine, famotidine, and ranitidine, all now available over-the-counter, but also the prescription drug nizatidine (Axid). Long prescribed for ulcers, these medicines can relieve heartburn and help heal mild esophagitis.

Drug class/ How sold	Generic and brand names	Action and effectiveness
Antacids Over-the-counter. Available as tablets and in liquid form. Relatively inexpensive.	• Aluminum (carbonate, hydroxide, or phosphate forms), found in such drugs as Rolaids, Amphogel, Maalox, and Mylanta.	Neutralize stomach acid on contact. Provide fast but short-lived relief from heartburn pain. Frequent doses may be necessary as symptoms recur.
	• Calcium (carbonate or phosphate forms), found in such drugs as Tums and Alka-2.	
	• Magnesium (carbonate, hydroxide, or other forms), found in such drugs as Gelusil, Maalox, Mylanta, Riopan, and milk of magnesia.	
	• Sodium bicarbonate, found in such drugs as Alka-Seltzer and Bromo Seltzer.	
Histamine H_2-receptor antagonists (Also called H_2-blockers) By prescription and also over-the-counter at half the standard prescription dosage. Nizatidine sold by prescription only. H_2-blockers are available as liquids, tablets, or capsules.	• Cimetidine (Tagamet) • Famotidine (Pepcid) • Ranitidine (Zantac)	Suppress acid production in the stomach. Can relieve heartburn and promote healing of mild esophagitis. Some types may be taken before meals to prevent heartburn. New nonprescription versions carry strict warnings limiting dosage and duration of use, often to no more than two weeks.
	• Nizatidine (Axid)	
Proton-pump inhibitors By prescription only. Relatively expensive.	• Lansoprazole (Prevacid)	Suppress acid production in the stomach. Highly effective in persistent cases. May be used over the long term to keep symptoms at bay.
	• Omeprazole (Prilosec)	
Prokinetics By prescription only. May be prescribed in combination with an H_2-blocker or proton-pump inhibitor.	• Bethanechol (Urecholine) • Metoclopromide (Reglan)	Encourage the movement of food through the digestive tract; speed emptying of the stomach; strengthen the lower esophageal sphincter. Limited effectiveness at treating heartburn and esophagitis, particularly when used alone.
	• Cisapride (Propulsid)	Effective both alone and in combination with other drugs for relieving heartburn and healing esophagitis.

Most common side effects and risks

Can constipate. May interfere with calcium absorption and interact with some antibiotics. Overuse or use by people with kidney problems may cause bone damage.

- Can constipate. Overuse may cause kidney stones or other kidney problems.

Can cause diarrhea. May interfere with calcium absorption and interact with some antibiotics. Overuse may cause kidney stones or drops in blood pressure.

- Can cause gas. High in sodium. Should not be used by people with high blood pressure.

Side effects are rare. May interact with such drugs as theophylline (for asthma), warfarin (for blood-thinning), or phenytoin (for seizures).

- Side effects are rare.

Side effects are rare. May interact with blood-thinning drugs.

- Side effects are rare.

Side effects are rare. May interact with the asthma drug theophylline

- Side effects are rare. May interact with such drugs as diazepam (for mood and sleep disorders), warfarin (for blood-thinning), and phenytoin (for seizures).

Can cause diarrhea. Sometimes may cause a range of more troublesome side effects, such as muscle spasms, restlessness, and drowsiness. May interact with alcohol and other depressant drugs

- Can cause diarrhea. Other side effects are rare. May interact with alcohol and many medications.

Another class of acid-suppressing drugs is proton-pump inhibitors, including omeprazole (Prilosec) and lansoprazole (Prevacid). Although very effective, these drugs are expensive and available only by prescription. They are generally reserved for extreme or persistent cases of esophagitis.

Other drugs that doctors may prescribe in severe cases, either alone or in addition to acid-fighting drugs, are prokinetics. Cisapride (Propulsid) is the newest of these agents, which speed stomach emptying and strengthen the lower esophageal sphincter.

While many of these drugs can help heal esophagitis and prevent further complications, there is no specific drug treatment for Barrett's esophagus. The usual medical response to this condition is to check for cancerous changes in the esophagus by means of endoscopy and biopsies every year or two.

While all these drugs can help in managing heartburn, GERD itself remains a long-term disease that generally requires taking medicine indefinitely to keep symptoms under control. For a small proportion of patients, complications persist despite ongoing drug treatment. Others, particularly younger people, find the prospect of life-long drug therapy troublesome. In such cases, doctors may recommend surgery to eliminate the problem for good. Various tests of sphincter function and swallowing abilities can help doctors determine whether surgery will benefit a particular patient.

The standard surgical treatment for reflux (and, often, hiatal hernia) is fundoplication, in which the surgeon wraps a fold of the stomach around the bottom of the esophagus to increase pressure on the lower esophageal sphincter. Some surgeons now perform this surgery using laparoscopic techniques, which involves inserting miniature instruments through tiny incisions. Compared with traditional surgery, this approach means less scarring and faster recuperation.

Even so, surgery for heartburn remains a last resort, largely reserved for patients whose symptoms do not respond well to medication. Simple lifestyle modifications—such as losing weight and altering diet—and judicious use of well-proven remedies are far more practical approaches for the vast majority of heartburn sufferers. •••

Gum disease is a serious threat to adult teeth. But with regular home care and dental visits, it can be controlled.

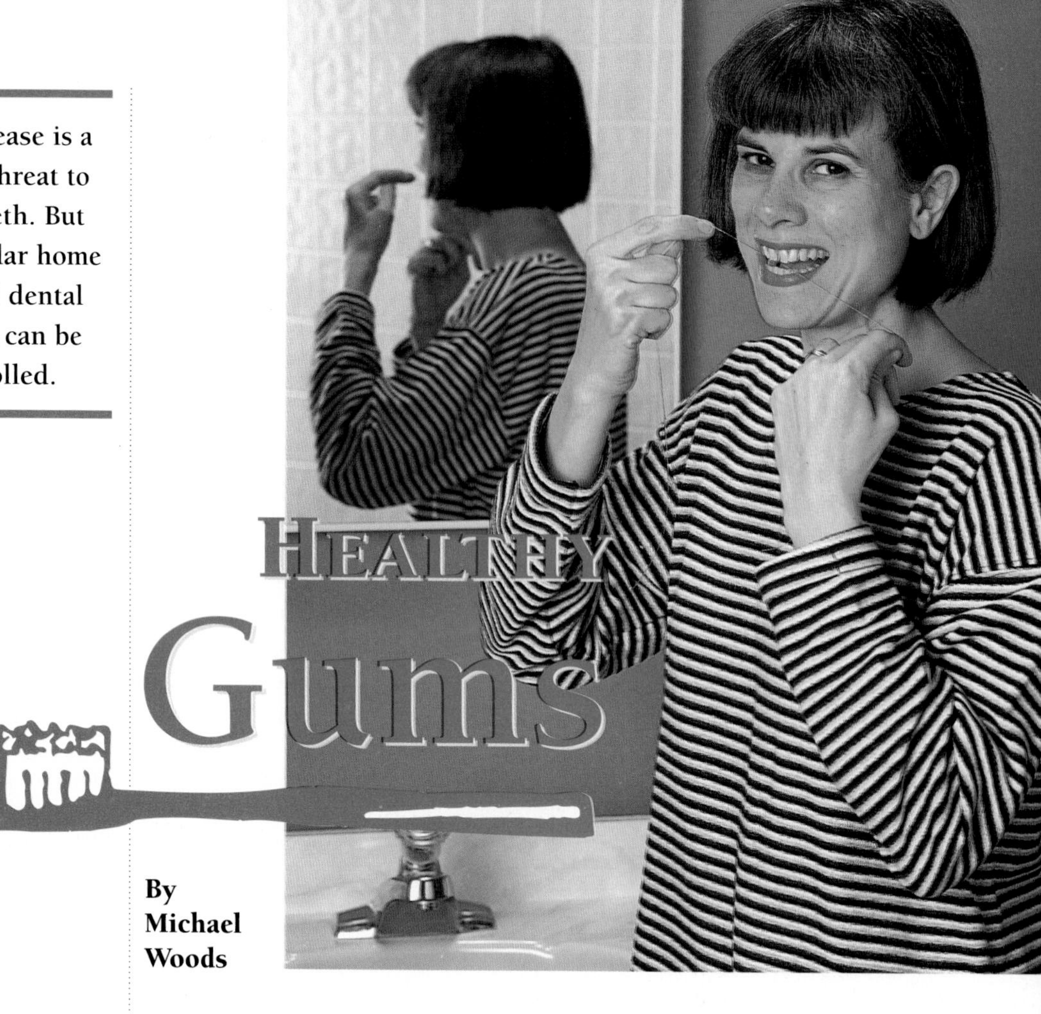

Healthy Gums

By
Michael
Woods

AFTER YEARS OF WORRYING ABOUT TOOTH DECAY, people are finally recognizing that gum disease poses a more serious lifelong threat to their teeth. Although tooth decay causes most tooth loss in children, gum disease is the number one threat to an adult's teeth—in fact, it is responsible for about two-thirds of all lost teeth in people over 50 years of age.

Store shelves now bulge with new types of toothbrushes, toothpastes, mouth rinses, and other products designed to fight gum disease. Dentists are using new techniques to detect and treat the problem. And people are taking the time to learn more about gum disease, sharing tips for keeping their gums healthy.

The new awareness is justified. Gum disease can develop in children as young as age 5, but the prevalence of the problem increases with age. Researchers estimate that at least half of American adults already have gum disease, and anywhere from three-quarters to nine-tenths will develop it sometime in their lives. Still, how severe the problem will be and when it will occur will depend on the care people take now to prevent problems from developing later.

Healthy gums are coral-pink and firm; they do not bleed when brushed. They form a tapered, "knife-edged" margin next to each tooth and come to a fine point between each front tooth.

What is periodontal disease?

Dentists call gum disorders *periodontal diseases*—commonly, infections of the periodontium, the tissues that surround the teeth and hold them firmly in the jaw. These include not only the visible gums, but also the bones and ligaments beneath the gums that anchor the teeth in place.

Common forms of periodontal disease are caused by bacterial *plaque*, a sticky, often invisible film that constantly forms on the teeth. Plaque consists mostly of hundreds of different kinds of bacteria—some more harmful than others. These bacteria get their energy from the food people eat and from body fluids, and they release products that can damage the gums and underlying structures. If not removed daily, plaque can harden into a stonelike material called *calculus* or *tartar*. Tartar also collects under the gums, causing difficulty in brushing and flossing and thus allowing plaque to grow undisturbed.

Gum disease comes in two common forms. The mildest and most prevalent is gingivitis—a term that comes from a Latin word for *gums* and the suffix *-itis* meaning *inflammation*. Its visible signs are red gums, rounded gum margins alongside the teeth, and gum swelling between the teeth. The first symptom often is a pink stain on the toothbrush that comes from bleeding of the gums during brushing.

Left untreated, gingivitis can progress into the more serious type of gum disease, periodontitis. Whereas gingivitis affects only the gums, periodontitis typically involves the ligaments and bone that support the teeth. The gums pull away from the teeth, leaving gaps or pockets that contain plaque and calculus. Infection deepens and may eventually erode so much ligament and bone that teeth loosen until they fall out or must be removed. Periodontitis can reach an advanced stage painlessly, causing few symptoms beyond those of gingivitis. Or it may produce such signs as bad breath, gums that shrink or recede to expose the tooth root, and loose teeth.

Periodontitis usually occurs in adults and progresses slowly. But sometimes it starts in adolescents or young adults and develops rapidly. Dentists call this form of the disease early-onset periodontitis.

Many factors can increase a person's chances of developing gum disease. Smoking increases calculus build-up, irritates the gums, and

Warning signs of gum disease

Gum disease is usually painless, but there are signs to watch for. Any of the following clues can indicate gum disease:

- Gums that bleed when you brush.
- Red, swollen, or tender gums.
- Gums that have pulled away from the teeth.
- Pus between teeth and gums that appears when you press the gums.
- Loose teeth.
- A change in the way your teeth come together when biting.
- A change in the fit of partial dentures.
- Persistent bad breath.

Source: American Dental Association.

interferes with the immune system's response to the bacteria responsible for gum disease. Poor diet can lower resistance to infection. Teeth-grinding, nail-biting, and even improper use of toothpicks can damage gum tissues and make them more susceptible to disease. Poorly fitting dental bridges and faulty dental work can create hiding places for plaque. And some medications can reduce the amount of saliva in the mouth and may make the gums more prone to infection in various ways. These drugs include certain tranquilizers, muscle relaxants, decongestants, antihistamines, antidepressants, and antispasmodics. Other medications, such as cancer drugs, blood pressure drugs, and calcium channel blockers can cause swelling of the gums.

In pregnant women and women taking birth control pills, hormonal changes can make gums more sensitive to irritants and more prone to swelling and bleeding. Also at higher risk for gum disease are people with certain medical conditions, including diabetes and AIDS. People whose close relatives have experienced severe gum disease are more likely to develop it, too. This association may suggest a genetic factor in gum disease, or it may simply mean that people living in the same home tend to learn and practice the same kinds of oral care. And, as Canadian and Dutch researchers found in a 1993 study, an individual with gum disease may transmit particular strains of harmful mouth bacteria to family members, increasing their risk of developing problems.

Diagnosing periodontal disease

Dentists typically diagnose periodontal disease by looking at the teeth and gums, taking X rays to check for bone loss, and probing the periodontium. Probing is by far the most important method and involves inserting a tiny measuring gauge into the gum pockets to check the gum's attachment to the tooth. Pockets in healthy gums normally are less than an eighth of an inch (3 millimeters) deep.

These techniques have their limitations, however. They provide no way for a dentist who spots signs of gum disease to know whether the disease is still active or how fast it is progressing unless the dentist has tracked the patient's condition at regular intervals over a long period. In 1992, the American Dental Association (ADA) began a major effort to encourage early detection of periodontal disease by tracking the condition of patients' gums. The program established a technique called Periodontal Screening and Recording (PSR), in which the dentist uses visual examination and probing to produce a numerical "gum health score" for the patient. A score of 0 means good periodontal health; 1 to 2 means that early disease is present; and 3 to 4 means more advanced disease that requires further examination. The ADA predicted that following this approach at every routine dental checkup could decrease gum disease in the 1990's as dramatically as fluoride reduced tooth decay in the 1960's.

Another limitation of visual inspection, X rays, and probing is that

The author:

Michael Woods is science editor of *The Toledo Blade* and the author of many articles on scientific and medical topics.

The plaque attack

Gum disease begins with a build-up of *plaque,* a sticky film made up mostly of bacteria. Substances the bacteria release can damage the gums. If not removed daily, plaque can harden into tartar. Tartar collects under the gums and makes brushing and flossing difficult, allowing plaque to grow undisturbed. Left untreated, the mildest form of gum disease, gingivitis, can progress into the more serious type, periodontitis.

Healthy gums
Healthy gums are pink and firm and fit tightly against the teeth. They do not bleed when the teeth are brushed.

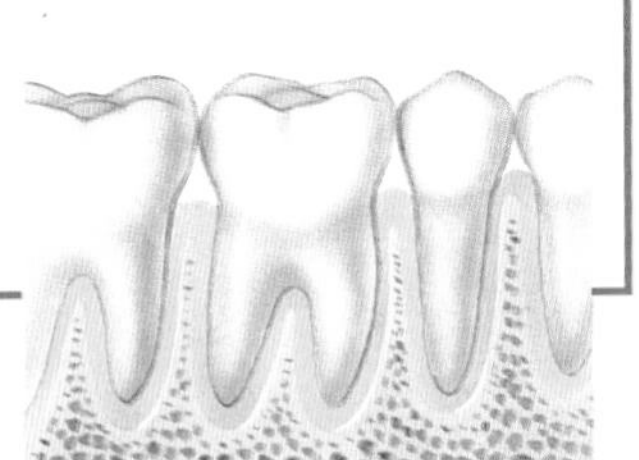

Gingivitis
Gingivitis is an inflammation of the gums that makes them red and swollen. A pink stain may appear on the toothbrush from bleeding of the gums during brushing.

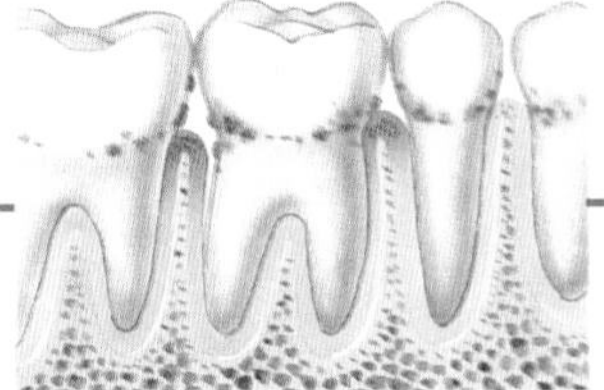

Periodontitis
Periodontitis is an infection that has spread from the gums to the ligaments and bone that anchor the teeth. The gums pull away from the teeth, leaving pockets that contain plaque and tartar. Teeth may loosen as the ligament and bone that support them erode.

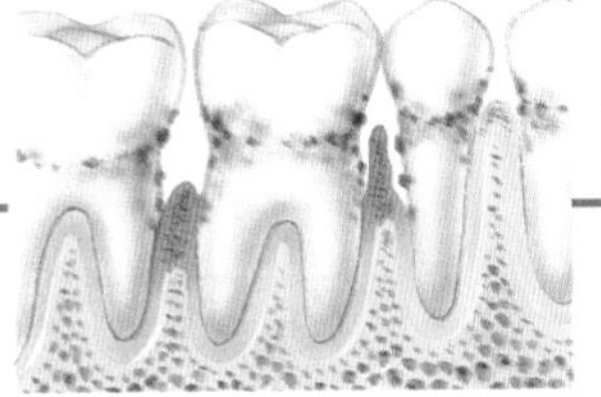

these traditional techniques can identify gum disease only after it has begun to destroy tissues. New tests, however, can help reveal the presence of active disease much earlier. To do so, the dentist uses a special piece of absorbent paper to take a sample of the plaque or fluid from the gum pocket. One test looks for the DNA—genetic material—of known disease-causing bacteria. Other tests identify chemicals released when bacteria destroy gum tissue. The presence of these chemicals shows that the gum is currently under attack. Some of these tests must be sent to a laboratory for results, but new types of tests can be done in the dentist's office.

Treating periodontal disease

The damage to gums from gingivitis need not be permanent. Early disease may require only the simple treatments of scaling and root planing, in which the dentist uses tiny instruments to scrape away calculus and smooth diseased root surfaces. Sometimes the dentist will carefully scrape small bits of infected tissue from periodontal pockets, a procedure called *curettage.* Once the irritants and infected

Scaling back

With regular visits to the dentist, gum disease can be detected early, when a thorough cleaning with scaling, root planing, or curettage may be enough to restore gum health.

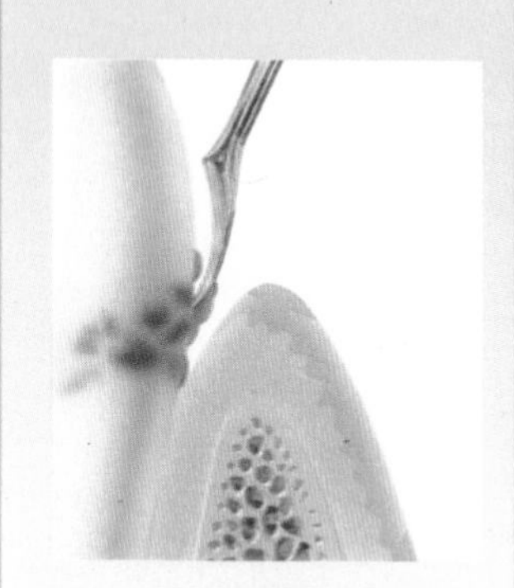

Scaling involves scraping away deposits of tartar that have formed on the teeth.

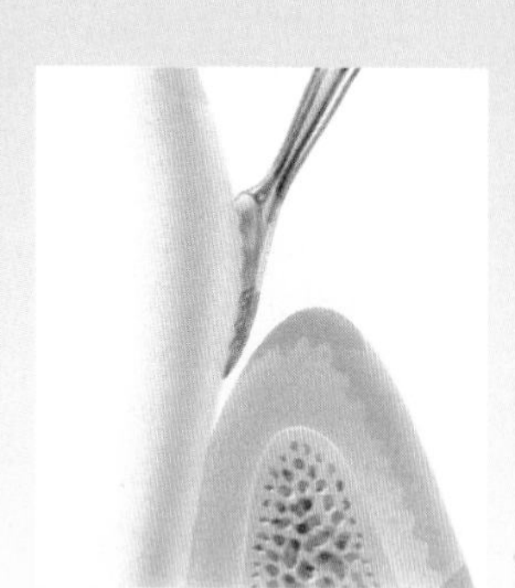

Root planing involves smoothing tooth and root surfaces to permit gum tissue to reattach to the teeth.

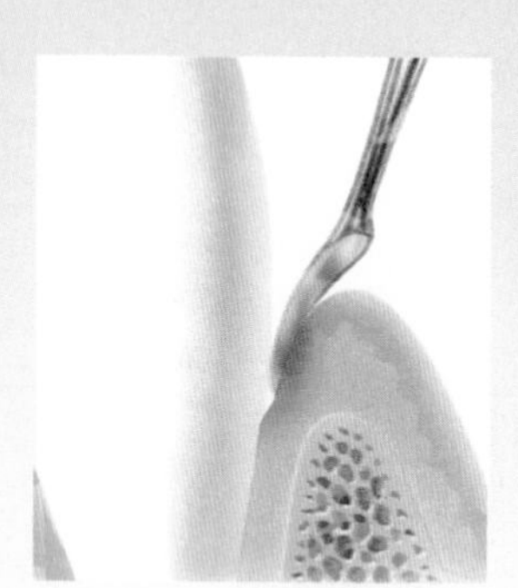

Curettage involves scraping small bits of infected gum tissue from periodontal pockets. This allows the gum tissue to heal and reattach to the teeth.

tissue are removed and the diseased surfaces smoothed, the gums can gradually heal and reattach to the teeth.

In more advanced disease, the pockets are often so deep that it is difficult for a dentist or hygienist to treat them using these measures—and virtually impossible for a patient to keep them clean. In such cases, surgery may be necessary to remove plaque and calculus, shrink the pockets, and reshape the gum tissue.

Gum surgery is usually done by a specialist called a periodontist. In one procedure, *gingivectomy*, the periodontist cuts diseased tissue from the pocket wall so that healthy gum tissue meets the tooth and can reattach. If pockets are very deep, a more involved procedure called flap surgery might be needed. Here, the periodontist lifts a small flap of gum tissue away from the tooth in order to remove all the plaque, calculus, and diseased tissue—and, if necessary, remove or reshape diseased bone near the tooth.

Traditionally, periodontists have then sutured the gum back around the tooth in the desired shape. This prevents further damage, but if any of the bone or ligament supporting the tooth has already been eaten away, that loss might be permanent. Today, newer techniques enable periodontists to stimulate the regrowth of eroded bone and ligament tissue. One method involves inserting grafts of

Emptying deep pockets

Simple cleaning techniques are no longer sufficient when gum disease is advanced and the pockets between gum and teeth have become deep. Surgery by a dental specialist called a periodontist may be necessary at this stage.

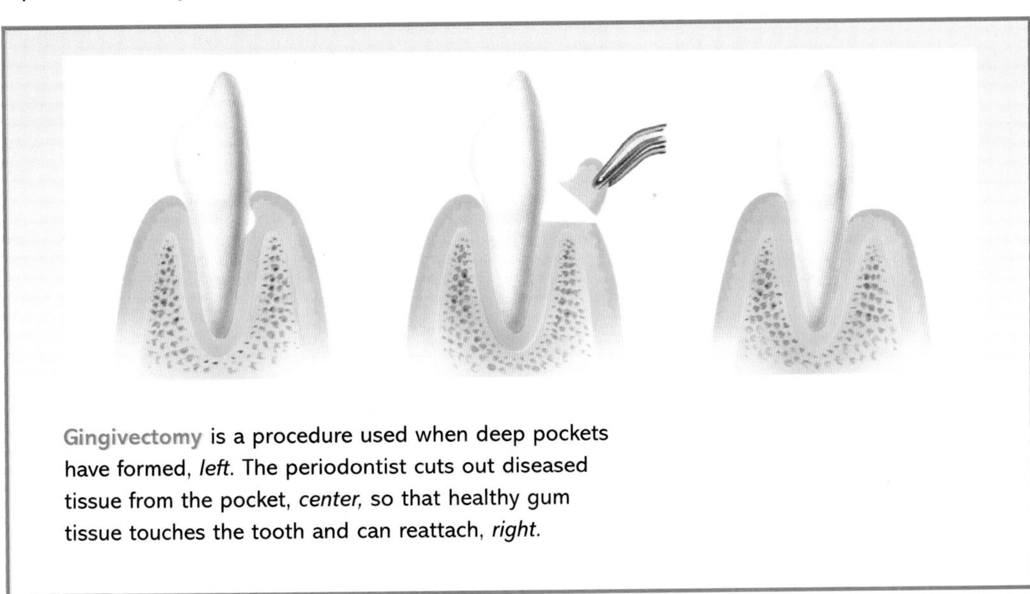

Gingivectomy is a procedure used when deep pockets have formed, *left*. The periodontist cuts out diseased tissue from the pocket, *center,* so that healthy gum tissue touches the tooth and can reattach, *right*.

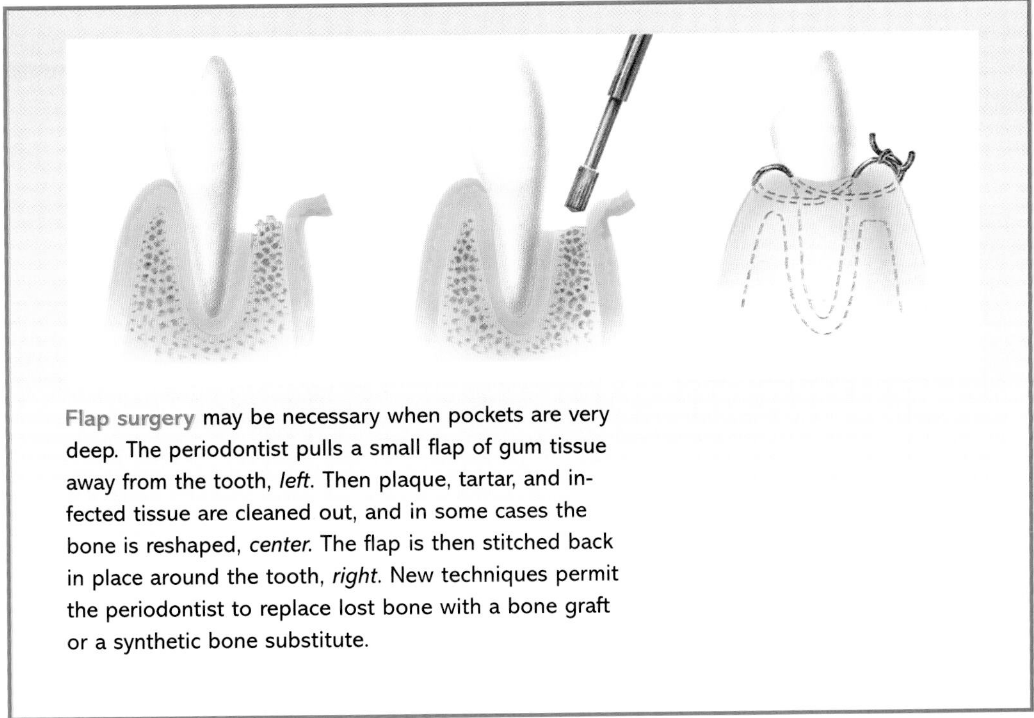

Flap surgery may be necessary when pockets are very deep. The periodontist pulls a small flap of gum tissue away from the tooth, *left*. Then plaque, tartar, and infected tissue are cleaned out, and in some cases the bone is reshaped, *center.* The flap is then stitched back in place around the tooth, *right*. New techniques permit the periodontist to replace lost bone with a bone graft or a synthetic bone substitute.

Staying in the pink

In addition to regular dental visits, brushing and flossing are the most effective weapons against gum disease. The American Dental Association (ADA) recommends brushing at least twice daily. The ADA says flossing at least once a day is also essential to remove plaque from areas your toothbrush can't reach.

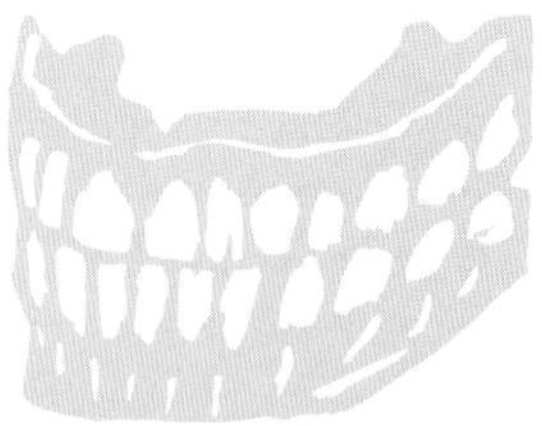

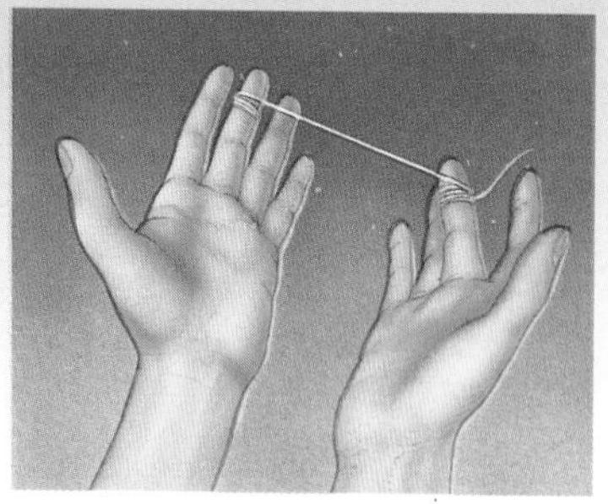

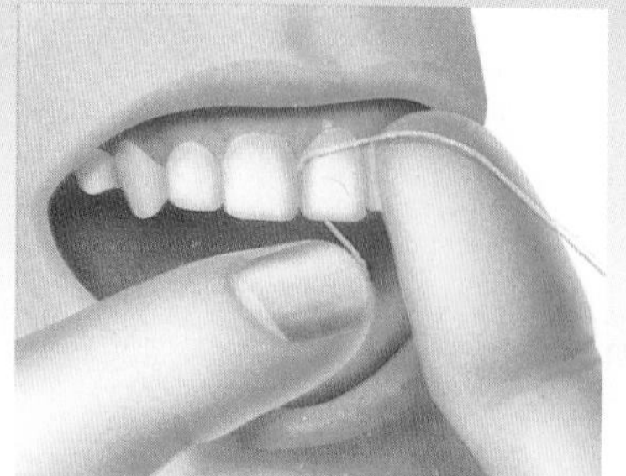

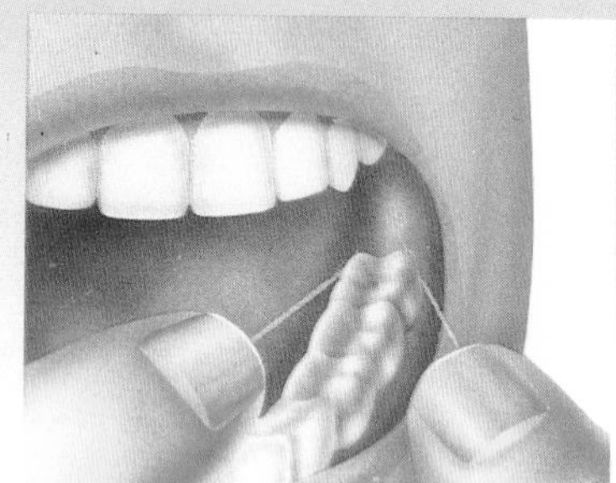

Proper flossing technique

Wrap a length of floss about 18 inches (46 centimeters) long around the middle finger of each hand, *left*. Holding the floss tightly over the thumb and forefinger, gently guide it between your teeth, *center*. At the gum line, curve the floss into a "C" shape against one tooth and gently slide it into the space between tooth and gum. Holding the floss against the tooth, rub up and down to remove plaque. Don't forget the back side of your back teeth, *right*.

bone taken from elsewhere in the patient's body or obtained from a tissue bank. Or the periodontist might pack gaps in bone with a synthetic "bone substitute" that provides a framework for regrowth of natural bone.

Another technique, *guided tissue regeneration* (GTR), involves covering the eroded area with tiny patches of a special fabric that protect bone and ligament as they grow back. This is helpful because it keeps gum tissues away from the healing site and allows cells from the bone and ligament to regenerate and form new attachments between the previously diseased root surface and newly formed bone. After a few weeks, the dentist removes the fabric to permit the gums to reattach to the new bone. Newer fabrics require no removal; instead, they are slowly absorbed into the gum when their job is done.

Although these surgical procedures are common, patients may be able to avoid the expense and trouble of surgery altogether. Periodontal disease usually progresses slowly, and in most people, experts say, there is no harm in delaying surgery briefly to try nonsurgical alternatives. For instance, if scaling and root planing prove insufficient, the dentist might suggest using antibiotics to battle the bacteria. Until recently this meant taking pills, which can cause wide-ranging side effects. In 1994, however, the United States Food and Drug Administration (FDA) approved the use of antibiotic fibers that can be placed directly into infected periodontal pockets. The fibers release the drug at the site, giving infected gums more than 100 times the dose possible with traditional oral antibiotics while avoiding the drugs' systemwide side effects.

Two prescription mouth rinses, PerioGard and Peridex, also combat gum disease. Their active ingredient, chlorhexidine, can cause

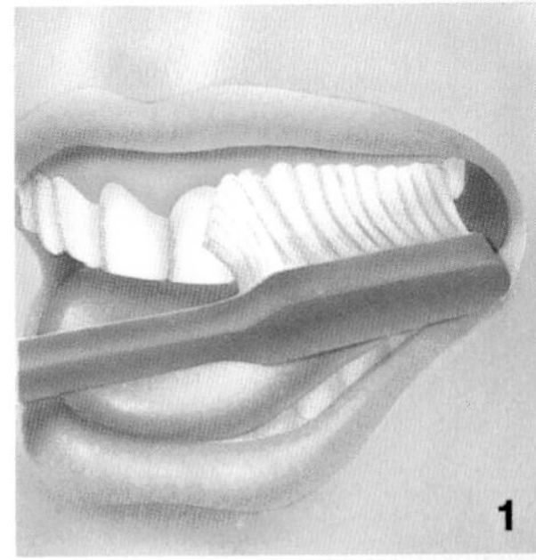
1

Proper brushing technique

The ADA recommends brushing with a soft-bristled toothbrush. It recommends the following steps: (1) Place the brush at a 45-degree angle against the gums and gently brush back and forth with short strokes. (2 & 3) Brush the outer and inner surfaces as well as the chewing surfaces and (4) use the brush to reach the inner surfaces of the front teeth. (5) Also brush the tongue to remove the coating of food debris and bacteria.

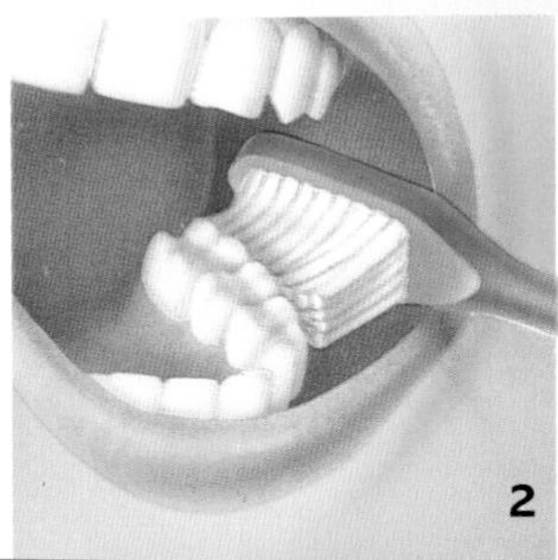
2

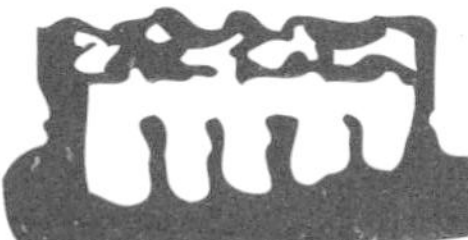

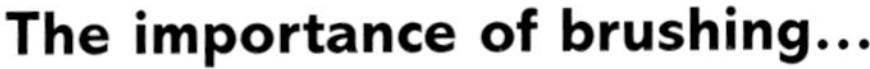

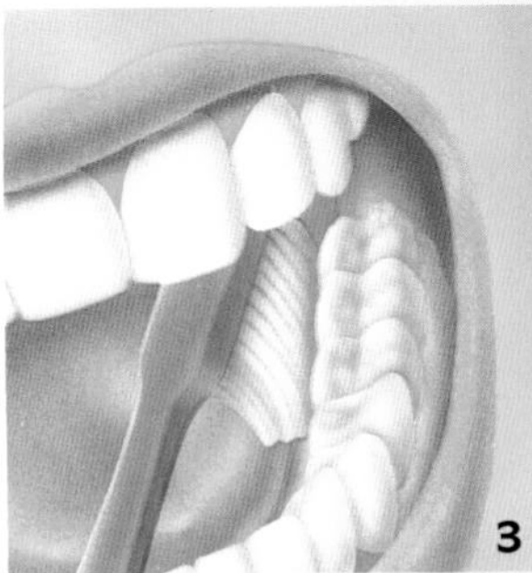
3

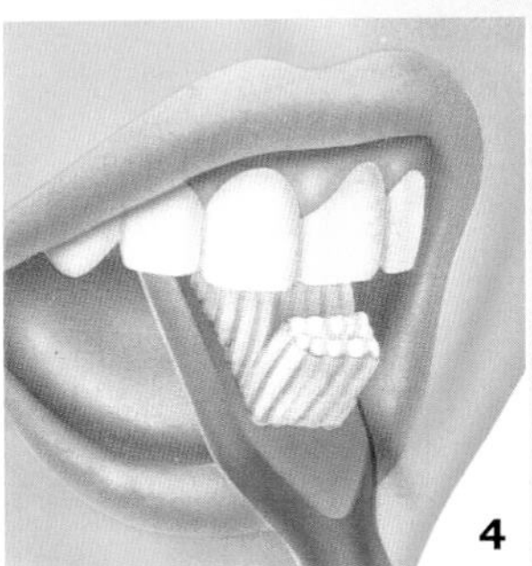
4

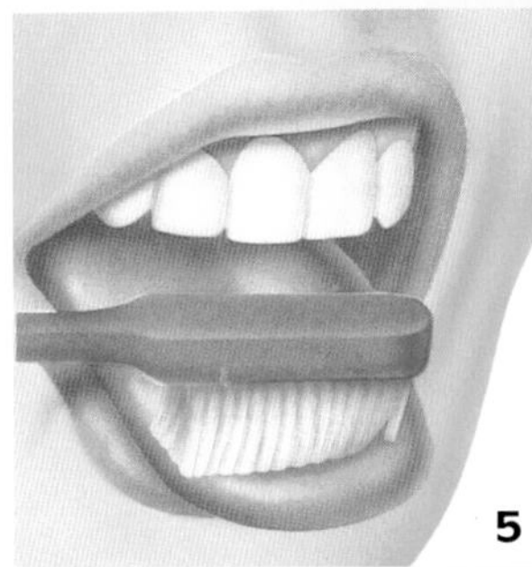
5

brown stains on the teeth, but dental hygienists can remove the stain during routine cleanings. The ADA also recognizes that the ingredients in certain nonprescription mouth rinses, such as Listerine, help reduce plaque and gingivitis, though studies indicate that their effect is less powerful than the prescription products.

The importance of brushing...

Of course, the purpose of these approaches—surgical or nonsurgical—is to treat damage that has already occurred. Ideally, people should avoid gum disease in the first place. And if their gums do require professional treatment, they need to take prompt action to keep the problem from recurring.

The key to both of these goals is proper oral care and maintenance. The ADA recommends brushing twice a day with a soft-bristled toothbrush. New high-tech toothbrushes have improved handles, sculpted bristles designed to clean between teeth and under the gums, and heads made to reach the back teeth. Still, long-term studies have not yet indicated whether these special brushes really are more effective in preventing gum disease.

Proper brushing technique may differ from what many of today's adults learned as children. Dentists now recommend placing the toothbrush at a 45-degree angle against the gums and moving the brush back and forth gently in short tooth-wide strokes. It's important to brush outer, inner, and chewing surfaces of the teeth, as well as the tongue, to remove the coating of food debris and bacteria.

An electric toothbrush may help some people clean more thoroughly, according to the ADA. Current models have tufts that rotate thousands of times per minute. Before buying an electric toothbrush, however, people might consider the results of a 1992 reader survey by *Consumer Reports* magazine, which found that 72 percent of readers who owned electric brushes preferred to use a manual brush instead.

Choosing toothpaste has also become more complicated, with a bewildering variety of products available. Most dentists recommend that you select an ADA-accepted toothpaste containing fluoride, which hardens tooth enamel and helps prevent decay. Tartar-control toothpastes usually contain another active ingredient, pyrophosphate. These pastes really are effective, according to the ADA; some studies have shown that they reduce calculus formation by as much as 36 percent. Some tartar-control toothpastes contain stannous fluoride, which may reduce plaque-forming bacteria. The ADA says, however, that there is no conclusive evidence that baking soda toothpastes reduce gum disease.

...and flossing

Flossing at least once a day is essential, dentists say, to remove plaque from areas your toothbrush can't reach. Gently guide floss between the teeth. At the gum line, curve it into a "C" shape against one tooth and gently slide it into the space between tooth and gum. Hold the floss firmly against the tooth and rub up and down to remove plaque. Repeat on each tooth.

There are a variety of alternative products for cleaning between the teeth for people who have difficulty manipulating floss. These include special tiny brushes and picks or sticks made from wood or plastic. Some people find that a floss holder—a rod with floss stretched across a forked end—helps them clean between hard-to-reach teeth. And a device called an irrigator can flush water or mouth rinses directly into gum pockets.

Some periodontists emphasize using a light touch for gum care, particularly after treatment for gum disease. Brushing too vigorously or forcing floss too deeply between the tooth and gum can discourage healing gums from reattaching to the tooth.

Regular visits to your dentist for professional cleaning and a gum checkup are also essential in battling the plaque plague. Most people miss some areas of plaque despite thorough brushing and flossing. Once the plaque hardens into calculus, only a dentist or hygienist can remove it. Make your concern about gum disease clear to the dentist. Be sure you get periodontal probing at each visit, and ask the dentist to keep track of your PSR score. Office visits are also a good time to get advice about the confusing variety of gum-care products.

New hope for gum disease treatment

Dental researchers are studying many new ways of diagnosing, treating, and preventing periodontal disease. New test kits may make screening for active disease a routine part of every adult's dental checkup. Already under development are tests that instantly identify especially dangerous types of plaque bacteria.

Research on a group of natural body chemicals called *tissue growth factors* shows special promise for better guided tissue regeneration techniques. These chemicals speed the regrowth and healing of damaged periodontal bone and ligament.

Gene therapy may provide new preventive measures, according to the National Institute of Dental Research (NIDR) in Bethesda, Maryland. Gene therapy is the use of pieces of DNA as a medicine to treat or prevent disease. NIDR researchers are seeking ways to insert plaque-fighting genes into a person's salivary glands. The glands then would produce saliva containing substances that control plaque bacteria.

While these developments offer great promise for the future, much of the knowledge we need to control gum disease already exists. Reducing gum disease's toll can be as simple as raising public awareness of the dangers posed by plaque and encouraging regular home care and dental visits. ●●●

For more information:

American Dental Association
211 East Chicago Avenue
Chicago, Illinois 60611
(312) 440-2500

American Academy of Periodontology
737 North Michigan Avenue
Suite 800
Chicago, Illinois 60611
(312) 787-5518

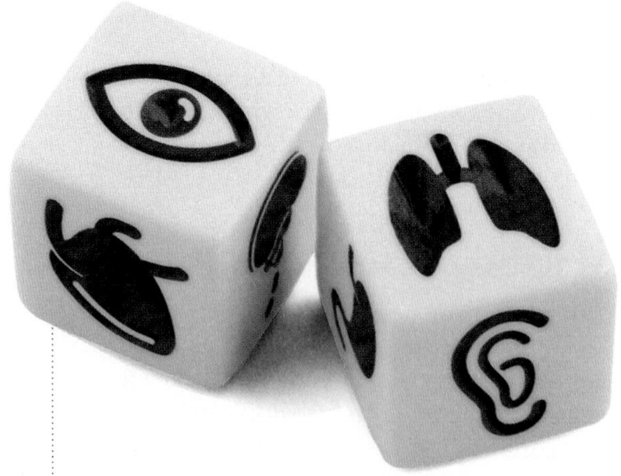

With headlines warning of new health threats daily, it's helpful to know which risks to pay attention to.

Evaluating Health Risks

By Meira Ben-Gad

The author:

Meira Ben-Gad is a free-lance writer.

PERIODICALLY THE HEADLINES APPEAR: "Power lines tied to cancer risk," or "Can your hairdryer give you cancer?" At issue are electromagnetic fields (EMF's), a form of radiation generated by electric power lines, household appliances, and the like. If EMF's do raise cancer rates, it would indeed be major news. In 1992, two Swedish studies that aimed to settle this long-standing question found that leukemia rates rose with exposure to EMF's. But a 1993 Danish study failed to link EMF's and leukemia, and a Finnish study that year found no increased risk of cancer at all. A 1994 study in Canada and France again uncovered an elevated leukemia risk. This was followed, in 1995, by a North Carolina study that suggested a link with brain tumors but not leukemia.

The stream of conflicting research findings about EMF's is but one instance of contradictory scientific evidence that has caused public confusion. Consider a few other examples: Pesticide residues—first a cause of breast cancer, then not. Hair dyes—linked to leukemia, then not. Margarine—a safe alternative to butter, then tied to heart disease. The issues grab headlines, frighten and perplex the public, and then fade out of view until the pendulum of scientific opinion swings the other way.

Scientists are, in fact, less at fault for the confusion than they appear. The real culprit may be a combination of overeager reporting on the part of press agents and journalists and the nature of scientific inquiry itself. A single scientific study is rarely definitive. It can take years of gathering evidence piece by piece before experts reach consensus on a health issue. And the process affords numerous opportunities for dead ends and wrong turns.

Scientists can collect evidence about potential health risks from three main types of studies: laboratory experiments, clinical trials, and observational studies. In laboratory studies, researchers use lab animals or cell cultures as stand-ins for human beings. For instance, by giving lab animals—usually mice or rats—varying doses of a compound such as a pesticide, scientists can determine how great an exposure is needed to induce cancer or another disorder in them. Scientists then calculate the likely risk to human beings exposed to small amounts of the compound over long periods. In test tube experiments, researchers try to uncover the mechanisms by which toxic agents affect the body—for instance, the ways in which *carcinogens* (cancer-causing agents) produce the genetic damage that can lead to cancer. Once they understand the biological mechanisms by which chemical compounds cause disease, researchers can more accurately predict the effects of these agents on human health.

Despite the value of laboratory research, it falls short as a means

The risk of breast cancer

Women repeatedly hear that their odds of developing breast cancer at some point are 1 in 8. But that is true only if they live to at least age 95. The odds for younger women are much lower.

By age	Odds
25	1 in 19,608
30	1 in 2,525
35	1 in 622
40	1 in 217
45	1 in 93
50	1 in 50
55	1 in 33
60	1 in 24
65	1 in 17
70	1 in 14
75	1 in 11
80	1 in 10
85	1 in 9
95 or older	1 in 8

Source: National Cancer Institute.

Keeping risks in perspective

To give people some idea of which hazards of daily life are worth worrying about, John Paling, a former biology professor at Oxford University in England, developed a risk scale. Paling says he got the idea after watching a woman who was smoking while inquiring about a water purification kit.

Event	Annual risk
Extra risk of cancer from eating a charcoal-broiled steak once a week	1 in 4 million
Being killed by lightning	1 in 3 million
Drowning in a bathtub	1 in 800,000
Extra risk of cancer from cosmic rays in Denver versus New York City	1 in 100,000
Extra risk of cancer from eating a peanut butter sandwich every day	1 in 90,000
Dying in childbirth	1 in 15,000
Becoming a murder victim	1 in 12,000
Dying in a crash while driving a car	1 in 8,000
Dying from any form of cancer	1 in 400

Source: *Scientific American*.

of measuring health risks fully. In animal experiments, for instance, animals are exposed to compounds in huge doses, making it easier for researchers to discern any ill effects. But critics argue that the body's defense mechanisms may be able to minimize the impact of small doses while being overwhelmed by large ones. And what happens in mice and rats, or in a cell culture, may only partially represent what happens in a living person.

Worth worrying about?

Two studies in 1995 and 1996 reported that taking certain oral contraceptives—so-called third-generation pills—rather than second-generation pills raised a woman's risk of developing blood clots by 50 percent to 100 percent. But early news stories failed to note that only 2 in 10,000 women taking second-generation pills develop blood clots—meaning that only 3 or 4 women in 10,000 on third-generation pills would be expected to do so. When risk is small to start with, doubling it won't make a big difference.

To seek information about human health directly, scientists often conduct clinical trials. In a clinical trial, the "gold standard" of medical research, researchers can manipulate the factor they want to test—a new drug treatment, say—while keeping other variables constant. Researchers randomly divide volunteers with similar characteristics, such as middle-aged men at risk for heart disease, into two groups. Members of one group receive the new drug, while those in the other group, called controls, receive a *placebo* (a substance with no active ingredients). At the study's end, the researchers determine the drug's effectiveness by comparing the rate or severity of illness in the two groups.

Clinical trials work well when scientists want to test drugs or treatments designed to improve people's health. But they are not so useful for studying factors that might be harmful to health. Scientists cannot ethically expose people to a potential carcinogen, for example, to see how many of them eventually develop cancer.

Another option exists for researchers who want to study potential health risks: the observational study. In these studies, scientists observe a selected population in an effort to uncover associations between disease and specific risk factors. For instance, researchers can identify people with some disorder and compare them with a control group of healthy adults similar in age, sex, and other characteristics. The researchers question the two groups about their diet, where they live and work, what they might have been exposed to, and the like, looking for factors that differentiate the sick individuals from the healthy ones. In another type of observational study, researchers follow a group of healthy people for many years to see who develops a particular illness—or who doesn't. They then look for factors common to those individuals.

Observational studies are a valuable part of medical research. However, these studies are limited in their usefulness. For one thing, they rely on estimates of exposures, instead of controlled dosages as in a clinical trial. How, for instance, can researchers accurately assess a person's exposure to EMF's, given the many possible sources at home, work, and elsewhere? Also, the studies depend on subjects' own reporting of their eating habits and other activities. But people's memories may not be reliable, especially when they are asked about their patterns of behavior.

Another problem is that these studies can show only an association between risk factors and disease—they cannot prove cause and

Words to watch for

The fruits of medical research are usually made known to scientists through publication in a medical or scientific journal. But the public learns of study results through news reports and press releases, which can make imperfect filters. Here are some words favored by journalists that may not say what they appear to.

"May"

This word is often treated as a synonym for "will." In fact, "may" means just what it says, suggesting that conclusions should be regarded with skepticism.

"Contributes to," "is linked with"

Most studies can only reveal associations—they cannot prove cause and effect. Some studies have shown a link between baldness and heart disease, for instance. But no scientist believes that baldness itself causes heart disease. More likely, physiological changes that can lead to baldness are the culprits.

"Doubles the risk"

This phrase, and others like it, are meaningless unless you know the level of risk you started out with. If the risk was 1 in 100,000, then doubling it still leaves a relatively remote 1 in 50,000. On the other hand, if the risk was 1 in 100, even a 50 percent increase raises your risk considerably, to about 1 in 67.

"Significant"

In scientific terms, *statistically significant* doesn't mean *important*. Rather, it indicates the scientist's level of confidence that a result is not likely to have occurred by chance. If a link between risk factor A and disease B is statistically significant at a 95 percent confidence level, there is at least a 5 percent chance the association is a statistical fluke.

"Proves"

Scientists rarely regard a single study as definitive. Most studies simply add a small piece to a large puzzle.

"Breakthrough"

Real breakthroughs in science are extremely rare. The discovery of antibiotics was one. A study that finds a risk factor which causes a 1-in-1,000 rise in cancer rates is not.

effect. Suppose, for instance, a study reveals that people who drink heavily are susceptible to a particular form of cancer. But heavy drinkers may also tend to smoke, to eat poorly, and to exercise infrequently. Perhaps one of these factors, or some combination of them, is responsible for the increased cancer risk.

With both clinical and observational studies, the validity of the results is dependent on how well a study was designed. Someone setting out to evaluate a clinical or observational study might ask the following questions:

- How many subjects did the study include? The smaller the number of participants, the more likely that any results are a statistical fluke—just as a coin is more likely to land on heads 8 times in 10 tosses than 800 in 1,000.
- Were the subjects drawn from the population at large or only

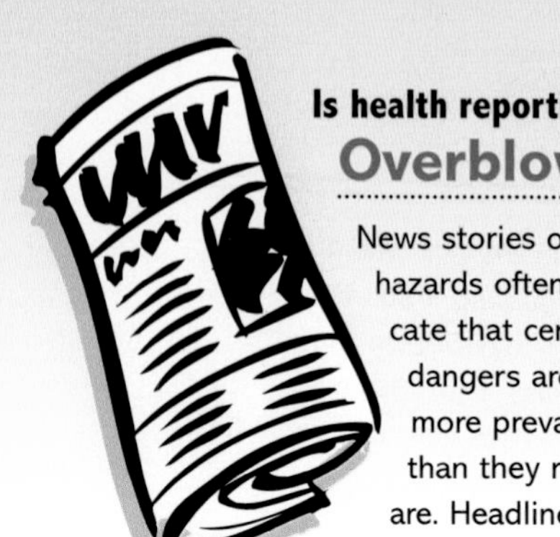

Is health reporting
Overblown?

News stories on health hazards often indicate that certain dangers are much more prevalent than they really are. Headlines trumpeting a supposed growing threat of rabies, for instance, may have unduly alarmed many people. Although it is true that rabies is a serious disease, people rarely contract it. No more than one or two Americans die of rabies each year.

Raccoon Rabies Called Permanent Threat in State

BEAVER ATTACKS BOY, 8, IN RIVER

CITY COUNCIL CANDIDATE ALARMED BY RABIES

Rabies and the indoor cat; Epidemic can strike pets almost anywhere

from a select group? For instance, did the participants include both men and women? A variety of ethnic and age groups? A study that includes few blacks might be applicable to the black population—or it might not. And compounds found safe for adults might pose risks for children.

- How long did the study last? Health effects can take many years to appear—20 years or more, in the case of cancer.
- Were the subjects already at risk for the disease under study? Finnish researchers found in 1994 that, contrary to expectations, giving subjects supplements of the nutrient beta carotene seemed to increase their risk of developing lung cancer. But the subjects were all long-term smokers who already were at high risk for lung cancer. Experts agreed that taking the supplements for a few years was unlikely to reverse the damage caused by smoking.
- In studies using controls, might some hidden factor distinguish the test group from the controls? One team of researchers discovered they had inadvertently skewed their control group by calling proposed subjects during the daytime, when poorer individuals—who might not have answering machines—were less likely to be home. As a result, when higher cancer rates appeared among the test subjects than among the controls, nobody could be sure some poverty-related factor was not responsible.
- Were the goals of the research decided on before the data were collected? In most kinds of research, investigators must say what they are looking for at the outset of the study. In any large set of data, odd-looking clusters—say, three brain tumor patients living within a few blocks—are almost bound to appear, tempting investigators to draw false inferences.
- Was the research published in a peer-reviewed scientific or medi-

cal journal? Journals rely on peer review, in which panels of experts read and comment on articles submitted for publication, to help weed out weak or poorly designed research. Peer review by itself does not insure that a study's conclusions are valid, however.

Even when a study is well done, its conclusions may not matter much to the average person. Often, the data that scientists produce about health risks is of little import compared with the many other risks that most people live with each day. For instance, knowing that a given activity "doubles" or "triples" your risk is meaningless unless you know the level of risk you started out with—which scientists call the baseline risk. Imagine two headlines, "Peanut consumption doubles the risk of XYZotis" and "Hamburgers raise ABCitis risk by 20 percent." Your first reaction might be to give up peanuts immediately, while you might be less concerned about hamburgers. But when you read the articles, you discover that XYZotis is a relatively rare disease affecting 1 in 10,000 people, whereas ABCitis strikes 100 people in 10,000. Thus, your risk of getting sick when you eat peanuts is only 2 in 10,000—60 times less than the 120-in-10,000 risk you incur when you eat hamburgers.

Another issue that can lead to misunderstanding is the notion of statistical significance. When most people say that something is significant, they generally mean important or noteworthy. But in science, the word refers only to a researcher's level of confidence that a result is real and not a chance occurrence. In most cases, the confidence level required for a result to be statistically significant is 95 percent, meaning there is only a 5 percent chance that what appears to be an association is in fact a fluke. This holds true whether the level of risk itself is large or minuscule.

In general, it helps to keep in mind that medical studies are best at revealing very strong associations, such as that between cigarette smoking and lung cancer. Smoking has been shown to increase a person's lung cancer risk by as much as 30 times, or 3,000 percent. But most purported risk factors raise an individual's risk by perhaps 2 or 3 times, and often by much less. Studies that make such claims should be treated with extreme caution, experts say, unless laboratory research can show a plausible biological mechanism by which a risk factor might cause disease. And even in that case, remember that the results may not be anything to be concerned about.

Scientific research, in short, is not a cut-and-dried process. Press releases and news reports may treat it as such by failing to give the public the information required to interpret a study's findings, or by failing to put the study in the context of past and current research. The solution is to treat every health report cautiously, and to try and minimize large and known risks while keeping small and uncertain ones in perspective. In other words: Wear your seatbelt, don't smoke, eat a healthy diet, and don't worry too much about the daily barrage of health news. •••

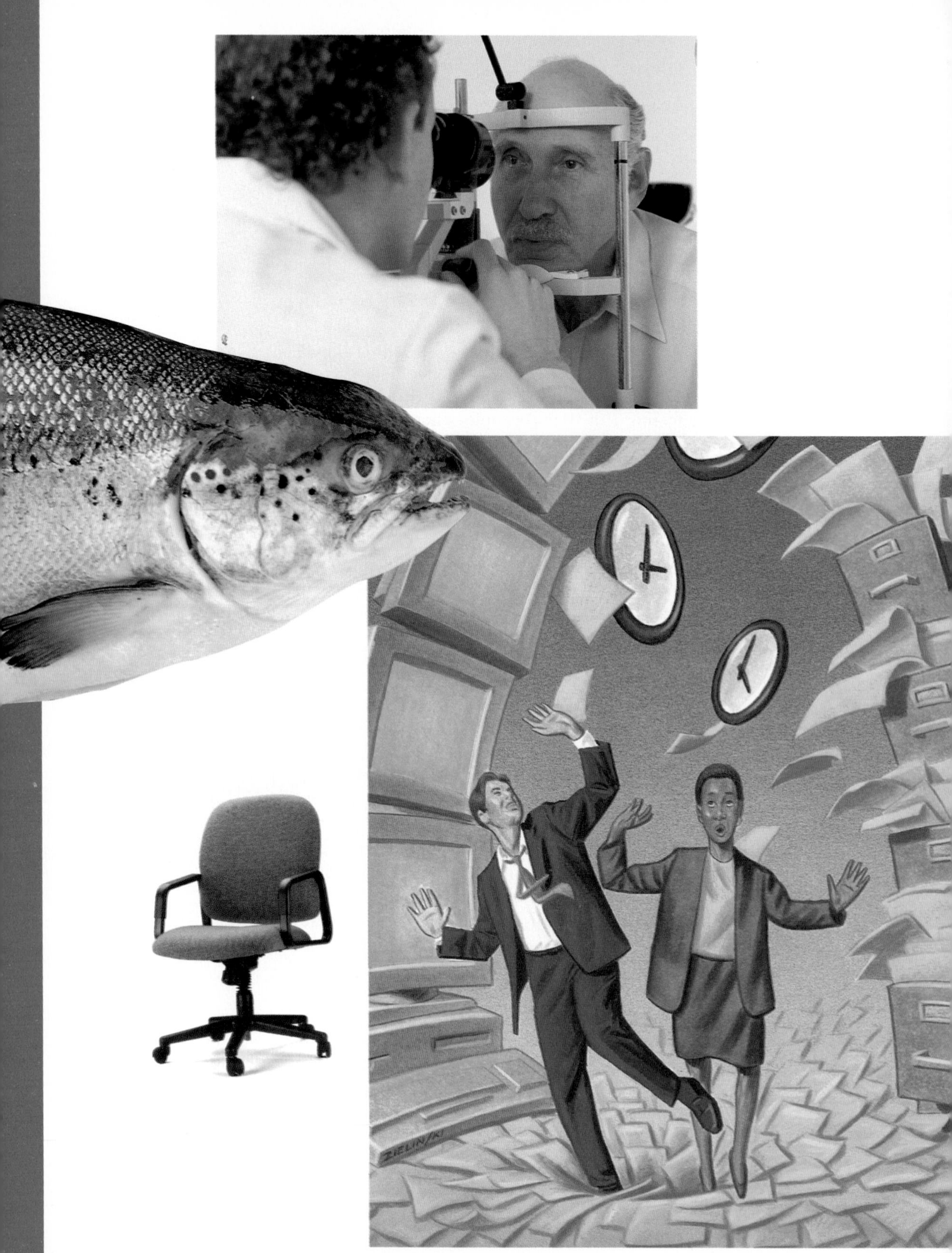

Medical and Safety Alerts

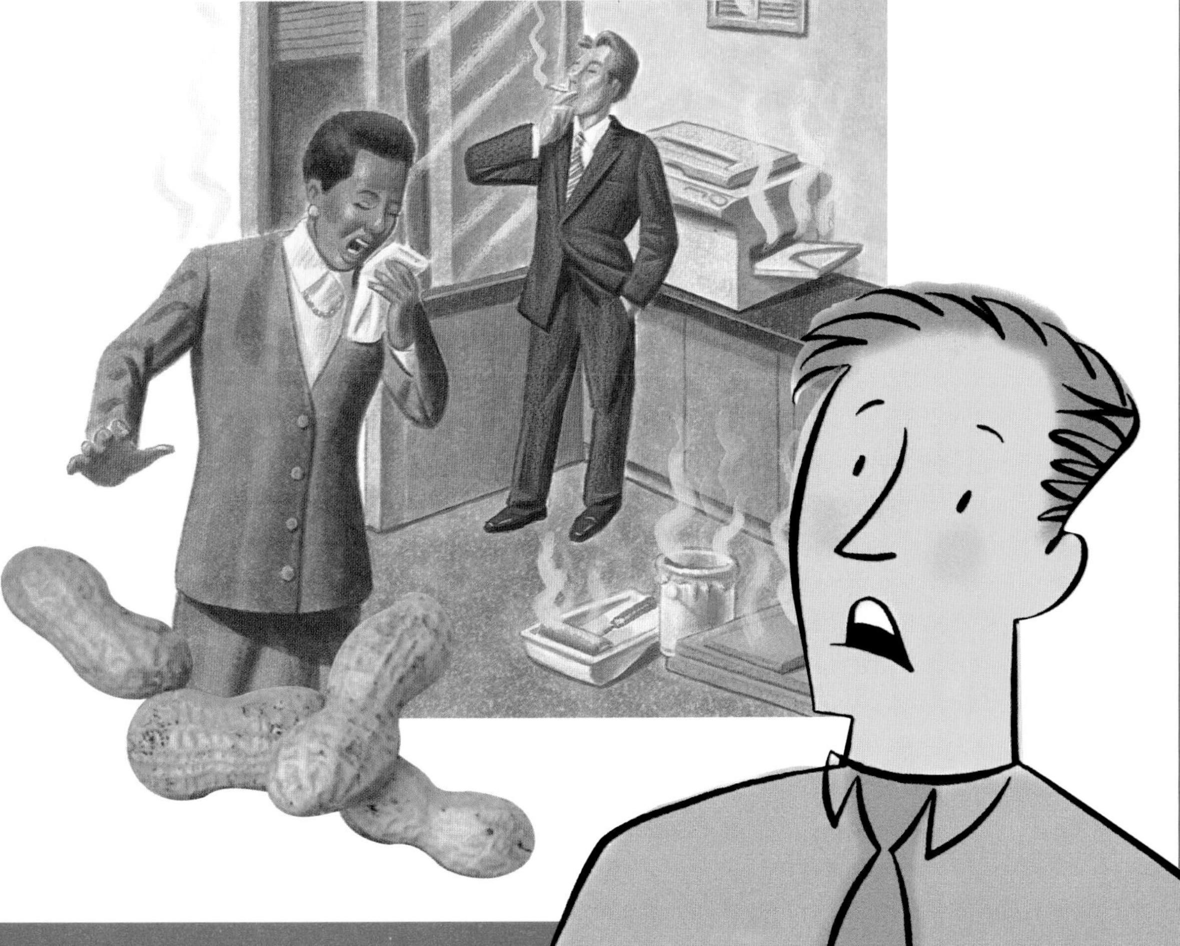

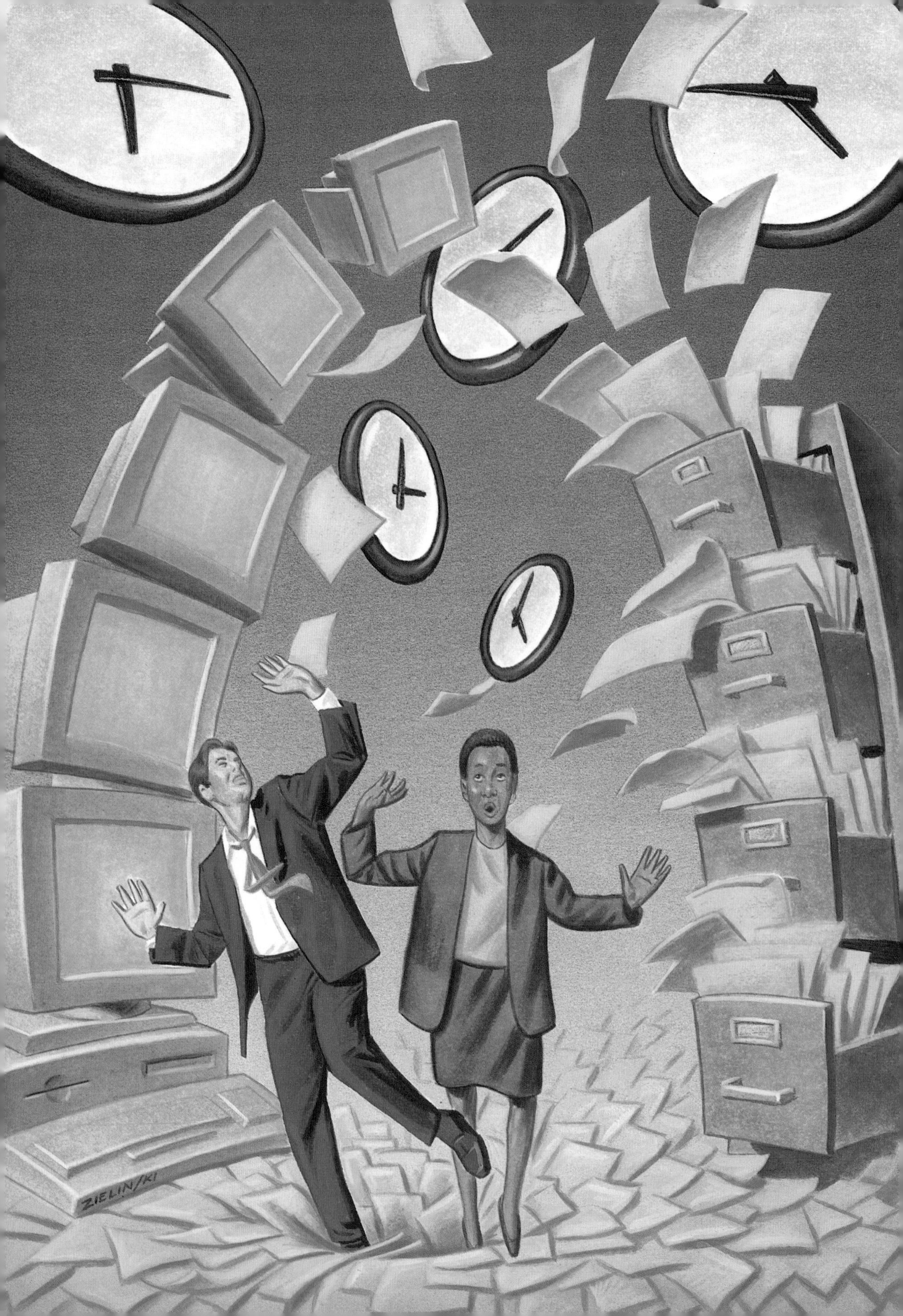
ZIELINSKI

Is the modern, computerized office as hazardous to health as yesterday's workplaces were to an earlier generation?

Health Hazards at the Office

By Jennifer M. Reese

EARNING ONE'S DAILY BREAD has involved hazards to health since hunters first chased animal herds across savannas. For millennia, farmers have lived with the physical effects of too much exposure to the sun in summer and too little of its warmth in winter. Miners have suffered serious lung disorders from breathing air fouled with the dusts of minerals. And hatters, since the early 1800's, have been the proverbial standard against which "madness" is judged—all because of occupational exposure to the poisonous fumes of mercury.

Today, more than half of all workers in industrialized nations toil in offices. According to the United States Bureau of Labor Statistics, white-collar workers—most of whom work in offices—make up 58 percent of the total labor force, up from 38 percent in the mid-1950's. While we tend to think of working in a modern office as relatively harmless, much of today's office work is ill-suited to the human body.

In offices across the country, workers sit for hours staring at a computer screen requiring their fingers to repeat the same motions countless times. Hours of sedentary concentration can lead to health problems. And then, there is the air itself.

The U.S. government estimates that one-third of all office workers in this country are exposed to indoor air that is appreciably more polluted than the air outdoors in the country's largest cities. So toxic have some buildings become that the Occupational Safety and Health Administration (OSHA) not only officially recognizes that buildings can be "sick"—and capable of making their inhabitants so—but also admits that the agency's own Washington headquarters once suffered from what has since been dubbed "sick building syndrome." OSHA is a U.S. Department of Labor agency that promotes safe and healthful working conditions.

Hazards of working at a computer

At the core of the contemporary business office—and of the way people feel at the end of the working day—is the computer terminal, which makes it possible to do one's job without ever getting up from a chair. Surprisingly, sitting exerts more pressure on the spine than standing does. To relieve this pressure, people typically slump forward in their chair, which simply transfers the stress to ligaments and joints. More than 75 percent of people who work at a computer terminal experience back pain, according to the National Institute of Occupational Safety and Health (NIOSH), an agency of the U.S. Department of Health and Human Services. NIOSH investigates working conditions to determine the causes of employee illness and accidents.

Prolonged sitting can also lead to circulation problems as pressure exerted on the buttocks by the chair seat cuts off the circulation of blood to the legs. This can cause legs and ankles to swell. The problem can be especially severe for those already at risk for swelling, including pregnant women and people who are overweight.

Long hours spent staring at a computer screen, especially if there is glare or poor contrast, can lead to dry, weary eyes. People engaged in other tasks normally shift their gaze, focusing on objects at various distances. However, someone working at a terminal may focus for long periods of time on a screen at a fixed distance. The eyes can tire from this fixed focal distance, a problem that age accentuates. Prolonged concentration can also slow the rate of blinking, producing dry eyes. According to another NIOSH study, 75 percent of all people who work at computer terminals experience occasional eye problems.

Bifocals can constitute an additional problem for those who work at computers. People who wear bifocals may lift their chin to view the computer screen through the lower part of their glasses. And they typically lean forward if the screen is too far away for the bifo-

The author:

Jennifer Reese is a freelance writer.

Unhealthy Office Equipment

More than half of American workers sit at a desk in an office. An office may seem to be an area with few health hazards, but poorly designed office furniture and other equipment can present health risks over the long term.

Eye strain

Eye strain can result if you focus your eyes at the same distance for long periods, as when staring at a computer screen. In addition, gazing at a computer terminal for long periods without blinking can dry your eyes, producing irritation. Bright light that reflects off light-colored surfaces can also cause eye strain or fatigue, as can light reflecting off a computer screen.

Neck strain

Neck muscles can become sore from holding your head still for extended periods, especially if your head is tilted up for viewing a terminal, which tightens your neck muscles. Neck and shoulder strain can also result when you balance a telephone receiver between your ear and shoulder.

Back strain

Sitting for long periods puts great pressure on the muscles that hold your back rigid. If your desk chair offers little support, back pain can result.

Repetitive-stress injuries

Any movement repeated often enough, such as typing, can result in injury to your muscles and other body tissues. Working at a computer keyboard can place you at risk for a repetitive-stress injury called carpal tunnel syndrome, in which tendons that pass through a channel in the wrist become swollen and press on a nerve.

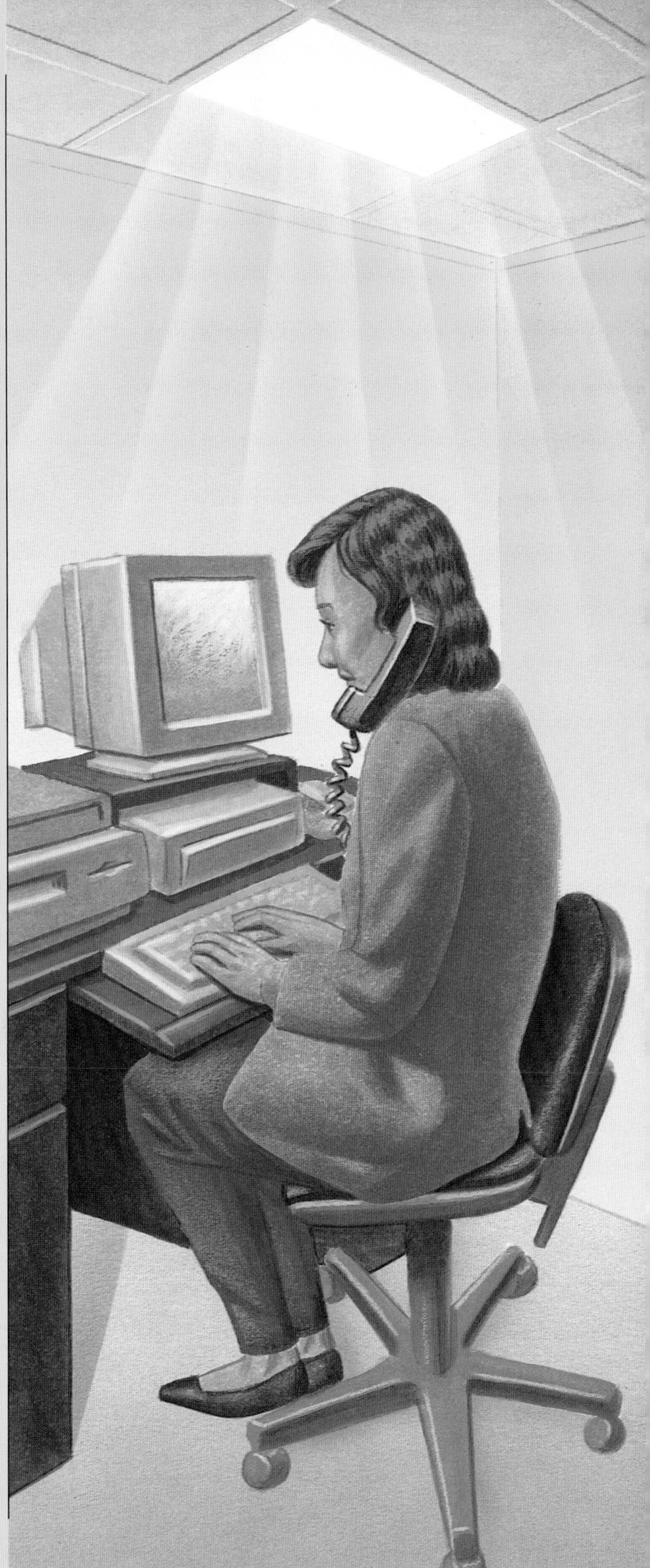

cals to work properly. Holding the head in this awkward posture often results in a stiff neck and sore back. The problem is compounded by progressive bifocals, which may have too narrow a field of vision for the wearer to scan the entire width of the screen. To compensate, people move their head from side to side but try not to move it up and down, so as to keep the screen in focus. This practice adds to neck and back pain.

These computer-related problems are relatively easy and inexpensive to prevent or correct. As a first step, employees should take frequent breaks. NIOSH recommends that people working at a computer break at least once every two hours, getting up from their work- stations and walking about. Walking loosens tight muscles and improves circulation. Tired eyes also get a break and a chance to focus on distant objects.

It's also a good idea to alternate computer work with tasks that require more movement—delivering a memo by hand, for example, or taking papers to the copying machine. Experts also suggest that people make a conscious effort to relax their shoulders and back while working at a computer. Setting the alarm on the computer clock can provide a reminder to take an hourly break.

A well-designed workstation

As a second step toward correcting computer-related problems, many employers have examined the immediate work environment for ways to make improvements. They have been helped in this task by experts in the relatively new field of *ergonomics*, which seeks to adapt the working environment to the human body, instead of the other way around. There are three key components to an ergonomically sound computer workstation: the chair, the keyboard, and the terminal or screen.

The key to an ergonomically designed office chair is solidity and adjustability. The height of the seat should permit the feet to rest flat on the floor and the thighs to form a 90-degree angle with the lower legs. The seat should be padded with a rounded edge; a sharp edge can cut off circulation. The chair should have a contoured back that extends almost to the shoulder blades and tilts backward slightly. Armrests can take some of the pressure off the lower back, but they should not prevent the chair from being pulled in close to the desk or work surface. Nor should they be so high that the shoulders are hunched.

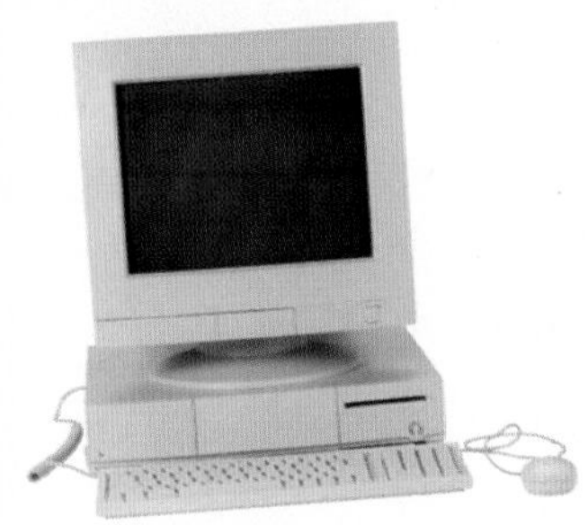

In your own office, after evaluating your chair, take a look at the computer keyboard. An ergonomically correct computer keyboard is detachable, so that it can be placed in a comfortable position—ideally, directly in front of you and stationed at elbow height or lower. This position allows you to keep your shoulders relaxed rather than elevated. The mouse or track ball should be kept in easy reach beside the keyboard. Finally, if the keys are sticky and have to be pounded to function, the keyboard should be replaced immediately.

Healthy solutions

Many of the potential health risks from working at a desk can be prevented or alleviated by ensuring that your workstation meets certain standards developed by experts in *ergonomics* (the relationship between people and their work environment).

To prevent eye strain

Keep your computer screen free of dust for clear viewing, and adjust the monitor so that there is no glare from artificial overhead light or sunlight. If the screen is still too bright, a tinted screen placed over it can reduce glare. Be sure that prescription eyeglasses are appropriate for reading from a computer screen, which is usually farther from the eyes than a book would be.

To prevent neck and shoulder strain

The top of the computer screen should be at or slightly below eye level. Receptionists, news reporters, and others who spend a lot of time on the telephone should use a headset to avoid cradling the telephone receiver.

To prevent back pain

Sit with your back straight and do not slouch. Adjust the height of your chair seat so that your feet rest flat on the floor or on a footrest. To prevent strain on lower back muscles, keep your knees level with your hips. The back of the chair should be firm but slightly flexible.

To prevent repetitive-stress injuries

Keep your wrists straight when typing. Limit the motion of your wrists as much as possible and do not rest them on the desktop. An adjustable keyboard tray can help set the keyboard at the right height.

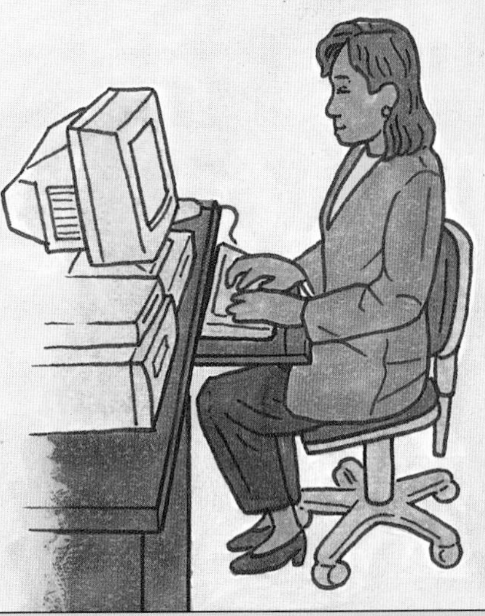

Preventing carpal tunnel syndrome

Carpal tunnel syndrome, characterized by numbness and tingling in the hand and forearm has become a common repetitive-stress injury as more people spend long hours at computer keyboards. The disorder is caused by pressure from a swollen tendon on a major nerve in an area of the wrist known as the carpal tunnel. Repeated wrist motions cause the tendon to swell. Taking frequent breaks and doing stretching exercises can reduce the risk of developing carpal tunnel syndrome.

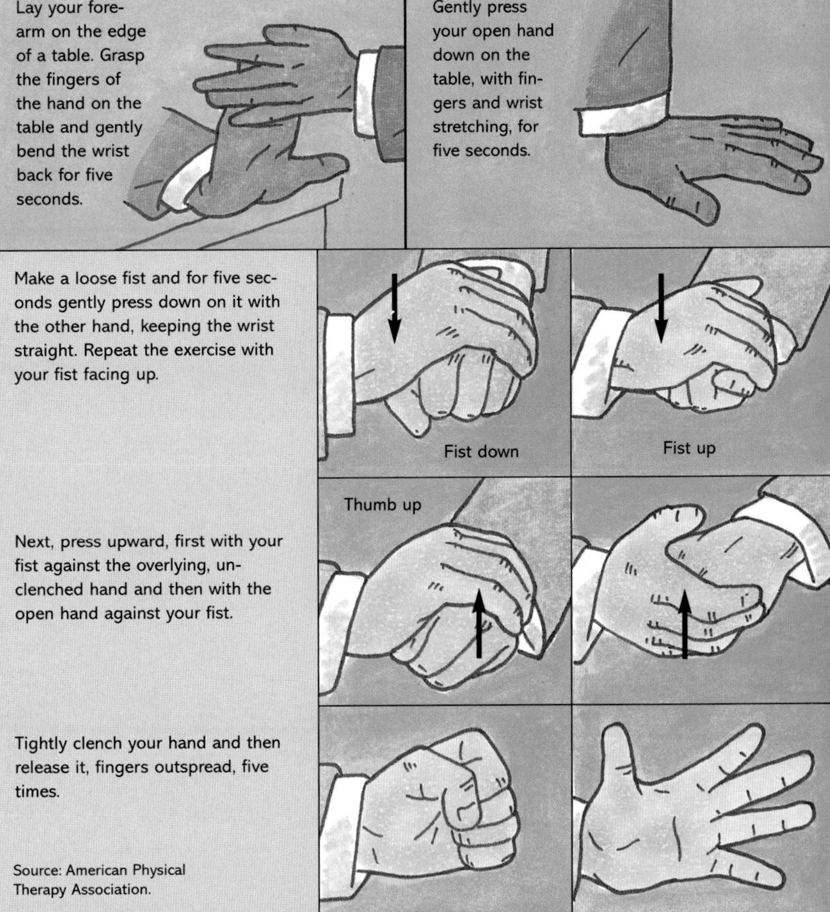

Preventing muscle strain

Sitting still for long periods strains many muscles in the upper body. Taking several breaks a day and doing exercises to loosen and stretch those muscles makes you feel better and helps prevent injuries.

- Sit straight in your chair, and tuck your chin down.
- Gently roll your head to the left, bring it back to the center, then roll it to the right.
- Repeat this sequence three times.

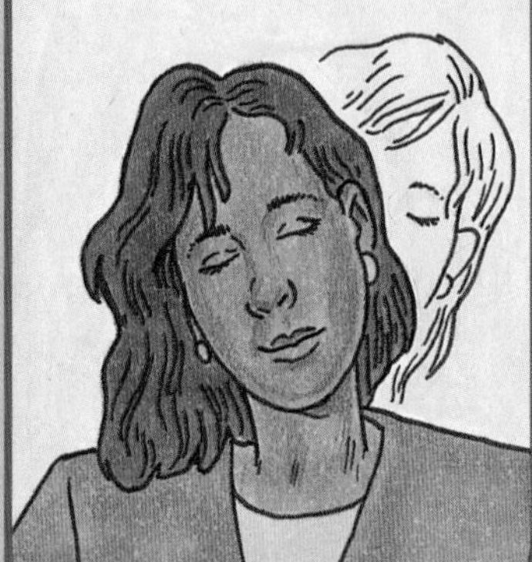

- Raise your hands and forearms at your side.
- Push your forearms back so that your shoulder blades squeeze together. Hold for several seconds.
- Relax the muscles and repeat three times.

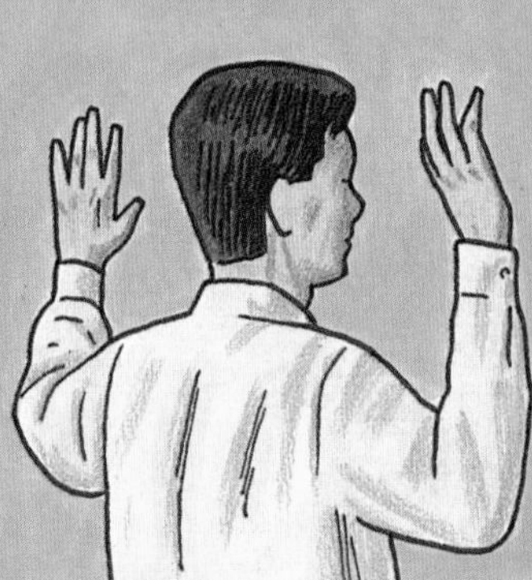

- Standing or sitting, drop your arms to your sides.
- Shake your arms and hands out gently for several seconds.
- Relax and repeat three times.

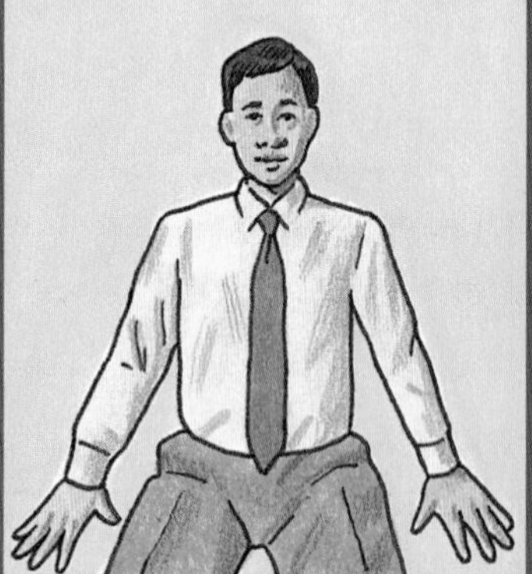

- Extend your arms out in front of you.
- Rotate your arms to make the backs of your hands touch each other.
- Hold for several seconds.

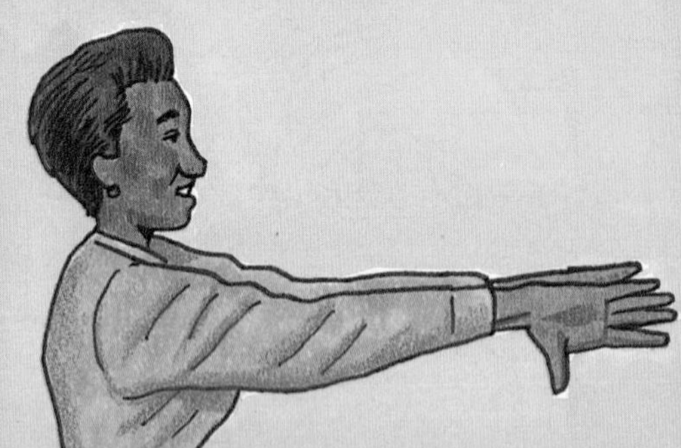

- With your arms still extended, rotate them so that the palms of your hands face up.
- Hold for several seconds.
- Relax and repeat both arm rotations three times.

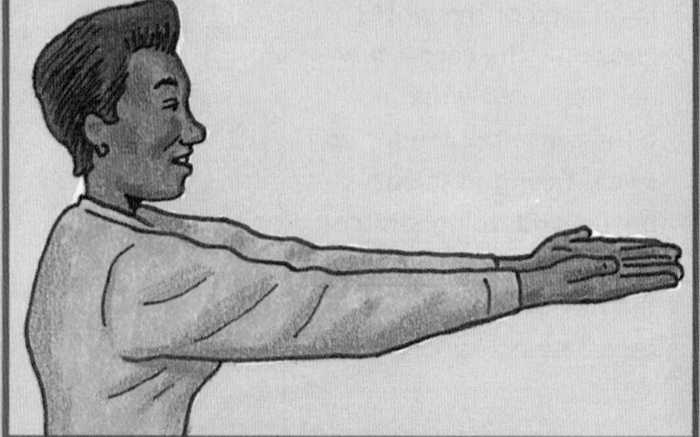

Typing should require no more than a light touch, and the mouse should move with a gentle push.

A few simple adjustments on or around the computer terminal can often prevent or remedy eye strain and back and neck problems. First, ergonomics experts say, adjust the light. Sources of light, whether natural or artificial, should be above or beside the screen, and artificial light should strike the screen at an angle to prevent glare and distracting reflections on the screen. If possible, have the screen fitted with an antiglare filter, preferably of glass. A flat screen is generally more desirable than a curved screen, as it creates less glare. Mounting the terminal on a stand that tilts and swivels allows you to make periodic adjustments to the position of the screen throughout the day as natural light shifts.

The computer terminal is too high if you have to look up at it. Place the terminal so that the top of the screen is at eye level and the line of sight for the rest of the screen is 10 to 20 degrees below eye level. Keep the screen at a distance of 18 to 24 inches (46 to 61 centimeters) from your eyes. The closer one gets to the screen, the more difficult focusing becomes. If the type on the screen is hard to read, enlarge it or change fonts. Finally, dust can blur the screen. Computer screens, like television screens, attract dust and require regular wiping with a damp cloth.

A tool that makes working at a computer easier is a document holder, a vertical stand against which papers can be propped or clipped in place. The holder should be placed at the same height as the screen and at the same distance from the viewer.

If vision problems persist after making these adjustments, schedule an appointment with an eye specialist. Vision problems unrelated to the computer may have developed. But there may be a simple solution. For example, a person who wears bifocals can be fitted with lenses designed for computer work.

Computers and repetitive-stress injuries

Repetitive-stress injuries (RSI's) constitute the most serious health hazard associated with computer work. RSI is a catchall designation for injuries to muscles, tendons, and other tissues caused by the wear and tear of a repeated motion. Doing any one task over and over, whether typing at a keyboard, tightening bolts on an assembly line, or slicing meat, can lead to an RSI. According to OSHA, repetitive stress injuries accounted for nearly 67 percent of all occupational illnesses in 1994. OSHA also said that the incidence of RSI's is growing at an alarming annual rate of 5 to 10 percent.

The RSI that most often troubles people working at a computer is carpal tunnel syndrome. The syndrome affects the median nerve, one of three nerves that control movement and sensation in the hand and fingers. It develops when this nerve is compressed as it passes through the carpal tunnel, a narrow passage formed by the bones of the wrist and the ligaments connecting them.

Airborne microbes

Microbes, including bacteria, molds, and fungi, can breed in a ventilation system and circulate through a building. Microbes can cause allergic reactions, respiratory infections, and other ailments.

Dry air

Indoor air, especially during winter months, can be very dry. The low humidity can irritate your eyes and mucous membranes, making them vulnerable to infections.

Dust

Rugs and carpeting absorb dust and provide an ideal environment for dust mites, microorganisms that can trigger asthma.

Tobacco smoke

While most institutions and companies no longer allow smoking, tobacco smoke remains a problem in some worksplaces. Nonsmokers can develop respiratory problems from breathing secondhand smoke.

Unhealthy office air

Modern office buildings are nearly airtight and depend upon mechanical systems to circulate air. Fresh outdoor air is limited in these buildings, and indoor contaminants can become trapped within the circulation system. Scientists have identified more than 1,500 microbes and chemicals that can pollute indoor air, and occupational-health experts estimate that the air in as many as 30 to 40 percent of all modern offices is substandard.

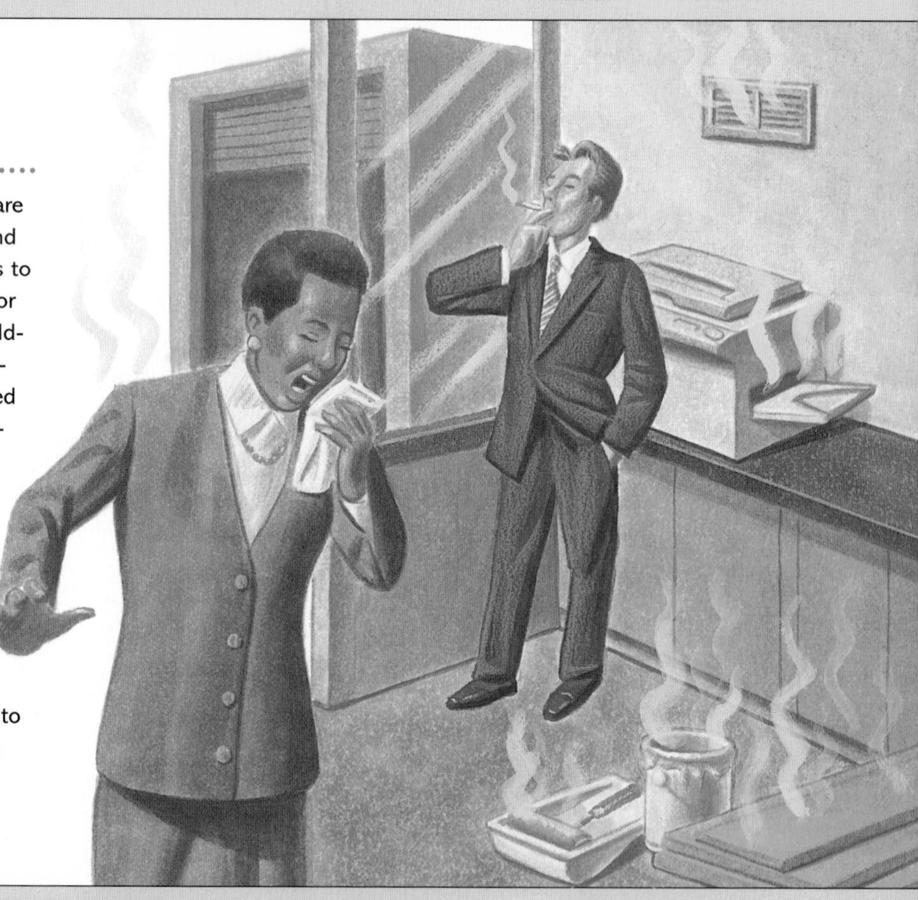

Inadequate ventilation

Many ventilation systems are turned off after hours and on weekends, so people working overtime lack fresh air. In addition, if remodeling is underway in a building, paint fumes and dust from drilling may circulate through offices.

Poor ventilation systems

Ducts that carry air through a building may be coated with fiberglass, which provides ideal conditions for the growth of molds and mildew. Also, air-intake vents are sometimes located near busy streets or loading docks, where exhaust fumes from automobiles and trucks may enter the system.

Airborne chemicals

Office workers may breathe fumes emitted by new floor coverings, contact cement, and cleaning agents. Formaldehyde is released by glues and particle-board furniture, and acetone is given off by paints and caulking. In addition, perfumes, pesticides, and everyday dust fill the air. FAX machines, printers, and photocopiers also emit gases.

Poorly maintained air conditioning

Inadequately maintained air conditioning systems can become damp, allowing disease-causing molds and mildew to flourish. Certain respiratory ailments can be transmitted through poorly maintained air conditioning systems.

Difficulty arises when tendons that surround the median nerve swell due to repeated flexing and extending of the wrist. Swollen tendons can be painful in themselves, but the problem worsens when the tendons press against the median nerve. At first, the pressure usually produces numbness and a tingling or "pins-and-needles" sensation in the arm and hand. The tingling sensation is typically replaced by burning and pain, often localized in the thumb and first two fingers as well as in the palm and wrist. Because symptoms often occur at night, when the wrists naturally bend during sleep, many people do not connect the discomfort to occupational tasks.

Carpal tunnel syndrome can be intensified by other conditions that place pressure on the median nerve. Either broken or dislocated bones, for example, can crowd the tunnel. Women seem more likely to develop the syndrome, possibly because they have narrower wrists—and hence less room in the carpal tunnel—than men. Fluid retention caused by pregnancy can produce pressure on the median nerve. Disorders such as diabetes and thyroid problems can also render people more vulnerable to carpal tunnel syndrome.

Manual dexterity can decrease if carpal tunnel syndrome goes untreated. Performing such everyday tasks as buttoning clothes or tying shoelaces often becomes difficult. Eventually, the muscle at the base of the thumb can weaken to the extent that the ability to clench the hand is lost. The more advanced the carpal tunnel syndrome, the more difficult it is to treat.

Treating carpal tunnel syndrome

Treatment of carpal tunnel syndrome usually begins with a lightweight splint to keep the wrist in a neutral position and reduce pressure within the carpal tunnel. The physician may recommend wearing the splint only at night or, rarely, during the workday as well. Anti-inflammatory drugs, such as aspirin and ibuprofen, can reduce swelling and relieve pain. If these measures fail to help, the physician may inject drugs called corticosteroids directly into the swollen tissue to lessen swelling.

Surgery is recommended only when conservative treatments do not improve the condition, pain is severe, nerve damage is occurring, or diagnostic tests show serious abnormalities in the tunnel. In the procedure, called carpal tunnel release, the surgeon cuts the ligament that encircles the passageway to make more room and relieve pressure on the nerve. The surgery is generally performed on an outpatient basis, and the patient wears a splint for a number of weeks after surgery, before gradually increasing activity.

If you spend long hours at a computer, you can best avoid carpal tunnel syndrome by taking regular breaks and making certain that the keyboard is positioned directly in front of you and at the correct height. While typing, be sure to keep your arms and wrists straight, with your elbows tucked in and your wrists above the keyboard.

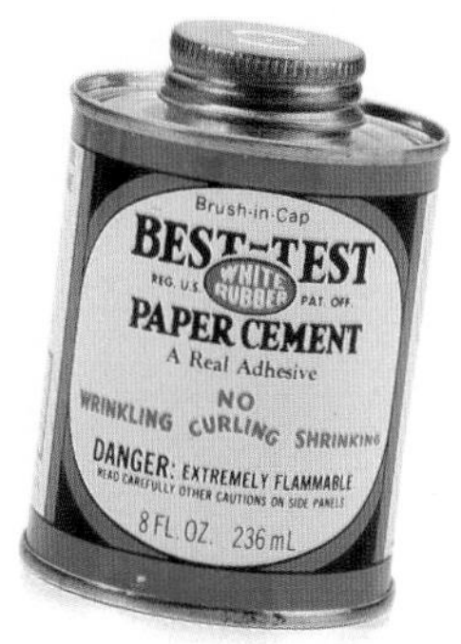

It is essential that your wrists do not bend upward during typing.

In the early 1980's, safety questions about computer screens arose after several clusters of miscarriages were reported among women who worked at computer terminals. In 1988, a study of 1,600 women in California indicated that women who worked in front of computer terminals for 20 or more hours a week had an increased incidence of spontaneous abortion. A health maintenance organization, the Northern California Kaiser-Permanente Medical Care Program, conducted the study. But a 1994 study by Great Britain's National Radiological Protection Board demonstrated "no significant association" between the use of computer screens and spontaneous abortions. Other studies were in progress in 1996.

Work-related stress

Americans consistently rank work as the number-one source of stress in their lives. A moderate amount of work-related stress can be beneficial and even lead to higher productivity. But too much stress can trigger health problems, including depression and sleep disorders, as well as such stress-related behaviors as overeating and drinking to excess.

Work-related stress seems to be particularly acute among office employees. Well over half of workers' compensation claims filed in California, for example, are for stress-related complaints. In part, the present high level of stress is due to the introduction of com-puters and other new technology. While computers can be liberating, providing users with access to nearly limitless sources of information and making many jobs much easier, they can also be con- fining. Typists and secretaries once had a certain amount of discretion over how they did their jobs, but today's human data proces-sors are subjected to electronic monitoring and increased pressure to perform, which can leave them feeling they have little control over their work.

Frank Landy, a psychologist and management consultant, attributes most job-related stress to three factors: unpredictability, lack of control over working conditions, and conflict. Layoffs and downsizing have created an environment of chronic unpredictability. New technologies have led to a generation of workers who feel they have little or no control over their jobs. And the influx of women into the workplace has blurred traditional male/female roles and created a population of employees torn between job responsibilities and family obligations.

Experts in occupational health say that on-the-job stress is a fact of modern life. But it has not gone unnoticed. Many companies, large and small, now offer stress-reduction programs. Noting that exercise is an effective stress antidote, some large companies have outfitted on-site fitness centers with exercise equipment and part-time trainers. However, offering strategies for managing the symptoms of job strain is only half the battle.

According to Landy, a company that is serious about reducing job strain—rather than just managing its symptoms—needs to be honest, forthright, and flexible with employees. Landy notes the need for more flexible working hours, for wider opportunities for working at home, and for office day-care centers so working parents are less torn between commitments. He also emphasizes the importance of providing employees with information about future company plans, including layoffs. Landy points out that anxiety decreases as information increases.

Until companies start making such changes, stress experts say, employees need to take action themselves. People basically cope with job-related stress in two ways, according to Arthur Brief, a psychologist at Tulane University in New Orleans. A person can deal with the actual problem or with the emotions evoked by that problem. Brief says that people who feel their jobs are being threatened often attempt not to think about the problem or try to distract themselves through shopping, alcohol, or other measures. But suppressing feelings of anxiety is usually far less effective than confronting those feelings. According to Brief, someone who is worried about losing a job can best confront that worry by immediately starting to look for a new job.

Brief applies this formula to other tense work situations. If there is conflict with a boss, he advises, search for a solution rather than avoiding the boss, and then calmly talk it out. Rather than resenting a rigid schedule that makes it impossible to take a child to the doctor, ask for flex-time. If a supervisor has not addressed rumors about a company restructuring, ask if the rumors are true. If a two-hour commute is exhausting or a crowded workspace triggers headaches, request permission to work at home one or two days a week. You may not get everything you ask for, but solving a work problem, however small, can make a significant difference to your psychological well-being.

Finally, Frank Landy emphasizes communication—that is, plain old talk with fellow workers—to reduce stress. The more isolated people feel, the more anxious and depressed they become.

Air quality in the modern office

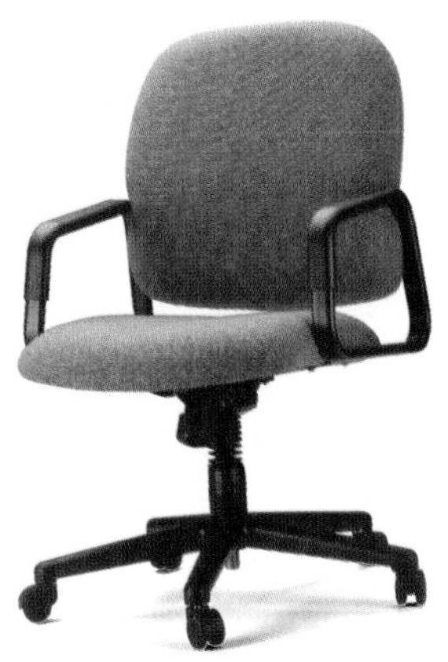

Office workers also are subject to a relatively new and increasingly disturbing source of stress in the workplace—poor air quality. The resulting problems range from the mildly irritating effects of low humidity to the debilitating symptoms produced by sick building syndrome.

One reason for the dry air in offices is the computer. Office computers produce heat, and the warmed air draws moisture from whatever sources are available—including the eyes, nose, throat, and skin of people working in offices. Most offices need to increase humidity to compensate for the drying effects of computers. This can easily be accomplished with humidifiers, though environmental scientists

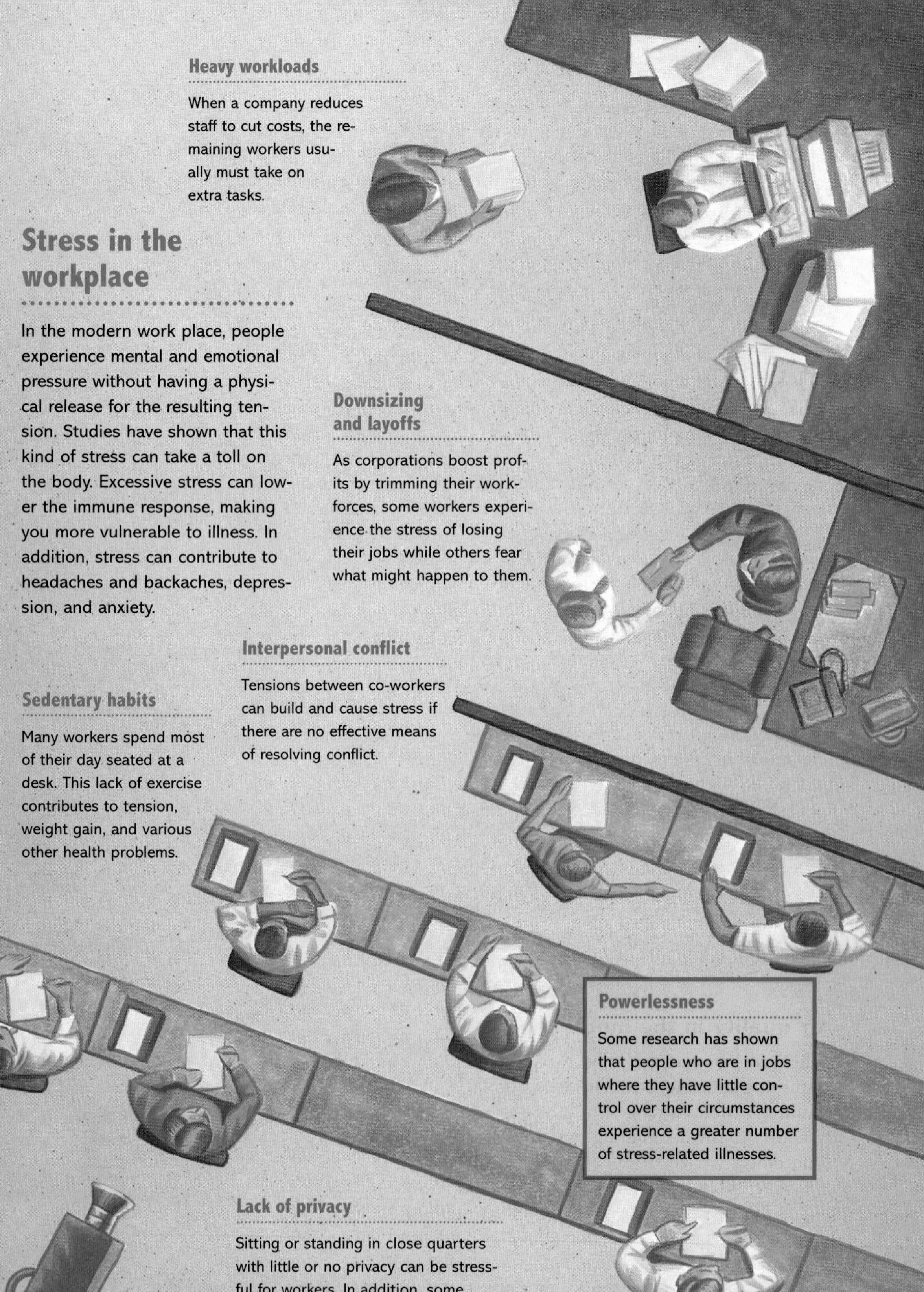

Stress in the workplace

In the modern work place, people experience mental and emotional pressure without having a physical release for the resulting tension. Studies have shown that this kind of stress can take a toll on the body. Excessive stress can lower the immune response, making you more vulnerable to illness. In addition, stress can contribute to headaches and backaches, depression, and anxiety.

Heavy workloads

When a company reduces staff to cut costs, the remaining workers usually must take on extra tasks.

Downsizing and layoffs

As corporations boost profits by trimming their workforces, some workers experience the stress of losing their jobs while others fear what might happen to them.

Interpersonal conflict

Tensions between co-workers can build and cause stress if there are no effective means of resolving conflict.

Sedentary habits

Many workers spend most of their day seated at a desk. This lack of exercise contributes to tension, weight gain, and various other health problems.

Powerlessness

Some research has shown that people who are in jobs where they have little control over their circumstances experience a greater number of stress-related illnesses.

Lack of privacy

Sitting or standing in close quarters with little or no privacy can be stressful for workers. In addition, some companies exercise their right to listen in on workers' phone calls or place surveillance cameras overhead.

warn that humidifiers pose their own dangers. They act as factories for mold and require regular cleaning.

But the major cause of poor air quality in an office is the nearly airtight modern office building. Many of these buildings went up in the 1970's and were designed to conserve energy by shutting out the elements. Windows were sealed, entrances were equipped with revolving doors that minimized natural ventilation, and air was recirculated through the building by mechanical systems.

In response to the energy crisis of the 1970's, the recommended standard for fresh air in office buildings was lowered by the American Society of Heating, Refrigerating, and Air-conditioning Engineers (ASHRAE), a professional organization based in Atlanta, Georgia. Building owners happily complied, and the reduction saved energy, which was patriotic and economical. In this energy-efficient environment, however, not only is the supply of fresh, outdoor air limited but contaminants become trapped indoors.

Approximately one-third of the 70 million Americans who work indoors breathe air that may be twice as polluted as the air outdoors, according to a 1995 U.S. government estimate. Although ASHRAE upgraded its fresh-air standard in 1989, the amount of fresh air circulated through many airtight buildings remains well below the new standard. A recent ASHRAE analysis of major European and U.S. studies of indoor air quality confirmed that buildings that effectively meet the new standard are much less likely to cause health problems.

Pollutants in modern offices

Scientists have identified more than 1,500 chemical and bacterial air pollutants in modern, sealed office buildings. These include chemicals from floor coverings, contact cement, and cleaning agents; formaldehyde from glues and particle-board furniture; acetone from paints and caulking; and perfume, pesticides, and everyday dust. Building systems are simply not designed to vent out fumes from these substances, according to the indoor-air division of the Environmental Protection Agency

On-the-job stress

Americans consistently rank work as life's number-one source of stress, which experts attribute to three factors:

- unpredictability
- lack of control over working conditions
- conflict

Coping with stress

People who handle on-the-job stress well—

- feel a sense of control on the job
- are committed to their work
- are challenged rather than threatened by problems and new developments
- view change as inevitable and normal, rather than a source of stress
- participate in activities outside of the workplace
- exercise regularly

(EPA), a government agency that sets and enforces standards for controlling pollution.

Gases given off by molds and fungi can also contaminate the air, researchers at the Georgia Institute of Technology have found. Molds such as aspergillus and mildew produce gases that "tweak the immune system into severe allergic reactions or a suppressed response to infection," says Charlene Bayer, director of Georgia Tech's Indoor Environment Research Program. Air conditioning systems serve as particularly fertile breeding grounds for molds and fungi. Such microorganisms are too small to be removed from the air by the inexpensive filters used in many air conditioning systems. The common practice of shutting office systems down over weekends produces what Bayer calls a "Monday morning cocktail"—a mixture of air contaminants all too familiar to office workers.

Many larger offices use fiberglass-lined ductwork to control noise. Dirt trapped in the fibers creates a rich breeding ground for microbes. "Add a little moisture and you can have a mold garden in your ductwork," says Bayer. "The microbes can grow and multiply and then get blown all over the building to infest other areas.

Sick building syndrome

In the media, issues of poor indoor air quality have revolved around sick building syndrome, a term coined in the 1970's to describe a variety of nose, throat, and skin complaints from workers in airtight buildings. OSHA lists the symptoms of the syndrome as eye, nose, and throat irritation; dryness of mucous membranes and skin; nosebleeds; skin rash; mental fatigue; headache; cough, hoarseness, and wheezing; nausea; and dizziness. These symptoms typically disappear when people leave the building. In 1986, the World Health Organization estimated that 30 percent of new and remodeled buildings could be "sick." (Sick building syndrome should not be confused with building-related illnesses, in which the outbreak of a specific disease can be traced to a particular building.)

Because office workers spend so much of their time indoors, air quality has become a major cause for concern. In 1980, only 6 percent of all requests for NIOSH investigations involved indoor environmental quality; in 1992, such investigation requests made up 44 percent of the total; in 1995, 75 percent of the total. Although air quality accounted for some 80 to 90 percent of these problems, experts prefer the term indoor environmental quality to indoor air quality. Noise, vibration, and lighting, they point out, can also play a role.

The myriad possible causes for sick building syndrome make finding and solving the problem difficult. In about 25 percent of cases, investigators can identify a single specific cause. But most of the time, problems with indoor air stem from several sources, experts say. Inadequate fresh air might not be a problem, but in combination with high temperatures and low-level chemical contamination, it could lead to symptoms.

Illness triggered by poor indoor air quality is not life-threatening, with the exception of a few very rare conditions. However, the EPA estimates that poor air quality does lead to enormous economic loss, as many as 13.5 million lost workdays annually. According to the EPA, someone who feels chronically ill and suspects that an indoor environment is responsible should first find out if others are experiencing the same symptoms. Recognition of a problem typically entails a complaint filed by more than one individual. If a building seems to be causing widespread discomfort, the issue should be raised with a manager. He or she can have the ventilation checked or bring in an industrial hygienist to study the air quality.

The source of the problem might be something obvious and easily remedied. For example, are surfaces cleaned and carpets vacuumed regularly to remove dust? Dust in offices (and in houses as well) causes more health problems than most people realize. Are shelves where office products are stored closed off to prevent fumes from circulating? Is the temperature kept between 72 and 76 °F (22 to 24 °C)? Finally, an individual who believes that he or she has a serious health problem related to the office environment should visit a primary-care physician, who can suggest a course of action and, if necessary, recommend an occupational specialist or allergist.

The tools of our jobs and how we use them can affect how we feel at the end of the day. Although health hazards at the office are not likely to be lethal, they can be serious—even crippling in the case of repetitive-stress injuries. And office-related health problems are becoming far more numerous as the number of Americans working in offices rises. Awareness of these problems is the first step toward combating them. •••

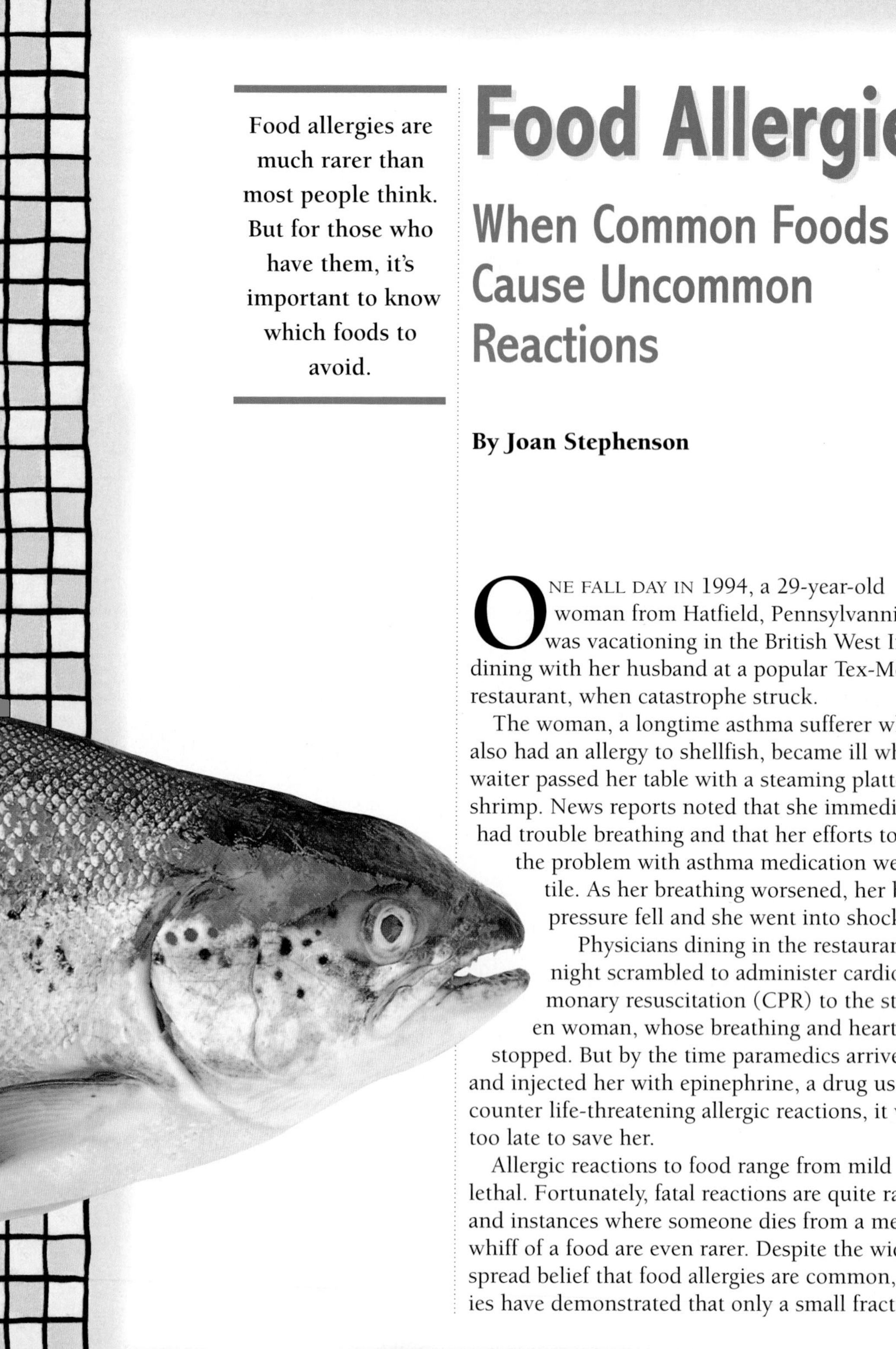

Food allergies are much rarer than most people think. But for those who have them, it's important to know which foods to avoid.

Food Allergies:

When Common Foods Cause Uncommon Reactions

By Joan Stephenson

One fall day in 1994, a 29-year-old woman from Hatfield, Pennsylvannia, was vacationing in the British West Indies, dining with her husband at a popular Tex-Mex restaurant, when catastrophe struck.

The woman, a longtime asthma sufferer who also had an allergy to shellfish, became ill when a waiter passed her table with a steaming platter of shrimp. News reports noted that she immediately had trouble breathing and that her efforts to ease the problem with asthma medication were futile. As her breathing worsened, her blood pressure fell and she went into shock.

Physicians dining in the restaurant that night scrambled to administer cardiopulmonary resuscitation (CPR) to the stricken woman, whose breathing and heart had stopped. But by the time paramedics arrived and injected her with epinephrine, a drug used to counter life-threatening allergic reactions, it was too late to save her.

Allergic reactions to food range from mild to lethal. Fortunately, fatal reactions are quite rare—and instances where someone dies from a mere whiff of a food are even rarer. Despite the widespread belief that food allergies are common, studies have demonstrated that only a small fraction of

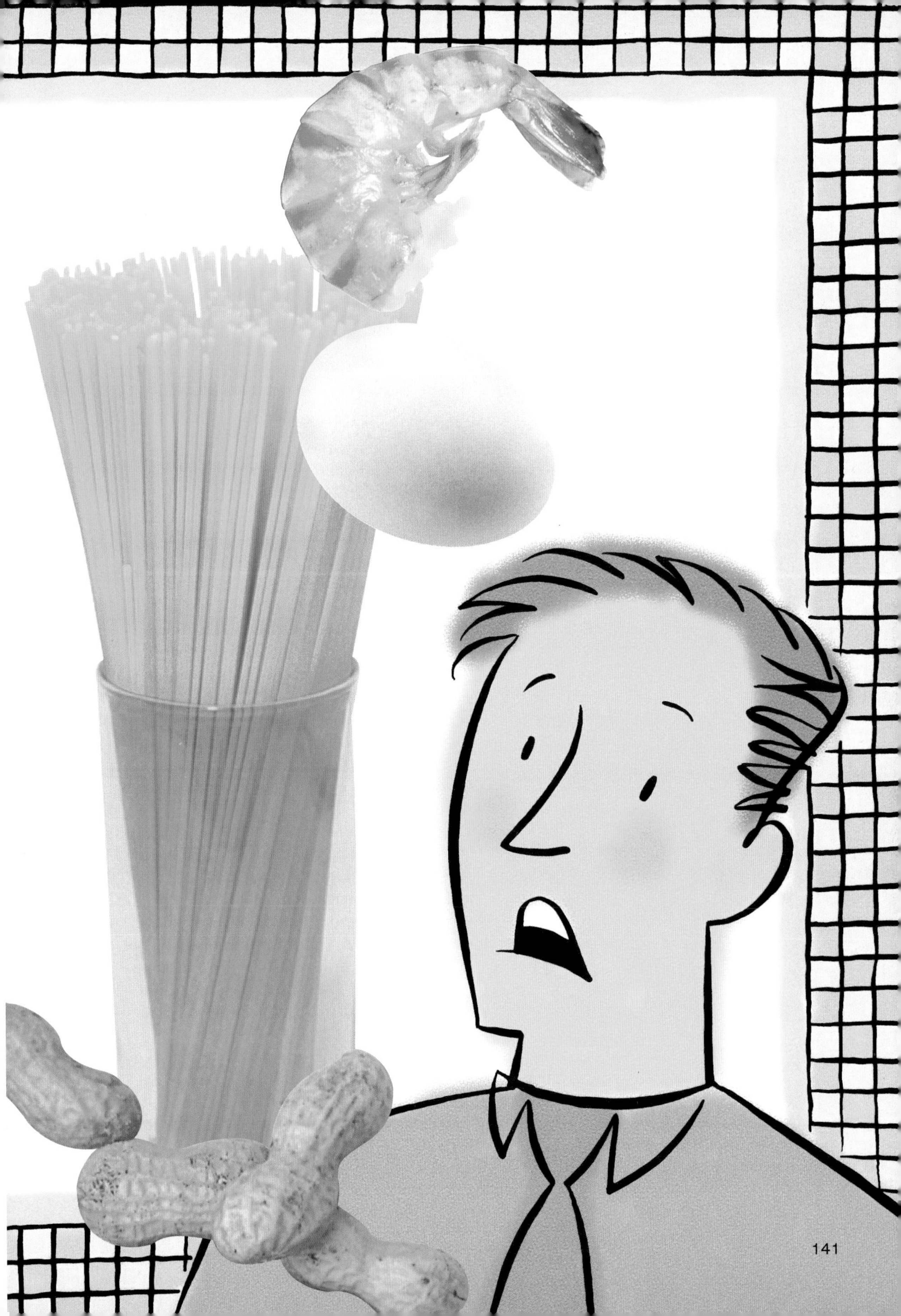

the population actually has a genuine allergic reaction to food.

Surveys have found that as many as one-third of all adults believe they have food allergies, a term that experts reserve for any abnormal reaction by the body's immune system to an otherwise harmless food or component of food. But this perception far exceeds the reality: Allergy researchers estimate that less than 2 percent of Americans—only 1 to 2 percent of adults and perhaps as many as 4 to 5 percent of young children—have a true food allergy.

Is it really a food allergy?

Authorities refer to any abnormal response to a food or a food additive (such as an artificial coloring or preservative) as an *adverse food reaction*. This category includes food allergies as well as food intolerances, which are exaggerated or abnormal reactions to foods in which the immune system is not known to play a role. Perhaps the most common example of a food intolerance is *lactose* (milk sugar) intolerance, which occurs when someone is deficient in *lactase*, an enzyme the body needs to digest the lactose in milk and other dairy products. As a result, the undigested lactose remains in the intestines, causing abdominal cramps, bloating, and diarrhea. Lactose intolerance is not a food allergy because it does not involve the immune system.

Another example of a food intolerance that people sometimes mistake for a food allergy is a reaction to chemicals found naturally in foods. For example, some people get a headache after drinking red wine or eating certain cheeses and other foods that contain a compound called tyramine. Other adverse reactions to food, allergy researchers suggest, may result from still-unidentified biochemical reactions in the body. In other cases, psychological factors play a role in the food intolerance, causing people to react to a particular food because of smell or memories.

Medical experts agree that it's important to clear up the confusion surrounding food allergies and intolerances, because the potential consequences of such confusion can be serious. While a food intolerance can be unpleasant, it's rarely dangerous. Individuals who have genuine allergies to foods, on the other hand, need to know which foods to avoid, how to recognize the symptoms of an allergic attack, and how to take steps to prevent or short-circuit a severe allergic reaction. And even with a nonallergic food reaction such as lactose intolerance, identifying the cause of the problem makes it possible to avoid the offending substance.

Identifying food allergies is also important because they can contribute to other health problems. Allergy-provoking foods can trigger asthma attacks in susceptible children, and failure to avoid such foods can prevent such youngsters from responding well to asthma treatment, according to a 1996 study by researchers at Johns Hopkins School of Medicine in Baltimore. Food allergies also appear to play a role in the recurrent ear infections that many children ex-

The author:

Joan Stephenson is an associate editor of the *Journal of the American Medical Association.*

perience, researchers at Georgetown University in Washington, D.C., reported in a 1994 study, and avoiding the offending foods may help prevent future episodes.

At the same time, it's important to rule out food allergies to avoid eliminating foods from the diet unnecessarily. A severely limited diet can result in poor nutrition, especially in young children. In one 1994 study, researchers found that some parents who mistakenly believed that their children had numerous food allergies drastically restricted the youngsters' diets, resulting in a growth-stunting condition that physicians call "failure to thrive."

Food allergies occur when the body's disease-fighting immune system mounts an attack on certain proteins in food. The substances that trigger this immune-system response are called *antigens* or *allergens*. The body's response to the antigen sets into motion the release of powerful chemicals that are responsible for the allergic symptoms. The chief chemical released in this process is histamine. (In hay fever, pollen grains rather than food allergens stimulate the release of histamine, and the result is sneezing, watery eyes, and other annoying symptoms of this condition.) In people who are extremely sensitive to a food antigen, like the woman who was allergic to shellfish, merely inhaling miniscule amounts of the food or touching the culprit is enough to trigger a reaction.

Symptoms of food allergies

Symptoms may appear within minutes or as long as several hours after eating the allergy-provoking food. They typically begin with itching and swelling of the lips, mouth, and, in some cases, the throat. The reaction may also include a flushed face, hoarseness, and bumps on the lining of the mouth. These symptoms, which doctors call oral allergy syndrome, may be the only reaction some individuals with a food allergy experience.

But for others with food allergies, additional symptoms occur when the offending food enters the stomach and intestines, where it can cause nausea, abdominal cramping and *distention* (swelling), diarrhea, vomiting, and gas. The skin may erupt in red, itchy swollen patches, commonly known as hives, or in widespread itching, redness, and swelling. Food-related allergies can also worsen a rash in children who have atopic eczema, a chronic condition of itchy, inflamed skin.

Other potential targets in the body's response to food allergens are the eyes and respiratory tract. The result can include red, itchy, watery eyes; a runny or stuffy nose; and sneezing, coughing, shortness of breath, wheezing, and other breathing problems. Food allergies also can aggravate asthma in people who suffer from the condition.

People with food allergies who also have asthma or hay fever appear to have an increased risk of a relatively rare but potentially fatal allergic condition called anaphylaxis. Anaphylaxis can affect several parts of the body at the same time, including the skin, the digestive

Potential effects of a food allergy

A food allergy is an abnormal reaction by the body's immune system to an otherwise harmless food or component of food. The body's response leads to the release of powerful chemicals, especially histamine, which cause the unpleasant—and sometimes dangerous—symptoms of food allergies. Doctors do not know what determines the specific symptoms an individual develops.

Respiratory tract symptoms can include a runny or stuffy nose, sneezing, coughing, shortness of breath, wheezing, or other breathing problems. People who suffer from asthma as well as a food allergy may find that the food allergy aggravates the asthma.

The lips, mouth, and **throat** may begin to swell within minutes of eating an allergy-provoking food. Tightness in the throat and hoarseness may also develop.

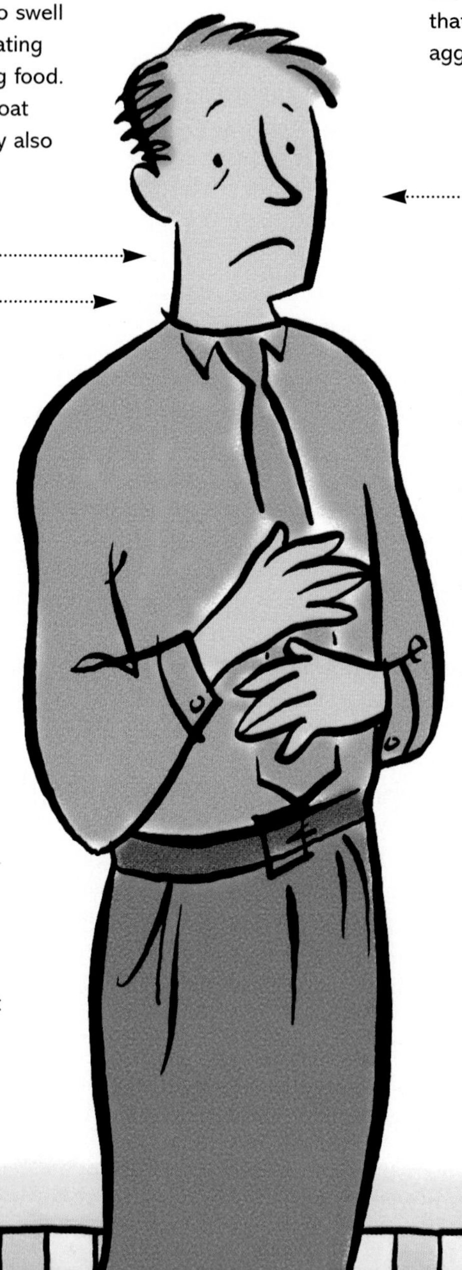

The skin may become hot and itchy or break out in a rash.

The stomach and **intestines** may become involved once the offending food enters them. Nausea, abdominal cramps and *distention* (swelling), diarrhea, vomiting, and gas can result.

The body may go into anaphylactic shock, a life-threatening allergic response that occurs in people who have an extreme sensitivity to a food. In addition to the other symptoms of a food allergy, it can lead to lightheadedness, a fast or irregular heartbeat, falling blood pressure, unconsciousness, and death.

Allergy: An immune system response

Allergies are inappropriate or exaggerated responses by the body's immune system to particular foods, plant pollens, dust, and other normally harmless substances. Immune responses are usually aimed at "foreign" invaders, such as bacteria, viruses, or parasites that could cause disease. When a properly functioning immune system detects proteins called antigens on the surface of these microbes, it responds to this perceived threat by producing defensive proteins called antibodies and sensitized white blood cells. The antibodies and sensitized cells recognize and attack the microbes bearing those antigens when they next encounter them.

In an allergic reaction, the immune system mistakenly identifies as harmful the antigens on molecules of food, pollen, or other substances, and it churns out antibodies to the antigen. These antibodies circulate in the blood and coat specialized immune-system cells called basophils and mast cells.

The next time the allergen enters the body, it attaches to the antibodies on mast cells. The mast cells respond by discharging a host of powerful chemicals, including histamine, that produce the allergic symptoms. The symptoms experienced—skin rashes, diarrhea, runny nose, or breathing difficulties, for example—depend on where in the body these chemicals are released. Mast cells are concentrated in tissues exposed to the outside world. Those tissues include the skin; the lining of the lungs, nose and throat, the gastrointestinal tract (stomach and intestines); and the reproductive system.

and respiratory systems, and the heart and blood vessels. In addition to producing the symptoms of food allergy already mentioned, anaphylaxis may lead to lightheadedness, a fast or irregular heartbeat, falling blood pressure, and eventual unconsciousness after the body goes into shock. As in the case of the asthma sufferer allergic to shellfish, anaphylaxis that is not treated with medication immediately can lead to death. This reaction usually occurs within minutes of consuming the food allergen, though reports indicate that it sometimes occurs hours later.

In some people, strenuous activity within hours of eating certain allergy-linked foods plays a role in provoking anaphylaxis. Researchers suggest that exercise helps trigger anaphylaxis in such individuals by increasing the absorption of food-related antigens into the bloodstream during digestion. Fortunately, people for whom exercise helps trigger anaphylaxis can avoid an attack by separating eating and exercising by at least four hours.

In most cases of anaphylaxis, the symptoms subside with treatment. Some fatal reactions develop quickly, while others begin with deceptively mild symptoms, only to progress during the next hour or two, causing the blood pressure to plummet and heart to stop. Estimates of the rate of fatal anaphylaxis due to any cause, including reactions to drugs such as penicillin, insect stings, and food allergens, range from 0.4 to 2 cases per million people per year. In the United States, this translates to some 100 to 500 deaths a year.

Which foods cause allergic reactions?

Although virtually any food can trigger an allergic response, most reactions are caused by eight foods: eggs, fish, milk, nuts, peanuts

Food Allergies: Myths and Misconceptions

Many people are confused about what food allergies are and aren't. Here are some of the more common myths about this widely misunderstood health problem:

Myth #1. Food allergies are extremely common. Although surveys show that as many as one-quarter to one-third of adults believe they have food allergies, most of them do not. Estimates vary, but studies indicate that less than 2 percent of Americans suffer from true food allergies, which involve the body's immune system. Other conditions, such as the absence of an enzyme needed to adequately digest certain foods, are responsible for some abnormal but nonallergic responses to foods.

Myth #2. Lactose intolerance is a food allergy. Unlike food allergies, which always involve the immune system, lactose intolerance is caused by an enzyme deficiency that prevents the body from digesting lactose, a sugar found in milk. This digestive problem causes nausea, diarrhea, and bloating, which are also common symptoms of food allergies.

Myth #3. Food allergies aren't serious. Although most food-related allergic reactions are fairly mild, a small percentage of people with food allergies develop a life-threatening reaction called anaphylaxis. More people die of allergic reactions triggered by foods than allergic reactions caused by insect stings.

Myth #4. Once you develop a food allergy, you'll have to avoid the offending food forever. Children, particularly infants, often outgrow food allergies. Studies also indicate that up to one-third of older children and adults can also lose their sensitivity to some allergy-provoking foods by avoiding them completely for a year or two. But people with allergies to certain foods, including peanuts, nuts, fish, and shellfish, rarely outgrow the problem.

Myth #5. "Just a little taste" of a problem food can't hurt. For people who are extremely allergic, even miniscule traces of the offending food—as little as one-thousandth of a teaspoon—can trigger a fatal allergic reaction. In rare cases, people have died after inhaling airborne allergens carried in the steam from cooking foods.

Myth #6. Most food allergies are caused by food additives, such as colorings and preservatives. Most allergic reactions are triggered by natural constituents of foods. The most common culprits include eggs, fish, milk, nuts, peanuts (which are legumes, not nuts), shellfish (especially shrimp), soy, and wheat.

(which are actually legumes, not nuts), shellfish, soy, and wheat. Milk, eggs, peanuts, soy, wheat, and fish trigger most of the food-related allergies seen in children, whereas the foods that most commonly pose problems for allergic adults are fish, nuts, peanuts, and shellfish.

Sometimes, an individual's allergic reaction to a particular food extends to other foods that contain similar antigens, a phenomenon called *cross-reactivity*. For example, someone who is allergic to peanuts may also have a problem with other legumes, such as soybeans or peas.

Cross-reactions also can develop between foods with antigens similar to those of other allergy-provoking substances, such as plant pollens. Researchers have found, for example, that some people who suffer hay fever symptoms when they inhale birch pollen also have an allergic reaction when they eat kiwi fruit or apples. Similarly, people with an allergy to avocados may also react to latex, a plant fluid used to make surgical gloves and other rubber products.

Furthermore, a 1996 study demonstrated that genetic engineering techniques aimed at improving food crops can unintentionally result in a formerly "safe" food becoming allergenic. When scientists inserted a Brazil nut gene to improve the nutritional content of soybeans, they discovered that the gene-altered soybean produced a strong allergic reaction in people who were allergic to the nut but not to regular soybeans. As a result, the company abandoned plans to market the "improved" soybean.

When do food allergies develop?

People can develop food allergies at any age, though the condition is more common in children, particularly in the first years of life. One reason infants are particularly vulnerable, researchers believe, is that their immune system and digestive tract are not yet fully developed. For this reason, allergy-provoking food antigens may more easily pass into an infant's bloodstream, increasing the likelihood of an allergic response from the immune system.

Food allergies are not necessarily a lifelong condition, however. Children, particularly infants, often outgrow food allergies, and studies indicate that as many as one-third of older children and adults can lose their sensitivity to some allergy-provoking foods by strictly eliminating them from their diet for a year or two. But people with allergies to certain foods, including peanuts, nuts, fish, and shellfish, rarely outgrow the problem.

Diagnosis of food allergies

Because unpleasant symptoms after eating can result from a number of health problems, medical experts advise people who suspect they have a food allergy or food intolerance to discuss their suspicions with their doctor, who in turn may recommend seeing an allergy specialist. In some cases, determining the nature of the problem is fairly straightforward: if, for example, someone always has the same reaction after eating a particular food. But most of the

Foods that commonly cause allergic reactions

Almost any food can cause an allergic reaction in a susceptible individual. But the most common culprits are the following:

- Fish, including cod, halibut, and salmon
- Nuts from trees, such as walnuts, cashews, and pecans
- Shellfish, including shrimp, lobster, and clams
- Soy, which is found in many processed foods, including soy sauce, tofu, meat extenders, and baked goods
- Cow's milk
- Peanuts
- Wheat
- Eggs

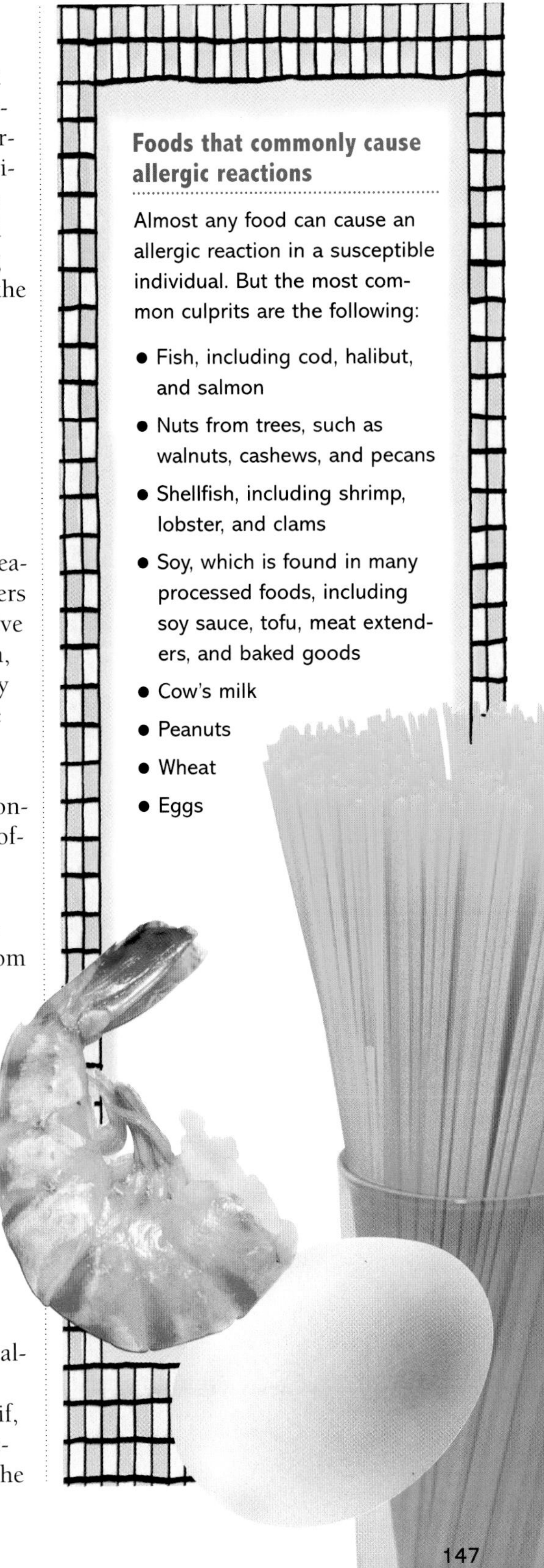

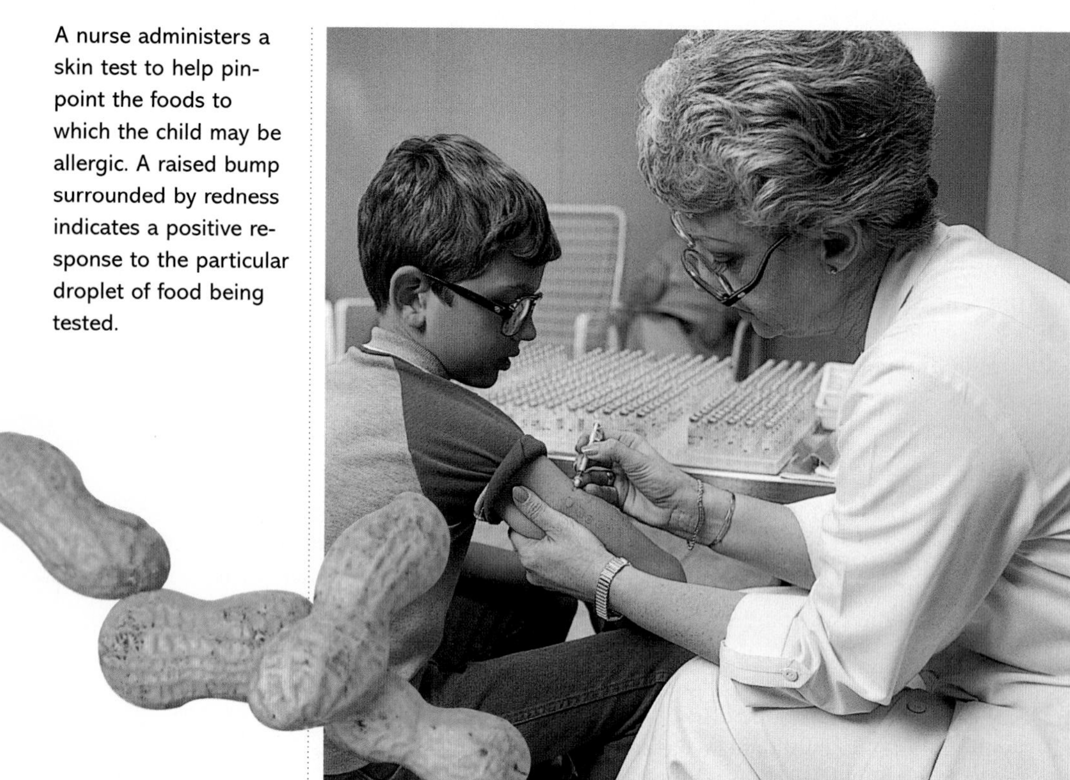

A nurse administers a skin test to help pinpoint the foods to which the child may be allergic. A raised bump surrounded by redness indicates a positive response to the particular droplet of food being tested.

time, some diagnostic detective work is necessary to verify that a person is really suffering from an adverse reaction to food and then to pin down the cause.

The first step is usually a thorough medical history and a physical examination to rule out other conditions, such as an infection, an intestinal disorder, or a side effect of medication, that might explain the symptoms. A medical history and family health history may shed some light, because allergic tendencies seem to run in families. Someone whose medical history includes other allergies, such as asthma or hay fever, is also more likely to have a food allergy.

If neither parent has allergies, allergy experts have found, an individual has only a 10 percent chance of developing one. The odds of developing an allergy rise as high as 30 to 35 percent if one parent is affected and jump to 50 to 60 percent if both are allergic. Experts say, however, it's the tendency to develop allergies that is inherited, not a specific allergy.

The doctor also asks detailed questions aimed at uncovering a possible relationship between the symptoms and the patient's diet. The questions cover which foods seem to cause problems, the kinds of symptoms experienced, the amount of time between consuming a suspect food and the development of symptoms, how often the reaction occurs, the amount of food needed to trigger a reaction, and other information.

A person with a suspected allergy may be asked to keep a food diary for a few weeks, recording in detail the foods eaten and the appearance and severity of symptoms experienced. While this diagnostic tool cannot prove that a particular food causes certain symptoms, it can indicate possible links between foods and symptoms that might otherwise go unnoticed. To reach a conclusive diagnosis, the doctor may recommend an *elimination diet* and certain diagnostic tests.

An elimination diet is one from which foods suspected of causing an allergic reaction are removed for as long as several weeks. The physician or a dietitian usually provides a list of foods that are permitted or forbidden during this time. If the symptoms thought to be triggered by suspect foods disappear or are significantly reduced, these foods may be reintroduced one at a time to see if the symptoms recur, a process called a *food challenge*. However, people with histories of severe reactions are rarely challenged with the suspected triggers because the procedure itself could be life-threatening.

An elimination diet and food challenge can point to an adverse food reaction, but it doesn't distinguish between food allergies and food intolerances. Several tests, however, can help determine whether a person's immune system reacts to a particular food.

Skin testing can help pinpoint which foods trigger allergic reactions in people who have a true food allergy. It can also help rule out a food allergy when the problem is actually a food intolerance. In a

When children have a food allergy

Studies have found that children are more likely than adults to develop food allergies. But they're also more likely to outgrow food allergies. Children are most likely to react to milk, eggs, peanuts, soy, wheat, and fish.

In some cases, the immune system response that triggers the allergy is the same as that in adults. However, adults are spared another type of food allergy that strikes only infants and young children. This condition, called food-induced enteropathy or gastrointestinal food hypersensitivity, is a temporary one that disappears with age. Foods that have been linked with it include chicken, cow's milk, eggs, fish, rice, and soy protein.

Researchers link this allergic disorder with a still-developing immune system and digestive tract, which make it more likely that food antigens pass from the intestines into the bloodstream, where they trigger the allergic response. The disorder sometimes develops after a digestive-tract infection, a situation that further increases the likelihood that antigens will slip into the circulation.

Symptoms of this disorder include vomiting and diarrhea, and they usually appear during the first three months of life. Children with the condition can develop chronic diarrhea, and changes that occur in the intestinal lining can prevent them from absorbing nutrients.

The treatment is the same for both types of food allergy: avoidance of the offending foods. Fortunately, many children lose this kind of food allergy as they get older. Studies show that most children who have cow's milk enteropathy, for example, are no longer allergic by their second birthday.

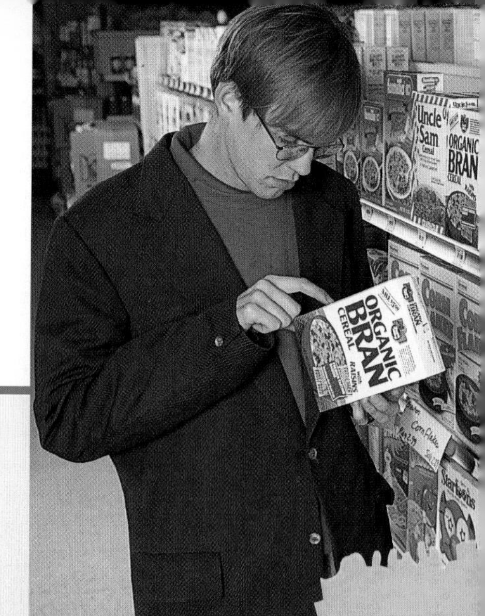

Choosing foods wisely

People with food allergies must be very careful about what they eat because allergy-causing foods and food ingredients may be hidden in a variety of prepared products and restaurant dishes.

Food families: Relatives to avoid

Some foods are related in their chemical composition and can produce similar allergic reactions. Knowing which foods are related can help people with food allergies avoid foods that may trigger an allergic response.

If you are allergic to	you may also be allergic to
Peanuts	Soybeans, peas, lentils, lima beans, kidney beans
Apples	Pears
Plums	Peaches
Beets	Spinach
Onions	Garlic, asparagus, chives, shallots
Strawberries	Raspberries, blackberries
Cucumbers	Melons
Carrots	Celery
Buckwheat	Rhubarb
Sunflower seeds	Lettuce, chicory, endive, escarole, artichokes
Cashews	Pistachios, mangos
Avocados	Cinnamon, bay leaf, sassafras
Allspice	Guavas, cloves, pimentos

skin test, the physician places a droplet with an extract of the suspect food on the skin, and then punctures or scratches the top layer of skin through the droplet. If a raised bump surrounded by an area of redness, like a mosquito bite, forms within 15 to 20 minutes, the skin test is positive. However, a positive response does not necessarily mean that the person has a food allergy. Although it's very uncommon for someone with a food allergy to have a negative result in a skin test for the allergen, many people who have a positive test result experience no allergic symptoms when they eat the food.

Skin tests are not appropriate for everyone with suspected food allergies. For example, the procedure might not be feasible for someone with a skin inflam-

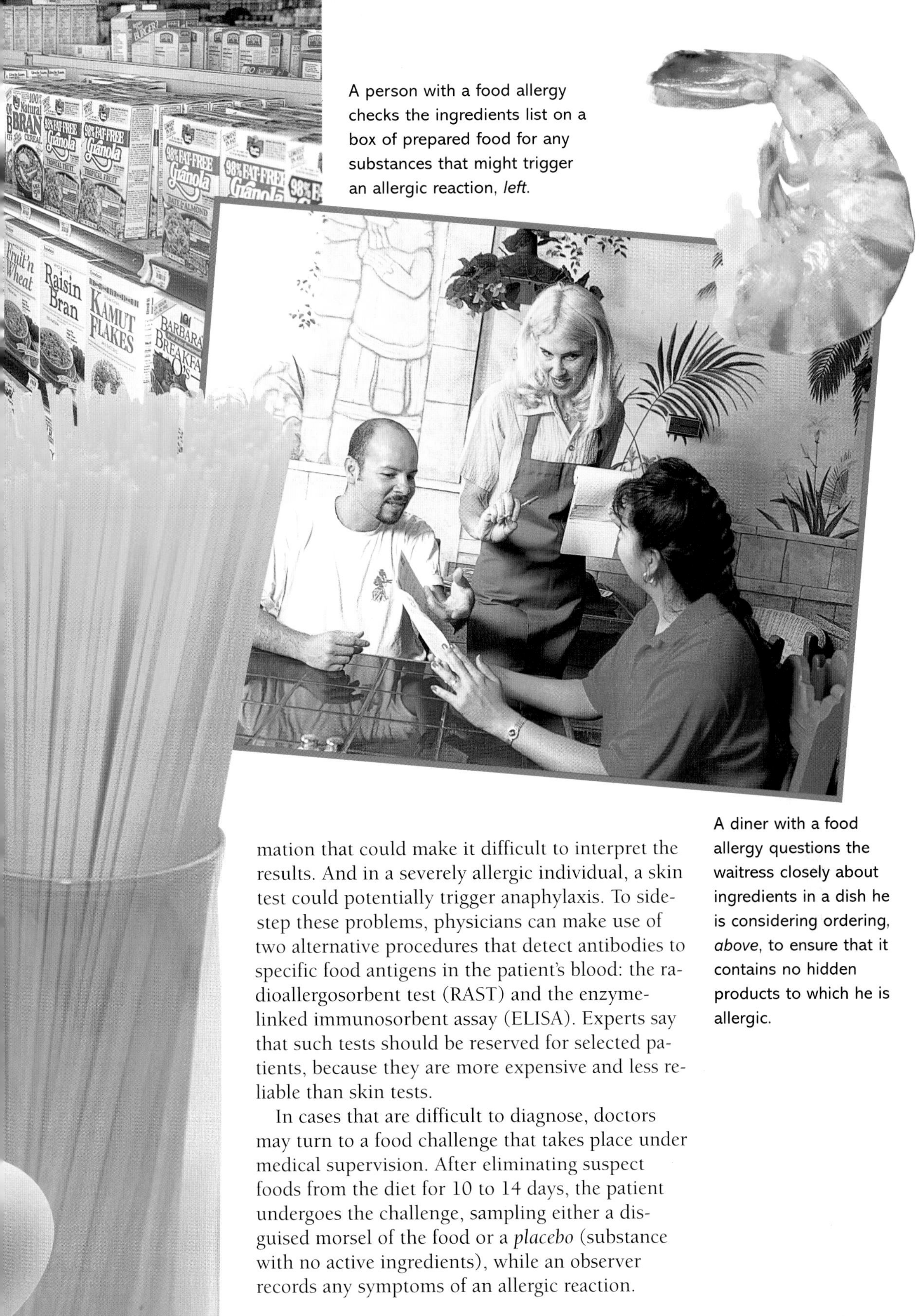

A person with a food allergy checks the ingredients list on a box of prepared food for any substances that might trigger an allergic reaction, *left*.

A diner with a food allergy questions the waitress closely about ingredients in a dish he is considering ordering, *above*, to ensure that it contains no hidden products to which he is allergic.

mation that could make it difficult to interpret the results. And in a severely allergic individual, a skin test could potentially trigger anaphylaxis. To sidestep these problems, physicians can make use of two alternative procedures that detect antibodies to specific food antigens in the patient's blood: the radioallergosorbent test (RAST) and the enzyme-linked immunosorbent assay (ELISA). Experts say that such tests should be reserved for selected patients, because they are more expensive and less reliable than skin tests.

In cases that are difficult to diagnose, doctors may turn to a food challenge that takes place under medical supervision. After eliminating suspect foods from the diet for 10 to 14 days, the patient undergoes the challenge, sampling either a disguised morsel of the food or a *placebo* (substance with no active ingredients), while an observer records any symptoms of an allergic reaction.

Increasing doses of the suspect food are given until the patient either develops symptoms or tolerates a normal portion. Ideally, neither the patient nor the observer can distinguish the food from the placebo, thus ruling out the possibility that the patient's or the observer's expectations are influencing the results.

Medical experts advise people to avoid two controversial methods sometimes touted for diagnosing food allergies: cytotoxic blood tests and sublingual provocation food testing (in which a dose of a food extract is placed under the tongue). According to the American Academy of Allergy, Asthma, and Immunology—a professional organization of physicians—these unproven methods are "expensive and unreliable in detecting true food allergy and should be avoided."

Treating food allergies

Once an allergy is diagnosed, strict avoidance of the offending food (or foods) is the only proven method of managing the allergy. The physician may arrange for a consultation with a registered dietitian, who can help design a food plan, suggest alternative foods or ingredients to replace forbidden ones, and provide instruction on reading food labels. People with food allergies and intolerances need to read the ingredient list on these labels carefully to check for foods that are off-limits and to detect "hidden" food allergens. That means learning the lingo used in listing ingredients. For example, people with egg or wheat allergies need to know that the terms *albumin* or *gluten* are tipoffs that the contents include egg white or wheat, respectively. Because food manufacturers sometimes change ingredients without warning, it's important to read the food labels every time you buy the product.

People with severe food allergies also need to be aware that tiny amounts of allergens left on pots, pans, and cooking utensils can contaminate other foods. The importance of such vigilance is illustrated by a recent episode in which a person with a severe peanut allergy nearly died after eating cookies lifted from a cookie sheet by a spatula previously used to remove cookies containing peanuts. To avoid this kind of danger, people with severe food allergies are advised to make certain that pots, pans, and utensils are carefully washed with soap and water after each use to remove any traces of forbidden foods.

Despite precautions, people with histories of significant food reactions sometimes unknowingly consume a food to which they are allergic, particularly when they eat at a restaurant, school, or social function. Although oral antihistamines may help control mild reactions, prompt administration of the drug epinephrine is often essential to treat anaphylaxis.

Doctors advise people with severe food allergies always to carry a self-injecting device loaded with epinephrine, called an Epi-Pen, or a kit containing a needle and syringe and to inject themselves at the first sign of symptoms to check a potentially life-threatening reaction. A person who is having a reaction also needs to seek medical attention immediately, because the problem may suddenly worsen, even after treatment with epinephrine.

Family members should also be familiar with the device, so they can quickly administer the drug if the allergy sufferer is unable to do so. Allergy experts urge parents of an allergic child to make certain that teachers and day-care providers are aware of the child's allergies and know how to administer epinephrine if the need arises. Medical emergency necklaces or bracelets describing the allergy can help alert emergency personnel and others when someone with an allergy is unconscious.

There is evidence that food allergies occur less frequently, or at least develop later, in babies who are breast-fed exclusively during the first several months of life. This protective effect is greatest when a nursing mother avoids certain foods—after consulting with her doctor or the baby's pediatrician—that contain common antigens, because the antigens can make their way into breast milk. Scientists believe that postponing an infant's exposure to cow's milk, soy, and other common allergy triggers until the digestive tract and immune system fully develop can reduce the likelihood that the baby will become sensitized to food allergens. For these reasons, some doctors advise mothers from allergy-prone families to breast-feed their babies and avoid giving the babies solid foods during the first six months of life.

For those who have food allergies, either temporary or lifelong, researchers are looking for better ways to diagnose and treat the problem. For example, the development of drugs could make it less risky for people with food allergies to eat away from home. In the meantime, the only option is avoiding problem foods and being prepared to treat severe reactions. For most people with food allergies, this policy means sparing themselves a little discomfort. But for others, their very lives may depend on it. •••

For more information:

American Academy of Allergy, Asthma, & Immunology
611 East Wells Street
Milwaukee, WI 53202
(414)272-6071

Food Allergy Network
4744 Holly Avenue
Fairfax, VA 22030-5647
(703)691-3179 or (800)929-4040

Physicians' Referral and Information Line
(800)822-2762

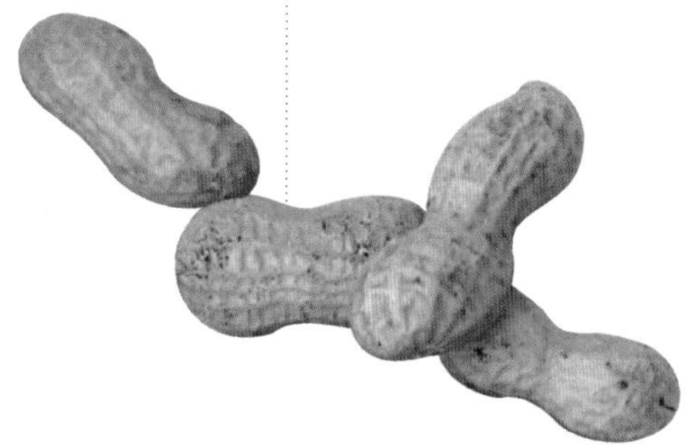

Glaucoma steals the sight of some 3 million Americans each year—but early detection and treatment of glaucoma can prevent vision loss.

Glaucoma Watch

By Jacob T. Wilensky

GLAUCOMA IS ONE OF THE LEADING CAUSES OF BLINDNESS in the United States and the world. More than 3 million Americans lose some or all of their vision to glaucoma each year, and eye specialists estimate that at least half of them don't even realize what is happening. This "sneak thief of sight" usually begins very gradually, with only a slight loss of vision along the edges of sight. But unless it is detected early and treated immediately, glaucoma causes vision loss that can never be regained.

It may be difficult to understand how people can lose part of their vision and remain unaware of it, but the most common form of glaucoma produces no obvious symptoms: no pain, blurred vision, swelling, or redness. And *peripheral* (side) vision usually disappears so slowly that it goes unnoticed, while the central field of vision remains unchanged.

Glaucoma develops when a natural fluid in the eye builds up. This fluid, known as aqueous humor, circulates in the front part of the eye between the *iris* (colored part of the eye) and its clear covering, the cornea. Aqueous humor brings nutrients to the cornea and lens, and it flows out of the eye through a drainage system of spongy tissue known as the trabecular meshwork.

In an eye with glaucoma, the flow of aqueous humor is blocked. As a result, the fluid, which the eye is constantly producing, fails to leave the eye as rapidly as it is produced. As the fluid builds up, pressure increases inside the eye. This pressure eventually leads to the death of nerve cells in the optic nerve at the back of the eye, permanently damaging vision. Exactly how the increased pressure causes nerve cells to die is still not understood.

Types of glaucoma

Ophthalmologists—physicians who specialize in diseases and disorders of the eye—classify glaucoma into two main types, primary and secondary, depending on its original cause. In primary glaucoma, pressure builds up inside the eye because of problems in the structure of the eye itself. In secondary glaucoma, pressure rises because of injury to the eye, a tumor, inflammation, or other disorder.

In both types of glaucoma, the outflow of aqueous humor can become blocked at one of two places: within the trabecular meshwork itself or just in front of it—in the angle between the iris and cornea. An obstruction in the trabecular meshwork resembles a clogged drain in a sink. It allows some fluid, but not all, to trickle through. An obstruction in front of the trabecular meshwork, however, resembles a plugged drain that completely blocks the flow of fluid.

The more common form of glaucoma involves blockage in the trabecular meshwork. It is called open-angle glaucoma because the angle between iris and cornea, which the trabecular meshwork occupies, remains open. Because the obstruction is only partial, *intraocular* (within the eye) pressure rises very gradually over a period of months or years. Both the cause and the exact nature of the obstruction are still unknown. Open-angle glaucoma usually occurs in both eyes. About 90 percent of all primary glaucoma cases are of the open-angle variety.

In the less common form of the disorder, angle-closure glaucoma, access to the trabecular meshwork becomes blocked. The pressure of aqueous humor as it tries to move past the iris causes the iris to suddenly bow forward and touch the back of the cornea. This motion closes off the angle that normally exists between iris and cornea and blocks the passage to the trabecular meshwork.

When this passage becomes blocked, intraocular pressure increases extremely rapidly, usually within an hour. The cornea swells and becomes cloudy, blurring vision or causing halos to appear around electric lights. As the cornea swells, the eye reddens and tears a lot. Other symptoms of angle-closure glaucoma can include headache, nausea or vomiting, and severe eye pain that may be sharp or dull. This acute form of glaucoma can cause rapid loss of vision leading to total blindness within hours or days.

The author:

Jacob T. Wilensky is professor of ophthalmology at the University of Illinois at Chicago and director of the glaucoma service at the university's Eye and Ear Infirmary.

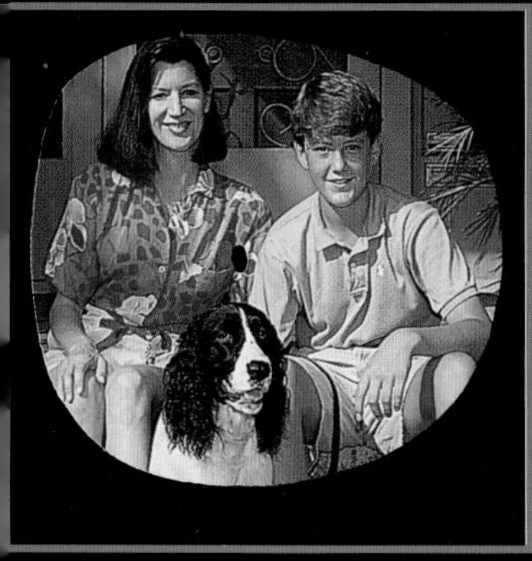

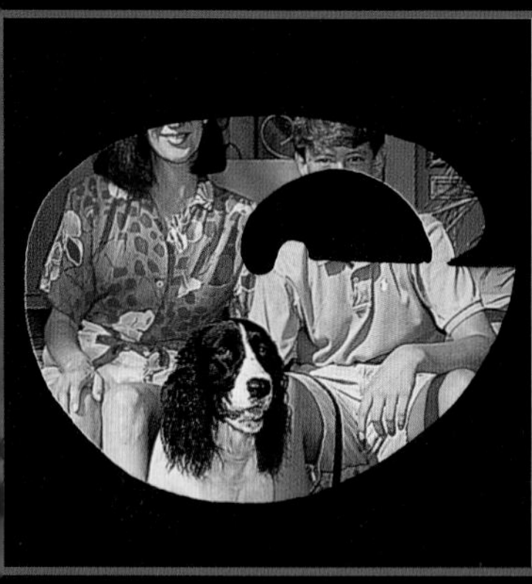

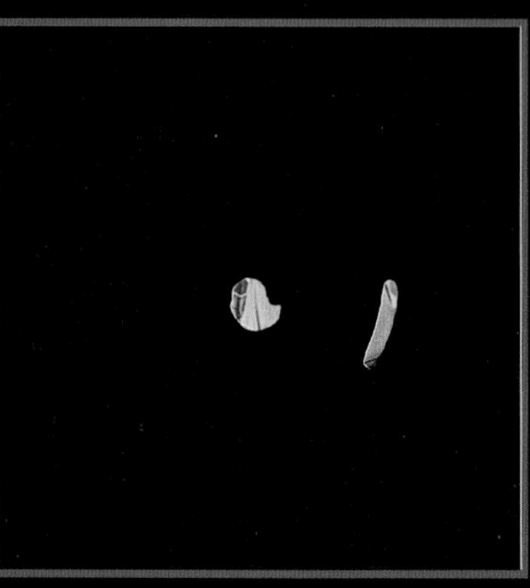

How a scene looks to someone with normal vision appears at the *top*. As peripheral vision deteriorates because of glaucoma, the field of vision narrows, *middle*. As the disease advances, most vision is lost, *bottom*. People who retain some central vision may still be able to read, however.

Angle-closure glaucoma tends to occur in only one eye. It is also more common in individuals who are far-sighted, though doctors are still not certain why this is so. They speculate that because far-sighted eyes are generally smaller and shorter than normal eyes, a narrower space is left between the iris and cornea.

Treating glaucoma

Sight lost because of either form of glaucoma can never be regained. However, treatment, if it is begun promptly, can prevent further loss of vision. The immediate treatment for both open-angle and angle-closure glaucoma involves the use of eye drops that decrease the pressure inside the eye.

In treating open-angle glaucoma, doctors may prescribe drops that reduce the amount of aqueous humor produced in the eye or drops that help the trabecular meshwork drain the aqueous humor more efficiently. The drugs most often prescribed for reducing the production of aqueous humor are called beta-blockers. Beta-blockers, administered in the form of eye drops, need to be applied once or twice daily and are effective for most people. As with other eye drops, some of the medication may enter the bloodstream and affect other body systems. Beta-blockers, for example, may slow the heart rate, and they can trigger serious problems in individuals with certain heart conditions, such as congestive heart failure. Beta-blockers also can cause breathing problems for people with asthma, and they may cause fatigue or reduced stamina.

Physicians can prescribe other drugs if beta-blockers are unable to control the open-angle glaucoma or if an individual has heart or respiratory problems and cannot take beta-blockers. Drugs called carbonic anhydrase inhibitors, which may be taken in pill or eye drop form, also reduce the amount of aqueous humor produced. The drops produce fewer and less severe side effects than the pills, which can cause loss of appetite, fatigue, and depression. The pills can also promote the formation of kidney stones and, in very rare cases, lead to severe anemia—a sharp reduction in the number of red blood cells.

Another group of drugs, called adrenergics, helps the trabecular meshwork drain the aqueous

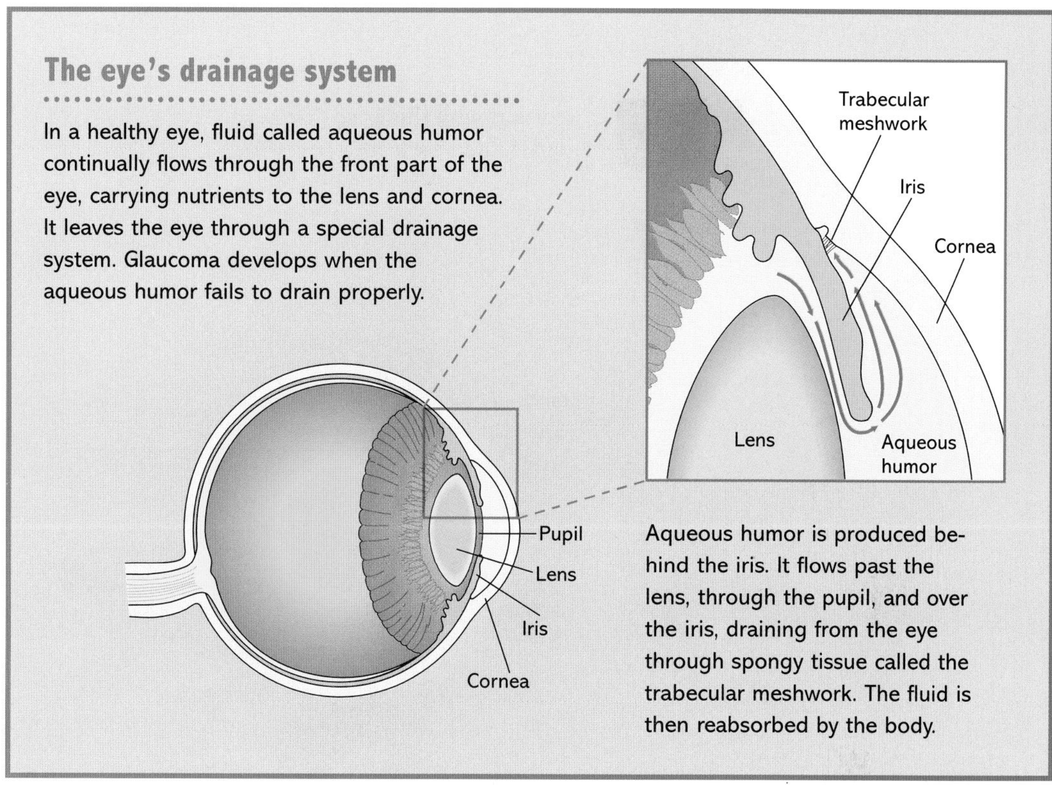

humor more efficiently. These eye drops are less effective than beta-blockers, however, and sometimes provoke an allergic reaction in the eyes. Nevertheless, they are useful for people who cannot take beta-blockers or carbonic anhydrase inhibitors.

In treating angle-closure glaucoma, doctors generally prescribe eye drops called miotics and oral medications called osmotics. Miotics make the pupil smaller by tightening the muscles around it. As the pupil becomes smaller, it pulls the iris away from the trabecular meshwork, stretching the porous drainage system and allowing the aqueous humor to flow out of the eye. Osmotics speed the flow of aqueous humor and enable it to drain into the bloodstream, thus relieving intraocular pressure.

In most patients with open-angle glaucoma, eye drops can successfully control the condition and prevent further loss of vision. In a minority of patients, however, eye drops are ineffective or cause serious side effects, and surgical procedures may be necessary to create an artificial drain and keep the pressure in the eye at a level that prevents further loss of sight.

Surgery using a concentrated beam of light from a laser is usually the next step. In the customary procedure, called argon laser trabeculoplasty, the ophthalmologist fires short bursts of laser light that create from 50 to 100 tiny laser burns in the trabecular meshwork. This treatment improves drainage, though exactly how it does so is

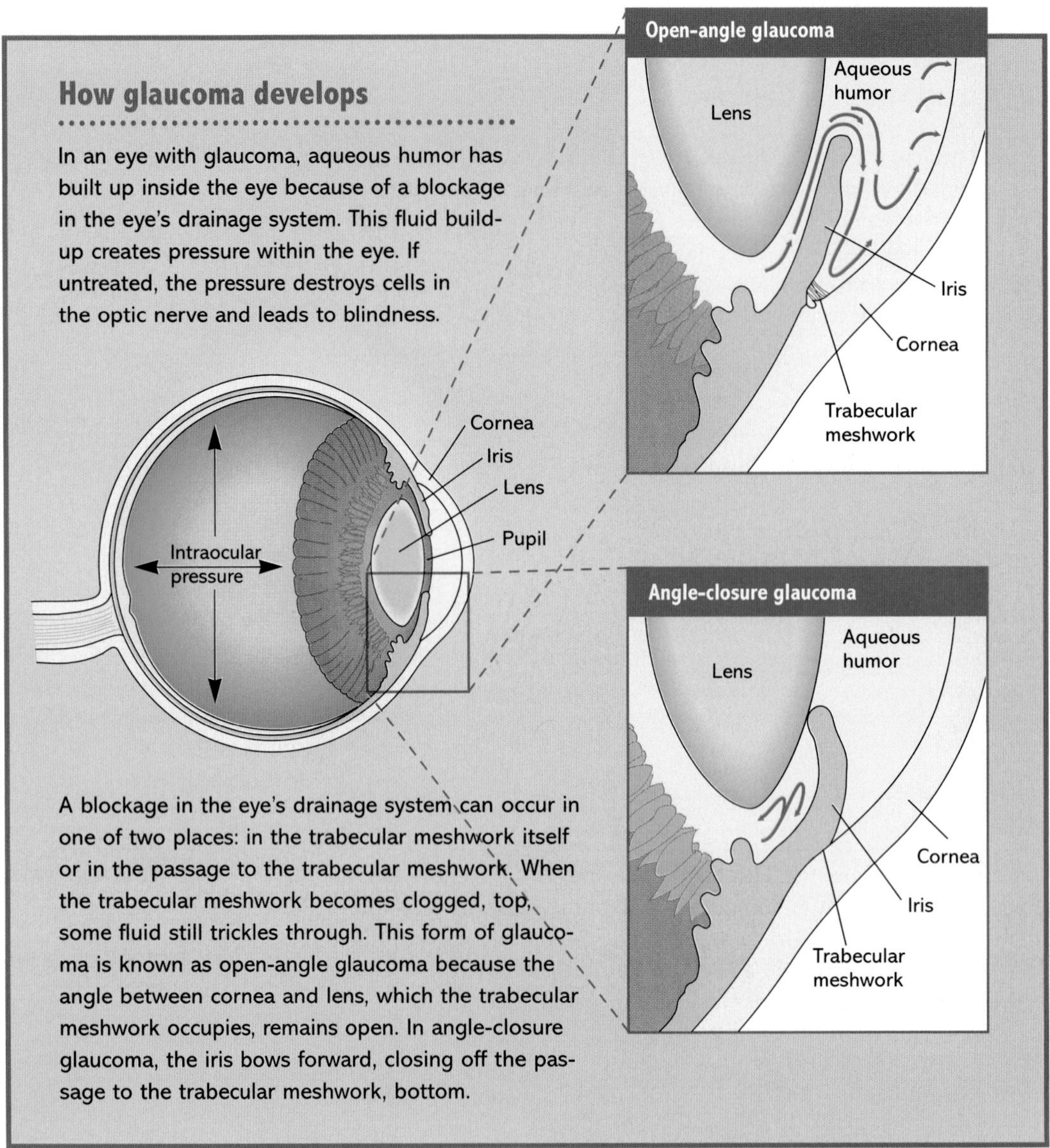

still unclear. Because laser surgery involves no cutting, unlike conventional surgery, it also carries less risk of infection or other complications. Laser trabeculoplasty can usually be performed in the doctor's office or at an outpatient facility, using local anesthetic.

Ophthalmologists turn to conventional surgery to treat open-angle glaucoma when neither medication nor laser treatment can control the rise of intraocular pressure. In a procedure called filtration surgery, the surgeon makes a hole in the *sclera* (white part of the eye) and creates a pocket beneath the membrane that covers the sclera. The aqueous humor then flows through the hole into the pocket, where it can be reabsorbed by the body. The procedure is usually performed on an out-patient basis.

The types of glaucoma

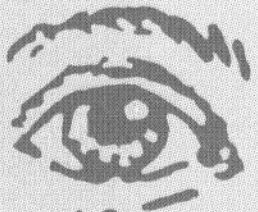

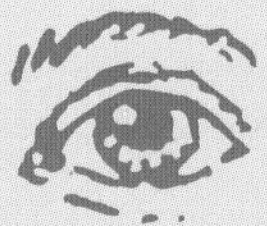

Glaucoma that develops because of problems in the structure of the eye is called primary glaucoma. Secondary glaucoma develops as the result of an injury, a tumor, or another disorder. Both primary and secondary glaucoma occur in one of two forms, which differ in the following respects:

Open-angle glaucoma

- Develops slowly.
- Develops because of a blockage in the trabecular meshwork that slows the drainage of the aqueous humor.
- Causes a gradual loss of *peripheral* (side) vision as its only noticeable symptom.
- Is treated with medication, laser surgery, or conventional surgery to prevent additional loss of sight.

Angle-closure glaucoma

- Develops rapidly, often within an hour.
- Develops because the iris bows forward, preventing the aqueous humor from draining through the trabecular meshwork.
- Can cause blurred vision, the appearance of halos around lights, severe eye pain, headache, nausea, and vomiting.
- Is treated temporarily with eye drops, but either laser surgery or conventional surgery is necessary to prevent loss of sight.

In angle-closure glaucoma, eye drops or pills can stop the rise of intraocular pressure only temporarily. The permanent treatment requires making a hole through the iris, usually by means of a laser. Fluid can then pass through the hole, relieving the pressure that is pushing the iris forward against the cornea. In some patients, laser treatment is ineffective or cannot safely be used because of other health problems. Ophthalmologists then surgically remove a piece of the iris to restore the flow of aqueous humor.

A delay in treating an attack of angle-closure glaucoma can allow the iris and cornea to become permanently stuck together. Once this occurs, neither laser treatment nor traditional surgery can relieve the intraocular pressure, and blindness results.

Who is at risk for glaucoma?

Although ophthalmologists still do not fully understand what causes primary glaucoma, they have noted that both the open-angle and angle-closure forms run in families. Approximately half the people who develop primary glaucoma have a close relative with the dis-

An ophthalmologist measures the pressure inside a patient's eye with an instrument called a Goldmann tonometer. After numbing the eye with a drop of medication, the doctor guides the tip of the tonometer to the eye. The tonometer determines the amount of pressure required to indent the eye slightly.

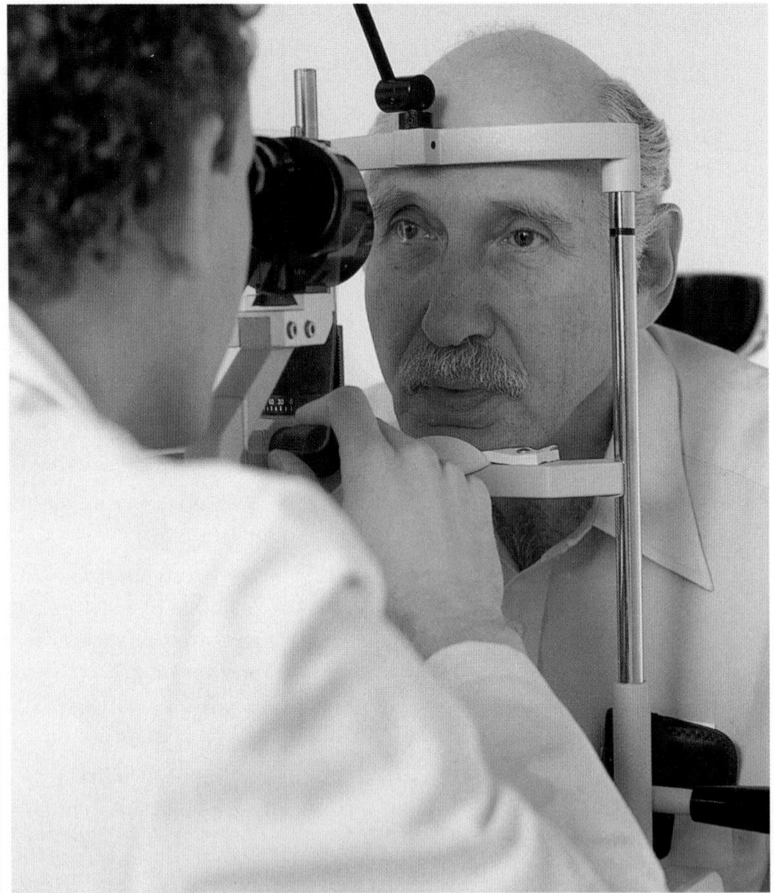

ease. The children and siblings of people with glaucoma have about 1 chance in 10 of developing the condition, compared with less than 1 chance in 100 for people who have no such family history. When glaucoma is hereditary, individuals usually develop only the form of the disease that runs in their family.

For unknown reasons, certain groups have a greater likelihood of developing glaucoma than others. In the United States, open-angle glaucoma is two to four times more common among African Americans than among Caucasians, whereas angle-closure glaucoma is more common among Caucasians. The population group with the highest incidence of angle-closure glaucoma is the Inuit. Angle-closure glaucoma also is much more common in women than in men.

Being severely nearsighted may also place people at greater risk for developing glaucoma. The larger size of the eye and the thinness of the eye's covering in nearsighted individuals may make the eye more susceptible to damage from stretching when intraocular pressure rises.

Glaucoma is predominantly a disease of older people. Angle-closure glaucoma affects people in their early 60's on average, while open-angle glaucoma is typically diagnosed in a person's late 60's or early 70's. The likelihood of developing the disease increases with age. Only about 1 percent of people aged 40 to 49 experience vision loss because of glaucoma, compared with at least 20 to 30 percent of people over the age of 70.

Despite these numbers, glaucoma can occur at any age. Some uncommon forms of glaucoma are present at birth or become apparent during the first years of life. Other rare forms develop during the teens or 20's or at other stages of life.

Testing for glaucoma

Even though glaucoma cannot be cured, it can be treated. The key to preventing vision loss from glaucoma is early diagnosis. The American Academy of Ophthalmology recommends that people without any symptoms of glaucoma have a comprehensive examination for glaucoma at age 40, followed by eye examinations every two to four years from the ages of 40 to 64 and every one to two years after age 65. African Americans, who as a group are at higher-than-average risk for glaucoma, and people with a family history of glaucoma or severe nearsightedness should have more frequent eye examinations, every one to two years after age 40 and every year after age 60.

Ophthalmologists use several techniques in checking for glaucoma. Tonometry measures intraocular pressure. Many doctors once used an instrument that released a puff of air at the eye and then measured the force necessary to indent the eye. Air-puff tonometers are still used, but most doctors prefer to use a more accurate instrument, the Goldmann tonometer, for measuring this force. After numbing the eye with a drop of medication, the ophthalmologist then applies pressure to the eye with the tip of the tonometer.

In another test, the physician uses a viewing device called an ophthalmoscope to examine the optic nerve for any signs of damage resulting from glaucoma. Usually, the doctor first *dilates* (enlarges) the pupils with eye drops, so that the back of the eye, where the optic nerve is located, can be seen more clearly. The eye drops may blur a patient's vision briefly and increase the eyes' sensitivity to light. However, since no instrument touches the eye, the ophthalmoscope does not cause any discomfort.

Treating glaucoma

Prompt treatment can halt vision loss from glaucoma, though it cannot restore vision already lost. In treating open-angle glaucoma, physicians turn to surgery if drugs prove ineffective or cause serious side effects. But surgery is necessary for treating angle-closure glaucoma.

Treatments for open-angle glaucoma

- Medications, primarily beta-blockers and carbonic anhydrase inhibitors.
- Laser surgery called trabeculoplasty, which improves drainage through the trabecular meshwork.
- Filtration surgery, which creates a hole in the *sclera* (white part of the eye) and a pocket beneath the sclera's covering, allowing the aqueous humor to drain.

Treatments for angle-closure glaucoma

- Medications such as miotics and osmotics, which temporarily stop the rise of pressure.
- Laser surgery called iridotomy, which creates a hole in the iris, allowing the aqueous humor to drain.
- Surgical removal of a piece of the iris, called iridectomy, which allows the fluid to drain.

Determining glaucoma risk

If left untreated, both open-angle and angle-closure glaucoma can result in permanent vision loss. The best way to prevent such loss is through regular eye examinations, which are especially important for people at higher-than-average risk for glaucoma. People can determine their risk by adding up the weighted numbers that apply to them and checking their score below.

Risk factor*	Category	Weight
Age	Younger than 50 years	0
	50 to 64 years	1
	65 to 74 years	2
	Older than 75 years	3
Race	Caucasian/other	0
	African American	2
Family history of glaucoma	None or only in relatives other than parents or siblings	0
	Yes for parents	1
	Yes for siblings	2
Most recent complete eye examination	Within the last two years	0
	Two to five years ago	1
	More than five years ago	2

Level of glaucoma risk	(Total score)
High	4 or greater
Moderate	3
Low	2 or less

*Other factors such as nearsightedness or diabetes may also contribute to an increased risk for glaucoma. They are not strong enough to be weighted in this table, but an ophthalmologist will consider them when assessing an individual patient's risk.

Source: American Academy of Ophthalmology.

A third test, perimetry, checks for blind spots and loss of peripheral vision. The patient sits in front of a machine called a perimeter and peers at a small circle or dot inside the machine. A light flashes on in various locations within the machine, and the patient signals upon noticing the light. By moving the light, the ophthalmologist tests all areas of the person's field of vision and locates any blind spots. Doctors also repeat perimetry at regular intervals to assess the success of treatment in preventing further vision loss in patients diagnosed with glaucoma.

In secondary glaucoma, the elevated pressure in the eye results from injury or other condition, such as inflammation or a tumor. In some cases, treating the underlying problem eliminates the glaucoma. But in others, the glaucoma persists and requires the standard therapy for primary glaucoma, though the underlying condition sometimes renders these treatments less effective or even unsafe. In such cases, doctors must evaluate all of the patient's medical problems and choose the treatments which best control the most dangerous conditions.

Individuals who are taking medication for glaucoma must exercise great care in taking any other drugs, even over-the-counter products. Some nonprescription eye drops for red or itchy eyes and some cold or sinus medications contain ingredients that *constrict* (narrow) blood vessels. Such drugs can cause the pupil to dilate and bring on an angle-closure glaucoma attack in susceptible people. These drugs can be used safely by people with open-angle glaucoma, however.

Other cold remedies and some drugs that combat nausea or motion sickness contain ingredients called antihistamines. Certain antihistamines can raise intraocular pressure in susceptible individuals, though most open-angle glaucoma patients are able to use these medications safely. Glaucoma patients or those with a family history of glaucoma should discuss with their ophthalmologists which of these drugs they can use and which ones they should avoid.

Although glaucoma is a progressive disease and the damage it causes to the eyes is irreversible, early diagnosis and treatment can prevent any further vision loss and preserve the sight that remains. By scheduling regular eye examinations with an ophthalmologist, it's possible to outwit the sneak thief of sight. •••

For further reading:

Eden, John. *The Physician's Guide to Cataracts, Glaucoma, and Other Eye Problems.* Consumer Reports, 1992.

Gayton, Johnny L., and Ledford, Jan R. *The Crystal Clear Guide to Sight for Life: A Complete Manual of Eye Care for Those over 40.* Starburst, 1996.

For more information:

Glaucoma Research Foundation
490 Post Street, Suite 830
San Francisco, CA 94102
800-826-6693

Prevent Blindness America
500 East Remington Road
Schaumburg, IL 60173
800-331-2020

Glaucoma 2001
Foundation of the American Academy of Ophthalmology
655 Beach Street, P.O. Box 7424
San Francisco, CA 94120-7424
800-391-EYES

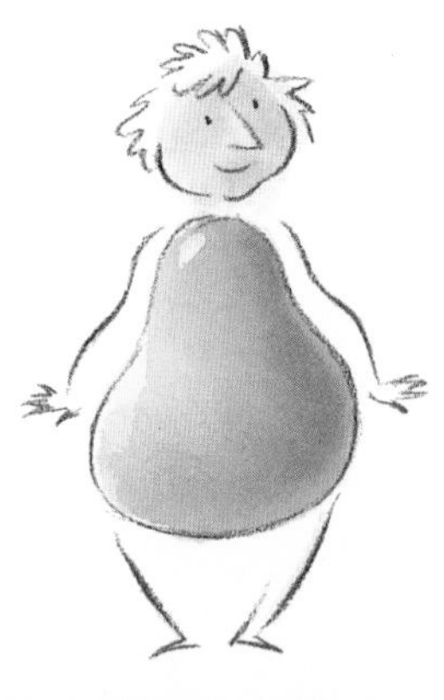

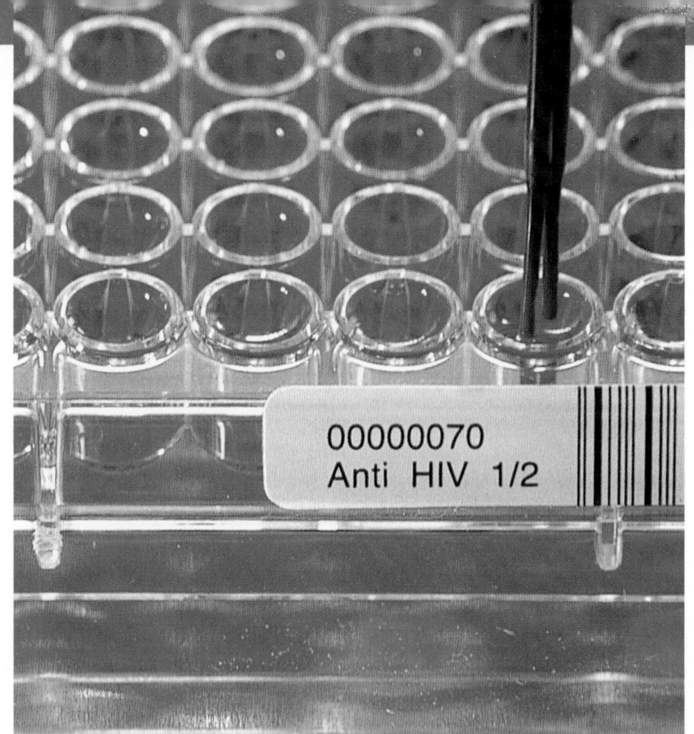

00000070
Anti HIV 1/2

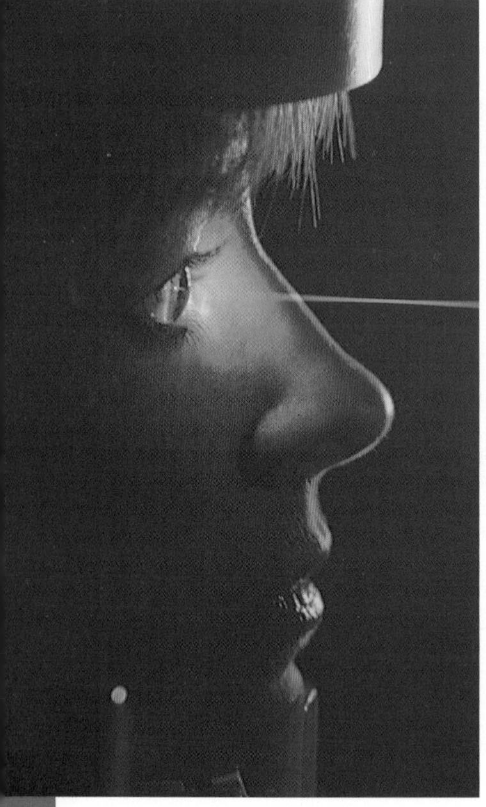

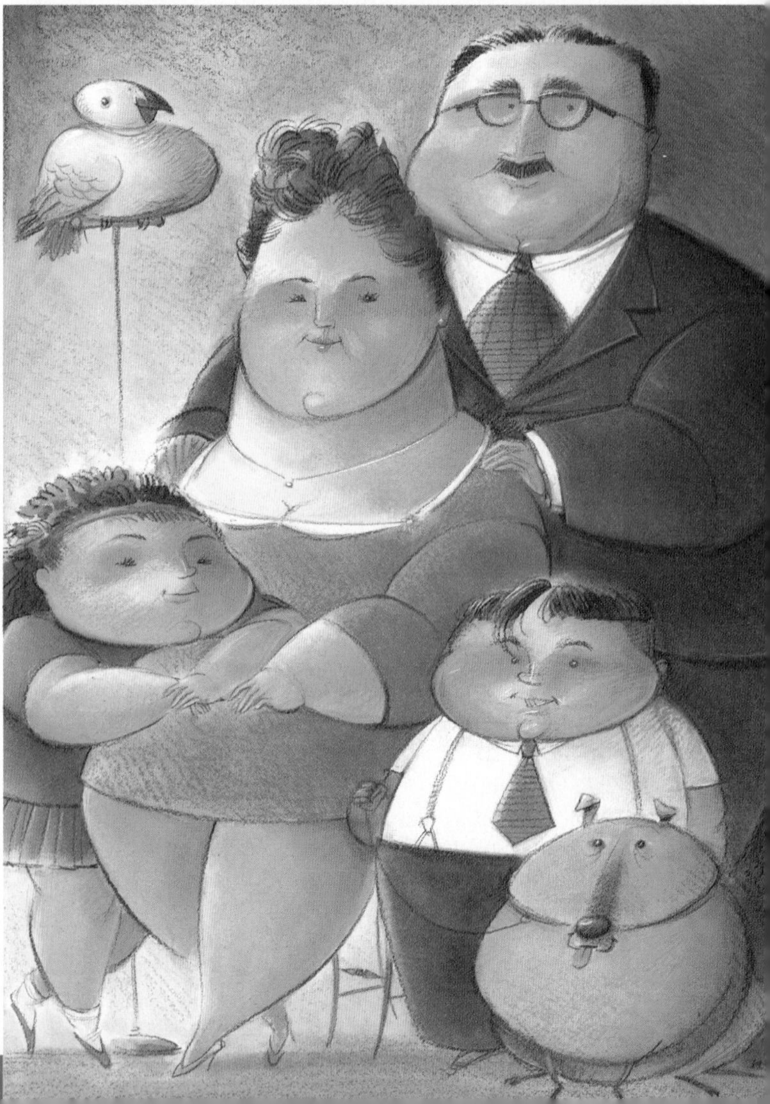

On the Medical Frontier

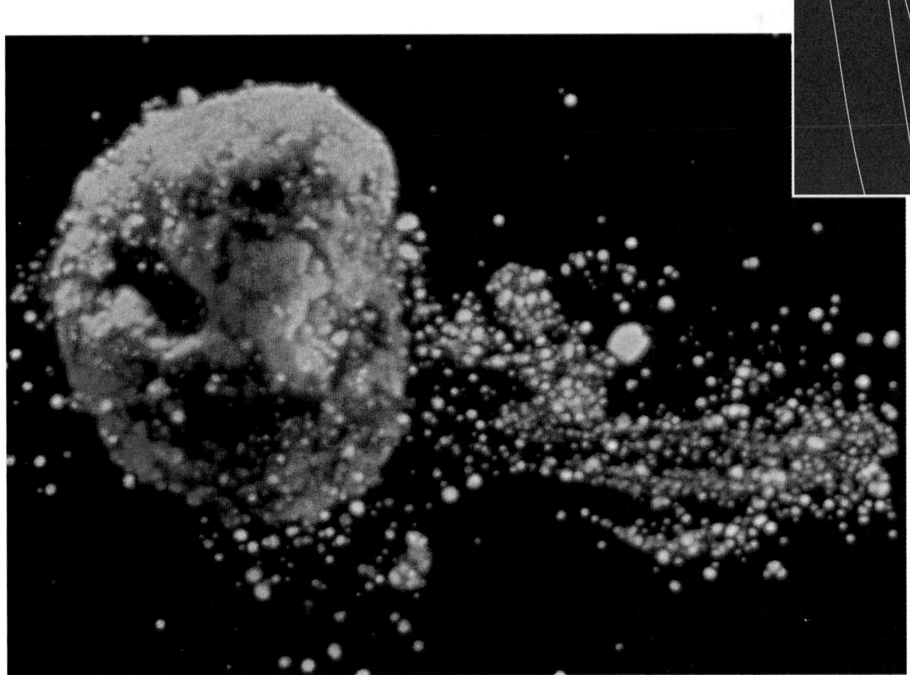

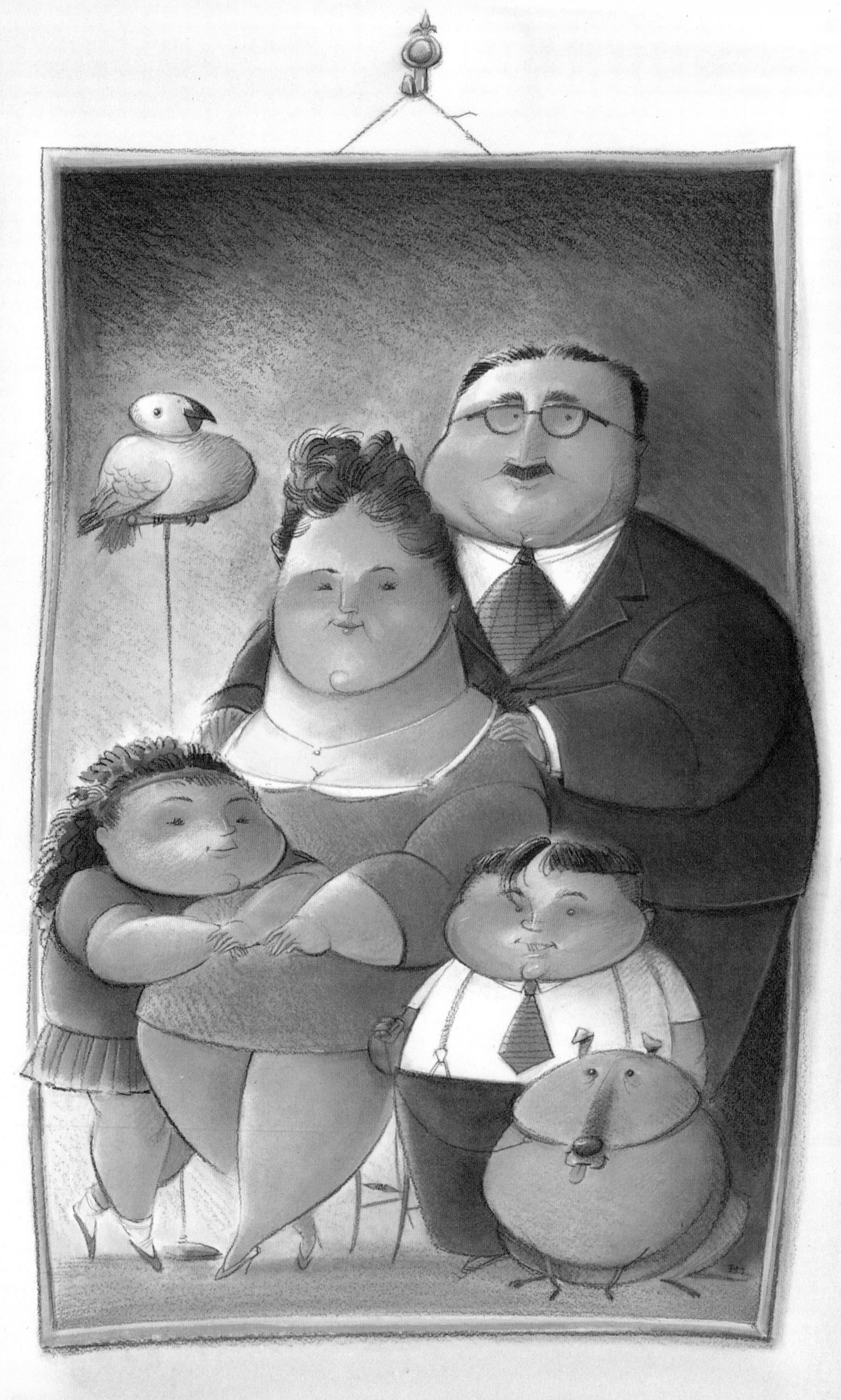

Research on the genetic basis of obesity may help explain why losing weight is so difficult for some people—and it could lead to new weight-loss drugs.

New Weapons in the War Against Weight

By Richard Trubo

EACH MORNING AS THEY STARE AT THE BATHROOM SCALE, millions of Americans fret about how they're ever going to win the battle of the bulge. Hungry for the latest weight loss miracle, they may jump from weight-loss clinics to "fat farms" to endless diet books—but often all that ends up thinner is their self-esteem and their wallet.

Based on a nationwide survey conducted from 1988 to 1991 and reported in 1994, the Centers for Disease Control and Prevention (CDC) estimated that about 58 million American adults were overweight. Overweight was defined as weighing more than recommended for one's height, as indicated in tables published by the U.S. Department of Health and Human Services and the Department of Agriculture. These tables are reevaluated every five years.

Physicians generally reserve the term *obese* for those who weigh at least 20 percent more than their recommended weight. But weight-loss experts agree that obesity really means an excessive amount of body fat, and a simple height and weight chart cannot accurately interpret how much body fat a person is carrying. Muscle and bone weigh more than fat, so people who are muscular or have large frames can weigh more than the charts recommend and yet not be obese.

Weight-loss experts consider a calculation called body mass index (BMI) a more accurate indicator of obesity. BMI also reflects body fat more accurately than a standard height and weight chart, because it is derived from statistics on deaths and illnesses caused by conditions associated with obesity. A simple method of determining BMI is to consult a chart like that on page 175.

A genetic link to obesity

Those who lead lives of diet desperation can be at least somewhat encouraged by scientific discoveries since 1994 that may eventually provide new weapons in the fight against fat. Most of the attention was directed at a gene called *ob* (for its ties to obesity), which scientists isolated in 1994. The ob gene is active only in fat cells, and a defective or missing ob gene appeared to play a key role in obesity.

Researchers came closer to understanding the gene's function in 1995, when they discovered the protein the ob gene produces in mice. (Genes are made of DNA, the master molecule of life. Genes contain instructions for the production of proteins, which carry out the functions of a cell.) The protein in this case is also a *hormone* (chemical messenger), which the researchers named *leptin* after the Greek word for *thin*. Leptin appeared to play a role in the process that regulates fat storage in the body, though how it does so was still under study. After the discovery of leptin, researchers uncovered several more pieces of the obesity puzzle.

These discoveries went a long way toward driving home the point that obesity is not necessarily the result of a personality flaw or emotional problems, as many people have thought. And while scientists realized that one particular gene or protein would not provide an explanation for every individual's inability to lose weight, they hoped that the breakthroughs would lead to the development of drugs that could be the answer to a healthier weight for millions of people.

The first breakthrough came from a study on obese mice. In December 1994, scientists at Rockefeller University in New York City reported that they had isolated the ob gene in mice and found a very similar gene in human fat tissue.

The scientists hypothesized that the ob gene produces a protein that travels through the bloodstream to the brain. The protein, the theory continued, carries a message telling the brain how much fat the body has stored. When the fat stores reach a certain level, signaled by the amount of hormone that reaches the brain, the brain releases a hormone producing a sensation of fullness that prompts the person to stop eating. In some people, however, the brain does not receive the message, and thus they do not experience satiety. The absence of that signal may explain why they continue to eat.

In July 1995, three groups of researchers—the team from Rockefeller University and teams at two pharmaceutical companies—isolated the protein, leptin, that the ob gene produces in mice. Using biotechnology techniques, the scientists manufactured sufficient lep-

The author:

Richard Trubo is a freelance medical writer.

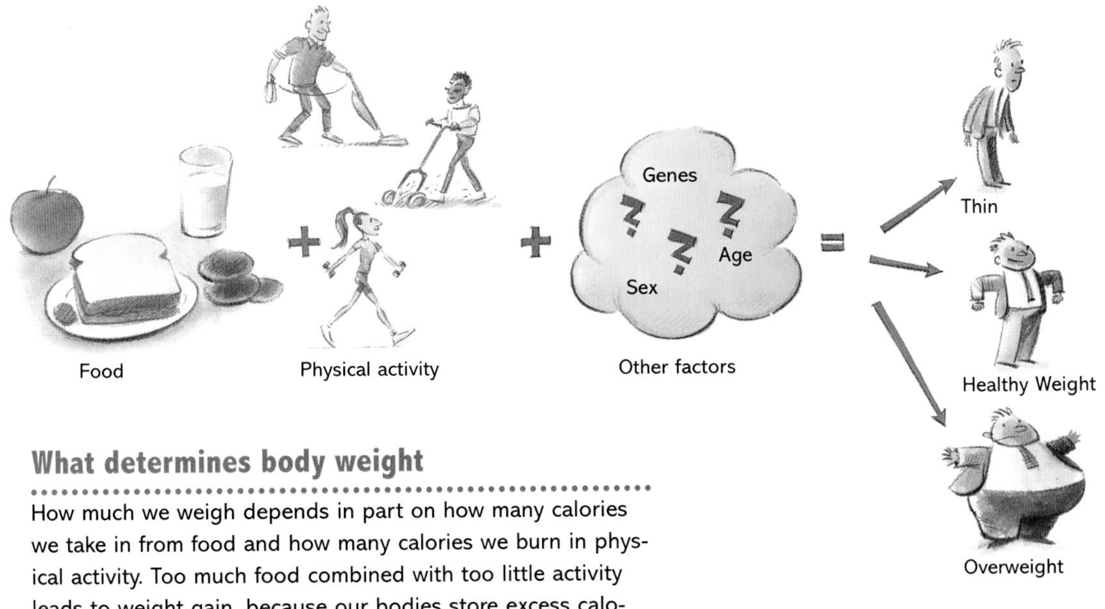

What determines body weight

How much we weigh depends in part on how many calories we take in from food and how many calories we burn in physical activity. Too much food combined with too little activity leads to weight gain, because our bodies store excess calories as fat. But this isn't the whole story. Other factors influence whether we are overweight, thin, or in between. These include our age, sex, and the genes we inherit.

tin for their experiments. They then injected the hormone into a strain of obese mice that had a defective ob gene, which prevented them from producing leptin. After the injection of leptin, the mice ate much less, their *metabolism* (the process by which food is converted to energy) accelerated, and their weight dropped by 12 to 40 percent, mostly through reductions in body fat.

Of course, the fact that this experiment worked in mice provided no guarantee that it would succeed in humans, and by mid-1996, there was still no evidence that injections of human leptin would help obese people lose weight. Some research had already raised doubts about leptin as a magic potion to turn fat people thin.

A study reported by a team at Thomas Jefferson University in February 1996 evaluated leptin levels in the blood of 136 volunteers of normal weight and in 139 obese volunteers. The scientists found that 90 to 95 percent of the obese people had plenty of leptin—an average of over four times more than the people of normal weight. As a result of this finding, the researchers speculated that the problem in the overweight men and women might be an inability to use leptin properly, rather than a scarcity of the protein, though they did not offer a theory on the possible cause of a leptin insensitivity.

An editorial in the *New England Journal of Medicine* of Feb. 1, 1996, accompanying the Jefferson University study suggested another possibility. Leptin, the authors said, appears to act on a chemical that stimulates appetite in a part of the brain called the hypothalamus. In animal experiments, rats of normal weight that received large infusions of this chemical, called neuropeptide Y, overate and became obese. Low levels of neuropeptide Y in the rats acted as an appetite depressant. In 1996, scientists were investigating the possibility that leptin may decrease the production of neuropeptide Y. If so, administering leptin might help obese people lose weight.

The discovery of a genetic link with obesity was no surprise to weight-control experts. Earlier evidence that genes might play a role in determining weight had come from studies of adopted children. If genes do play a role, then adopted children should resemble their biological parents in body weight more often than they resemble their adoptive parents. A widely cited Danish study compared the weights of 540 adoptees with those of their biological and adoptive parents. The study found that the adoptees were much more likely to be-

A genetic basis for obesity

Several discoveries that stem from research on mice have led scientists to formulate a theory on how a faulty gene might contribute to obesity in humans.

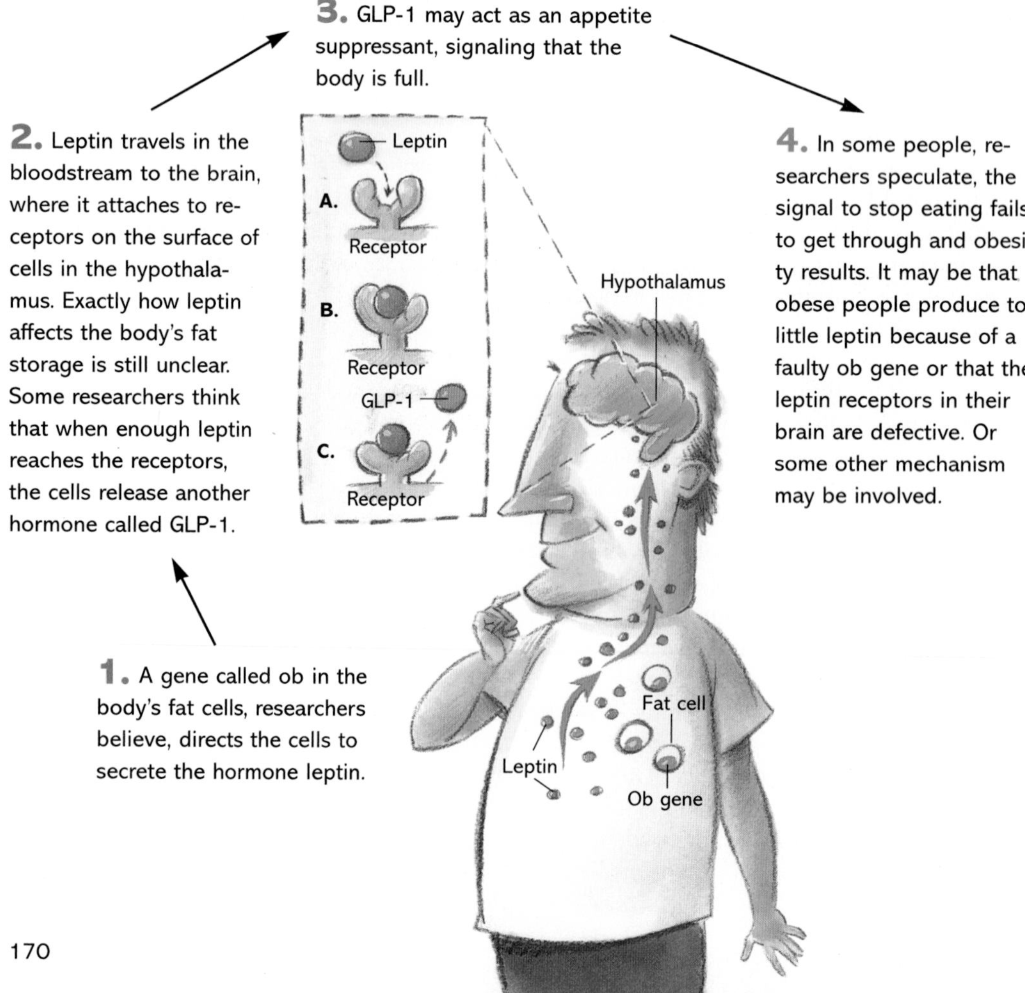

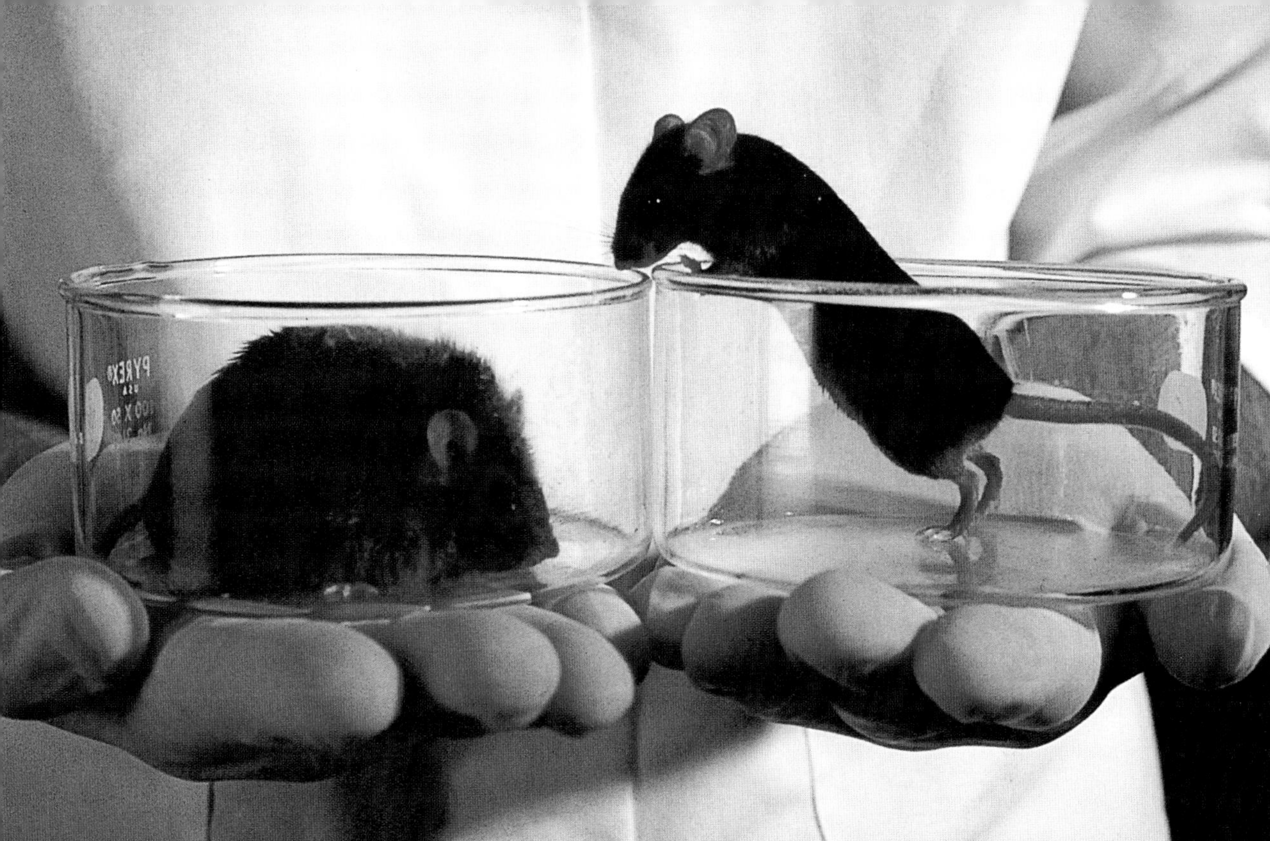

Mice provide major clues

A strain of obese mice helped scientists identify the ob gene and isolate the hormone leptin that the gene produces when working normally. Both of the mice have flawed ob genes, but the once-obese mouse at the right slimmed down after receiving leptin injections. The other mouse received no injections.

come obese if their biological parents were obese than if only their adoptive parents were obese. Similarly, studies of identical twins who were reared apart suggest that genetic makeup has a much stronger influence on body weight than environment does.

Other factors that influence weight

A biological predisposition, however, does not doom someone to obesity, weight-control experts maintain. Other important factors help determine weight. One of these is what the person chooses to eat. Another is metabolism. When someone consumes more energy in calories than the body burns off in exercise and daily activities, the body stores the leftover calories as fat. The kinds and amounts of foods people choose determine the number of calories they take in. Fat has more than twice as many calories per gram as the two other groups of nutrients, carbohydrates and proteins. Fat contains nine calories per gram, while carbohydrates and proteins each have four.

Many Americans, apparently, are choosing fatty foods more often than they should. A 1992 survey of 4,000 households showed that Americans dine out an average of nine times each week. About three-fourths of respondents named fast-food restaurants as their favorite places to dine. People choose high-fat food more often than healthier fare in these establishments.

A sedentary lifestyle also contributes to weight gain, and the typical American way of life has led more and more people to become sedentary. Consider the conveniences that keep us from burning calories—automobiles, elevators, television, power lawnmowers, and snowblowers—and it's not surprising that we're paying the price with ever-expanding waistlines.

Psychological, emotional, and behavioral factors also contribute to eating habits. Weight-loss experts say that, as children, many people learn to associate calorie-dense foods with love, perhaps because their mother always had a dish of ice cream or a plate of cookies at the ready to soothe them during times of distress or disappointment. As a result, they may be programmed to reach for those same foods as adults whenever they feel the need for love or comforting.

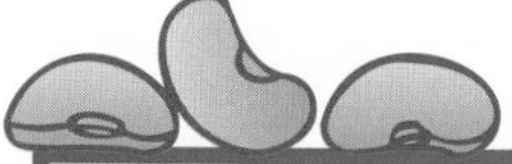

What really works

Although losing weight is difficult, it is not impossible. Weight-control experts agree that a combination of healthy eating habits and increased physical activity works best. They recommend the following:

- Be sure that any changes you make in your diet and exercise habits comfortably fit your lifestyle. Radical changes that you cannot maintain over the long term make losing weight and keeping it off more difficult.
- Set reasonable goals. Aim to lose about 1 to 2 pounds (0.5 to 0.9 kilogram) per week and maintain the loss.
- Change your eating habits. Replace sugary treats and fatty foods with whole grains, beans, fruits, and vegetables.
- Get enough exercise. Try to accumulate at least 30 minutes of moderate physical activity on most—preferably all—days of the week.

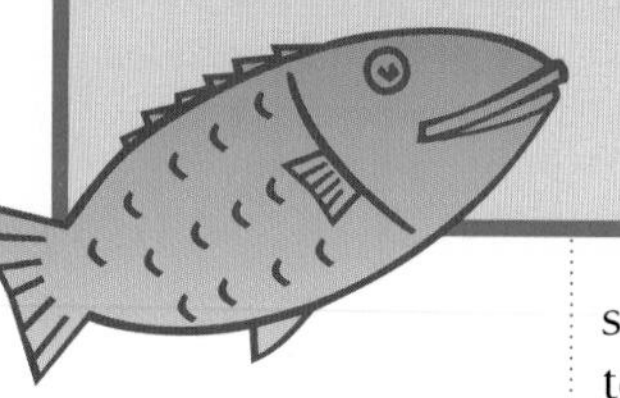

Weight-loss experts have long known that people eat for a variety of reasons besides hunger, grabbing food to relieve depression, stress, loneliness, or simple boredom. Some studies suggest, however, that there is a biochemical basis to such behavior. Researchers speculate that a chemical in our brain called serotonin curbs appetite by causing a feeling of fullness and satiety, and that certain fatty foods—such as chocolate—increase the level of serotonin in our brains. (Antidepressant medications also achieve their effect by elevating serotonin levels in the brain.) Thus, it may be that someone who reaches for a chocolate bar when unhappy is really trying to achieve the feeling of satisfaction that higher serotonin levels bring. Still, not everyone picks up the chocolate habit.

The set-point theory

Even before the genetic studies, it had become clear to many weight-loss experts that losing weight was not as simple a proposition as burning more calories than you consumed. For years, a number of experts speculated that another mechanism was involved. According to their hypothesis, the hypothalamus has its own idea of how much fat a person should store—called the set point—and it tries to maintain that level despite a person's efforts to reduce.

Someone who is obese, the theory says, may simply have a higher set point than someone who is thin. If the person goes on a diet and starts to shed pounds, the hypothalamus senses that body fat levels have fallen below the set point and takes action: It slows metabolism, reducing the amount of fat calories burned, so that body weight stays put.

Some drugs used to treat obesity

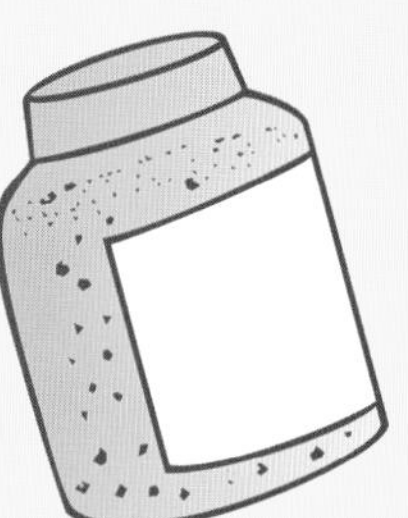

Doctors agree that no "magic pill" can take off fat and keep it off. But they sometimes prescribe drugs that can speed weight loss for individuals whose obesity poses a serious health risk. A number of drugs were available and others were in development as of mid-1996. Sibutramine awaited FDA approval, orlistat had reached the last stages of clinical trials, and clinical trials of leptin had begun.

Generic (brand) name	Action
Over-the-counter drugs	
Benzocaine (Permathene and other brand names)	Diminishes appetite by reducing sensation in taste buds
Phenylpropanolamine hydrochloride (Dexatrim, Acutrim, and other brands)	Suppresses appetite.
Prescription drugs	
Amphetamine (Dexedrine, Desoxyn, and others)	Stimulates central nervous system, accelerates metabolism, and suppresses appetite.
Benzphetamine hydrochloride (Didrex)	Suppresses appetite.
Dexfenfluramine (Redux)	Suppresses appetite.
Diethylproprion (Anorex, Tenuate, Tepanil)	Suppresses appetite.
Fenfluramine (Pondimin)	Suppresses appetite.
Mazindol (Sanorex, Mazanor)	Suppresses appetite.
Phendimetrazine tartrate (Plegine and other brand names)	Suppresses appetite.
Phentermine (Ionamin and other brand names)	Suppresses appetite. One study found that phentermine and fenfluramine are more effective when used in combination (fen/phen).
Drugs under development	
Leptin	Suppresses appetite.
Orlistat (Xenical)	Limits the absorption of dietary fat.
Sibutramine (Meridia)	Suppresses appetite and accelerates metabolism.

Critically reviewed by Hal Seim, M.D.

A study reported in March 1995 in *The New England Journal of Medicine* provided support for the set-point theory. Researchers at Rockefeller University placed both obese and nonobese adults on a liquid diet through which they lost 10 to 20 percent of their weight. The researchers then checked the amount of energy each of the study participants burned when at rest and found that everyone's body burned fewer calories after they lost weight.

Another stage of the study had participants eat as much as they wanted of whatever foods they chose until they weighed at least 10 percent more than their usual weight. The researchers found that the regulatory mechanism continued to work in all of the individuals. Their bodies compensated for the weight gain by burning calories at a faster rate to restore their weight to its previous, lower level.

Little wonder that losing weight and keeping it off is so difficult. But it is not impossible. Studies have shown that people can adjust their set point by changing their eating and exercise habits. However, these changes must be permanent to maintain the new, lower set point.

Does dieting really work?

For many years, articles on weight control claimed that 95 percent of dieters regained their lost weight within a few years. However, scientists at the Yale Center for Eating and Weight Disorders and other researchers note that this figure may be too pessimistic, since it came from a study conducted in the 1960's at a hospital clinic, a

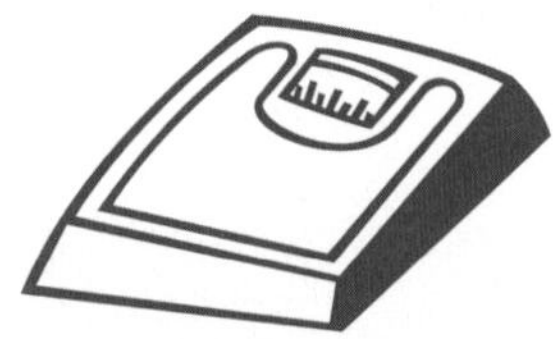

Latest guidelines for healthy weight

In 1995, the federal government issued new guidelines for healthy weight. Women—who generally have less muscle and bone than men—should aim for the lower end of the range, while men—especially those who are muscular or have a large frame—can weigh in the higher end of the range. The table is based on height without shoes and weight without clothes.

Source: U.S. Department of Agriculture.

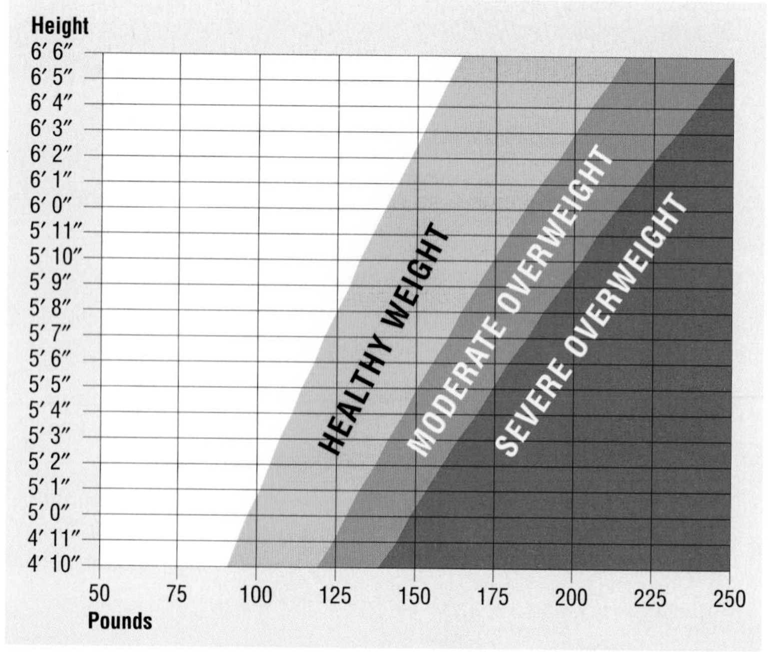

Body mass index

Most weight-loss experts prefer a calculation called body mass index (BMI) to a standard height and weight chart. The BMI is derived from statistics on deaths and illnesses associated with obesity, and it provides a more accurate reflection of body fat. Doctors consider a BMI of 19 to 25 an indication of a healthy weight. A BMI of 27 to 29 signals borderline overweight. And a BMI higher than 30 generally indicates a health risk from obesity.

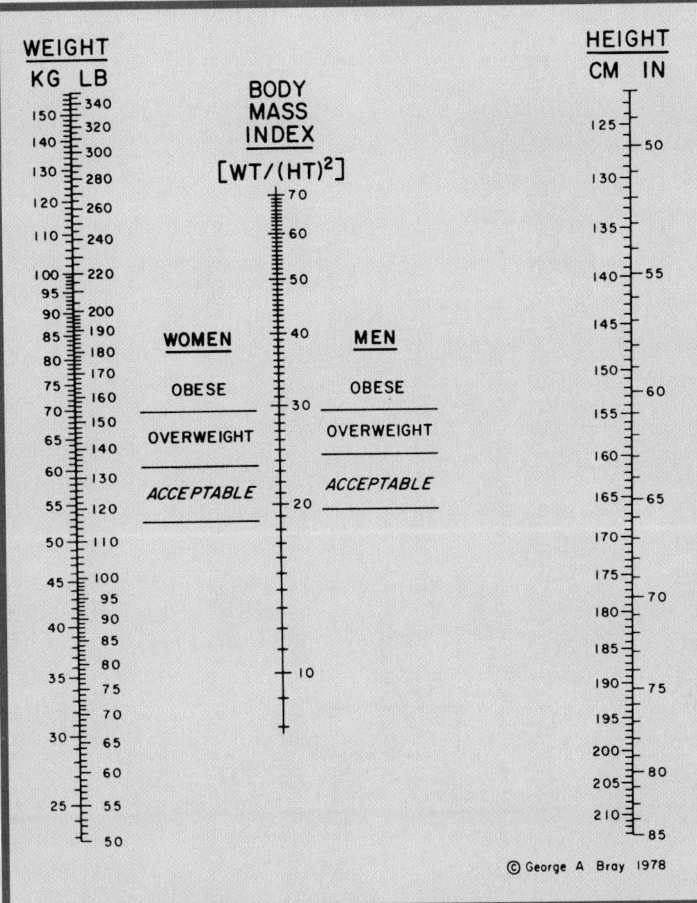

Finding your body mass index

Find your weight in the column at the left and your height in the column at the right. Draw a line connecting those two numbers. The point at which the line intersects the middle column is your BMI.

Body mass index and risk of premature death

Risks for a woman who is 5 feet 5 inches tall.

BMI	Weight	Increase in risk
Less than 19	Less than 120 lbs.	Lowest risk
19-24.9	120-149	+20%
25-26.9	150-160	+30%
27-28.9	161-175	+60%
29-31.9	176-195	+110%
Greater than 32	Greater than 195 lbs.	+120%

Sources: JoAnn E. Manson, M.D./*New England Journal of Medicine*; Associated Press.

Is gaining a little weight really dangerous?

A study published in September 1995, which tracked the weight of more than 115,000 nurses over the course of 16 years, found that women who gained 22 pounds or more after age 18 increased their chances of dying from heart disease or another medical condition associated with obesity. Women with a BMI of less than 19 were least likely to die prematurely. The risk of premature death increased with BMI by the percentages shown at the left.

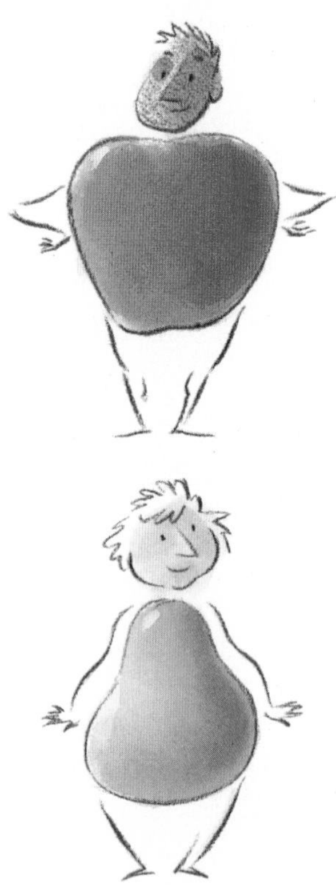

Are you an apple or a pear?

Where people store fat also affects their health. People who carry excess fat in the abdomen—primarily men—are said to have an apple-shaped figure. Studies have found that they are at greater-than-normal risk for such conditions as coronary artery disease and stroke. People who carry excess fat in the hips, buttocks, and thighs—primarily women—are said to have a pear-shaped figure and are at less risk for these conditions.

setting that tends to attract people with a history of diet failures.

A survey of dieters in organized weight-loss programs, conducted by the National Institutes of Health (NIH) and reported in 1992, found that dieters regained one-third to two-thirds of their lost weight within a year and nearly all the lost weight within five years. But a *Consumer Reports* survey cited by the Yale Center was more optimistic: 25 percent of 90,000 people who dieted on their own or through organized programs kept the weight off over the long term.

The best way to lose weight by dieting, most weight-loss experts agree, is to substitute low-fat foods for those high in fat; to eat more fruits, vegetables, and whole grains; and to set a goal of losing no more than 1 to 2 pounds (0.5 to 0.9 kilogram) a week. Such a diet is relatively easy to maintain in the long term and the body can adjust to it easily. Furthermore, consistently eating a low-fat diet helps keep the body's set point at a lower level so that lost pounds stay off.

Dieters who want to lose weight quickly may turn to fad diets that strictly limit the foods allowed or to extremely low-calorie diets. However, while the initial weight loss on such diets is encouraging, people who follow them generally end up regaining the weight they have lost. Neither type of diet can be maintained, and neither offers the opportunity to develop sensible, sustainable eating habits.

Diets that are extremely low in calories—fewer than 800 calories a day—can also cause serious health problems, according to the American Dietetic Association. A panel assembled by NIH in 1992 determined that diets of 800 calories or fewer should only be undertaken with medical supervision. In the short term, the NIH panel said, these diets can cause such symptoms as fatigue, hair loss, and dizziness. Over the long term, the diets increase the risk of gallstones and gallbladder disease.

Additional health risks of extremely low-calorie diets were reported by researchers from St. Luke's-Roosevelt Hospital Center and Columbia University College of Physicians and Surgeons in New York City in October 1993. The risks they named included liver problems, because the ultralow-fat diets rapidly deplete fat stores in the liver; irregular heartbeat and other circulatory system problems, because the diets cause water loss and with it the loss of key minerals that affect heart rate; and elevated levels of uric acid, which can contribute to kidney stones and gout. For these reasons, a physician should monitor the dieter's condition and prescribe supplements as needed to prevent or minimize such consequences.

Exercise can help

In addition to diet, exercise is important in lowering the level of body fat that the set point defends, according to an editorial that accompanied the Rockefeller University set-point study. And an October 1993 review of weight-loss studies in the *Annals of Internal Medicine* pointed out that, while exercise alone—with no change in diet—typically results in a weight loss of only 4 to 7 pounds (2 to

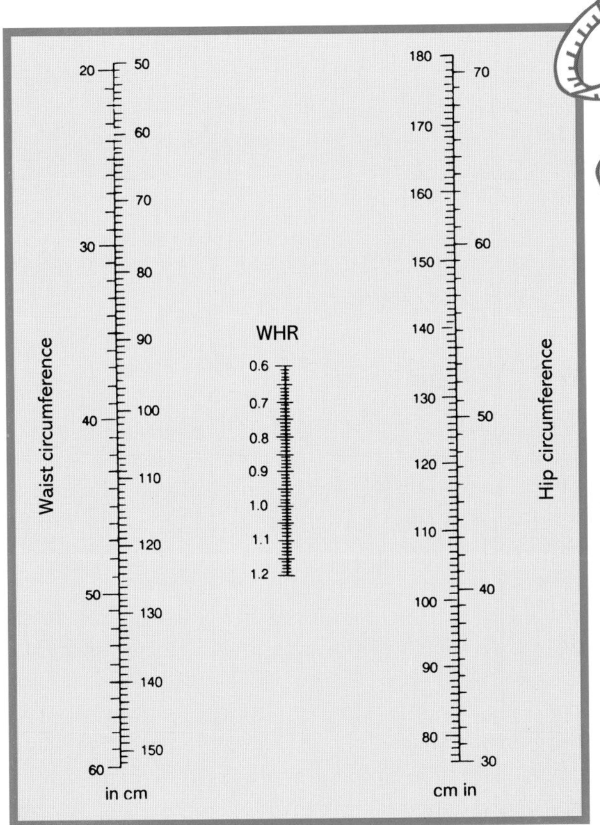

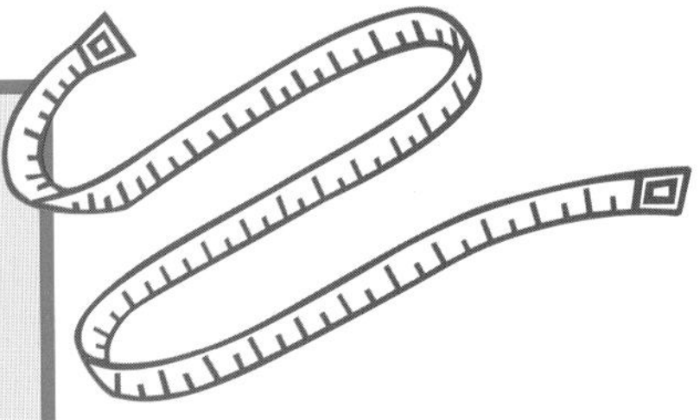

Waist-to-hip ratio

Your waist-to-hip ratio indicates how much fat you are storing in your abdomen. To calculate it, measure your waist at the narrowest point between your ribs and your navel and find the figure in the column at the left. Measure your hips around the widest part of the buttocks and find the figure in the column at the right. Draw a line between the two points. The point at which the line intersects the middle column is your waist-to-hip ratio (WHR). Doctors generally agree that a healthy WHR is less than 1.0 in men and 0.8 in women.

Source: National Research Council.

3 kilograms), exercise serves other important weight-control functions. It increases muscle mass, and muscle cells need more calories to maintain themselves than fat cells do. Therefore, exercise can help keep weight off in the long term more effectively than dieting alone can. Even more important, according to the *Annals* article, exercise changes the distribution of body fat.

For years, doctors suspected that where people carry fat can be just as significant as how much fat they carry. Our bodies store fat in two distinct areas: the abdomen and the hips and thighs. People who store excess fat at or above the waist, in the abdomen, have an "apple" shape, while those who store fat below the waist—in the hips, buttocks, and thighs—have a "pear" shape. Men are more likely to have an apple shape, and women to have a pear shape.

Studies have shown that the apple shape is associated with a higher-than-average risk for high blood pressure, heart disease, stroke, and diabetes. The pear shape poses a smaller health risk than the apple shape does. Because fat in the hips, buttocks, and thighs is stored just under the skin, researchers think that it has less effect on body organs than the deeper abdominal fat does.

Exercise can help to shift fat from the more dangerous area of the abdomen and thus improve an individual's overall health. The minimum amount of exercise that the Centers for Disease Control and

Prevention and the American College of Sports Medicine recommended in 1995 for all adults was at least 30 minutes of moderate exercise a day, preferably on all days of the week. "Moderate" exercise is about equal to a brisk walk and allows people to maintain their weight or to lose a small amount of weight. To shift fat from the abdomen, weight-loss experts recommend more vigorous exercise, including a 30- to 60-minute aerobic workout three to five times per week and muscle-strengthening exercises, such as weight training, two or three times per week.

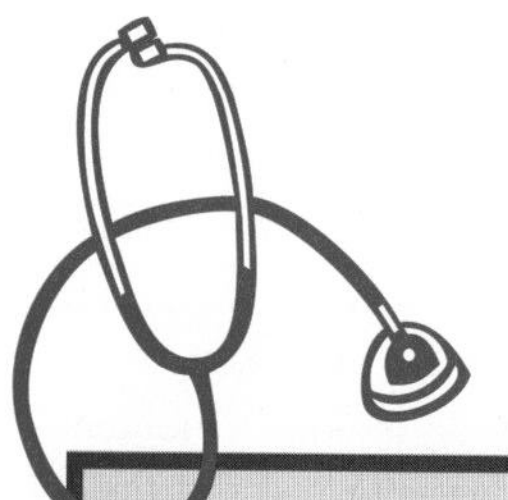

Some health risks associated with obesity

People who weigh 20 percent more than the recommended weight for their height face a higher-than-average risk of developing the following medical conditions:

- Certain cancers, such as colon cancer
- Diabetes
- Gallstones
- Gout
- Heart disease
- High blood pressure
- Lower-back problems
- Osteoarthritis
- Sleep disorders, such as sleep apnea
- Stroke

Source: *Annals of Internal Medicine*, Oct. 1, 1993.

Weight-loss drugs

While long-term changes in diet and exercise are most often recommended for weight loss, they can be daunting. Out of frustration, some people look to weight-loss drugs for deliverance. Among the medications tried over the years are a group of drugs called amphetamines. Amphetamines, which include Benzedrine and Dexedrine, and amphetamine derivatives, such as phenylpropanolamine, stimulate the central nervous system, accelerate the metabolic rate, and minimize appetite. Physicians warn that these drugs are potentially dangerous because they can elevate blood pressure, quicken the heart rate, and cause dependency in some people. Also, people who regularly take amphetamines need to increase the dosage over time to achieve the same effects.

Many patients in the mid-1990's began to ask their physicians to prescribe a combination of two appetite suppressants, fenfluramine and phentermine (fen/phen). Fenfluramine inhibits uptake of the brain chemical serotonin, leaving more of it in the system. Therefore, the patient feels full longer. But the drug can cause drowsiness, nausea, vomiting, diarrhea, and dizziness. Phentermine acts upon two chemicals in the brain, dopamine and norepinephrine, and appears to increase metabolism without the risk of addiction that amphetamines carry. But it can cause insomnia, nausea, and vomiting. Although doctors had prescribed these two drugs since they were approved by the Food and Drug Administration (FDA) in the 1970's, it was only in 1992 that a study showed that the drugs were more effective and had fewer side effects when used together than when used alone.

In the study reported in 1992, doctors at the University of Rochester divided 121 obese patients into two groups, giving one group fen/phen and the other a *placebo* (substance with no active ingredients). All the people in the study weighed from 30 to 80 percent more than their recommended body weight. Both groups also participated in the same behavior-modification program, which included exercise and calorie restriction. After 8½ months, those receiving fen/phen had lost an average 16 percent of their initial weight, compared with an average of 5 percent for those receiving the placebo. Some participated in the study for 3½ years with few side effects. The most frequent side effect reported was a dry mouth. However, as with many weight-loss drugs, once people stopped taking fen/phen, they tended to put their lost weight right back on.

Patients with a BMI of 30 or greater might benefit from a new drug approved by the FDA in 1996, according to the NIH. Dexfenfluramine, sold as Redux, triggers the release of serotonin, decreasing the appetite. Though year-long tests on 900 obese men and women showed that Redux helped people lose less than 10 percent of their body weight, some doctors believed that the drug was still important, since even a 10 percent loss improves the health of a severely obese person.

What lies ahead?

The hopes of many overweight people by the mid-1990's rode on leptin and other newly recognized components of the body's weight-regulating mechanism, and pharmaceutical companies rushed to begin their own research. Some researchers looked toward a leptin pill that might suppress appetite by tricking the brain into thinking that the stomach was full. At least one drug manufacturer began human testing of a leptin drug in 1996.

Whether leptin would provide the answer was still unclear. One study found that some obese people already have high levels of leptin, while other researchers pointed out that these individuals may be less responsive to leptin than other people and thus require even larger amounts of the hormone to transmit the message of fullness effectively. For those individuals whose genes do not produce leptin, a leptin drug might well be the answer.

Drug companies also were studying leptin receptors—docking sites—on nerve cells in the brain. Leptin enters a cell by first attaching to a receptor on the cell's surface, and defective leptin receptors might prevent the transmission of the message leptin carries. But the receptor mechanism that scientists had studied by mid-1996 seemed to work well in obese people, and researchers speculated that the problem might lie elsewhere in the hypothalamus and involve other elements still to be uncovered.

Any drug that scientists may develop as a result of the latest genetic research would still require years of testing before gaining FDA approval. And scientists caution that weight loss may never become as easy as swallowing a pill. Until we learn more about the body's complex mechanisms for regulating fat storage, doctors say that eating a prudent diet and exercising regularly is probably the best prescription for getting weight under control. •••

Once considered exotic technology, lasers are becoming standard tools for many types of surgery.

Laser Surgery Comes into Focus

By Jeff Hecht

A PATIENT SITS QUIETLY IN A DARKENED ROOM as an eye surgeon peers through an optical microscope in an attempt to find tiny abnormalities deep within the patient's eye that threaten her vision. Satisfied, the surgeon moves back from the eyepiece, slips on a pair of colored goggles, and pushes a button that fires a carefully controlled pulse of laser light into the patient's eye. This delicate procedure is over in 30 minutes. Every year, hundreds of thousands of people in the United States undergo laser surgery for a variety of reasons, from the treatment of eye disorders and enlarged prostate glands to the smoothing of wrinkles and removal of tattoos.

Physicians began using lasers in surgical procedures in the early 1960's. The first laser surgeries involved the eyes or skin alone, but researchers have since discovered many more procedures that lasers can successfully perform. In 1996, nearly 20,000 lasers were in medical use in the United States, and lasers had become the standard tools for dozens of surgical procedures.

A laser is a device that produces a narrow, powerful beam of light. Unlike the light from a light bulb, which scatters in many directions over a wide area, light from a laser is highly concentrated and aimed in a single direction. Most lasers used in medicine produce visible

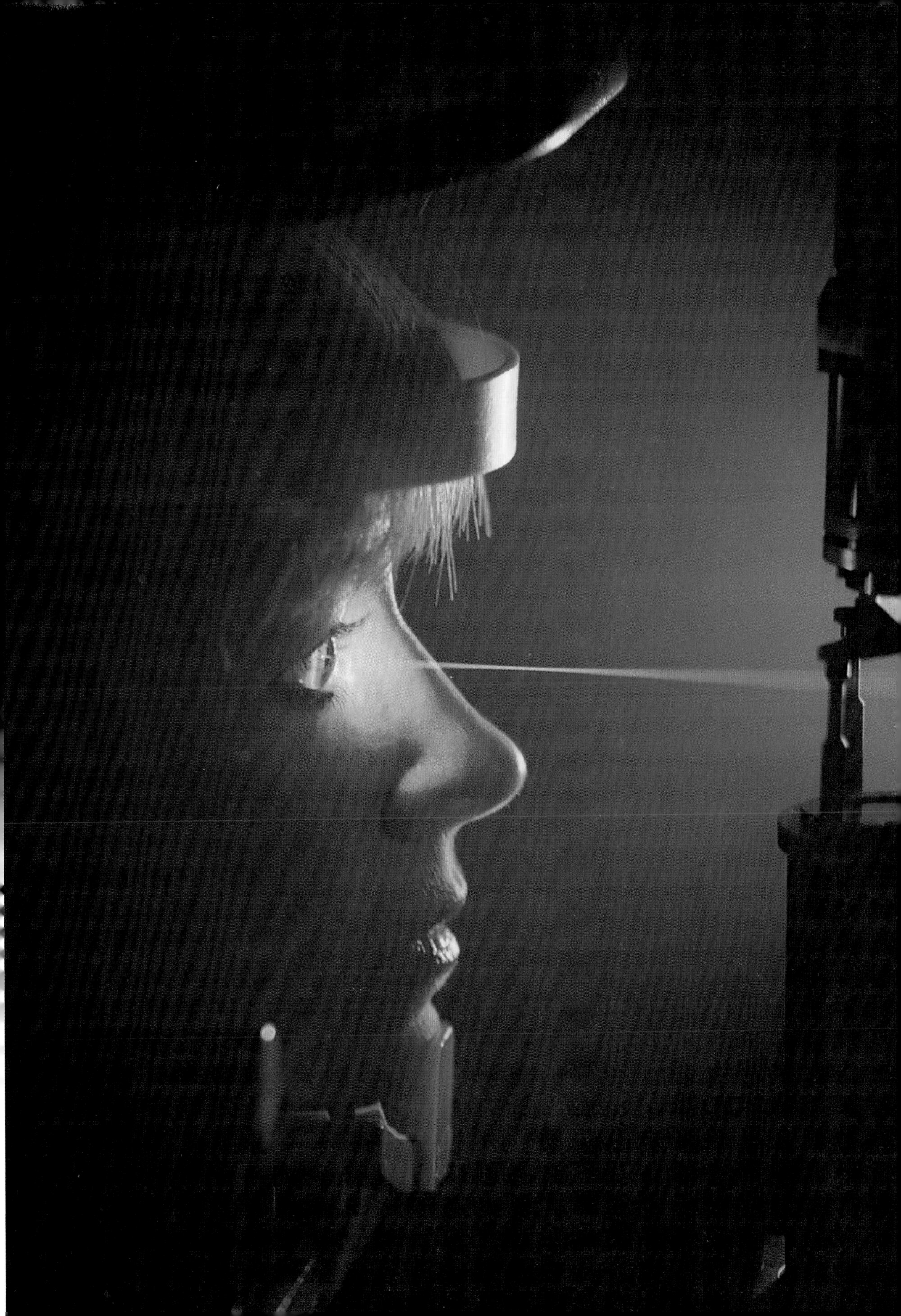

How lasers work

Lasers are devices that produce a highly concentrated beam of light. Mirrors inside the laser *amplify* (strengthen) the light, and a lens focuses it into a narrow beam that a surgeon can aim with great precision. The intense heat created within the targeted tissue when it absorbs laser light destroys the tissue's cells.

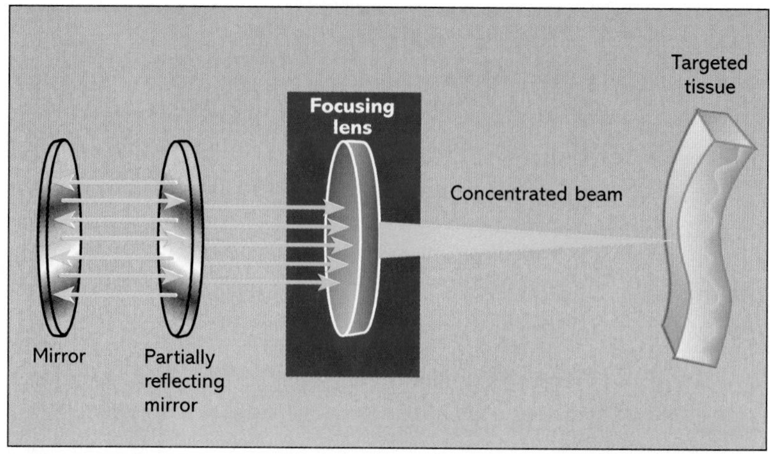

light, though some produce invisible light in the form of infrared and ultraviolet radiation.

All laser surgery depends on the absorption of laser light by the body's cells. The light heats the cells—killing or, in some cases, even vaporizing them. Lasers work most effectively when the targeted cells fully absorb the laser energy. Because body tissues vary in their ability to absorb different wavelengths of light, the choice of laser wavelength is critical for successful treatment. (The wavelength of light determines its color.) Cells in the light-sensitive retina, for example, absorb green light better than surrounding tissues do, so surgeons can treat damaged retinas with green light without harming other parts of the eye.

Lasers excel at delicate surgery, especially in hard-to-reach places. Because lasers produce such a narrow beam of light, they permit great control and precision. Thus, a laser can make a far smaller incision than a scalpel and cause less damage to surrounding tissue. In addition, less blood is lost during laser surgery because the heat produced by the laser quickly seals blood vessels after the laser cuts through them. Furthermore, with the aid of extremely thin threads of plastic or glass known as optical fibers, lasers can deliver their energy to joints and to organs deep inside the body, thus avoiding the need for a large incision.

Lasers are not suitable for all types of surgery, however. Most medical lasers are designed to slice through a very thin film of tissue, and removing a large tumor or polyp with a laser would be extremely time-consuming. Moreover, using a laser to burn away a cancerous tumor could in many cases endanger the patient by scattering cancer cells into nearby tissue or into the bloodstream.

Nor have lasers proved successful in every procedure for which they have been tested. Experiments using lasers to clear fatty deposits from arteries, for example, have been largely unsuccessful because the heat produced by the laser can damage artery walls. And the success of a laser procedure to correct nearsightedness depends

The author:

Jeff Hecht is an editor of *Laser Focus World* magazine and the author of the book *Understanding Lasers.*

on how well the eye heals. Because the healing process varies from person to person, it is difficult to predict how precise the correction will be.

Lasers in eye surgery

Lasers are most often used for treating disorders inside the eye. The ability to aim a laser with great precision at a tiny target makes it especially well-suited for this kind of surgery. But precision is not the laser's only advantage in treating eyes. Even before lasers came into medical use in the 1960's, *ophthalmologists* (eye specialists) used sunlight and intense light from flash lamps to treat a vision-threatening disorder in which the retina becomes detached from the back of the eye. The light burned the retina, and when the burned area healed, scar tissue helped weld the retina back in place. The light was targeted at such a small area of the retina that vision was not affected. Today, laser surgery is the standard method for reattaching detached retinas.

Treating diseases of the retina

The leading cause of blindness in people from the ages of 20 to 64 has long been diabetic retinopathy, a common complication of diabetes. In people with diabetes, blood sugar builds to abnormally high levels. This build-up can harm eyesight by causing blood vessels that nourish the retina to leak, close up, or proliferate. As a result, blood may enter the clear, jellylike fluid that fills the eyeball, making the fluid opaque and gradually obscuring vision.

If diabetic retinopathy is detected early, laser surgery can destroy the abnormal vessels before blood leaks into the fluid. For less than a second, the surgeon fires the laser at a spot on the retina, then moves to another spot. This procedure causes virtually no pain. Patients typically receive 200 to 300 laser pulses in each of several sessions in the physician's office. These pulses cover the affected part of the retina and kill the cells of the abnormal blood vessels.

Laser treatment for diabetic retinopathy is now routine. Although lasers do not permanently stop the spread of these abnormal vessels, they can slow the process, granting people extra years of

Advantages of laser surgery

For many procedures, lasers have advantages over traditional surgery. These advantages include:

- Less damage to surrounding tissue because of a laser's precise aim. This results in shorter healing time and less scarring.
- Minimal bleeding because lasers seal off blood vessels as soon they they are cut.
- Reduced risk of infection because lasers sterilize as they move through the body.

sight. Even in advanced stages of the disease, laser surgery can spare some patients a far more invasive surgical procedure to remove the blood-stained fluid.

Lasers can also treat some cases of macular degeneration, a cause of vision loss that primarily troubles older people. Those who have the disorder lose the ability to see objects in their direct line of sight, though *peripheral* (side) vision remains unaffected. Most cases result from a breakdown or thinning of the tissues of the *macula*—the central part of the retina responsible for sharp vision. There is no treatment for this form of the disease.

In about 10 percent of macular degeneration cases, leakage of fluid from blood vessels within the macula blurs central vision. Laser treatment can seal the vessels and prevent or delay severe vision loss in such cases, but only if treatment begins as soon as vision problems are noticed.

Lasers for eye disorders

Lasers are especially well-suited for delicate eye procedures because their narrow beam can be aimed with great precision. Eye disorders commonly treated with lasers Include:

- Cataract complication, a blurring of vision that sometimes occurs after the removal of a *cataract* (clouded lens). Lasers open a hole in the lens capsule to let in light.
- Detached retina, a condition in which the retina pulls away from the back of the eye. Lasers weld the retina back in place.
- Diabetic retinopathy, a complication of diabetes characterized by abnormal growth of tiny blood vessels on the retina. Lasers slow the spread of these vessels.
- Glaucoma, a condition characterized by elevated pressure of the fluid in the eye. Lasers open drainage canals so that fluid flows from the eye, lowering pressure.
- Macular degeneration, a deterioration of the central part of the retina caused by leaky blood vessels. Lasers seal the leaks.

Fighting cataracts and glaucoma

Lasers are also helpful as a follow-up to cataract surgery. A cataract is a clouding of the lens of the eye that blurs vision. The lens is a clear structure about the size and shape of an aspirin tablet. It helps bend incoming light rays so that they meet on the retina and produce clear vision. The gradual clouding from a cataract occurs most often in older people and once doomed them to blindness. Ophthalmologists can now restore vision by removing the jellylike interior of the natural lens and implanting a plastic replacement.

After cataract surgery, a thin membrane just behind the lens holds the artificial lens in place. This membrane clouds over in about 30 percent of cataract patients. By firing laser pulses lasting just a few billionths of a second at an area only $\frac{2}{1,000}$ inch (0.05 millimeter) across, an ophthalmologist can slit the membrane, permitting light to pass through it and enabling the patient to see again.

Another sight-destroying disorder than can accompany aging is glaucoma, a condition in which fluid builds up inside the eye. In people who have glaucoma, the fluid that nourishes the front of the eye does not drain properly, and pressure increases inside the eye as a result. This pressure can damage the optic nerve and lead to blindness.

Using lasers to treat diabetic retinopathy

Lasers are useful for treating a complication of diabetes known as diabetic retinopathy in which tiny blood vessels proliferate on the retina at the back of the eye.

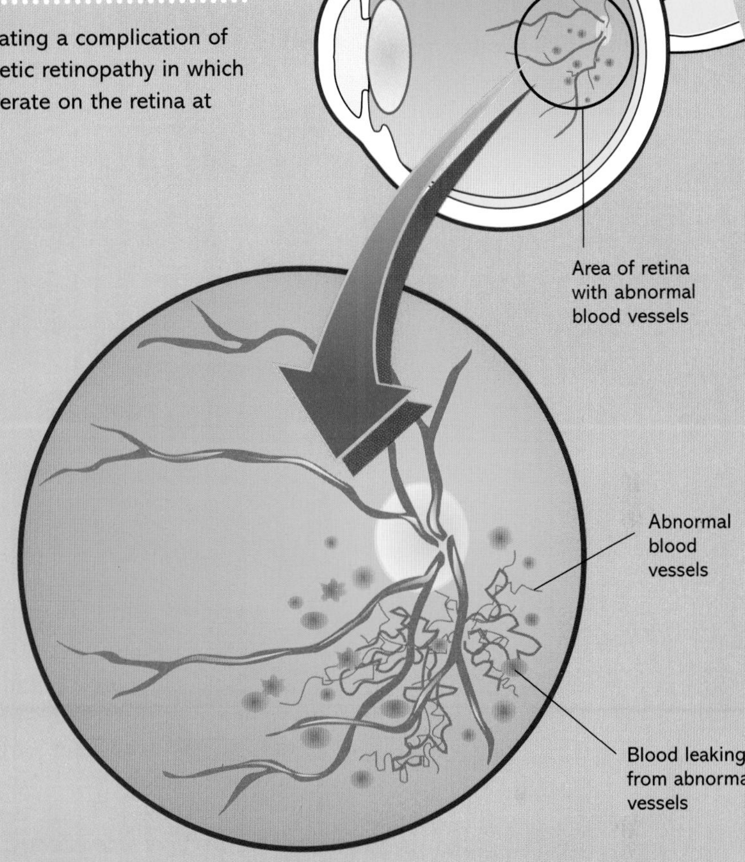

These abnormal vessels are fragile and may leak, blurring vision and, in severe cases, leading to blindness. The leaks may occur suddenly as a result of sharp movements of the head, or they may develop slowly over years.

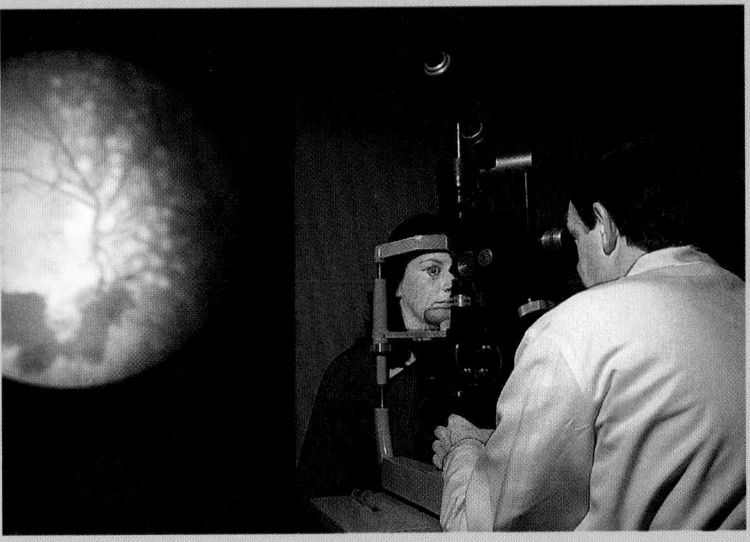

A surgeon views a patient's damaged retina through the optical microscope of a laser system. The two red splotches indicate leaks from blood vessels, and the numerous orange spots mark areas where the surgeon has burned tiny holes in the retina with a laser to stop the bleeding.

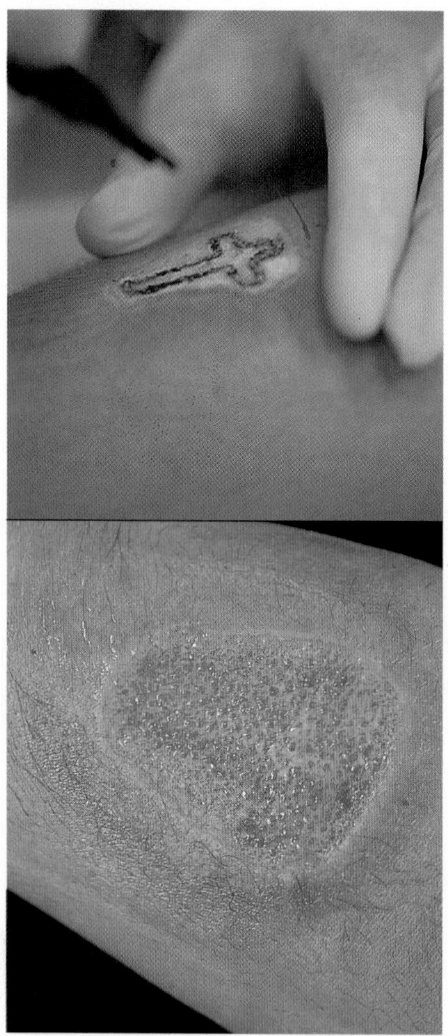

Laser removal of tattoos can require as many as 20 treatments. Some pigments are easier to remove than others because they absorb laser light more readily. The first treatments gradually lighten the tattoo, *top*, but the skin may need several weeks to heal following tattoo removal, *bottom*.

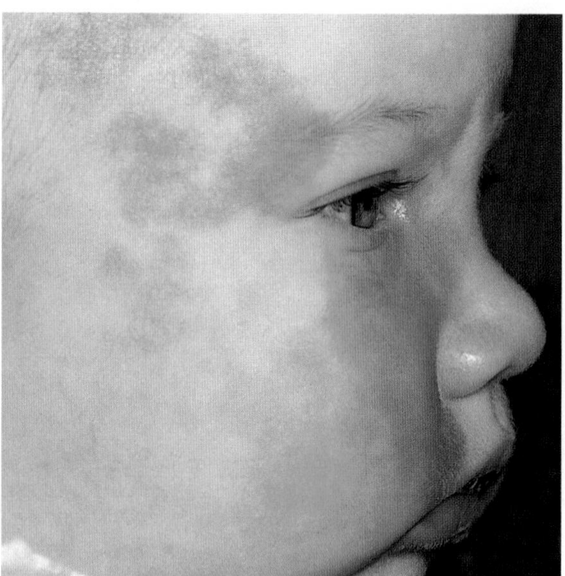

Using a laser, an ophthalmologist can open up the spongy tissue that normally drains the eye so that fluid flows through the tissue more readily and pressure inside the eye is reduced.

Eye drops can control many cases of chronic glaucoma as effectively as surgery can. Surgeons tend to recommend laser surgery only when the condition develops suddenly or when eye drops have either failed to lower the pressure in the eye or caused severe side effects. These side effects can include elevated blood pressure and breathing difficulties.

Surgeons cannot guarantee how long the laser treatment for glaucoma will remain effective. But the procedure can be repeated if the eye's drainage system clogs up again. Conventional surgery cuts a new channel in the eye to improve drainage. Although the procedure permanently lowers pressure in the eye, it also carries about a 5 percent risk of significant loss of vision. Laser surgery carries virtually no risk of vision loss.

Laser surgery for nearsightedness

Far more people need glasses to see clearly than suffer from potentially blinding vision disorders. Laser surgery is now being offered as an alternative to glasses for correcting vision. In October 1995, the United States Food and Drug Admin-

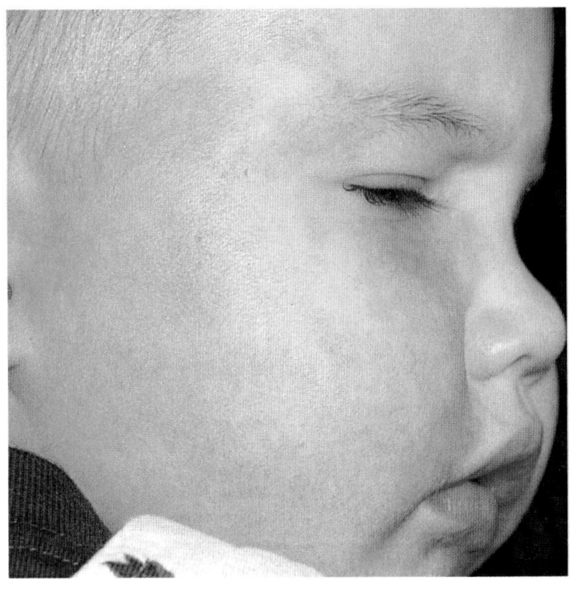

Lasers are especially successful at bleaching birthmarks such as this infant's port-wine stain, *opposite page*. The laser lightens or removes the birthmark by destroying blood vessels just below the skin that produce the darkened patches, *left*.

istration (FDA), which regulates medical devices, approved a highly automated laser system that corrects vision by reshaping the cornea. The procedure is known as photorefractive keratectomy (PRK).

The eye's ability to focus light on the retina is a requirement for sharp vision. Ideally, the lens and the cornea should work together in focusing light onto the retina, but in many people they do not. When light focuses in front of the retina, a person is *myopic* (nearsighted) and distant objects appear out of focus. When light focuses behind the retina, a person is *hyperopic* (farsighted) and near objects appear blurred.

Glasses and contact lenses bend incoming light to compensate for the eye's defects. Laser surgery reshapes the cornea to accomplish the same goal. The procedure involves shaving a sliver of cells from the outermost layer of the cornea. By mid-1996, the FDA had approved PRK only for mild to moderate myopia, and researchers were still testing the procedure's ability to correct hyperopia and severe myopia.

In PRK, the surgeon first peels back a surface membrane covering the cornea. The surgeon programs the computer-controlled laser system to the desired optical correction. The system measures the surface of the eye and calculates how much tissue should be removed to achieve the desired

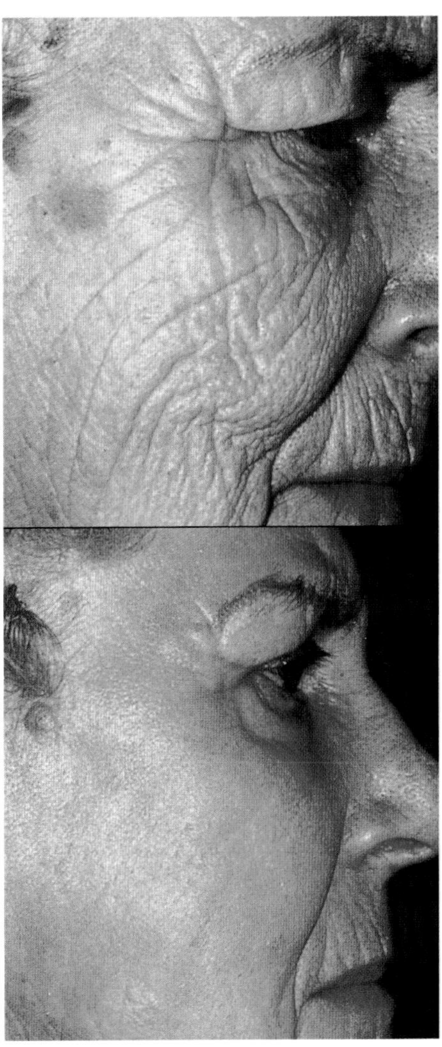

Lasers can smooth away facial wrinkles by removing a layer of skin cells. Deep wrinkles line this woman's face before laser treatment, *top*. Several months after treatment, new skin cells have grown in that are firmer and less inclined to wrinkle, *bottom*.

Where lasers are most effective

Although lasers are most commonly used to treat skin problems and disorders of the eye, the concentrated light from a laser can treat disorders in other parts of the body as well.

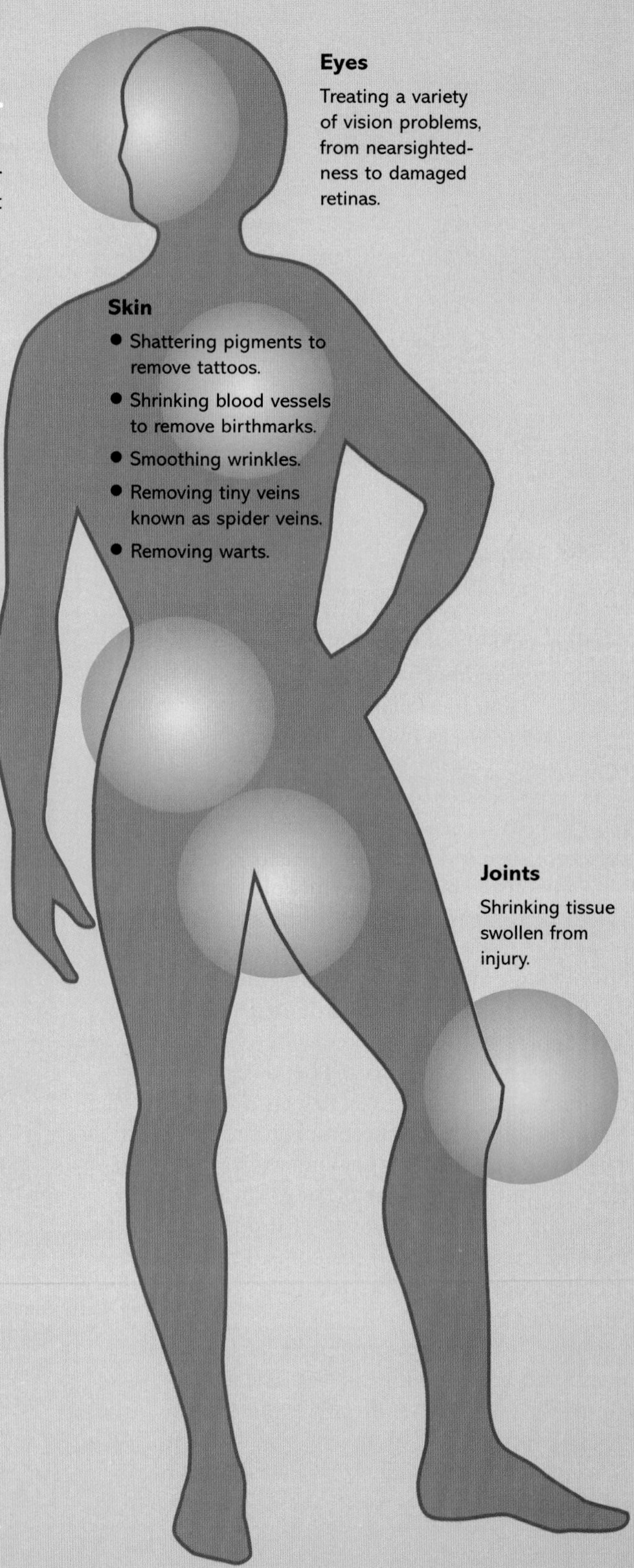

Eyes

Treating a variety of vision problems, from nearsightedness to damaged retinas.

Skin

- Shattering pigments to remove tattoos.
- Shrinking blood vessels to remove birthmarks.
- Smoothing wrinkles.
- Removing tiny veins known as spider veins.
- Removing warts.

Digestive and urinary tract

- Healing bleeding *ulcers* (sores) in the stomach.
- Shrinking hemorrhoids by cutting off their blood supply.
- Trimming an enlarged *prostate* (gland surrounding the urethra in men).
- Breaking up hard objects called kidney stones in the *urethra* (tube through which urine leaves the body).

Female reproductive system

- Removing cancerous and precancerous growths from the vagina and cervix.
- Removing genital warts.
- Removing tissue that has spread from the *endometrium* (lining of the uterus) to other areas of the abdomen.

Joints

Shrinking tissue swollen from injury.

correction. Then it aims pulses of ultraviolet light, each lasting 10 billionths to 20 billionths of a second, at the exposed cornea. The surgeon monitors the laser as it removes a thin sheet of surface tissue from an area of the cornea at least ¼ inch (6 millimeters) wide.

The aftereffects of the surgery can be painful for a few days, but medication can usually control the pain. However, PRK patients may experience fluctuations in their eyesight for six months to a year, before their vision finally stabilizes. Studies have shown that in 95 percent of patients PRK improves vision to 20/40 or better. (A score of 20/20 on a vision test is considered perfect.) Someone with 20/40 vision sees sharply from 20 feet (6 meters) an eye chart that a person with perfect vision can see equally sharply at 40 feet (12 meters). For some people, 20/40 vision may constitute a sufficient improvement. Others may be disappointed.

PRK is not for everyone with mild to moderate myopia. The developers of the procedure say only adults whose vision has not changed significantly for at least a year should consider it. As with eyeglasses, a stronger correction may be needed if eyesight worsens. And ophthalmologists stress that PRK does not eliminate the need for reading glasses in people over age 40. Furthermore, by 1996, researchers had followed the effects of the laser treatment for only three years, so long-term changes and possible side effects remain unknown.

Treating skin problems

The qualities that make lasers valuable tools in treating eye disorders also make them well suited for treating skin problems. Precise control enables *dermatologists* (specialists in skin disorders) to take off only the top layer of skin without harming tissue underneath. This property makes lasers useful in smoothing out wrinkles. The new skin cells that grow in after the procedure are presumably tighter than the old cells and thus less inclined to wrinkle. And lasers can aim large amounts of energy at a small area to remove birthmarks and warts.

One of the most effective uses of lasers in dermatology is in bleaching pink, red, or purple birthmarks on the face or neck. About 3 in every 1,000 people are born with these so-called port-wine stains, which are caused by clusters of large blood vessels just beneath the surface of the skin.

Lasers can remove port-wine stains by destroying the blood vessels that produce them. Researchers have found that the hemoglobin molecules in red blood cells absorb more yellow light than skin cells do, and so lasers that emit yellow light are used to lighten port-wine stains. Successful treatment may require six or seven sessions, each lasting about 15 minutes.

As tattoos have grown in popularity among young people, so has the demand for removing these sometimes embarrassing reminders of youthful indiscretions. To remove a tattoo, dermatologists fire laser pulses lasting 10 billionths of a second at the skin, selecting wavelengths absorbed by the particular tattoo pigments. The pulses shatter pigment grains into particles small enough for scavenger cells in the blood to carry off.

Some pigments are easier to remove than others because they absorb laser light more effectively. Blue and black tattoos are easiest to remove; purple and green are harder; and red, yellow, and orange are the most difficult. Dermatologists may use several lasers to target different pigments. Tattoo removal typically requires from 10 to 20 laser sessions, spaced a month or more apart. Even then, the procedure may leave traces of pigment behind. It may also lighten the skin color around the tattoo.

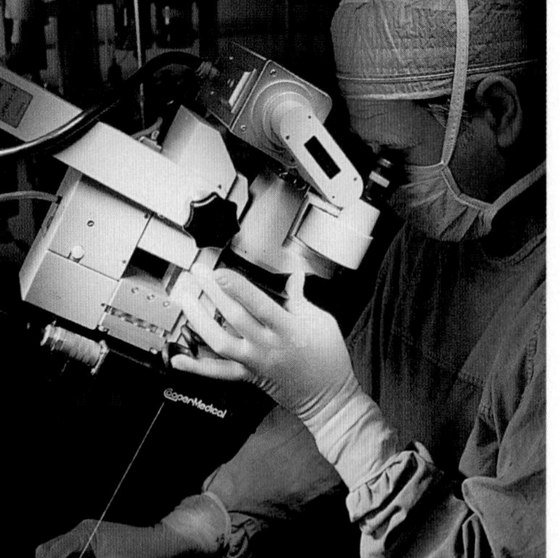

A surgeon directs a pulse of laser energy into a patient's ear. Laser surgery provides easier and safer access than conventional surgery with a scalpel to delicate internal areas of the body, such as the inner ear, the reproductive system, and the vocal cords.

Aiming inside the body

Treatments for the eye and skin are not the only procedures that exploit the laser's ability to remove tiny amounts of surface tissue. *Gynecologists* (physicians who treat disorders of women's reproductive organs) have found lasers to be useful tools for a number or procedures. Not only do lasers burn off surface tissues, they also seal blood vessels, limiting bleeding in the blood-rich organs of the female reproductive tract. Precancerous growths on the surface of the *cervix* (neck of the uterus) can be burned off by laser. Lasers also can destroy genital warts, a viral condition that can affect both men and women.

Lasers make some gynecologic procedures less invasive, sparing patients major surgery. For example, lasers can burn off clusters of cells from the *endometrium* (lining of the uterus) that spread inside the pelvic cavity. This potentially painful condition, known as endometriosis, can impair fertility.

Gynecologists perform the laser procedure by making small incisions in the abdomen through which they insert the laser probe and a viewing device called a laparoscope that is equipped with a tiny television camera.

Because of their exact aim, lasers can perform microsurgery—surgery on tiny structures—in hard-to-reach places such as the *larynx* (voice box). Singers and other people who strain their vocal cords can develop small growths called polyps on the larynx, impairing their voice and sometimes causing internal bleeding. Although physicians can view the polyps through optical instruments, polyp removal by conventional surgery is difficult, and a slip of the hand wielding a scalpel could have disastrous consequences.

Surgeons can aim a laser beam more precisely and steadily with optical fibers than they can direct a scalpel in this small space. After

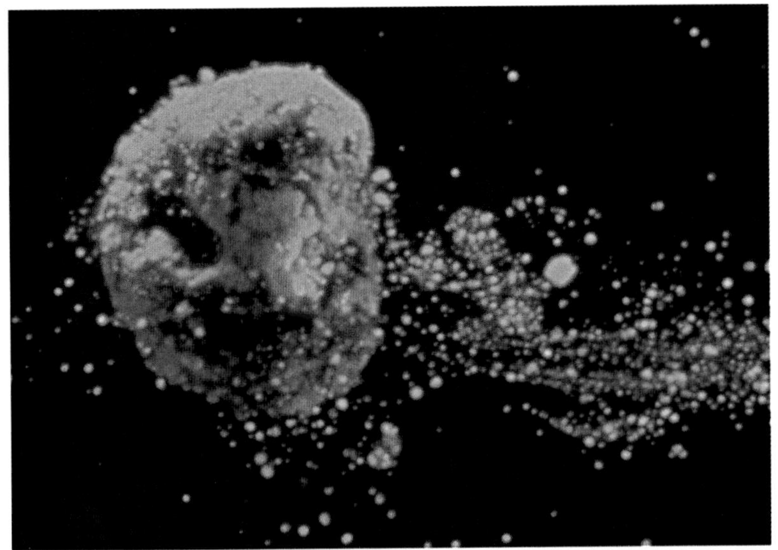

A laser shatters a kidney stone into tiny pieces. Surgeons can deliver pulses of laser light to kidney stones through thin optical fibers that are threaded through the urethra. The small pieces can then pass easily out of the body.

aligning the laser with the target, the surgeon vaporizes the polyp with laser pulses.

One new use of fiber-optic laser surgery is in breaking up "stones" that can form from dissolved minerals in the kidney or bladder. These stones range in size from microscopic to about as large as a golf ball, and they can block urine flow and cause acute pain if they pass into the *urethra* (the tube that carries urine from the bladder). Lasers can break these stones into fragments small enough to pass easily through the urethra.

To shatter the stone, the physician first threads an optical fiber through the urethra and aims the fiber at the stone. Pulses of laser light fired through the fiber heat the stone, eventually producing a shock wave that breaks the stone into fragments small enough to pass easily through the urethra. Drugs and focused *ultrasound* (high-frequency sound waves) are other methods used to break up kidney stones. The heat generated by ultrasound may damage tissues in the kidney and in the tubes called ureters that connect the kidneys with the bladder.

Shrinking enlarged prostates

In March 1996, the FDA approved a laser technique for treating enlargement of the prostate. The prostate is a walnut-sized gland that surrounds the urethra in men. In about half of men over age 50, the prostate gradually expands until it closes the urethra, making urination difficult and painful. Each year, about 400,000 American men undergo surgery for enlarged prostates.

The traditional surgical procedure shrinks the prostate with an instrument called a resectoscope, which the surgeon runs through the urethra to the area where excess tissue has grown. The resectoscope

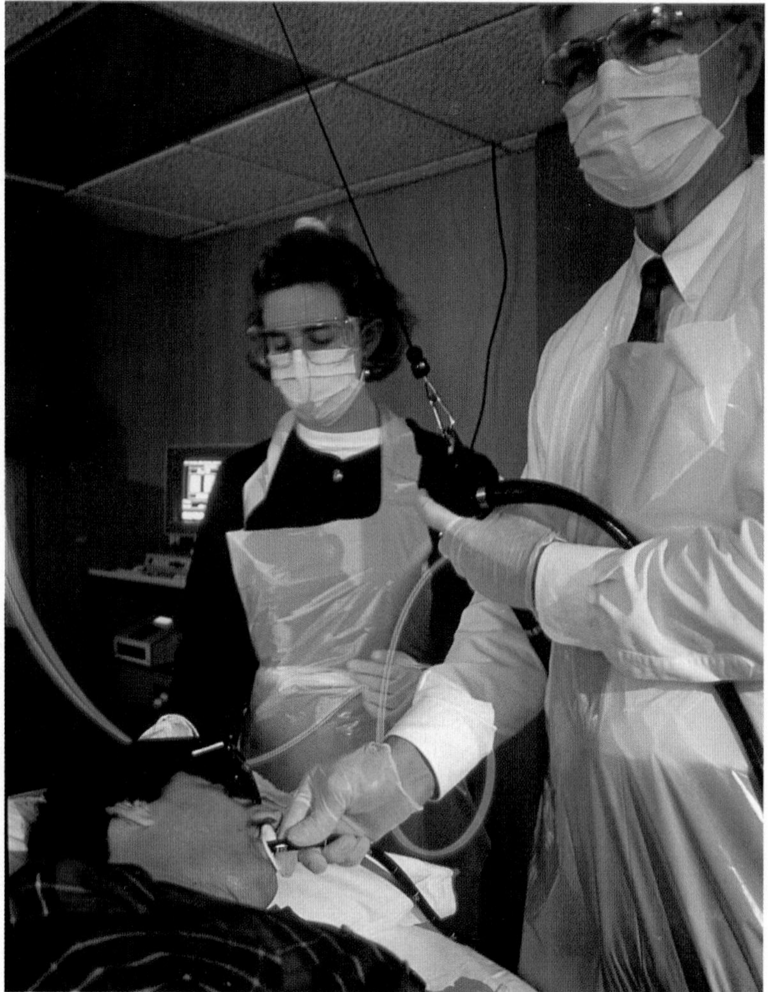

A laser is used in combination with special drugs that absorb certain wavelengths of light in a new treatment for advanced cancer of the esophagus. The drug first coats the tumor, and a surgeon then guides an optical fiber down the patient's throat to the tumor site. The optical fiber delivers laser light to the tumor, and the light activates the drug.

cuts or burns off pieces of overgrown tissue, which are flushed out through the instrument with water. The procedure requires general anesthesia, two to five days of hospitalization, and a recovery period as long as six weeks. From 2 to 10 percent of men who undergo this surgery experience complications, which can include *incontinence* (inability to control urination).

The laser procedure replaces electric current with light energy, delivered through an optical fiber. The surgeon threads the optical fiber through the urethra and into the prostate. The surgeon then bombards the prostate with laser light to kill excess tissue. The bloodstream reabsorbs the dead cells in the body's natural scavenging process. Tissue removed by the laser may clog the urinary tract for several days, requiring the patient to urinate through a thin tube called a catheter inserted in the urethra.

The main benefits of laser surgery over the conventional resectoscope procedure for an enlarged prostate are reduced bleeding, faster recovery, and far less chance of incontinence than with the standard resectoscope procedure. Laser surgery, unlike conventional surgery, can also be performed as an outpatient procedure. However, the two procedures are equally effective at increasing the rate of urinary flow.

On the horizon

Prospects for new laser treatments loomed bright in the mid-1990's. One experimental therapy, called photodynamic therapy, used laser light in combination with a drug that collects in cancer cells and is sensitive to certain wavelengths of light. Only one such drug had received FDA approval by 1996, however: a light-sensitive drug for treatment of advanced cancer of the esophagus. This deadly disease kills about 90 percent of people who have it within five years. In advanced stages of the disease, patients have tumors so large that they can no longer swallow.

After the light-sensitive drug is administered to the patient and time is allowed for it to collect in the tumor cells, the physician guides an optical fiber down the patient's throat to the tumor. Laser light beamed through the fiber activates the drug and triggers chemical reactions that destroy the tumor cells and the blood vessels that nourish them. Photodynamic therapy does not offer a cure, because by the time esophageal cancer has reached the advanced stage, it has spread to other organs. However, it can enable patients to eat and swallow, making their remaining days more tolerable.

Photodynamic therapy also has serious side effects. The drugs travel through the body, and healthy cells can absorb enough of them that exposure to light could trigger an attack on other body tissues for some days after treatment.

While some people view lasers as space-age gadgets too advanced for everyday use, lasers are rapidly becoming the standard tools for many surgical procedures. Even though they have not proved their worth for every surgical procedure, they have saved the eyesight of millions of people and made certain types of surgery easier and safer for millions more. As surgeons continue to find new uses for lasers, there is little doubt that many more people will benefit from laser surgery. •••

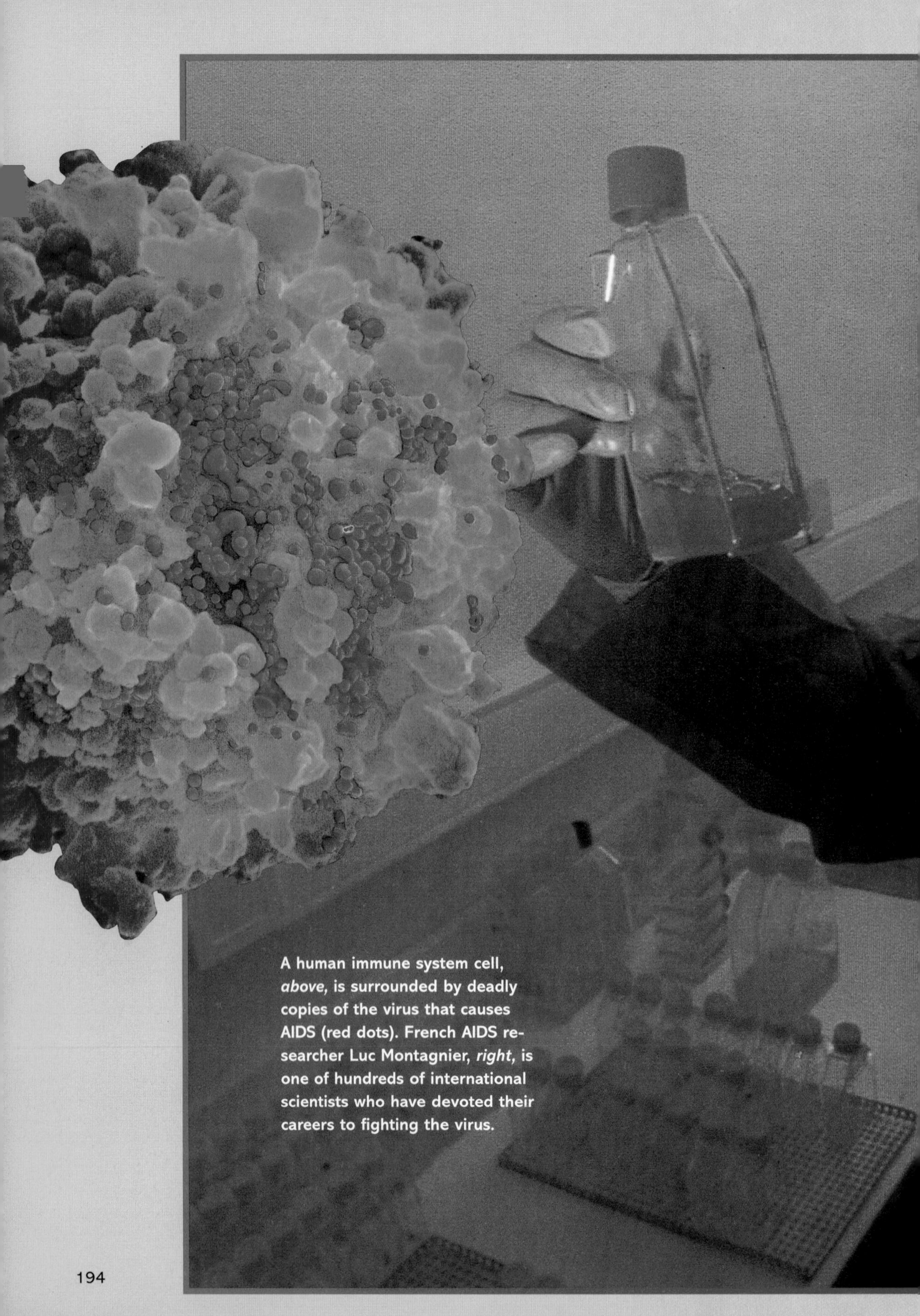

A human immune system cell, *above*, is surrounded by deadly copies of the virus that causes AIDS (red dots). French AIDS researcher Luc Montagnier, *right*, is one of hundreds of international scientists who have devoted their careers to fighting the virus.

Medical researchers trying to create a vaccine or cure for AIDS are struggling against an unexpectedly wily foe.

Science Versus the AIDS Virus

By June E. Osborn

FROM THE OUTSET, MEDICAL RESEARCHERS SUSPECTED that this was a disease unlike any other. When the illness was first recognized in 1981, it was clear that it killed in a strange manner—by causing apparently healthy people to succumb to diseases the body normally had no trouble resisting. A common fungus in the environment caused a fatal pneumonia in some patients. In others, cancerous tumors quickly spread across the skin. Something, it seemed, was destroying the patients' disease-fighting immune system. But few similar ailments were known to medical science, and most of those were rare inherited disorders.

The disease's unusual nature—along with an ominous increase in the number of cases—soon sparked thousands of medical research projects in the United States, Europe, and other parts of the world. Less than three years after physicians first reported the illness, laboratory researchers had named it acquired immune deficiency syndrome (AIDS) and had identified a previously unknown virus, which we now call the human immunodeficiency virus (HIV), as the cause. Early studies showed that the virus itself was unusual, a member of a little-known group of microbes called retroviruses.

By the mid-1990's, more was known about HIV than about any infectious agent of humankind. Scientists had quickly learned how the virus was transmitted—through sexual intercourse, transfusion of infected blood, injection of drugs using HIV-contaminated needles, or birth to an infected mother. Researchers had produced dozens of drugs for the treatment of HIV infection and AIDS.

Yet today, despite the dramatic increase in basic knowledge about the new illness, we have neither an effective vaccine nor a curative treatment. Meanwhile, the virus continues to spread. Experts predict that by the year 2000, more than 100 million people worldwide will have become infected with HIV.

Why has more than a decade of all-out research failed to produce the hoped-for results? The answer to that question has much to do with the unusual nature of AIDS and the oddities of the deadly microbe that causes it.

Glossary

AIDS (Acquired immune deficiency syndrome): The final stage of HIV infection, typically diagnosed when the patient's number of immune system cells falls below a certain level or when the patient develops certain opportunistic infections.

CD4 lymphocytes: Human white blood cells that are the primary target of HIV infection. The loss of these immune system cells leads to AIDS.

HIV (Human immunodeficiency virus): The virus that causes AIDS.

Opportunistic infection: An infection that tends to occur in people with weakened immune systems.

Protease inhibitors: A class of drug that fights HIV by preventing copies of the virus from being assembled in an infected human cell.

The author:

June E. Osborn, a former chairperson of the National Commission on AIDS, is professor of epidemiology at the University of Michigan School of Public Health in Ann Arbor and professor of pediatrics and communicable diseases in the university's medical school.

How HIV causes infection and AIDS

HIV, like other viruses, is considered "nonliving" because it must use the energy and materials of a living cell to reproduce. HIV's preferred host cell is a particular type of human white blood cell called CD4 lymphocytes. These cells are vital to human health because they coordinate most of the work of the immune system.

When HIV infects a person, the tiny virus attaches to and then enters a CD4 cell in the bloodstream. Once inside the cell, HIV does something unusual, even for a virus. It converts its genetic material into a form compatible with the genes of the cell. (Genes, which are the chemical instructions for making proteins, control the structure and function of viruses and all living cells.)

The infection that leads to AIDS

AIDS is caused by a microbe called the human immunodeficiency virus (HIV). The disease process begins when the virus enters the bloodstream—typically through having unprotected sexual intercourse, injecting drugs, being given a transfusion of infected blood, or being born to an infected mother.

HIV

Human CD4 cell

The first stage of infection occurs when HIV enters a type of human white blood cell called a CD4 cell. The cells are a crucial part of the human body's disease-fighting immune system.

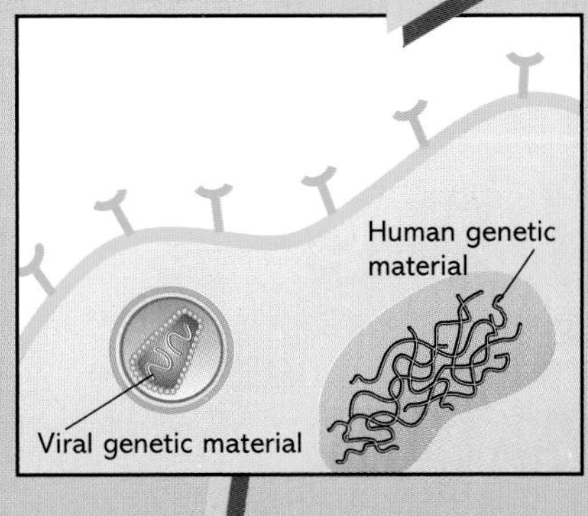

Once inside the cell, the virus inserts a copy of its genes into the genetic material of the human cell. By doing so, HIV "programs" the human cell to manufacture and assemble multiple copies of the virus.

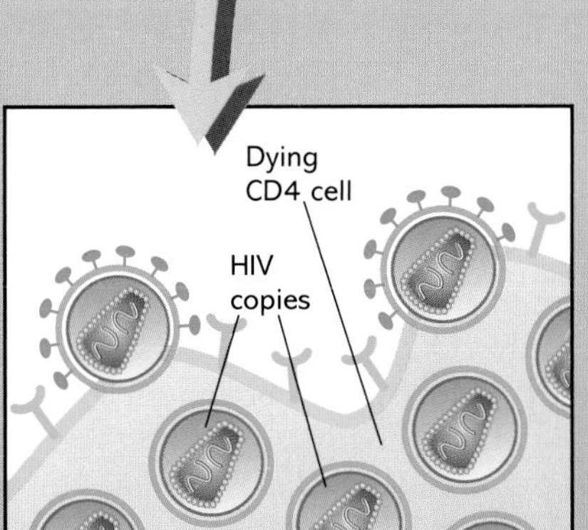

Eventually, the copies of the virus leave the human cell in a process called budding. The human cell dies, but the virus copies infect more cells, replicate inside them, and kill them.

By about 7 to 10 years after infection, most of the CD4 cells have died, crippling the infected person's ability to fight any kind of disease. With the drop in CD4 cells and the appearance of other illnesses, the person has developed AIDS.

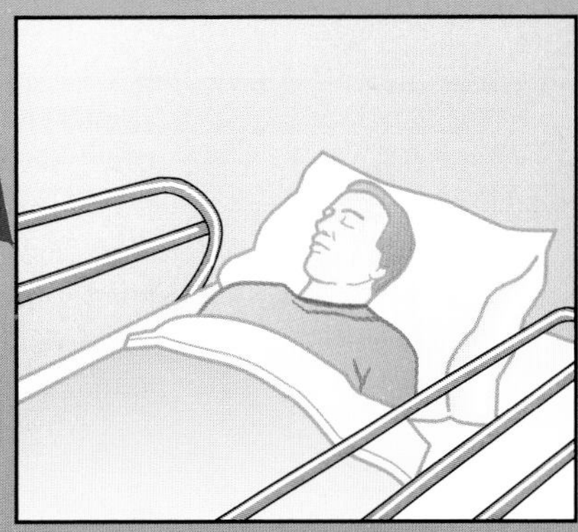

After HIV translates its genes, they are inserted into the human genetic material. That action permanently alters the human cell so that the cell does the virus's bidding—making more viruses. Over time, the CD4 cell will create and assemble thousands of copies of the original virus. The new copies will leave the cell in a process called budding and flow into the bloodstream to infect other cells and multiply anew. Meanwhile, the CD4 cell dies as a result of the virus's activity.

There follows a sort of race between the body, which strives to replace the dying immune cells, and the virus, which continues to multiply and infect the replacements. Little by little, the body's capacity to keep producing new CD4 cells is worn down until, after several years, an infected person runs out of them. At that stage, the patient falls prey to the diseases that characterize AIDS, such as the form of pneumonia called PCP and the cancer called Kaposi's sarcoma. (An HIV-infected person is considered to have AIDS when the number of CD4 cells drops below a certain level or when these AIDS-related illnesses begin to appear.) Physicians can treat some of these diseases successfully for a while, but in the long run, the AIDS patient dies.

Most of the harm done by HIV happens because of the death of CD4 cells. However, HIV can cause illness in a more direct fashion as well, by infecting another type of white blood cell called a macrophage. These cells are not so readily killed as CD4 cells, and some of the infected macrophages move through the bloodstream to settle in different parts of the body, particularly the brain. Many people with advanced AIDS have trouble thinking clearly or remembering because of the build-up of these HIV-infected cells in the brain.

Searching for a drug to kill the virus

As soon as HIV was discovered, researchers began searching for a drug that could kill the virus before the infection led to illness and death. At the same time, physicians treating people with AIDS devised drug therapies to extend the life of their patients by combating AIDS-associated diseases. Perhaps the most important of these advances was the finding in the early 1990's that when CD4 cell counts drop to low levels, drug treatment directed against the fungus *Pneumocystis carinii* can defer or completely prevent the occurrence of PCP. In the 1980's, that form of pneumonia had been the cause of death for 60 percent of AIDS patients.

Scientists developed other drug regimens to prevent or treat many other AIDS-associated infections, and intensive research produced promising new treatments for Kaposi's sarcoma. In addition, physicians in 1991 learned that HIV infection in women may cause rapid development of cancer of the *cervix* (the neck of the uterus). Doctors now know to monitor their female HIV patients carefully for changes that indicate cervical cancer, which can be treated effectively in its earliest stages.

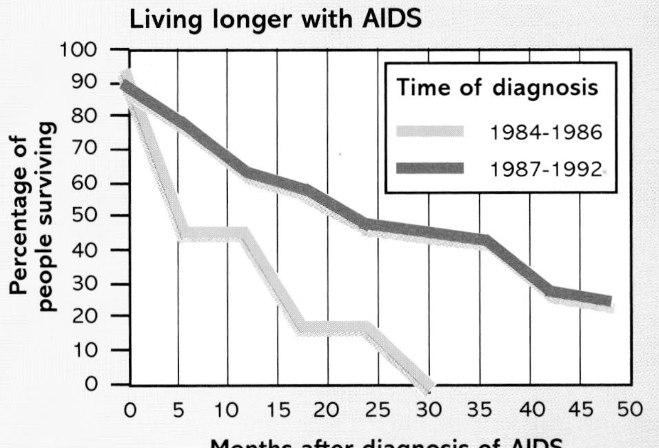

Modest progress in combating AIDS

Although researchers have not found a cure for HIV infection, they have made progress in developing therapies. Patients diagnosed with AIDS today can expect to live significantly longer than those diagnosed before 1987, *left,* And drug treatment has sharply reduced the likelihood that a baby born to an HIV-infected women will develop AIDS, *below.*

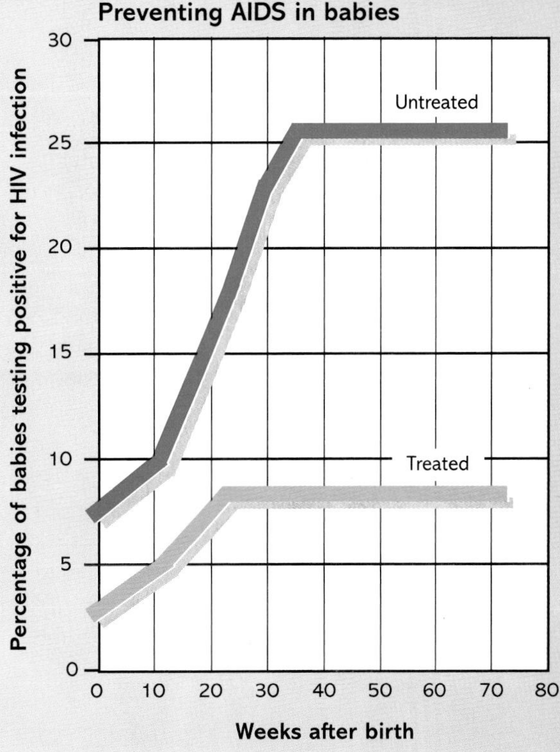

These developments translated into additional years of life for people infected with HIV. In the early 1980's, AIDS was often recognized so late in the process of CD4 cell destruction that most newly diagnosed patients died swiftly. By the mid-1990's, the life expectancy of AIDS patients had been extended considerably, both because physicians had learned how to prevent infections such as PCP and because pharmaceutical researchers had found new treatments for cancerous tumors such as Kaposi's sarcoma.

None of those treatments is an AIDS cure, however, and that continues to be the prime goal for many laboratory researchers. But it has proved difficult to find a compound that can kill the virus without harming the vital CD4 cells in which it resides.

At first, scientists hoped they might be able to develop a drug that could block HIV's entry into the lymphocytes. The virus gets into these cells by latching onto a molecule called a CD4 receptor on the cell's outer surface. But drugs designed to attach to the CD4 receptor to block the virus's entry have so far not proved effective in halting the HIV infection.

Other scientists reasoned that the virus might be attacked at the point when it translates its genetic material into a form compatible with the genes of a human cell, a step crucial to the virus's ability to reproduce. Their thinking was correct, and this line of inquiry has yielded most of the drugs currently in use against HIV.

The first of those new drugs was called zidovudine (AZT). In

1987, researchers found that the drug was a major help to people with AIDS, often improving their physical well-being and even reversing some of the damage to the brain caused by HIV infection. As physicians gained experience with AZT, however, they discovered that the drug's beneficial effects seemed to wear off after patients took the drug for 18 to 24 months.

The problem of drug resistance

Why was AZT no longer effective in those patients? Scientists trying to answer that question discovered another distinctive feature of HIV: The virus develops resistance to drugs in an unusually short period of time. Drug resistance, which also occurs in microorganisms such as bacteria, stems from the fact that an infection involves large numbers of microbes reproducing very quickly. That situation makes it highly probable that some microbes will be formed with one or more random errors in their genes. Such an error, called a *genetic mutation*, may enable a microbe to withstand a drug that kills off its normal cousins. Over time, the mutant will reproduce to form a large number of drug-resistant microbes.

HIV is particularly good at developing drug resistance because the process by which its genetic material is translated is unusually prone to errors. The random mutations eventually produce some viruses that are not harmed by AZT. Over the course of several months, AZT will kill most of the normal HIV in an infected person, but by then, any AZT-resistant microbes will have given rise to vast numbers of similarly resistant ones. Normal doses of AZT will no longer help keep the patient's infection in check.

One strategy for dealing with drug resistance is to develop a varied arsenal of drugs, so that a virus with a mutation that allows it to withstand one drug may nonetheless be felled by a drug with a slightly different method of action. Researchers in the 1980's and early 1990's developed several other drugs that act in the same fashion as AZT, including didanosine, stavudine, and zalcitabine. The drugs can be used in some instances by themselves, and several research studies show that combining one or another of the newer drugs with AZT may delay the problem of resistance.

Meanwhile, some medical researchers took an entirely different approach to drug therapy against HIV by targeting a key step in the cell's production of virus copies. This research, which has yielded a new class of drugs called protease inhibitors, began to pay off in the mid-1990's, when compounds called indinavir, ritonavir, and saquinavir appeared effective in killing HIV without harming CD4 cell's.

In addition, combination therapy, in which a patient takes AZT-like drugs as well as protease inhibitors, reduces the amount of HIV in the body much more dramatically than does taking just one of the drugs alone. Because the two types of medicines attack HIV by completely different mechanisms, the virus is far less likely to develop drug resistance to both medicines.

Strategies for an AIDS cure

Scientists have been exploring several avenues that may lead to drugs capable of stopping HIV infection. Each strategy targets a different step in the virus's infection and replication process. The greatest hope may lie in developing anti-HIV "cocktails" consisting of two or three different types of drugs. Such a regimen promises to combat HIV's ability to adapt to any single drug and render it ineffective.

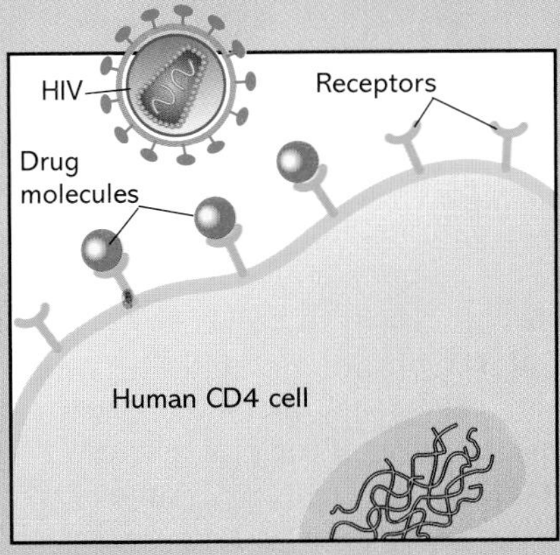

An early avenue of research involved drugs that prevent HIV from infecting cells. Scientists hoped the drugs would block molecules called receptors that the virus latches onto before entering a cell. But so far, no such drugs have proved effective.

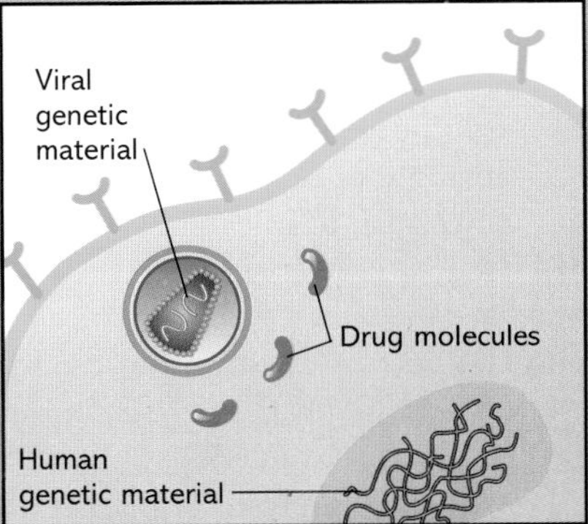

A more promising line of research deals with drugs that prevent HIV from incorporating its genes into the human cell. AZT and most other currently prescribed anti-HIV drugs use this approach. Unfortunately, HIV becomes resistant to these drugs relatively quickly.

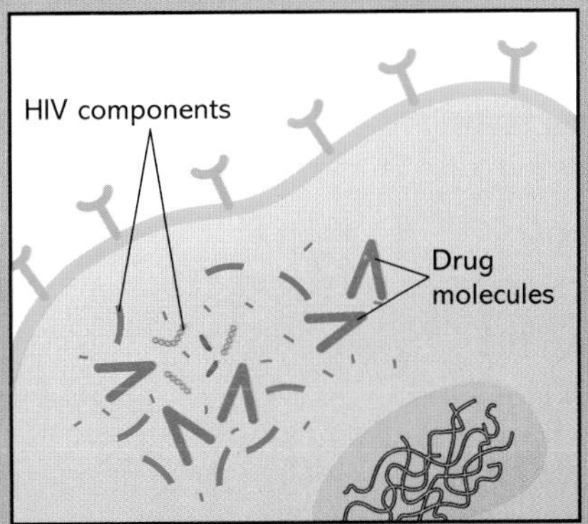

One of the newest areas of research focuses on drugs that prevent HIV copies from being assembled in the cell. These drugs are called protease inhibitors. When used with AZT-type drugs, they may help avoid the problem of drug resistance.

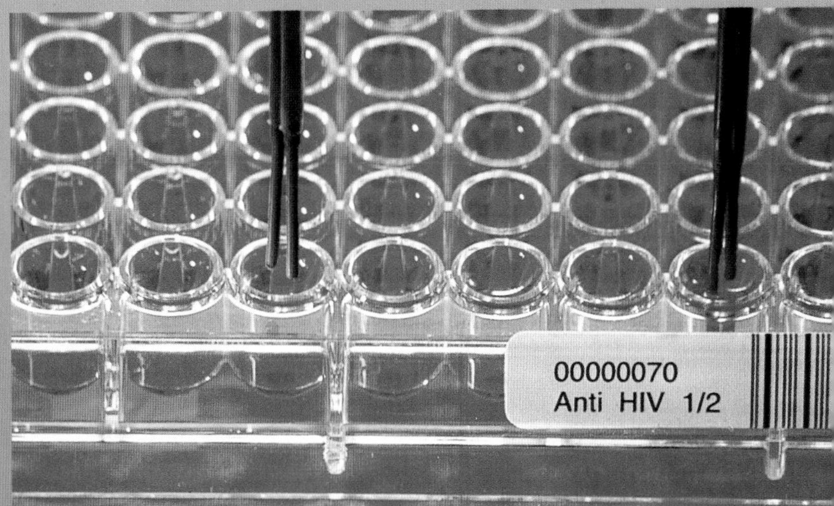

Tiny tubes containing cultured cells are used to test compounds for their possible usefulness as anti-HIV drugs.

Researchers in 1996 were actively developing drugs that function in an entirely different way—by boosting normal responses of the human immune system. If this strategy pans out, it may be possible to use combinations of three different types of drugs to completely block the virus from its avenues of change.

If HIV infections could be recognized very early, researchers believe, such combination-treatment strategies might give the patient an advantage in the race between virus multiplication and CD4 cell replacement. The early results of tests with protease inhibitors and newer drugs offer no long-term guarantees of effectiveness, however, and few scientists expect that they represent the hope of a true cure—that is, the complete elimination of HIV from the body.

Thus far, the greatest success of AIDS drug research has been the prevention of HIV infection in some babies born to infected mothers. Throughout the 1980's and early 1990's, more than 25 percent of all infants born to infected mothers were themselves infected with HIV. To try to lower that percentage, researchers in eight American cities in 1994 carried out a clinical trial in which pregnant women with HIV took AZT from the second half of pregnancy through delivery. Their babies then received the drug for the first six weeks of life.

For the treated group of infants, the likelihood of being infected with HIV dropped sharply—to slightly more than 8 percent. The results of this research were so convincing that physicians now strongly recommend that pregnant women be tested for HIV and, if infected, be treated with AZT to reduce the risk to the baby. By doing so, hundreds of newborns have been spared AIDS since 1994.

Frustrating quest for a vaccine

An HIV vaccine could offer such protection to any uninfected person, and that is why such famous scientists as the late Jonas Salk, who developed an effective polio vaccine, turned their attention to developing an AIDS vaccine in the 1980's. Even if pharmaceutical researchers can never find an antiviral medicine to kill HIV, halting the spread of AIDS to uninfected people could nonetheless be helped by the availability of an effective vaccine. That strategy has helped control several viral diseases, including smallpox, yellow fever, influenza, polio, measles, rubella, mumps, hepatitis B, and chickenpox.

Most vaccines work by causing the immune system to develop disease-fighting proteins called antibodies, which circulate in the bloodstream ready to target the virus for destruction. The body normally produces antibodies to a particular virus after the virus enters the system. The antibodies give what is called protective immunity from a second attack by the microbe. That is why people who have had the measles or chickenpox will never get the disease again, even if they are exposed to the virus by being around infected people.

Some of the vaccines now used to prevent viral infection are made of weakened viruses, which are reproduced under laboratory con-

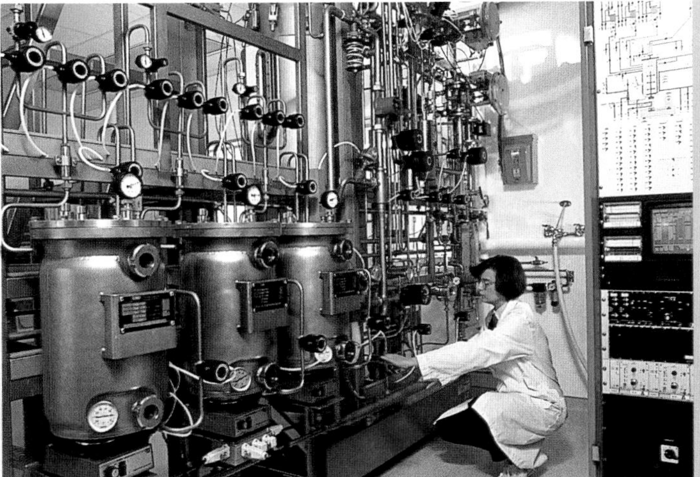

A worker at a biotechnology firm in Meriden, Connecticut, monitors the elaborate equipment used to manufacture an experimental HIV vaccine.

ditions to lessen their capacity to cause disease. When injected into a human being, the weakened viruses provoke protective immunity that enables the body to mobilize quickly and effectively in the event of a later invasion by the full-strength virus.

Other vaccines are created by "killing," or inactivating, the virus so that it can no longer infect human cells and reproduce. A more advanced technique is to create a vaccine out of only part of the original virus—often a key protein on the virus's outer surface. Those preparations are called subunit vaccines.

Unfortunately, researchers have found that developing a vaccine against HIV is much more difficult than creating a vaccine against measles or smallpox. The first problem is the lack of an example of natural protective immunity that scientists could seek to imitate. The vast majority of people infected with HIV do not recover from the infection but rather develop AIDS and die.

However, as the AIDS epidemic has progressed, physicians have identified a few individuals who have maintained relatively healthy levels of CD4 cells for 10 or more years after becoming infected with HIV. Among AIDS experts, such people are referred to as long-term nonprogressors or long-term survivors. Using laboratory tests, scientists

On the trail of an AIDS vaccine

Researchers working on an anti-HIV vaccine have tried to follow the methods used to create effective vaccines against other viral diseases, such as polio or measles. Those vaccines work because they provoke the human body to produce disease-fighting proteins called antibodies. If the same microbe tries to cause infection in the future, the antibodies will be ready to target it for destruction. So far, however, the unusual nature of HIV has made vaccine development extremely difficult.

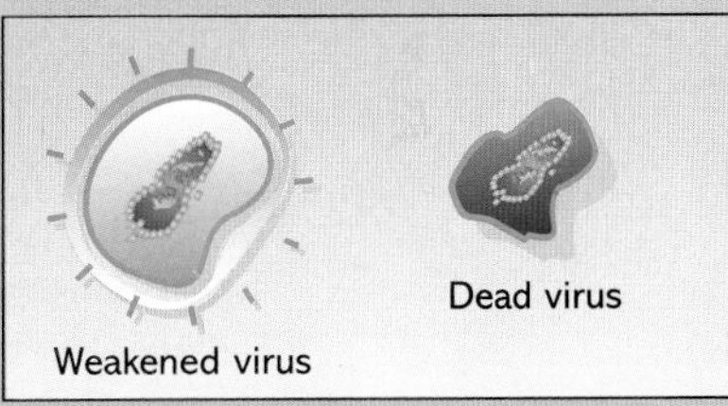

Most vaccines are injections of whole viruses that have been weakened or "killed" in the lab so that they cannot cause infection. But because HIV can insert its genes into human genetic material, scientists fear that even "killed" HIV will have the potential to cause AIDS if its genes are intact.

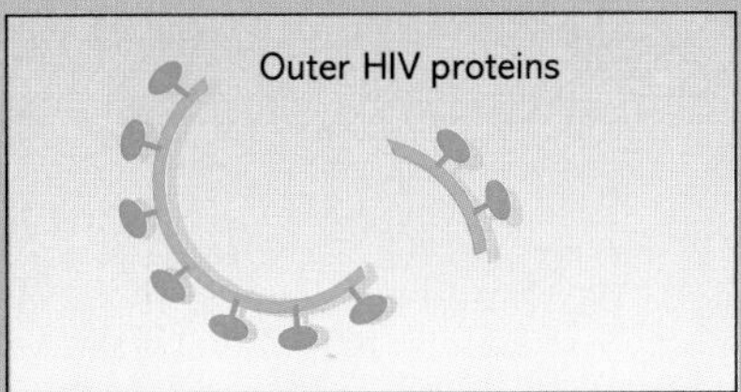

For safety's sake, the vaccines being developed for HIV contain just a portion of the virus's outer protein coat. Unfortunately, such vaccines are not very potent, and different subtypes of HIV have different proteins. A vaccine that works against one subtype would not be effective against others.

have looked for special or unusual features of the survivors' immune responses. Finding something unusual about their immunity or about the specific strain of virus that infected them might point the way toward an effective vaccine. As of mid-1996, however, such studies had not detected anything significantly different about the immune response in long-term survivors.

A second problem for vaccine researchers relates to HIV's unusual method of establishing infection in human cells. Since HIV can insert its genes into human genetic material—unlike many other viruses—experts fear that even the weakened HIV used for a vaccine might regain the ability to produce disease. Most researchers are therefore reluctant to use the weakened vaccine strategy that has worked so well with other viruses, and they consider even the idea of using completely inactivated HIV quite risky as long as the virus's genetic material is still intact.

How HIV evades vaccines

To date, researchers trying to produce HIV vaccines have all relied on the subunit approach, using just the proteins on the outside of the virus. By the mid-1990's, this line of research had proved frustrating, partly because subunit vaccines tend not to be very potent, and partly because of the adaptable nature of HIV. During the long course of an infection, copies of the virus may arise with different surface proteins, due to the same process of random genetic mutation that leads to drug resistance. While antibodies and other features of the immune system may hold HIV in partial check for years after infection, any mutated virus with a variation in its surface proteins will be able to reproduce without interference.

If a vaccine could prevent HIV infection entirely, such mutated viruses would never be formed. Unfortunately, the capacity of HIV to change through mutation suggests that a person who was successfully immunized might still be susceptible to infection by "newer" versions of the virus circulating among the human population.

HIV's ability to change has led to its classification by subtypes. Researchers have known since shortly after HIV was identified that there are two major classes of the virus—HIV-1, which is causing the worldwide epidemic; and HIV-2, which is common only in west Africa. As of mid-1996, researchers had also discovered 12 subtypes of HIV-1, labeled A through L. Only one subtype dominated in the United States—subtype B—but others had made an appearance.

The various subtypes all spread and produce disease in the same way, but they differ enough in their outer proteins that a vaccine effective against one subtype would not protect against the others. The problem of making different vaccines for a potentially growing number of subtypes adds another level of complexity to the difficult task of vaccine development.

When AIDS was first identified, many researchers hoped that studying the disease process in animals would provide clues for developing a vaccine. Unfortunately, HIV is a species-specific virus—that is, a virus that infects only one species or that produces different patterns of illness in other species. HIV is known to infect only one other species, chimpanzees, but it seems to cause far less damage to the chimp immune system than to the human system.

That being the case, researchers turned to studying viruses that produce AIDS-like illness in other animals. Many experts have focused on a virus called simian immunodeficiency virus (SIV), which infects several species of monkeys and leads to AIDS-like disease in some of them. From those studies, scientists thus far have not developed any major new strategies for dealing with HIV. It seems likely, however, that animal research, along with continued efforts to understand how long-term survivors hold HIV at bay, could be the source of new insights to break the HIV-vaccine impasse.

Despite these difficulties, by mid-1996, researchers had created dozens of candidate vaccines against HIV in the laboratory, and several had been tested in small numbers of people to be sure the preparations were safe and to find out what dosage was necessary to provoke immune responses. However, none of the vaccines was considered potent or promising enough to be tried in larger numbers of people at high risk for HIV infection in the United States.

Ethical and practical difficulties in testing vaccines

One vaccine trial was getting underway in Thailand in 1996. The HIV epidemic was growing so swiftly in that country that public health officials felt justified in trying even a weakly effective vaccine. Experts said the trial would be important to watch but quite complicated to evaluate. The problem is that in Thailand, two different subtypes of HIV are spreading, and the vaccine being tested protects against only one of them. Thus, researchers have to take into account which HIV subtype has infected an inoculated person before determining whether or not the vaccine was a success.

Researchers also caution that even if this vaccine or some other one were to appear very promising, more experimental trials would be required before it could be licensed for general use. At least some of those trials would have to be done in the United States before the vaccine could be used in this country.

That fact raises ethical problems as troubling as the scientific ones. To achieve results in a reasonable period of time, the participants would need to come from a population that has a high incidence of HIV infection—a rate of about 2 infections among every 100 people each year. Where people are becoming infected with such frequency in the United States—among the urban poor, for example—the rate of infection is so high in part because people lack access to AIDS information, to treatment for drug addiction, and to health care in general.

It is widely agreed that it would not be ethical to study a vaccine's effectiveness in such communities without offering them the stan-

In a medical research trial, a health-care worker gives an injection of an experimental HIV vaccine to a man infected with the virus in the hope that it improves his ability to fight HIV.

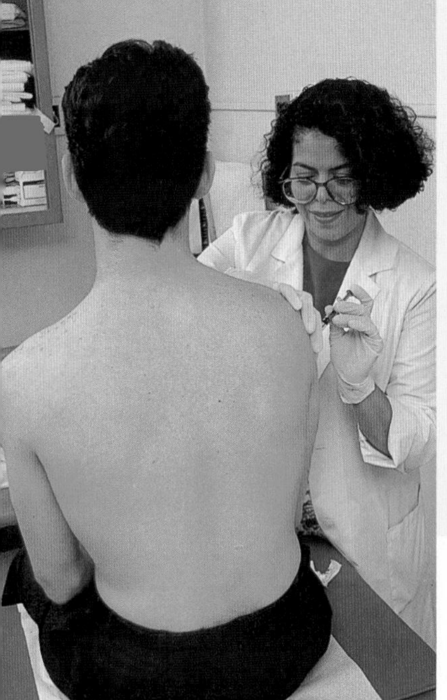

Highly experimental AIDS treatments

With a cure or vaccine still on the distant horizon, some AIDS patients and researchers have turned to much more experimental treatments.

Treatment	First used	Concerns and drawbacks
Giving vaccines of inactivated HIV to people who are already infected with the virus. Such vaccination is designed to improve the immune system's ability to combat the virus.	1991	The vaccine may accidentally encourage a patient's immune system to focus on fighting the inactivated microbe, rather than targeting the disease-causing HIV already in the body.
Transplanting baboon bone marrow into AIDS patients in the hope of boosting the patients' blood levels of immune system cells.	1995	The procedure could introduce baboon viruses into the human population, causing new infectious diseases with unforeseen consequences.
Developing gene therapy treatments, in which HIV infected patients would receive genetic material designed to make CD4 cells more resistant to further HIV infection.	Projected to be several years in the future	Gene therapy has not yet proved effective for controlling any disease. Although researchers are optimistic, the possible hazards of the treatment are not well understood.

dard of care available to others. That concern creates a catch-22 situation: Those interventions by themselves might prevent some people from getting HIV, thus making it difficult to gauge the vaccine's effectiveness.

These issues have prompted the U.S. government's National Institutes of Health in Bethesda, Maryland, to create safeguards for upcoming vaccine trials. One of the most important would involve participation and guidance in the design and completion of the trial from people belonging to the community where a vaccine was to be tested. Such procedures are intended to help ensure that the needs and rights of the participants are respected.

Finally, a highly experimental area of vaccine research involves giving HIV vaccines to people who are already infected. Medical researchers hope that the vaccine will boost the human body's immune response against HIV to tip the balance in favor of the person instead of the virus.

Some experts fear that this approach might do more harm than good, however. Theoretically, that could happen if the body expends so much energy attacking the inactivated HIV in the vaccine that its fight against the full-strength HIV already in the body is compromised. By 1996, experiments with these vaccines had not produced clear-cut results in either direction.

Other experimental treatments

Without a cure or vaccine yet in sight, some AIDS researchers have turned their attention to other experimental means of saving lives. The most publicized experiment occurred at the University of California in San Francisco in December 1995, when physicians transplanted bone marrow cells from a baboon into Jeff Getty, a San Francisco man with AIDS. Researchers hoped that the baboon cells, which are resistant to HIV infection, would "take" in Getty's body, providing him with blood cell replacements for the immune system cells destroyed by the virus. As of mid-1996, however, scientists had not detected any surviving baboon cells in the man's bloodstream.

A concern about this line of research is that such transplants are risky, not just for the recipient, but also for the human population as a whole. Most species have their own sets of viruses that apparently infect only that species because of the difficulty of getting into a different host species. By injecting cells or tissue from another primate into a human being, a researcher might unwittingly enable a virus to leap that barrier. The result, theoretically at least, could set the stage for baboon viruses to infect human beings. That prospect made the Getty transplant extremely controversial, even after the experiment received approval from the U.S. Food and Drug Agency.

Another experimental avenue for HIV treatment is gene therapy, in which patients receive injections or other preparations that contain genetic material. As envisioned for AIDS treatment, the genes received by an HIV-infected person would be taken up by blood cells that would then become resistant to further HIV invasion or replication. As of 1996, such treatments had not moved into clinical testing, but the slow progress of other efforts to find a cure made it important to pursue these avenues.

While we wait for more answers, public health experts stress that the chief goal of vaccine research—preventing the spread of HIV—is already possible. Unlike influenza and other viruses that are transmitted through the air, HIV can be avoided by curtailing risky behaviors such as unprotected sexual intercourse and injected drug use.

As international public health officials try to spread the word about these "low-tech" methods of avoiding AIDS, it may seem that high-tech medical researchers are doomed to be thwarted regularly by HIV. Yet scientists have already gained deep insights into the nature of this unusual virus and its complex relationship with human beings. And the more scientists understand about HIV, the closer they are to finding and exploiting its weaknesses. Amid the human tragedy that is AIDS, the extent of their progress is the surest basis of hope. •••

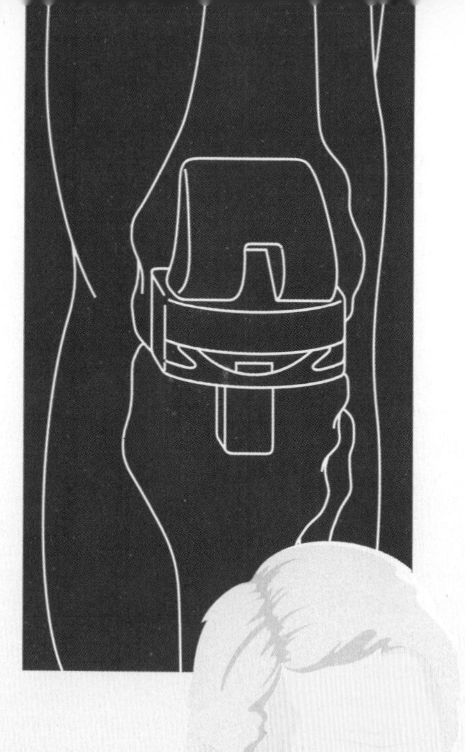

Artificial joints can relieve pain and make life more enjoyable for many people. But they don't last forever.

Active Lives with Artificial Joints

By Steven I. Benowitz

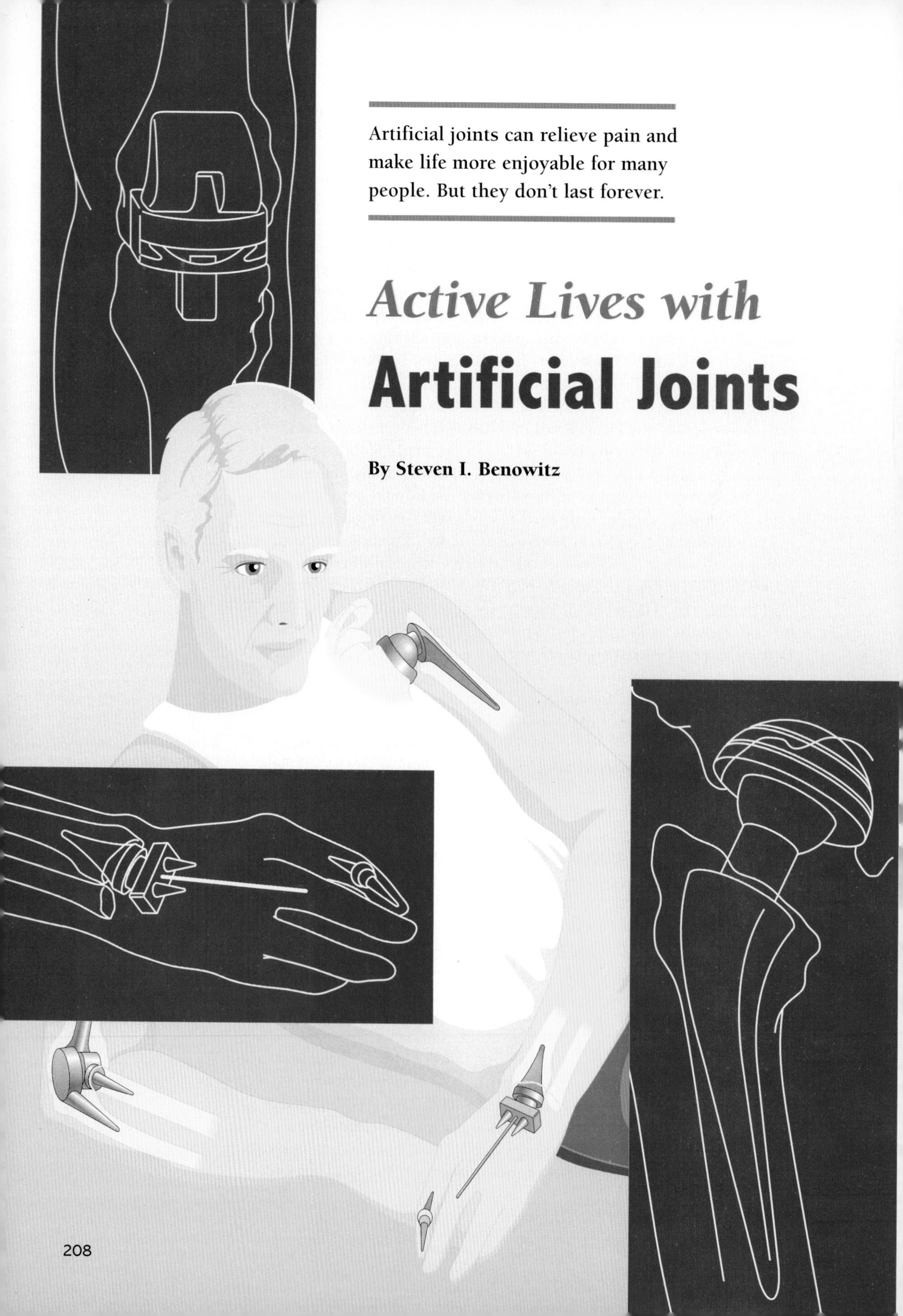

NEARLY EVERYONE KNOWS or has heard of someone who has had a hip, knee, or other joint replaced with a metal and plastic substitute. A grandmother or uncle, or perhaps the film star Elizabeth Taylor or a professional athlete such as baseball player Bo Jackson or quarterback Joe Namath. By the mid-1990's, joint replacement had become one of the most common surgical procedures in the United States.

Hip replacement has been hailed as one of the triumphs of modern spare-parts surgery. Not long ago, people with damaged joints had to make do with pain medication, applications of heat, and perhaps a cane or a walker. But surgeons have replaced more than 1 million hips in the United States since the late 1960's, demonstrating the ability of artificial implants to relieve pain and improve mobility. Surgeons replaced about 250,000 knees and 300,000 hips in the United States in 1993 (the last year for which estimates were available), according to the American Academy of Orthopedic Surgeons.

Various conditions can cause joints to deteriorate. They include fractures, repeated dislocations, bone tumors, and certain rare degenerative disorders. But 90 percent of the time, the damage that leads to joint replacement stems from arthritis.

Arthritis comprises a number of conditions characterized by inflammation of the tissues in a joint. Joints are special structures where two bones meet. The bones are held together with ligaments and tendons and capped with a protective tissue called cartilage. In healthy joints, cartilage acts as a cushion for the bones, preventing them from rubbing against each other.

The most common forms of arthritis—osteoarthritis and rheumatoid arthritis—lead to the destruction of the protective layer of cartilage. Osteoarthritis is the leading cause of joint deterioration, and it accounts for about 70 percent of all replaced joints. Rheumatoid arthritis accounts for most of the remaining surgery, but implants are sometimes necessary to replace badly fractured hips in older people.

In osteoarthritis, cartilage deteriorates as a result of injury, intense physical activity or overuse, or simple wear and tear over many years. Some evidence suggests that inflammation of the cartilage may also contribute to osteoarthritis. Once the lining of cartilage wears away, bare bone grinds against bone, resulting in pain. Aside from the odd automobile accident or athletic injury that might speed up the process, the rate at which osteoarthritis wears down cartilage depends largely on a person's genetic inheritance. Having a parent with osteoarthritis increases the likelihood of developing it. People who are overweight increase their chances of osteoarthritis by the added pressure they put on their joints. Osteoarthritis most often occurs after age 60, and anyone who lives long enough will develop it to some degree.

Rheumatoid arthritis is an inflammatory disease in which immune system cells mistakenly identify body tissue as "foreign" and attack it. The result in the case of rheumatoid arthritis is the eating away of cartilage and damage to tendons and ligaments at the joints.

Whichever form arthritis takes, it causes chronic pain, swelling, and stiffness in the affected joints. Despite the range of medications available to treat arthritis, there is no cure for the disease, and damage to affected joints often worsens as arthritis sufferers age.

Measures to try first

Before someone considers joint replacement, doctors usually recommend other measures to manage arthritis pain and improve mobility. Anti-inflammatory drugs such as ibuprofen and aspirin can relieve pain, and exercise can help keep the joints supple. A physician may also suggest losing weight when appropriate, because fewer pounds pressing on joints often means less discomfort from arthritis.

Surgeons are generally reluctant to recommend joint replacement for people under 50 years of age. Most artificial joints wear out after 10 to 15 years, and people younger than 50 are typically more active than their elders and tend to wear out an artificial joint more rapidly.

A surgical procedure called an osteotomy can postpone the need for an artificial joint. This procedure, which is most often performed on the knee, realigns the joint bone to change the pattern of wear and stress on the joint. Osteoarthritis or injury can deform the knee so weight that once had been evenly distributed across the joint shifts to one side. Eventually, the uneven distribution of weight destroys the cartilage on that side. In the hip, osteoarthritis or injury can wear away cartilage on the end of the *femur* (thighbone) at an uneven rate.

In an osteotomy, surgeons cut and reposition bones in the knee or hip so that only areas still covered with cartilage bear weight. The procedure can delay the need for an artificial joint by as long as 15 years. Eventually, however, the remaining healthy cartilage deteriorates as well.

Another surgical option is to have an arthritic joint fused. Surgeons fuse joints using surgical pins or plates that join adjacent bones and immobilize them. Fusion prevents the motion at the joint that causes pain. Ankles and wrists are better candidates for fusion than hips and shoulders. A fused hip takes as long as a year to heal and limits mobility. A fused shoulder also greatly reduces that joint's mobility. Fused wrists and ankles heal relatively quickly and still allow significant hand and foot function.

When arthritis is severe, pain relievers and exercise may be insufficient to relieve pain. If osteotomy is not an option and the patient does not wish to have the joint fused, an artificial joint can provide a solution. Joint replacement is not for everyone, however. Surgeons recommend joint replacement primarily for people aged 65 or older, who weigh less than 200 pounds (90 kilograms), have no chronic infections (which might interfere with the healing process), and have enough bone mass in which to implant the artificial joint.

The author:

Steven I. Benowitz is a free-lance science and medical writer.

Types of artificial joints

There are several kinds of artificial joints, but they are all designed to permit the type and range of movement that the original joint provided. The hip and shoulder are ball-and-socket joints, which permit the greatest range of motion, pivotal motion as well as movement up and down. Knees and elbows are modified hinge joints, which permit some pivoting motion, though their basic motion is in a single plane. Most replacement joints are of the ball-and-socket or modified hinge type and are typically made of plastic and a metal such as chromium or cobalt.

Hips and knees are the joints most often replaced. Although arthritis affects other joints as seriously, people can usually function with a painful elbow or swollen fingers. But an arthritic knee or hip can be incapacitating.

Hip and knee replacement

To replace a hip, the surgeon pulls the femur out of its socket in the pelvis and then cuts off the rounded head of the bone. The next steps include drilling a cavity in the femur to receive the stem of the implant, deepening the pelvic socket, and lining the socket with a plastic cup. The surgeon inserts the stem into the partially hollowed femur and fits the ball at the end of the stem into the plastic cup.

Recovery from hip replacement surgery takes three months or more and depends on the patient's physical condition and diligence in performing rehabilitation exercises. Some patients experience almost immediate relief from pain and begin physical activity soon after surgery.

Doing too much too soon can be dangerous, experts warn. The muscles and tendons in the area of the hip need about six weeks to heal, and too much stress can tear muscles that help hold the joint in place, allowing the ball to slip out of the socket. This complication can occur in up to 8 percent of cases. Most of the time, the surgeon can put the joint back in place without further surgery, much as he or she would reset a dislocated joint. Physicians generally recommend that patients avoid high impact activities such as jogging, tennis, and skiing after hip replacement surgery.

Why joints are replaced

Joints are replaced chiefly because of damage that results from arthritis—a condition that involves pain, swelling, and stiffness in one or more joints. When arthritis is severe, the joint may no longer function properly, limiting motion or mobility. Osteoarthritis and rheumatoid arthritis are the two most common forms of the disorder.

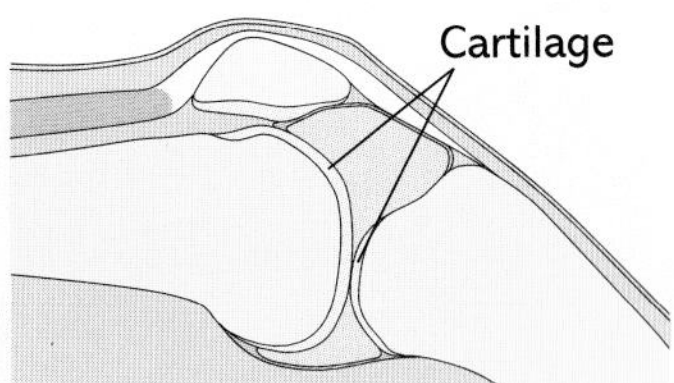

A joint is the meeting place of two bones. In a healthy joint, a rubbery tissue called cartilage covers the ends of the bones and prevents them from rubbing against one another.

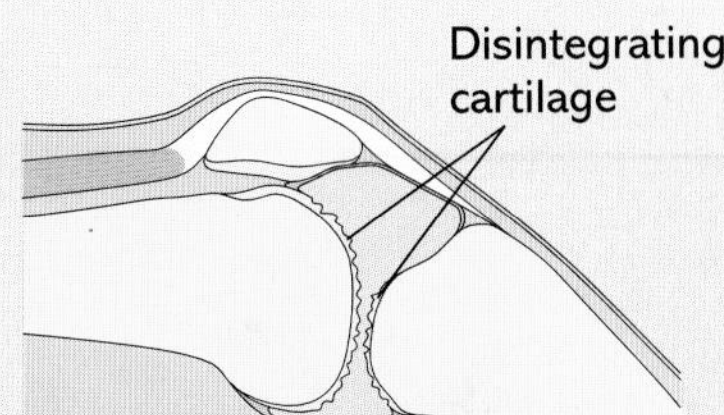

In osteoarthritis, the cartilage disintegrates and the bones rub against each other. Osteoarthritis primarily troubles older people.

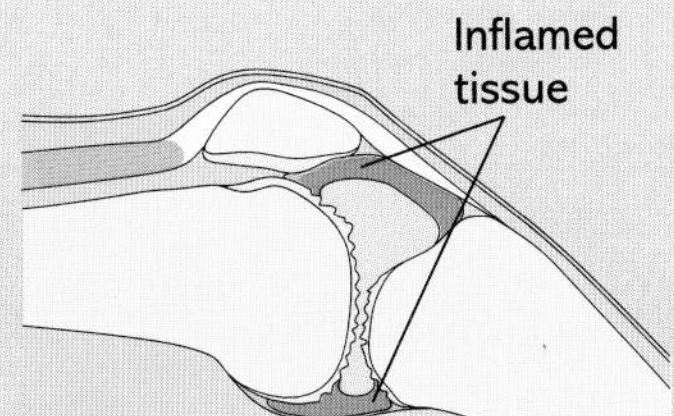

In rheumatoid arthritis, inflammation of the joints leads to the erosion of cartilage and bone. Rheumatoid arthritis strikes most often between the ages of 20 and 40, though it can affect people of any age.

Which joints are replaceable?

Almost all of the movable joints in the body can be replaced, though the only common procedures are knee, hip, finger, and shoulder joint replacement. The design of the artificial joint depends on the type of movement the joint allows. Ball-and-socket joints, such as the hip and shoulder, permit the greatest range of motion. Other joints, such as the knee, finger, and elbow, act as modified hinges.

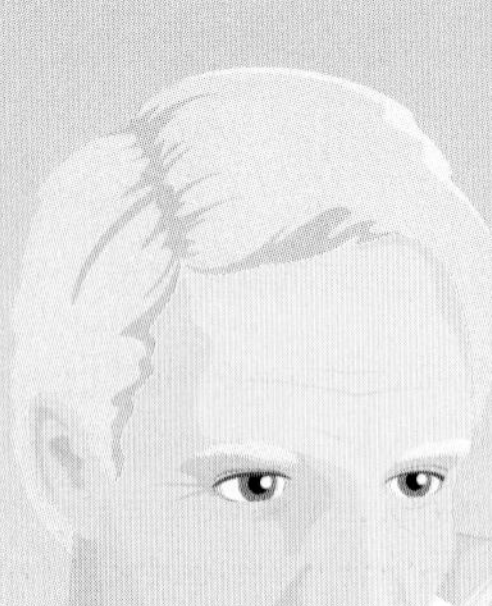

Shoulders

An artificial shoulder joint consists of two parts. A shaft with a ball attached to the end fits into the upper arm bone. The ball fits into a cup-shaped socket that is inserted into the shoulder blade.

Hips

An artificial hip joint consists of two parts—a shaft with a ball at one end, which fits into the thighbone, and a cup-shaped socket that fits into the pelvis. The ball swivels freely inside the socket.

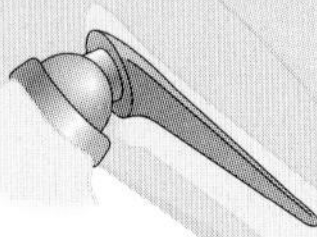

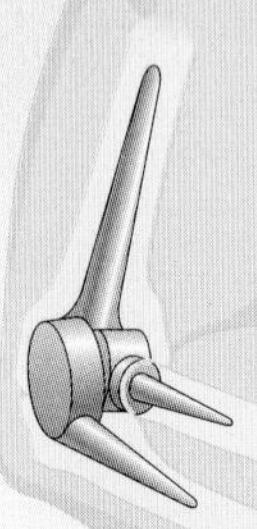

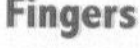

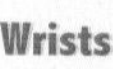

Elbows

An artificial elbow joint consists of two parts—a shaft that fits into the upper armbone and a circular plastic or metal base inserted into each of the bones in the forearm.

Fingers

An artificial finger joint is a piece of plastic hinge that separates and aligns the bones of the fingers and acts as a hinge.

Wrists

An artificial wrist joint consists of several pieces—a cylindrical metal shaft that fits into one of the bones in the forearm and a metal or plastic piece that fits into the hand. A metal rod anchors the implant into a finger bone. The implant allows movement sideways and up and down.

Who is a good candidate for an artificial joint?

Joint replacement is major surgery and should be undertaken only after careful consideration. In general, physicians consider people with the following characteristics best suited for joint replacement:

- People willing to work hard at rehabilitation. Physical therapy is needed after joint replacement to rebuild muscle strength. Therapy can be painful and strenuous, and those who do not adhere to the regimen may find that their artificial joints are less effective than they had wished.
- People for whom other measures, such as medication and exercise, have not eased pain sufficiently or restored sufficient movement.
- People who suffer from severe, chronic pain or from greatly restricted movement as the result of a damaged joint.
- People over age 60 who have a less active lifestyle. Artificial hips and knees can wear out after 10 to 15 years and tend to wear out sooner in active or younger people.
- People in generally good health. Surgery may pose a risk for people with severe heart disease or AIDS.

Source: The Arthritis Foundation.

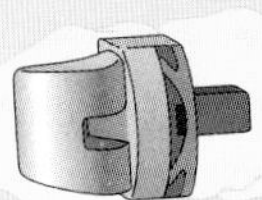

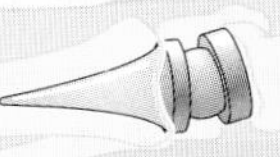

Toes
An artificial toe joint is a piece of plastic that separates and aligns the bones of the toes and acts as a hinge.

Ankles
An artificial ankle joint consists of two parts. A metal cap attaches to the ankle bone and fits into a plastic base at the end of the leg bone.

Knees
An artificial knee consists of three parts—a rounded metal cap that fits over the lower end of the thighbone and a plastic base inserted onto the top of the lower leg bone. The back of the kneecap is covered with a plastic cap.

Knee replacement is a slightly more complicated procedure because the knee joint is a complex type of hinge. In knee replacement, the bones are resurfaced in a way that preserves the ligaments and tendons of the joint. The surgeon shaves off a small amount of cartilage from the end of the femur and places a polished metal cap on the end of the bone. Similarly, a small amount of bone and cartilage is cut away from the *tibia* (shin bone) and replaced with a metal-backed plastic liner. Surgeons may also remove a bit of bone from the back of the kneecap and cover the surface with a plastic cap. By using metal and plastic, surgeons try to mimic the frictionless contact of the original surfaces.

Implanting the joint securely

Any implanted joint must bond securely to the existing bone to be effective. Bonding can be done with or without cement. Most orthopedic surgeons agree that both methods can be equally effective for their intended purpose but that neither method is perfect.

In a cemented implant, the surgeon anchors the joint with a special cement that serves the same function as mortar between bricks. Cementing came into popular use in the late 1960's and early 1970's and remains popular today for both knee and hip replacements because the cement is strong, provides a good fit, and sets quickly. Cementing remains the preferred method for holding knee implants in place, and it is also common in hip replacements. More than 90 percent of knee implants are cemented, and about 75 percent of artificial hips are anchored at least in part by cement.

Cement works well for a time, but the bond between bone, cement, and metal inevitably loosens, and the cement develops cracks. Cracked cement can cause serious problems for patients with artificial joints, including loosening of the implant. These patients may choose to have a new implant through a procedure called a revision. During a revision, the surgeon first has to remove any remaining cement from inside the bone, a process that is tricky. In a hip revision, the inside of the femur has many tiny holes, making the bone well-suited for absorbing cement and bonding with it. Scraping out the inside of the bone to remove leftover cement creates a larger cavity and exposes a smoother, less porous layer of bone that does not adhere as well to cement. As a result, the next implant requires a larger stem and, in many cases, a bone graft. The bone for grafts comes mainly from donations to bone banks.

The cementless joint

To circumvent the limitations of cemented joints, surgeons have turned to other methods of binding implants to bone. In the late 1970's, surgeons and biomedical engineers at Dartmouth Medical School in Hanover, New Hampshire, introduced a cementless coating for implant surfaces. The coating, which typically consists of tiny cobalt or titanium beads, is applied to the implant, forming ridges and grooves on the implant's surface. Once the implant is in place, bone or soft tissue grows in and around the raised surface and bonds with the metal. Today, about 25 percent of the approximately 300,000 artificial hips implanted annually in the United States are anchored solely with a porous metal coating.

Surgeons recommend cementing the implant in place for patients over age 75. Because older people's bones are less dense, they are weaker than younger people's bones and not as well suited to cementless fixation. Cementless implants require strong bone to function properly.

For people between the ages of 65 and 75, a hybrid hip implant may work best. In the hybrid, cement anchors the stem in the femur while the plastic cup to which the femur head attaches is pressed firmly into place without cement. Experts say that most patients in the 65 to 75 age range still have enough healthy bone in the pelvis to support a cementless socket but that bone growth in the femur may be insufficient to bond well with a cementless joint.

Cemented and cementless joints both have their proponents. A cementless implant is slightly more expensive because it requires an exact fit. On the other hand, a cementless implant is easier to remove and replace, if necessary.

Potential complications

Artificial joints carry other risks besides the loosening of a cemented implant. These include infection of the artificial joint and possible breakage.

Infection in the tissues around the implant strikes only 0.5 to 1 percent of joint replacement patients, according to orthopedic specialists. But it is a serious complication when it occurs. Nonsterile surgical instruments or a nonsterile implant can lead to infection while the patient is still in the hospital. Most patients who become infected in this way have a weakened immune system or are taking drugs such as corticosteroids that suppress the immune system.

Infection can also develop years after surgery. For reasons that researchers do not fully understand, the immune system is less effective at fighting infections near plastic or metal implants. Antibiotics can be mixed with bone cement in an effort to prevent infection, but this practice weakens the cement.

If bacteria lodge in tissue around a joint implant, the implant must be removed. Since bacteria can travel to the implant in the bloodstream, people with artificial joints should take antibiotics as a precaution when they face possible bacterial contamination of the blood. One such occasion is a dental visit, where teeth cleaning or surgery may allow bacteria in the mouth to enter the bloodstream. Implant patients also should seek immediate treatment for bacterial infections of the skin, urinary tract, or other sites.

Another risk comes from the removal of weight on the femur.

How a hip joint is replaced

Hip replacement has become a standard operation for people whose hip joints are disabled by arthritis or injury. An artificial hip consists of a metal ball and shaft and a socket made of metal or plastic. Hip replacement surgery can take several hours, and rehabilitation often lasts three months or more.

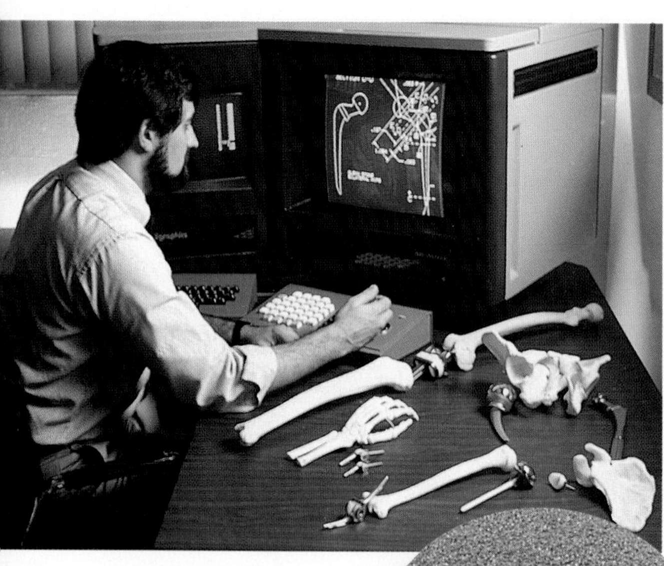

A technician uses computer software to help design joint implants, *above*. Designers try to fashion implants that will withstand wear and stress as long as possible.

An artificial hip joint consists of a stem with a metal ball at the top. The stem fits into the *femur* (thighbone). The ball fits into a plastic, cuplike socket that the surgeon presses into a hollowed out space inside the pelvis. An artificial hip joint is clearly visible in an X ray, *right*.

Pelvis

Socket

Femur head

Femur

The surgeon pushes aside or cuts muscles and tendons to expose the hip joint. The head of the femur is removed from its socket within the pelvis.

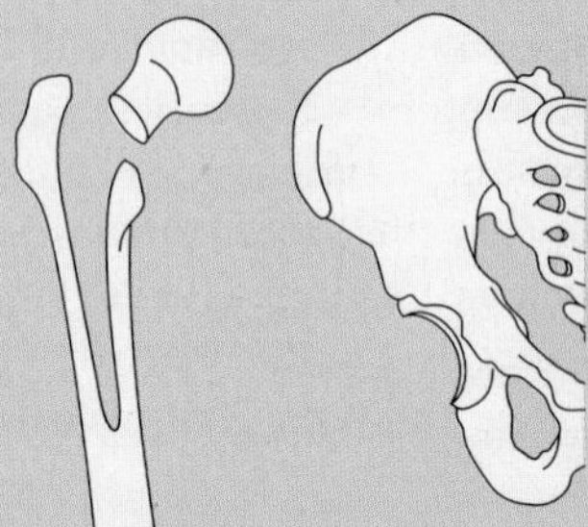

The surgeon cuts off the head of the femur and hollows out a space in the pelvis for the socket. A space for the shaft is also hollowed out in the femur.

The components of the artificial hip are set in place with a special cement that binds them to the bone. A replacement hip can also be cementless, which allows the patient's pelvis and femur to adhere naturally to the new joint. The ball is placed into the socket, the muscles are reattached to the femur, and the incision is closed.

Tissue in bone constantly dissolves and rebuilds. The bone-building process is stimulated by weight-bearing pressure on the bone, and too little pressure weakens the bone. Once an artificial hip is cemented in place, the implant absorbs most of the body weight that would normally bring pressure on the femur. As a result, bone tissue in the femur begins to thin. The removal of weight from a bone, an occurrence called stress shielding, mainly affects hip implants.

Severe stress shielding can weaken the femur to the extent that it breaks. If the femur breaks, extra weight shifts to the metal stem inside the bone, potentially causing the stem to break as well. Doctors monitor the extent of bone loss in the femur through X rays. If the X rays show a significant weakening of the femur, the artificial hip may need to be replaced. Stress shielding occurs mostly in cementless joints.

Blood clots are another potential complication of joint surgery, especially knee replacement surgery. During the surgery, the flow of blood to the leg stops. Some blood remains in the leg, where it can *coagulate* (thicken) and form a clot. Although blood clots can cause chronic swelling and pain in the leg, the vast majority produce no symptoms. In rare cases, clots break loose and travel through the bloodstream. They become dangerous when they lodge in the lung or block a blood vessel. As many as 50 percent of knee implant patients develop blood clots during surgery, according to experts. Most of these clots produce no symptoms, however.

Surgeons combat clots through blood-thinning drugs administered after surgery and through the use of compression stockings and boots during and after surgery. These devices squeeze the legs and feet tightly to promote blood flow and reduce swelling.

The problem of particle disease

A major problem for many implant patients is a condition known as particle disease. Particle disease occurs when tiny pieces of plastic or metal from an implant break loose and irritate the surrounding tissue, causing it to become inflamed. As part of the inflammation process, white blood cells called macrophages travel to the site and release infection-fighting chemicals. These chemicals can destroy bone, causing the implant to loosen.

Particle disease affects from 30 to 40 percent of hip-replacement patients within 10 years of surgery, according to a June 1995 report by a national panel of orthopedic surgeons and other specialists, and it occurs regardless of whether the implant was cemented or cementless. The report, which was sponsored by the National Institutes of Health (NIH), said that particle disease often produces no symptoms until it becomes serious and urged physicians to check patients' implants at least annually for the condition. If particle disease is detected, the implant may have to be replaced, depending on how badly the bone has been damaged. Several studies were underway in 1996 to determine how many artificial hips are dam-

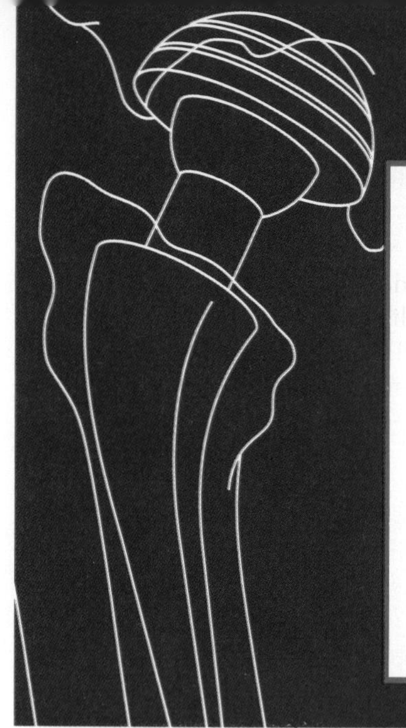

Benefits of joint replacement

For most people who decide on joint replacement, the benefits far outweigh the drawbacks. These benefits include:

- Pain reduction or elimination. Many people report almost immediate relief from arthritis pain after a joint replacement.
- Increased mobility. Surgery may not restore the full motion of a joint, but it will likely increase the range of motion and decrease stiffness in the joint.
- Improved appearance. Damage from arthritis can severely deform joints. In addition to restoring motion, artificial joints reduce deformity.

aged severely enough by particle disease to require replacement.

Although particle disease occurs with knee replacements, it usually poses less of a problem, because the particles that flake from artificial knees tend to be bigger than those from hips. Researchers believe that macrophages, the immune system's scavenging cells, may be unable to absorb the larger particles and thus do not begin the chemical attack that leads to bone loss in hips.

All joint implants will eventually fail, orthopedic surgeons say, though the joint may outlive the recipient. The two most common reasons for failure are stress shielding in cementless joints and cracked cement in cemented joints. Most studies show that artificial knees last somewhat longer than hips.

Researchers at the Mayo Clinic in Rochester, Minnesota, studied 9,000 knee replacements installed between 1971 and 1987. They found that 91 percent of new knee joints were still intact after 5 years, 80 percent after 10 years, and 69 percent at 15 years. The study found that patients with a cemented implant had the best results—some 98 percent still worked at 5 years, and 91 percent after 10 years. Patients older than 60 years and patients with rheumatoid arthritis tended to do better, probably because they were less active and put less stress on their knees. Orthopedic specialists agree that improvement in artificial joint design, materials, and cementing techniques for both knees and hips in the 1990's should allow new implants to outlast those installed in the 1970's and 1980's.

When an implant fails

An implant that fails causes chronic pain and stiffness and may need to be revised. Surgeons do not replace every failed implant, however. The age of the patient is a key consideration. If the patient is over 75 or 80 and not in too much pain, the surgeon is likely to leave the implant in. Few people require a revision, because the average age of people receiving hip and knee implants is about 70. But younger, more active patients are more likely to require revision. As the age of implant patients continues to decrease, orthopedic specialists say that revisions will probably become more common. Although the operation was not widely publicized, baseball player Bo Jackson required a hip revision just three years after the original surgery due to the heavy stress he placed on his artificial joint by playing professional baseball.

The importance of rehabilitation

People who are contemplating joint surgery should ask their surgeon for a detailed description of the procedure and a thorough explanation of its risks and benefits. To avoid disappointment later, the patient should also have a clear understanding of what to expect

Drawbacks of joint replacement

People considering joint replacement should be aware of some of the possible drawbacks of the surgery:

- A slow and painful recovery period. The recovery period for hip replacement surgery, for example, is at least three months, and patients may need to use a cane or walker during part of that time. Physical therapy, which can be painful, is part of the recovery process.
- A longer recovery time for obese people. People who are greatly overweight may not gain the full benefit from an artificial hip or knee joint. The extra weight adds to the strain on weight-bearing joints, which can lengthen recovery time and wear out the replacement joint more quickly than usual.
- The possibility of infection. In some cases, the area around the artificial joint becomes infected. If infection occurs, the implant will need to be removed and replaced again or the bones can be permanently *fused* (joined) at the joint.
- Particle disease. Particles from the implant can flake off, causing inflammation that damages the bone. If this happens, the new joint may need to be replaced.
- Stress shielding. The implant may absorb too much of the body's weight, causing bone around the implant to weaken and possibly fracture. Or the implant may fracture from absorbing too much weight.

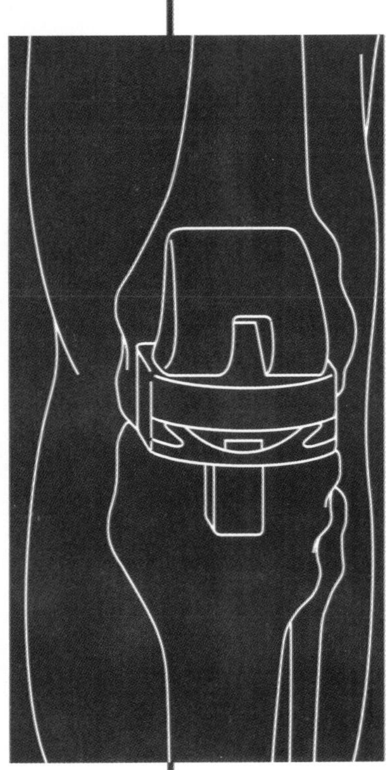

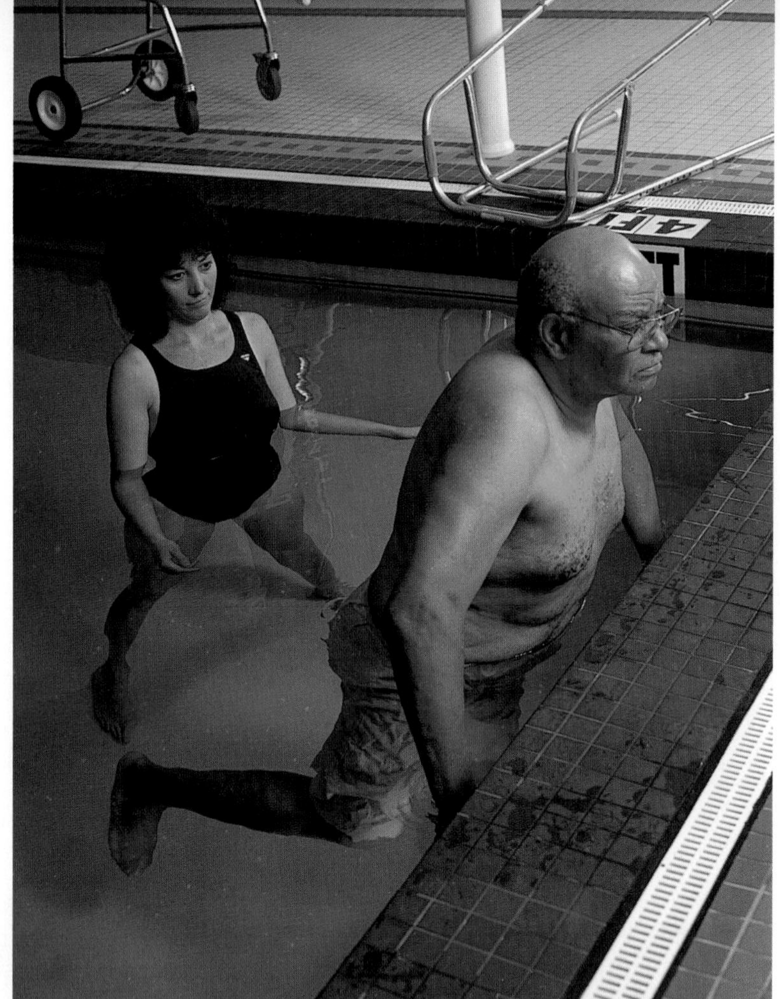

A physical therapist helps a patient exercise as part of physical therapy after his joint implant surgery. Physical therapy is essential to help rebuild strength and flexibility after joint replacement surgery.

from the new joint. Other questions might concern advance preparation and rehabilitation after surgery. In most cases, for example, physicians ask surgery patients not to take aspirin or any other anti-inflammatory drug for several days before surgery, because such drugs may increase bleeding during surgery.

Patients should also understand what rehabilitation entails, including the length of the recovery period and the amount of physical therapy involved. At least three months of physical therapy is standard after hip or knee replacement. But recovery time varies from individual to individual and depends on physical condition prior to surgery and dedication to rehabilitation after surgery. Recovery can also be painful, especially for knee patients.

The physical therapy regimen following joint replacement surgery is arduous. During rehabilitation, patients work with a physical therapist who recommends appropriate exercises and helps the patient through them. Most doctors recommend that hip and knee patients resume walking a day or two after surgery. Physical therapy usually begins at about the same time, and within a week, many are strong enough to go up and down stairs using a cane or crutches. For at least six weeks, they need to protect vulnerable muscles, and physicians may restrict a patient's activity to walking on a treadmill and light exercise on a stationary bicycle.

After about six weeks, hip patients begin to perform exercises designed to increase muscle strength in the hip. Knee patients perform bending and lifting exercises with weights attached to the ankle to strengthen knee muscles. Patients who are overweight may be asked to shed excess weight that puts added pressure on knee and hip joints. After three or four months on average, hip and knee patients have recovered almost completely.

How long do artificial joints last?

How long an artificial joint lasts depends mainly on how active a person is and how much he or she weighs. The more stress put on a joint, the sooner it is likely to wear out. Major artificial joints in a moderately active person can be expected to last:

- Hips: 10 to 15 years
- Knees: 10 to 15 years
- Shoulders: 10 to 20 years

Source: The American Academy of Orthopedic Surgeons.

Striving for better implants

Researchers continue to work on improving replacement surgery in the 1990's. Much of their work focuses on ways to improve the lifespan of implants.

Bioengineers at the University of Arizona in Tucson are experimenting with electronic sensors that could gauge the stress on joints. The sensor consists of a tiny electronic circuit board connected to wires, which is inserted in the artificial joint. The circuit board sends a weak electric current through the wire and measures the amount of resistance to the current in the wire. More resistance to the current indicates increasing stress on the joint. The circuit board then sends a signal to a device worn by the patient, alerting the wearer to reduce the amount of stress on the joint.

Researchers at New York University (NYU) Medical Center in New York City hope to increase the lifespan of implants through custom designs of hips and knees for revision surgery. Using modern computer technology, they design implants on a computer screen and then test them by applying a variety of simulated loads and muscle forces. By understanding the forces that affect joints, the researchers expect to design implants that withstand stress better. According to an orthopedic surgeon at NYU, proper size and fit can help distribute weight evenly between the implant and the femur and prevent stress shielding.

As older Americans make up an ever larger share of the population, artificial joints should become more and more common. And as baby boomers resist the effects of aging, they will challenge researchers to find new and better materials and techniques for joint replacement. •••

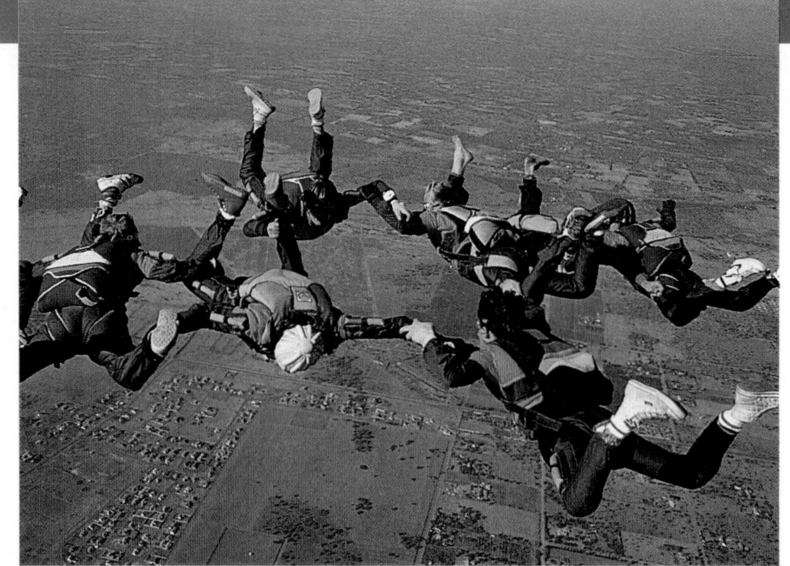

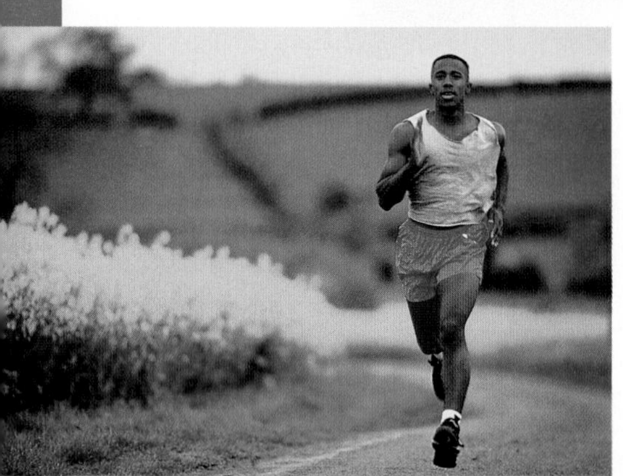

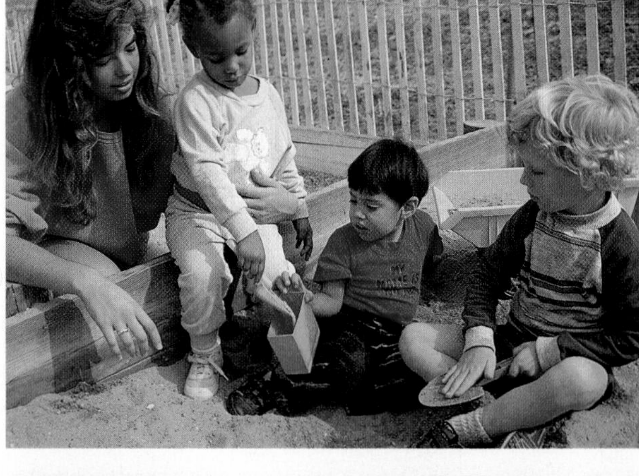

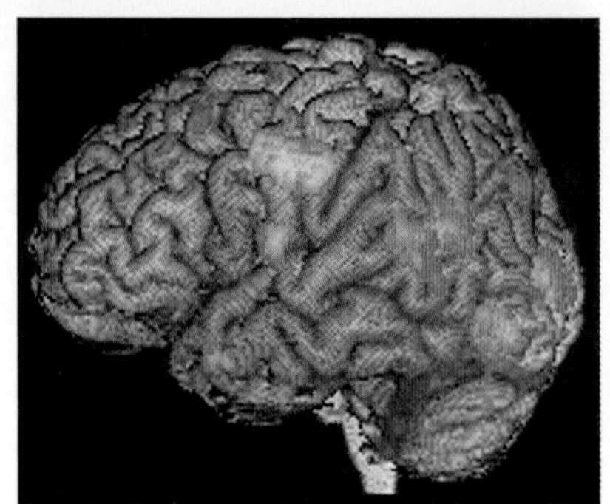

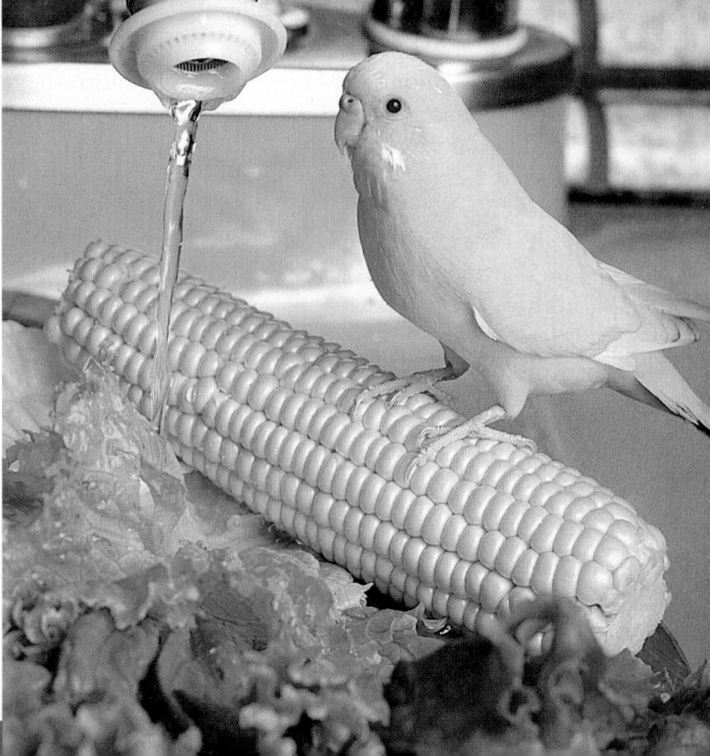

HEALTH UPDATES AND RESOURCES

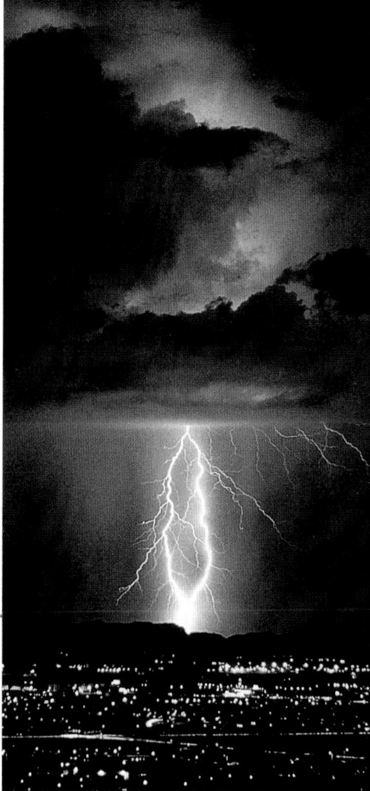

Aging

- Americans living longer and staying healthier
- Melatonin as sleep aid?
- Weight training and walking
- Health benefits of vitamins
- Alzheimer's disease and linguistic ability

Americans are living longer and with less chronic disease and disability, according to a February 1996 report. Investigators at Duke University in Durham, North Carolina, analyzed data from the National Long Term Care Surveys, a federal study that regularly surveys 20,000 people aged 65 and older. Survey participants were asked about their diseases and difficulties in caring for themselves. The researchers found that from 1982 until 1994, the number of older people with such chronic conditions as high blood pressure, arthritis, and emphysema steadily declined. Death rates from many ailments, including stroke and heart disease, also declined.

Researchers at the University of Southern California reported similar conclusions in February. From 1985 to 1996, they had studied 12,000 Americans aged 50 to 69. Study participants were asked whether physical or mental health interfered with their ability to work. (Inability to work is considered an indication of disability.) Over the course of the study, the number of people who reported being unable to work steadily declined.

The investigators suggested that higher education levels, which may lead people to choose healthy diets, give up smoking, and seek treatments for their diseases, contributed to the longevity and health of the people in the study. Medical advances in treating cataracts, joint diseases, and heart disease were also cited.

Melatonin as sleep aid? Melatonin, a natural hormone produced in the brain, may alleviate insomnia in older people. This finding was reported in August 1995 by researchers in Israel at two medical centers, a pharmaceutical company, and Tel-Aviv University.

In a study of 12 people aged 68 to 93, participants were given either a 2-milligram tablet of melatonin or a *placebo* (inactive substance) two hours before bedtime every night during a three-week period. The individuals all had long-standing insomnia and had been taking sleep medications. After a week in which no treatment was administered, subjects who had received melatonin were given placebos; those who had been taking placebos were given melatonin.

The researchers found that melatonin improved sleep quality significantly, without adverse effects. They concluded that because melatonin production is impaired in older people, melatonin supplements may help alleviate insomnia. But health professionals cautioned that people should take melatonin only under the direction of a physician.

Weight training and walking. Exercise programs that include weight

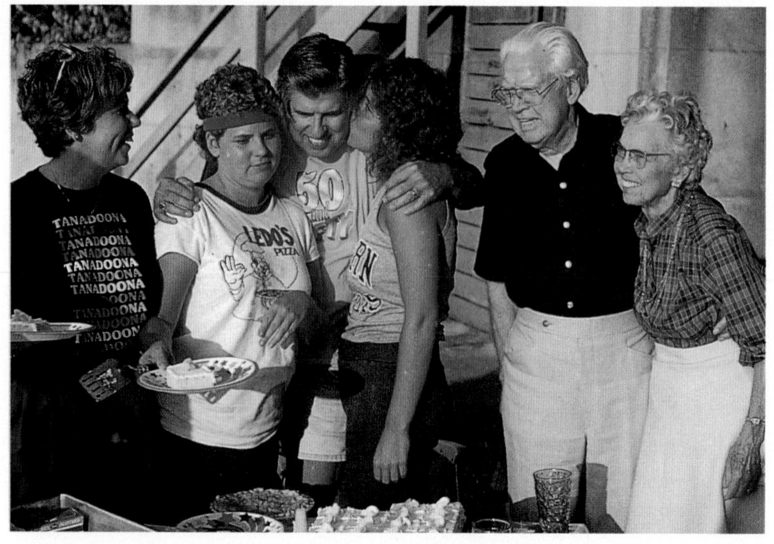

Birthday boomers

Between 1946 and 1964, a period known as the baby boom, 76 million Americans were born. On January 1, 1996, the first baby boomer turned 50. Four million boomers will hit the 50 mark each year until 2015. Because Americans are living longer, more parents are able to celebrate the 50th birthdays of their children. But some people worry that the large number of baby boomers will spur a "retirement crisis" and strain such systems as social security.

training may improve muscle strength and the ability to walk in elderly people. Researchers at the University of Vermont College of Medicine reported these findings in March 1996.

Study participants were 24 healthy men and women 65 years of age or older. One group of participants performed weight training three days a week. The training consisted of seven exercises done on an exercise apparatus, including arm and leg extensions and curls, bench presses, and squat exercises. Participants who were assigned to a second group did not alter their daily activities. After 12 weeks, the weight-training group exhibited a 38-percent increase in walking endurance. The other group showed no improvement.

Health benefits of vitamins. A study reported in September 1995 by researchers at the University of Iowa Hospitals and Clinics in Iowa City tested the theory that vitamin A may reverse macular degeneration, a common eye disorder in older people that leads to blindness.

The researchers focused on a family with a history of Sorsby's fundus dystrophy, a disorder that resembles macular degeneration but is easier to study. Family members of various ages who had experienced vision loss were given 10 times the normal dietary requirement of vitamin A. Two family members, both at early stages of the disease, experienced improved vision. The investigators concluded that vitamin A supplements may prove beneficial in reversing macular degeneration in older people.

A May 1996 study found a link between vitamin E and heart disease in postmenopausal women. For seven years, researchers at the University of Minnesota recorded the vitamin E intake of nearly 35,000 postmenopausal women with no signs of heart disease. They discovered that the women who consumed the most vitamin E—at least 10 international units daily, the recommended daily allowance—were 62 percent less likely to die of coronary heart disease than those who consumed the least.

Alzheimer's and linguistic ability. A study published in February 1996 by scientists at the University of Kentucky found that people's writing styles in early life may be used to predict the likelihood of their developing Alzheimer's disease. The study involved 93 elderly nuns who were living in convents, mostly in the Milwaukee area.

Researchers studied autobiographical essays that the nuns had written when they were in their 20's. They discovered a strong association between poor linguistic ability in early life and the onset of the devastating brain disorder decades later. (See BRAIN AND NERVOUS SYSTEM; MENTAL HEALTH.) • Rein Tideiksaar

In the section A Healthy Family, see PLANNING YOUR HAPPILY EVER AFTER. In WORLD BOOK, see AGING.

STATISTICS

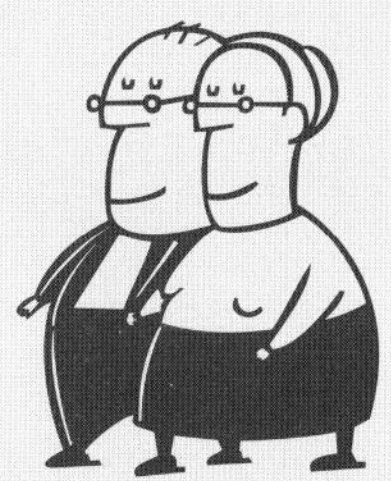

Elderly Americans live longest

Americans who reach age 80 live longer on average than people who reach 80 in England, France, Sweden, or Japan, according to statistics reported in November 1995 by researchers at Duke University in Durham, North Carolina. The research suggests that Americans may be receiving better health care than elderly people in other developed countries.

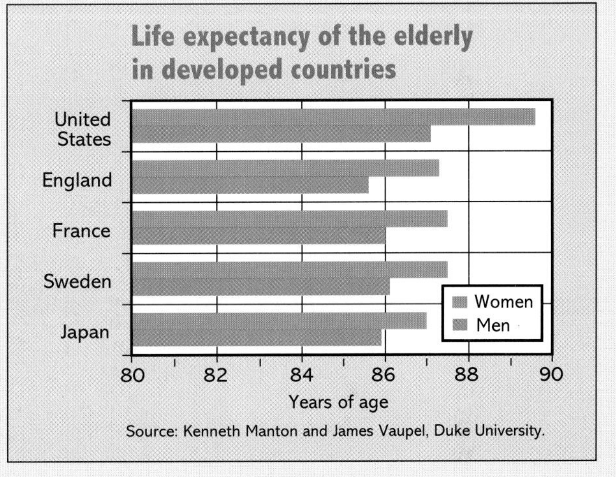

Source: Kenneth Manton and James Vaupel, Duke University.

AIDS

- AIDS statistics
- New AIDS drugs approved
- Vital cell-surface protein discovered
- Natural chemicals fight HIV
- Baboon cell transplant
- Risky sexual behavior
- Predicting AIDS progression
- Home testing for HIV

The number of new AIDS cases reported to the United States Centers for Disease Control and Prevention (CDC) in Atlanta, Georgia, in 1995 declined 7 percent from 1994. In a February 1996 report, the CDC said 74,180 new AIDS cases were diagnosed in 1995. The agency also reported that in 1994, the death toll from AIDS among men and women 25 to 44 years old rose 30 percent among white women, 28 percent among black women, and 13 percent among black men. The CDC said the rise in deaths among women and minorities was linked to intravenous drug use or sexual intercourse with drug users infected with HIV (human immunodeficiency virus), the virus that causes AIDS.

Since AIDS is mainly a young person's disease, deaths from AIDS have had the effect of halting the increase in life expectancy in the United States after a century in which it had climbed steadily. In August 1995, the Metropolitan Life Insurance Company reported that the life expectancy of a baby born in America in 1994 was 75.5 years, exactly the same as for 1993 and slightly less than for 1992, when life expectancy peaked at 75.8 years.

New AIDS drugs approved. The U.S. Food and Drug Administration (FDA) in 1995 and 1996 approved three drugs in a new class of medications called protease inhibitors. The drugs slow the progression of AIDS but are not a cure. They interfere with the activity of a substance that HIV uses to *replicate* (reproduce) itself in the body. In clinical trials, protease inhibitors were especially effective in patients who had not been helped by other AIDS drugs.

In December 1995, the FDA approved saquinavir (marketed as Invirase). In March 1996, the FDA approved ritonavir (marketed as Norvir). In an international study, about half of 1,090 patients with advanced AIDS were given ritonavir, and the rest were given a *placebo* (an inactive substitute). After seven months, the patients on ritonavir had about half the death rate of those taking the placebo and half the incidence of the severe illnesses that are the hallmark of AIDS. Ritonavir decreases the amount of HIV in the blood and boosts immune-system function.

Also in March 1996, the FDA approved what appeared to be the most potent of the protease inhibitors, indinavir (marketed as Crixivan). Clinical trials showed that when taken alone, indinavir cut the levels of HIV in patients' blood by 80 to 90 percent. In previous trials, indinavir in combination with two other AIDS medications—AZT and 3TC—reduced HIV in the blood by 99 percent, making it

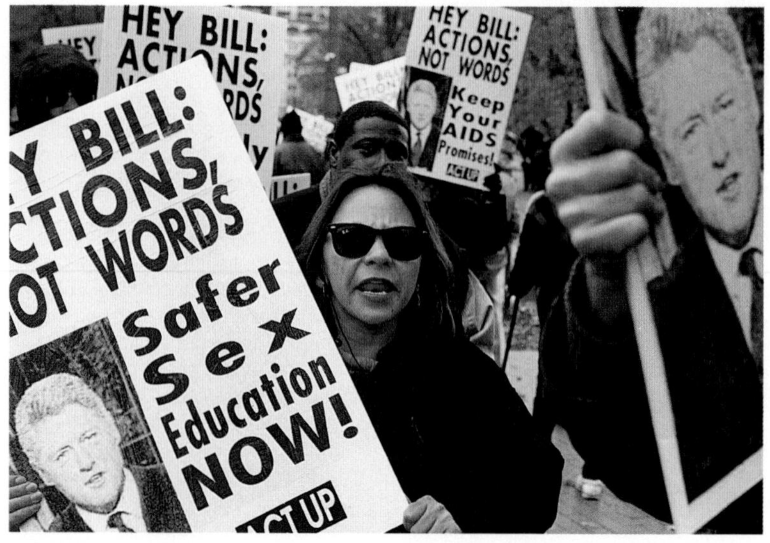

First White House AIDS conference

Activists outside the White House press President Bill Clinton for more action to combat AIDS as he held the first presidential conference on the disease in December 1995. President Clinton promised to protect funding for AIDS research, but the activists demanded that he consider a national needle-exchange program, housing assistance, and other actions to combat the disease and help its victims.

virtually undetectable. Scientists noted, however, that the virus can reside elsewhere in the body besides the blood.

Vital protein discovered. In May 1996, scientists at the National Institutes of Health (NIH) in Bethesda, Maryland, reported that they had discovered a protein on the surface of T cells that enables HIV to enter the cells. T cells, white blood cells of the immune system, are the primary target of the AIDS virus. According to the researchers, the protein, which they named fusin, must be present in order for the AIDS virus to attach to receptor molecules on the surface of T cells in the bloodstream. Fusin enables HIV to fuse with the surface of cells before it penetrates them.

Robert C. Gallo, a codiscoverer of HIV and head of the University of Maryland's new Institute of Human Virology in Baltimore, called the identification of fusin a milestone in AIDS research. He said it opened new doors for therapy and for developing vaccines.

Natural chemicals fight HIV. In December 1995, a research team led by Gallo reported the isolation of three natural chemicals, called chemokines, that interfere with the activity of HIV. The chemokines are secreted by white blood cells.

The researchers extracted the chemokines from HIV-infected white blood cells. They found that adding even a tiny amount of all three chemicals to HIV-infected cells in the laboratory prevented HIV from replicating. Adding the chemicals singly had no effect on the virus.

Researchers speculated whether the presence of chemokines was the reason some HIV-infected people have lived for many years without progressing to AIDS. Studies proceeded in 1996 to synthesize the substances for possible use as a treatment for HIV infection.

Baboon cell transplant. Jeff Getty, a 38-year-old AIDS patient with deteriorating health, underwent a controversial procedure at San Francisco General Hospital in December 1995, receiving a bone marrow transplant from a baboon. Baboon cells usually are not damaged by the most prevalent strain of the AIDS virus, HIV-1. Doctors hoped that the transplanted cells—the precursors of blood cells—would form an immune system parallel to Getty's own damaged system and fight off HIV.

However, tests on Getty conducted in February 1996 showed little evidence of baboon cell growth. Baboon cells made up less than 1 percent of his immune cells, a level thought to be inadequate to fight disease.

But surprisingly, Getty's health seemed to improve in the aftermath of the procedure. He gained 10 pounds (4.5 kilograms), and a test indicated his white-blood-cell count had almost tripled, though it was still

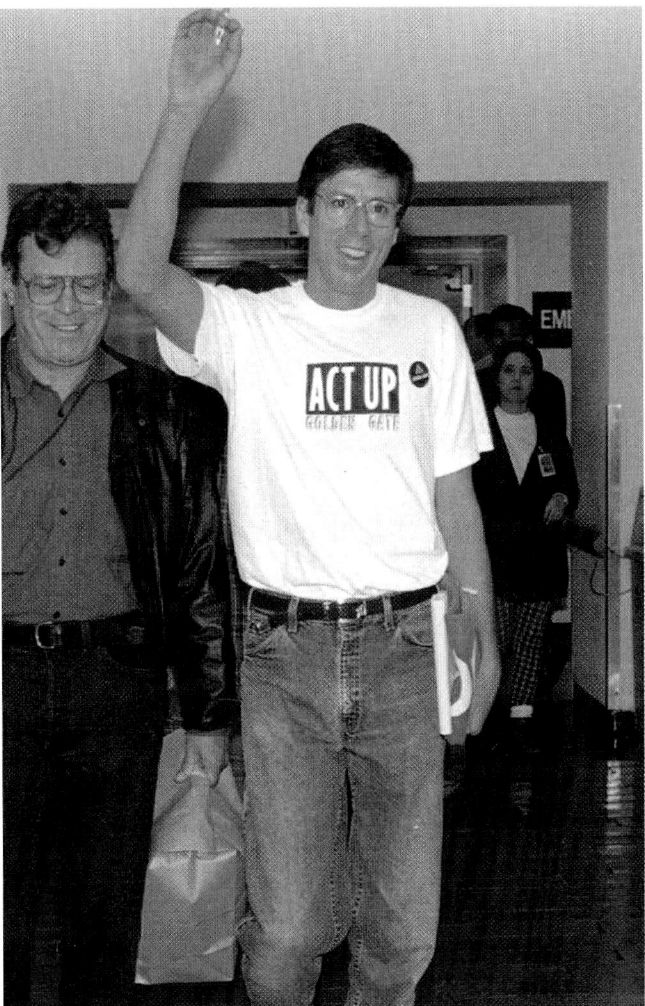

AIDS patient leaves hospital after transplant

Jeff Getty waves as he leaves San Francisco General Hospital, where he had received a transplant of baboon bone marrow cells in December 1995. Researchers at the hospital hoped the baboon cells, which are resistant to the primary strain of the AIDS virus, would rebuild Getty's immune system. Although the experimental procedure failed, Getty's health improved and he gained weight.

far below normal. Also, he had not developed any new infections. Getty's physician said the improvements were probably not due to any baboon cells but perhaps resulted from the intensive radiation and drug therapy Getty underwent in preparation for the transplant.

Risky sexual behavior. Oral sex may pose greater risks for contracting AIDS than was previously thought. That was the conclusion of a study reported in June 1996 by researchers at the Dana Farber Cancer Institute in Boston and Tulane University in New Orleans, Louisiana. The scientists deposited small amounts of simian immunodeficiency virus (SIV) on the tongues of seven healthy rhesus monkeys. SIV is closely related to HIV and causes AIDS in monkeys. Two of the monkeys in the experiment died of AIDS, four developed AIDS-like symptoms, and one remained healthy.

The monkeys did not have sores or cuts in their mouths through which SIV could have entered their bloodstream and caused infection. The doses of SIV were 6,000 times lower than those administered rectally that caused infection in other monkeys.

Oncologist (cancer specialist) Ruth M. Ruprecht, head of the research team, said further study was necessary to determine exactly how SIV entered the monkeys' bloodstream. She recommended that unprotected receptive oral intercourse be placed on the list of behaviors that put people at risk for HIV infection. She said no AIDS risk exists from kissing or the sharing of utensils.

Another study, reported in August 1995 by researchers at the University of Washington in Seattle, showed that the risk of HIV infection is high with unprotected sex. The scientists tested 100 semen samples from 16 HIV-infected men over a two-year period. The virus was detected 22 percent of the time, and the rate was the same for men taking AIDS drugs as for those who were not. Every blood test during the study period indicated the presence of HIV. The scientists warned that there is no way to determine when an infected man has HIV in his semen and thus may spread the infection to a sexual partner.

Predicting AIDS progression. A new test for HIV infections being evaluated in 1996 measures the amount of HIV in the bloodstream to predict the progression of the infection to AIDS or death. The test, called branched DNA, was developed by Chiron Diagnostics of Emeryville, California. Researchers at the University of Pittsburgh Medical Center reported in May 1996 that the test more accurately predicted the outcome of an HIV infection than measuring the level of T cells, which had been considered the most accurate test.

The Pittsburgh researchers studied 180 men who did not know when they first became infected with HIV. The scientists followed the men's progression to AIDS and death over a period of up to 10 years with both tests that measure T cells and the new branched DNA test. They found that the branched DNA test results more accurately predicted how each man's illness would progress than T-cell tests, because T-cell counts do not respond quickly to an HIV attack. T-cell counts can remain high even when the blood contains large amounts of HIV.

In June 1996, the FDA gave Roche Diagnostic Systems Inc. of Branchburg, New Jersey, approval to market a test that measures the amount of HIV in the blood as a means of monitoring the progression to AIDS. Roche had already marketed the test, called Amplicor HIV-1 monitor test, for more than a year in Europe and elsewhere.

Home testing for HIV. The FDA in May 1996 approved a new HIV screening test for home use, called Confide. An individual using the test would obtain a small blood sample from a finger, place it on a specially prepared test card, and mail the card to a testing laboratory. Results would be available in a week by calling a toll-free phone number and giving the identification number printed on the test card. The number was intended to ensure the anonymity of the person being tested. • Richard Trubo

See also DRUGS; SEXUALLY TRANSMITTED DISEASES. In the section On the Medical Frontier, see SCIENCE VERSUS THE AIDS VIRUS. In WORLD BOOK, see AIDS.

Marijuana was the most widely used illegal drug in the United States in 1995, according to a survey by the Substance Abuse and Mental Health Service Administration (SAMHSA), a federal agency. The survey found that some 10 million adults and teen-agers smoked marijuana, compared with 7.5 million in 1994. The survey found that one in five high school seniors smoked marijuana daily.

In February 1996, researchers at Harvard Medical School in Boston reported finding that heavy marijuana use is linked with "decreased mental flexibility and reduced learning ability." The study suggests that daily marijuana use has pronounced and lasting effects on the ability to sustain and shift attention.

Perceptions of drug use. In August 1995, investigators at the Center on Addiction and Substance Abuse at Columbia University in New York City reported the results of a telephone survey of students aged 12 to 17 and adults aimed at finding how they viewed drug use among American youth. Of the 400 young people in the survey, 32 percent named drugs as the greatest problem for people their age. More than half of the 10th-graders said they had friends who used marijuana and half had themselves been offered marijuana to buy or share.

Of the 2,000 adults surveyed, 82 percent thought youngsters could easily get cocaine or heroin. However, only 30 percent of the students thought those drugs were easily obtainable.

Growing abuse of inhalants. Glue, aerosol sprays, lighter fluid, and paint thinner, which contain substances that, when inhaled, produce feelings of euphoria, have grown in popularity among children and teen-agers. That was the finding of an annual survey of U.S. students conducted by the University of Michigan in Ann Arbor. The 1995 survey found that one out of five 13-year-olds reported using inhalants, an increase of 30 percent since 1991. Inhalants kill as many as 1,000 people each year, most of them in their teens.

Binge drinking. Alcohol use among 14-year-olds climbed 50 percent from 1992 to 1994, according to the University of Michigan study, and binge drinking—defined as having four or more drinks at one time—also increased. In 1995, one in five 10th-graders reported having been drunk in the 30 days prior to the survey. Two-thirds of high school seniors said they had a friend or acquaintance with a drinking problem.

Teen-agers who drink heavily during their high school years are likely

Alcohol and Drug Abuse

- Marijuana—the most widely used drug
- Perceptions of drug use
- Growing abuse of inhalants
- Binge drinking
- Heroin's new popularity
- Methamphetamine returns
- Drug newcomers
- Federal drug policy
- Drug abuse
- Needle-exchange programs

STATISTICS

High school drug use rising

Drug	1991	1995
Beer	56.2%	57.4%
Liquor	48.7%	51.5%
Cigarettes	35.2%	44.4%
Marijuana	16.9%	28.2%
Uppers	7.6%	9.3%
Hallucinogens	4.9%	7.7%
Inhalants	5.0%	7.5%
Downers	4.6%	5.5%
Cocaine	3.4%	4.5%

Source: National Parents' Resource Institute for Drug Education.

More high school students drank alcohol, smoked cigarettes, and used illegal drugs in 1995 than in 1991, according to the National Parents' Resource Institute for Drug Education (PRIDE) annual survey of 200,000 juniors and seniors, reported in November 1995. A PRIDE spokesperson attributed the big jump in smoking marijuana to a growing belief among teen-agers that the drug is harmless. The report urged parents to combat the upward trend by talking to their children about the dangers of using any drug.

Dealing with a father's alcoholism

Alcoholism in a parent can be painfully embarrassing to children. They see how drinking changes a loved one's behavior and causes fights at home. In *My Dad,* written by Niki Daly and published by Simon & Schuster, a brother and sister learn that their father's silliness every Friday night stems from his drinking. Their performance at a school concert turns into a crisis when Dad arrives, drunk and boisterous. They leave the stage, hurt and humiliated. For Dad, it is a turning point. He seeks help from Alcoholics Anonymous. The children learn that Dad's road to recovery will be long but are willing to join Mom in supporting him in his battle to beat alcoholism.

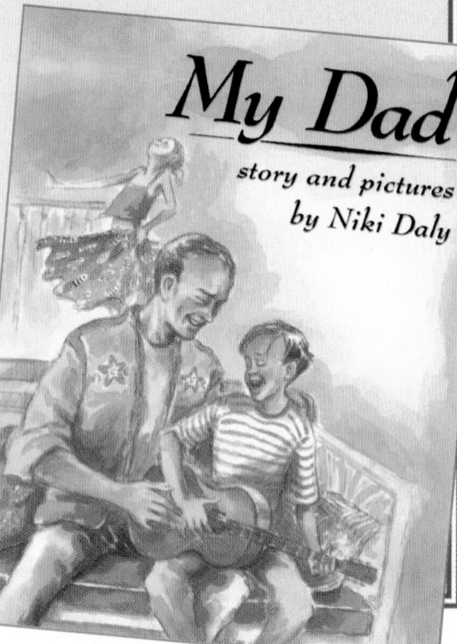

to drink even more in college, according to a study reported in 1995 in *Alcoholism: Clinical and Experimental Research.* The study found that alcohol consumption rose especially for students who drank heavily in high school and then joined fraternities and sororities in college.

Many colleges in 1995 and 1996 were attempting to tighten their policies on the use of alcohol on campus and stiffen penalties for intoxication. Still, a survey of 17,592 U.S. college students by the Harvard School of Public Health in Boston found that nearly half were binge drinkers.

Heroin's new popularity. The federal Office of National Drug Control Policy (ONDCP) reported in March 1996 that the number of "hard-core" drug abusers had tripled—to 2.7 million—since 1990. In particular, heroin use was surging among young, middle-class professionals and entertainers. The ONDCP characterized the heroin trend as a cultural rejection of the flashy cocaine culture of the 1980's. The agency also attributed heroin's popularity to the drug's higher potency than in the past and to the fact that it was cheaper and easier to buy than cocaine.

Rehabilitation centers and hospitals in 1996 reported treating an increased number of professionals and college students for heroin addiction, and emergency rooms saw a steady increase in heroin overdoses. Due to an increase in its purity, heroin was being "snorted" and smoked rather than injected. These modes of taking heroin increased its appeal to those who are reluctant to inject drugs for fear of contracting the AIDS virus from contaminated needles.

Methamphetamine returns. Abuse of methamphetamine was also on the rise in 1995 and 1996. The Drug Abuse Warning Network (DAWN), a survey conducted by the SAMHSA, showed a 144-percent rise in methamphetamine-related deaths between 1992 and 1994. Known as "crank" or "ice" on the streets, methamphetamine is a synthetic stimulant that produces euphoria, high energy, and a feeling of confidence. But use of the drug can also bring on violent and paranoid behavior. High doses cause seizure and death. In the late 1960's and early 1970's, the drug was often injected, but in the 1990's it was usually smoked, snorted, or taken orally.

Drug newcomers. Rohypnol, a legal tranquilizer in Europe commonly prescribed for severe insomnia, was slowly making its way into the American urban drug scene in 1996. Rock singer Kurt Cobain collapsed from an overdose of rohypnol and champagne a month before he committed suicide in 1994. In 1996, rohypnol, known as "roofies" and "rope" on the street, was in abundant supply in Florida and Texas. Rohypnol was sometimes called the "date-rape drug" because it seems to lower inhibitions and suppress short-term memory.

Another newcomer was Herbal Ecstacy, part of the new "natural" drug fad in the United States. Sold in health food stores under the trade names Cloud Nine or Ultimate Xphoria, these products consist primarily of the herb ephedra, an ancient Chinese remedy for upper-respiratory ailments. Ephedra's active chemical, ephedrine, is used in many over-the-counter decongestants sold in the United States. Herbal Ecstacy was being sold legally on the basis that it is considered an herbal substance under the 1994 Dietary Supplement Health and Education Act. But in 1996, the U.S. Food and Drug Administration (FDA) began an investigation of Herbal Ecstacy based on at least 15 reported deaths.

Federal drug policy. An official ONDCP priority in 1996 was to reduce drug use through treatment and prevention. The strategy was to prevent, or at least delay, people from getting started on drugs, get casual users to quit, prevent casual users from becoming hard-core users, and decrease the number of hard-core users. The ONDCP estimated that 180 million Americans had never used illegal drugs, 12.6 million were casual drug users, 2.7 million were hard-core drug users, and 65 million had used drugs at one time but subsequently quit.

The Senate on Feb. 29, 1996, confirmed U.S. Army General Barry McCaffrey as director of the ONDCP. McCaffrey had a mandate to invigorate the national drug strategy. He said effective treatment programs were essential to reduce the nation's drug consumption. And only by lowering drug use, he said, would it be possible to cut down the violence and property crimes long associated with the drug trade.

But the federal drug budget emphasized enforcement of antidrug laws over treatment and prevention. Of the $13.2-billion budget, approximately $8.8 billion was targeted for enforcement-related measures, including the interception of illegal drugs at the national borders. About $4.4 billion was allocated for treatment and prevention.

The strict enforcement of drug laws resulted in drug offenders becoming the largest and fastest-growing population in federal prisons, accounting for 61 percent of the nearly 83,000 inmates serving terms in 1996, according to the U.S. Bureau of Prisons. The 1996 Drug Strategies report from the ONDCP stated that although 52 percent of crack cocaine users were white, 90 percent of the inmates in federal prisons for crack cocaine offenses were black.

Drug-abuse treatment. The National Drug and Alcoholism Treatment Unit Survey by the SAMHSA had reported in early 1995 that almost 1 million people were in private and public substance-abuse treatment programs in 1993. Approximately 20 percent of those people were enrolled mainly for drug abuse, 45 percent for alcohol abuse, and 35 percent for combined alcohol and drug dependencies. Still, in 1996, drug-abuse experts estimated that another 2.6 million Americans were in need of drug treatment but were not enrolled in any program, due in part to inadequate public funding. Also, many addicts refuse treatment.

Needle-exchange programs. Support for needle-exchange programs remained controversial in 1995 and 1996. In needle-exchange programs, addicts can obtain clean needles to inject drugs in order to prevent the sharing of used needles, a known cause of the spread of deadly AIDS and other serious infections. Review panels at the National Academy of Sciences and at the Centers for Disease Control and Prevention in Atlanta, Georgia, had long supported needle exchange as a way to help stop the AIDS epidemic. But critics said that providing needles increases the amount of drug use.

Connecticut passed a law in 1992 that permitted pharmacies to sell 10 syringes at a time without a prescription. In 1995, Connecticut found that needle sharing among drug users fell 40 percent. • David C. Lewis

In World Book, see Alcoholism; Drug abuse.

Allergies and Asthma

- Airborne allergens
- Countering adrenal suppression
- Testing lung function
- Smoke and fetal development
- Latex allergy
- Dusty libraries and allergies
- Aspirin desensitization

A study reported in March 1996 by researchers in Italy found that almost 54 percent of 564 children treated for respiratory symptoms were allergic to at least one class of airborne *allergens*. An allergen is anything that causes an allergic reaction. Lung specialist Michela Silvestri and her colleagues at the University of Genoa tested the children for allergic reactions to dust mites, pollen, pet dander, and molds—four of the most common airborne allergens.

All of the 564 children, aged 5 months to 17 years, had received outpatient treatment during 1992 for respiratory symptoms of asthma or *rhinitis* (an inflammation of the membrane lining the nose) or both. The most common allergic reaction was to dust mites, microscopic organisms that are common in household dust. However, the older the child, the more likely he or she was to react to outdoor allergens, such as pollen, or to react to more than one of the allergens. The researchers said further studies would be required to learn the causes of age-related changes in reactions to airborne allergens.

Countering adrenal suppression. A spacer, or hollow chamber, attached to an asthma-treatment inhaler may reduce the chance of children experiencing an undesirable side effect called adrenal suppression. Pediatrician Shmuel Goldberg and his colleagues at the Shaare Zedek Medical Center in Jerusalem reported their findings in March 1996.

Inhaled drugs called corticosteroids reduce inflammation in the respiratory tract, keeping airways open and preventing asthma attacks. But they also cause adrenal suppression, a condition in which the drug tricks the body into thinking that the adrenal glands, which naturally produce corticosteroid hormones, are overworking. The brain then sends a message suppressing the work of the adrenal glands. Studies indicate that adrenal suppression may stunt a child's growth.

Goldberg and his associates studied the effect of attaching a spacer to the mouthpiece of a corticosteroid inhaler. A spacer filters off large particles of the corticosteroids that would end up in the mouth and throat and would be absorbed into the body rather than inhaled into the lungs. Monitoring the treatment of 39 children, the researchers found evidence of adrenal suppression among 47 percent of the the children inhaling corticosteroids directly without a spacer, but among only 8 percent of those using a large-volume spacer.

The investigators said that although inhaled steroids are important in the treatment of asthma, physicians should be concerned about possible adrenal suppression, especially in children.

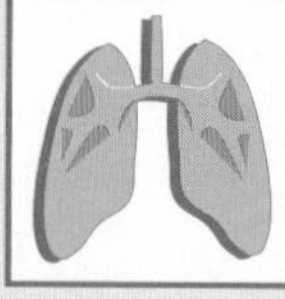

Everyone take a deep breath

The inability to relax the muscles around the breathing passages with deep breaths may be the cause of asthma. In an October 1995 report, researchers at Johns Hopkins University theorized that all people react to inhaled irritants with muscle contractions that close up the airways. A person without asthma is able to relax those muscles with deep breaths, but a person with asthma cannot. To test their theory, researchers asked nonasthmatic people to avoid breathing deeply when inhaling irritants. All of them developed breathing difficulties similar to an asthma attack.

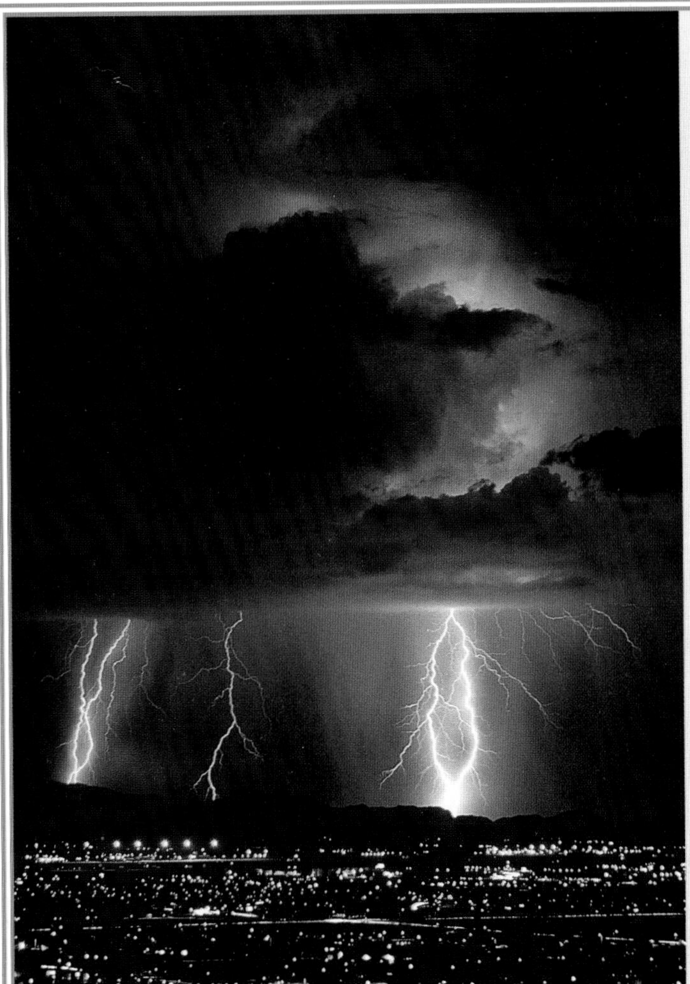

Struck by asthma

In a 1996 report, British researchers said a major outbreak of asthma was the result of a thunderstorm that occurred in the London area on June 24, 1994. During a 30-hour period, 640 people received emergency treatment for asthma, almost 10 times more than the number normally expected to need treatment. The demands were so great that many of the hospitals ran out of supplies and equipment.

The researchers offered possible explanations for how the thunderstorm could have caused the asthma epidemic. Gusting winds may have stirred up pollen, they said, or the storm may have carried allergens and deposited them with cold downdrafts. Also, the rainfall and humidity may have caused pollen to emit easily inhaled allergens.

Testing lung function. Despite the availability of reliable lung-function tests to evaluate the severity of asthma, many physicians do not use them to monitor treatment. Family physician Robert Fried and his associates at the Maine Medical Center in Portland based that conclusion, reported in August 1995, on surveys of 38 medical practices.

In 1991, the National Institutes of Health (NIH) in Bethesda, Maryland, recommended two tests for the diagnosis and management of asthma—spirometry and peak-flow rates. A spirometer measures the rate at which a person exhales air and the total volume of air exhaled. A peak-flow meter measures the maximum speed at which air can flow out of the lungs.

Over 70 percent of the practices surveyed reported having easy access to peak-flow meters and spirometers. A review of the practices' asthma-related visits, however, showed no spirometry testing for almost 70 percent of the cases and no peak-flow measurements for 55 percent of them.

The researchers expressed concern about the findings because the two tests provide more accurate information than other tests. For example, the maximum speed at which air can flow from the lungs can decrease 25 percent before a doctor can detect wheezing through a stethoscope. Inadequate measurements of lung function may cause delays in treatment for asthma that can increase the risk of serious illness or death.

Smoke and fetal development. A pregnant woman's exposure to secondhand cigarette smoke can increase her unborn child's chances of developing asthma. That conclusion was reported in May 1996 by researchers at the Hurley Medical Center in Flint, Michigan.

The investigators surveyed 22 mothers who had been exposed to secondhand smoke while pregnant and 25 mothers who had passed their pregnancy in a smoke-free environment. Mothers who had been exposed to smoke reported a much higher incidence of wheezing and other asthma symptoms in their young children than the other mothers did. Although the number of mothers surveyed was small, the study supported other research on the potentially harmful effects of secondhand smoke on fetal development.

Latex allergy. Two separate research groups reported in 1996 that 10 percent of health-care workers are allergic to the latex in protective gloves and many other medical products, such as blood-pressure tubing and stethoscopes.

Allergy specialist Jack Eades and his colleagues at the Vanderbilt Allergy Center in Nashville, Tennessee, concluded from survey results of 20 health-care workers that the length of time exposed to latex and the intensity of exposure appear to be risk factors for development of sensitivity to latex products.

In a study of 93 emergency medical service providers, Ghassan Safadi and his associates at the Cleveland Clinic Foundation found that 90 percent of the workers used latex gloves regularly, but most of the workers were unaware of possible latex allergies in themselves or their patients.

Safadi and his colleagues recommended educating health-care workers about possible allergic reactions to latex and providing alternative products for emergency medical use. Also, they said, anyone known to be allergic to latex should wear a Med-Alert label.

Dusty libraries and allergies. The dusty environment of many libraries has been implicated in the respiratory allergies common among library workers. Dust mites were the suspected culprit, but research reported in March 1996 by scientists at the Pontificia Universidad Javeriana in Bogotá, Colombia, suggested otherwise.

The investigators analyzed dust from 20 Bogotá libraries but found little evidence of mites or fungi. Moreover, only a few of the 108 library workers given skin tests were found to be sensitive to those allergens.

Since the study produced results different from the expected conclusions, the researchers planned further inquiries. They intended to study proteins present in the dust that may cause the allergic reactions.

Aspirin desensitization. In an aspirin desensitization program reported in March 1996, 65 people showed significant reductions in sinus inflammation, asthma attacks, and other allergic reactions to aspirin. Allergy and immunology specialist Donald Stevenson and his associates at the Scripps Clinic and Research Foundation in La Jolla, California, reported on the outcome of a treatment program lasting one to six years.

A hypersensitivity, or allergic response, to aspirin is often associated with asthma, nasal *polyps* (growths on the lining of the nose), and an intolerance to other anti-inflammatory drugs, such as ibuprofen. The National Asthma Education Program estimates that 5 to 20 percent of adults with asthma are sensitive to aspirin. For some people this condition is problematic if they need aspirin or related medications to treat other conditions.

A desensitization program is a carefully monitored treatment in which the patient is given aspirin in gradually increasing doses. Most patients will develop a tolerance to the drug instead of an allergic reaction if they continue to take it in a regular, daily program. The outcome of the program at the Scripps Clinic suggests that desensitization may be an appropriate and useful treatment for aspirin-sensitive asthma patients. • **Dominick A. Minotti**

In the section MEDICAL AND SAFETY ALERTS, see FOOD ALLERGIES: WHEN COMMON FOODS CAUSE UNCOMMON REACTIONS. In WORLD BOOK, see ALLERGY; ASTHMA.

Arthritis and Connective Tissue Disorders

- Bacterial DNA and systemic lupus erythematosus
- Inflammation and osteoarthritis
- New drug for osteoporosis
- Combination drug therapy for rheumatoid arthritis

Research continued in 1995 and 1996 on how DNA (deoxyribonucleic acid, the molecule genes are made of) from bacteria can modify immune cell activity. In an April 1996 report, Scientists at Duke University Medical Center in Durham, North Carolina, confirmed earlier research that bacterial DNA can protect against systemic lupus erythematosus (SLE) in mice.

SLE is an *autoimmune disease* (a disease in which the immune system attacks the body's own tissues) that primarily affects young women. It can cause serious kidney damage if *antibodies* (molecules produced by the immune system that normally protect us from disease) attack the kidneys.

In the late 1980's and early 1990's, scientists from several laboratories showed that DNA from bacteria can stimulate the immune system. To test whether bacterial DNA could modify the course of an autoimmune disease, the scientists studied mice that are highly prone to SLE.

The researchers injected some of the mice with bacterial DNA before the animals developed lupus and left other mice untreated. Although the treated mice eventually developed the high levels of antibodies that indicate the presence of SLE, they showed no evidence of kidney damage. Furthermore, when the scientists injected bacterial DNA into mice that had already developed lupus, they found that the DNA halted the progression of the disease.

The scientists did not know why or how the bacterial DNA protected the mice. However, they theorized that *cytokines* (hormonelike substances that regulate immune responses), which the DNA caused the immune system to produce, may have restored more normal functioning to the animals' immune systems. The results of this study suggested that bacterial DNA might be useful in the treatment of lupus and other human autoimmune diseases.

Inflammation and osteoarthritis. A protein that controls inflammation may contribute to the development of the joint disease osteoarthritis. That finding was reported in December 1995 by investigators at the Hospital for Joint Diseases Orthopaedic Institute and New York University Medical Center, both in New York City, and the University of Pittsburgh.

Osteoarthritis occurs frequently in older people and involves a loss of cartilage at the ends of bones. Cartilage helps to lubricate joints. While healthy cartilage is smooth, cartilage damaged by osteoarthritis becomes thinned, roughened, and frayed. Joints are less flexible and motion is painful.

Osteoarthritis is usually considered the result of wear-and-tear of the joints. However, some evidence suggests that inflammation may also play a part. To investigate that possibility,

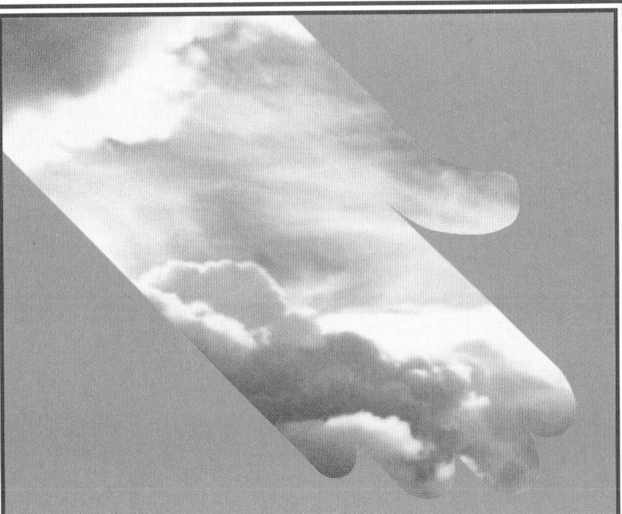

Can you really feel it in your bones?

A long-standing belief that people with arthritis feel more pain when the weather changes was challenged by a study published in April 1996 by internist Donald A. Redelmeier of the University of Toronto and psychologist Amos Tversky of Stanford University. The researchers followed 18 arthritis patients for 15 months, assessing the patients' pain regularly and noting the local weather conditions. They found no link between the weather and the patients' pain.

The explanation offered by the researchers was that people tend to see patterns where none exist. When arthritis pain is bad, the investigators said, patients look for causes—high humidity, rain, or increased air pressure. When the pain is less severe, they tend to ignore the weather. Even physicians have assumed that the severity of arthritis varies with the weather and have recommended that patients move to drier climates, but the researchers' results indicated that such a move would be unlikely to bring relief.

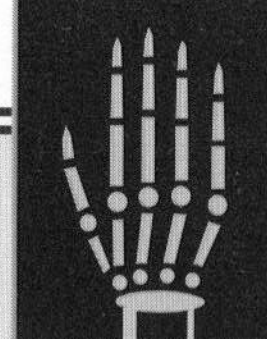

Guidelines for managing osteoarthritis

In 1996, the American College of Rheumatology released its recommendations for managing osteoarthritis of the hip and knee.

Lifestyle changes
- Exercise programs
  - Strengthen muscles
  - Increase mobility
  - reduce symptoms
- Weight loss
  - Reduces stress on afflicted joints
- Assistive devices such as canes, wall bars, and orthopedic inserts
  - Increase safety
  - Reduce stress on joints

Pain management and medication
- Physical and occupational therapy
  - Increase mobility
  - Improve function
- Acetaminophen, as first-line therapy
  - Provides safe and effective pain relief
  - Avoids gastrointestinal and renal risks of OTC nonsteroidal anti-inflammatory drugs (NSAID's)
- Prescription drugs, surgical treatment
  - Relieve more severe pain

Patient education
- Educational brochures and videos
  - Inform patients about disease
  - Encourage taking active role in care
- Am. Coll. of Rheumatology Arthritis Self-Help Course
  - Provides patients with tools and support to help overcome pain
- Discussions with professionals, family, and friends
  - Help patients adjust to situation
  - Empower patients to take control

the scientists studied nitric oxide (NO) in the body. NO is a gaseous molecule that helps regulate many processes in the body, including inflammation. An *enzyme* (a substance that speeds up biochemical reactions) called nitric oxide synthase (NOS)—of which there are several forms in different tissues in the body—produces NO.

The investigators found that cartilage from patients with osteoarthritis produces high levels of NO, but healthy cartilage does not. The researchers theorized that active inflammation may accompany osteoarthritis and may be responsible for the breakdown of cartilage.

Researchers said these findings could lead to new treatments for osteoarthritis. The study suggested that drugs that block NOS might improve osteoarthritis as well as rheumatoid arthritis, where the role of NO had already been shown.

New drug for osteoporosis. A powerful new drug may slow the progression of osteoporosis, a condition that causes the bones of many elderly people—especially women—to become fragile and break. According to a large international study reported in November 1995, a drug called alendronate sodium increases bone density in postmenopausal women and lowers the risk of fracture.

Bones are in a constant state of turnover. Cells called osteoclasts break down bone, while osteoblasts build new bone in its place. When this balance shifts in the elderly, a net loss of bone occurs and the bones become weak. Bone loss is most severe in women after menopause since estrogen, the female sex hormone, ordinarily slows down osteoclasts.

Alendronate sodium belongs to a class of drugs called bisphosphonates, which help to prevent osteoporosis by hindering the action of osteoclasts. Previous bisphosphonates affected the storage of minerals in bones and were difficult to use. But alendronate sodium is about 1,000 times more effective than older bisphosphonates, so it can be given daily at doses that block erosion without interfering with mineral storage.

Combination drug therapy for RA. Researchers at the University of Nebraska Medical Center in Omaha and the Omaha Veterans Affairs Medical Center reported in May 1996 that a new combination drug therapy is more effective in treating rheumatoid arthritis (RA) than the single drugs used in the past. The doctors studied more than 100 patients for a period of two years using combinations of three drugs and found that with the combination therapy, patients had fewer side effects and better results than with the single drugs.

Rheumatoid arthritis, a form of inflammatory arthritis that causes pain and swelling in joints, can destroy cartilage and bones and lead to crippling and deformity if left untreated.

To treat RA, doctors generally prescribe nonsteroidal anti-inflammatory drugs (NSAID's), such as aspirin or ibuprofen. These are usually followed by one of the disease-modifying drugs (DMARD's), such as methotrexate, hydroxychloroquine, and sulfasalazine, for patients who do not respond to NSAID's alone or who show evidence that their cartilage is being destroyed. DMARD's slow the progression of RA, but their long-term effectiveness remained uncertain.

The physicians taking part in the Nebraska study gave one group of patients methotrexate alone; another group, both sulfasalazine and hydroxychloroquine; and a third group, all three drugs. The doctors found that within nine months the patients who received all three drugs experienced a 50 percent improvement in their condition. They maintained that improvement for two years and suffered no major side effects. Though it was not clear how safe and effective the combination therapy would be in long-term treatment, the doctors concluded that it was a useful approach to alleviating arthritis, especially in patients who do not respond to single drugs alone. • David S. Pisetsky

See also DRUGS. In the section On the Medical Frontier, see ACTIVE LIVES WITH ARTIFICIAL JOINTS. In WORLD BOOK, see ARTHRITIS.

Birth Control

- Panel recommends FDA approval of abortion pill
- "Morning-after" pill
- The pill and strokes

An advisory committee to the United States Food and Drug Administration (FDA) recommended on July 19, 1996, that the FDA approve mefipristone, the so-called abortion drug more commonly called RU-486. Although the FDA is not bound by the panel's recommendations, it usually adopts them. FDA Commissioner David A. Kessler said a final decision on RU-486 would likely be made by mid-September 1996.

The Population Council, a nonprofit family-planning research organization in New York City, had received approval to start clinical trials of RU-486 in October 1994. The drug was first made and sold in France in 1988, but the French manufacturer did not want to enter the U.S. market because of the abortion controversy. The company donated its U.S. patent rights to the Population Council.

At the FDA panel hearing, the council presented preliminary data from its own trials, which involved 2,121 American women, but it relied mainly on results of a French study of 2,480 women. The women took two RU-486 pills in a doctor's office within seven weeks of their last menstrual period. The drug counteracts progesterone, a hormone needed to maintain a pregnancy. The women re-

Reliability counts

Consumers buying condoms find a large selection at most stores. Health experts advise that the most important feature should be reliability. In tests of condoms, the United States Food and Drug Administration (FDA) found that about 2 to 5 percent of condoms tear during use, but most breakage resulted from misuse rather than poor quality of the product. The FDA also found that condoms packaged as "stronger" tested poorer than those not promoted in this way, and products labeled as "thin" or "sensitive" were usually no different than others without such designations. However, health professionals stress that size is important. A condom that is too tight may break, and one that is too loose may slip off.

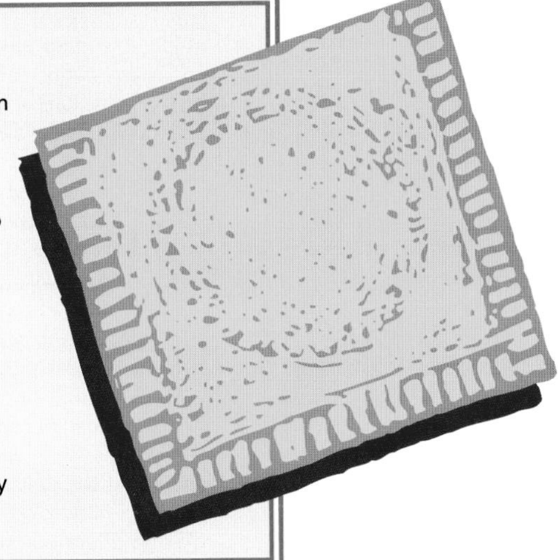

turned to the doctor 36 to 48 hours later to take misopristol, a drug that makes the uterus contract, causing it to expel a fetus. The study found that 95.5 percent of the women aborted. The most commonly reported side effect was pain from the contractions, reported by 82 percent of the women. Severe bleeding was reported by 1.4 percent.

The FDA said that if RU-486 is approved, the name of the manufacturer would be kept secret to avoid anti-abortion protests against that company. But the agency said it would reveal the name of the U.S. distributor.

"Morning-after" pill. Ordinary oral contraceptives might soon be marketed as "morning-after" pills. On June 28, 1996, an FDA advisory committee unanimously voted that birth control pills could be used up to 72 hours after unprotected intercourse to prevent pregnancy. At a date to be determined, the FDA said it planned to publish a notice in the Federal Register declaring that the pills can be safely and effectively used to block a fertilized egg from becoming implanted in the wall of the uterus.

The FDA has no power to approve a new use for a drug without a formal application from a manufacturer, according to FDA Deputy Commissioner Mary Pendergast. But, she said, the agency wanted to put the notice in the Federal Register to clarify any confusion about taking oral contraceptives as morning-after pills and to prompt manufacturers to apply for permission to market them as such.

Some doctors have long known that oral contraceptives work to block egg implantation. A 1995 Harris poll of 300 obstetrician-gynecologists found that 77.5 percent were very familiar with its morning-after effectiveness. Most said, however, that they would not prescribe it for that use unless a woman specifically asked for it. The doctors feared the possibility of malpractice suits stemming from prescribing a drug for a condition other than the one that gained FDA approval.

The pill and strokes. Healthy non-smoking women who take low-estrogen oral contraceptives do not increase their risk of stroke. However, women who smoke and take the pill face an increased risk for a heart attack. Those were the findings reported in July 1996 by researchers at the Kaiser Permanente Medical Care Program, a large health maintenance organization in California.

In the 1960's, oral contraceptives contained high levels of estrogen, which studies had linked with an increased incidence of stroke. Pills prescribed in the 1990's usually contained only 30 to 35 micrograms of estrogen. • Carol L. Hanson

In World Book, see Birth control.

Blood

- Hemoglobin as a blood pressure regulator
- New blood clot therapy
- Growing stem cells in the lab

A previously unknown function of hemoglobin, the major component of red blood cells, was reported in March 1996 by researchers at Duke University in Durham, North Carolina. The investigators found that as hemoglobin passes through the lungs, it picks up not only oxygen, but also a form of nitric oxide that helps make blood vessels widen. Thus, hemoglobin helps regulate blood pressure.

The body controls the flow of blood by contracting and relaxing smooth muscle cells in the blood vessels. Scientists had known since the late 1980's that the cells lining blood vessels release nitric oxide. The gas has a relaxing effect on muscle cells surrounding the vessels, thus increasing blood flow and reducing blood pressure. Without nitric oxide, the vessels would constrict and raise blood pressure. However, the iron atoms in hemoglobin quickly take up nitric oxide. So cell biologist Li Jia and his Duke co-workers wondered how the muscle cells obtain enough nitric oxide to function.

They found that a molecule in hemoglobin picks up a form of nitric oxide in the lungs that is different from the gas released by the cells lining blood vessels. The form is called super nitric oxide. Hemoglobin distributes super nitric oxide to the blood vessels and seems able to expand or contract the vessels as needed by regulating the amount of super nitric oxide it supplies to smooth muscle cells.

The researchers said the discovery could lead to new ways of controlling blood pressure, as well as to new treatments for heart attacks.

New blood clot therapy. The formation of blood clots in the vessels of legs and thighs is a serious problem for many patients that has required hospital treatment with blood thinners. However, according to two 1995 studies, clots can be treated on an outpatient basis using a special form of heparin, the drug traditionally used for this problem.

A clot in the lower extremities is dangerous because it can travel to the lungs and block blood flow, which can lead to the destruction of lung tissue. The situation turns life-threatening when a large segment of the lung is involved. The standard treatment for clots in the lower extremities has been to administer heparin intravenously in a hospital setting for up to 10 days, followed by treatment with oral blood thinners for three to six months. Patients have needed frequent laboratory tests while in the hospital to ensure that they were not receiving too much blood thinner, which can cause severe bleeding.

The blood thinner of choice for intravenous treatment has been a mixture of both low-molecular-weight and high-molecular-weight forms of heparin. The two 1995 studies involved only purified low-molecular-weight forms of heparin administered by injection.

Dutch researchers at the Academic Medical Center in Amsterdam, the Netherlands, reviewed the literature on heparin from 1984 to 1994 to compare the safety of the low-molecular-weight drug with the traditional form given intravenously. They found that patients on carefully controlled low-molecular-weight heparin had reductions in clot size, fewer recurrences of clots, and fewer major bleeding complications than patients receiving traditional intravenous heparin while hospitalized.

In the second study, Swedish doctors at Norrköping Central Hospital gave 102 patients with clots in the legs daily injections of low-molecular-weight heparin as an outpatient treatment. None of the patients reported serious problems. Furthermore, at six months, the recurrence of clots and problems resulting from clots, such as swelling of the legs, were no worse than for patients treated in the hospital with intravenous heparin.

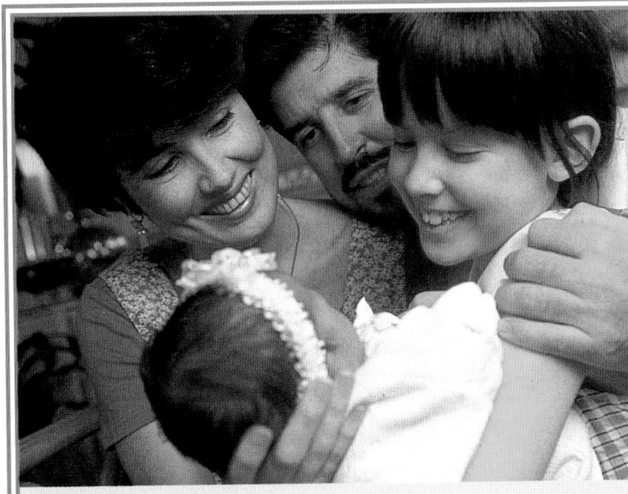

Infant donates blood

Tiny Mariajose Lebed is held by her parents and her sister Paulette, who suffers from leukemia. After her birth at a Miami hospital, doctors took three ounces of blood from the infant's umbilical cord and froze it for later extraction of stem cells to treat Paulette. The cord is a rich source of stem cells, which produce platelets and red and white blood cells when transplanted into patients with leukemia and other disorders of the blood and the immune system.

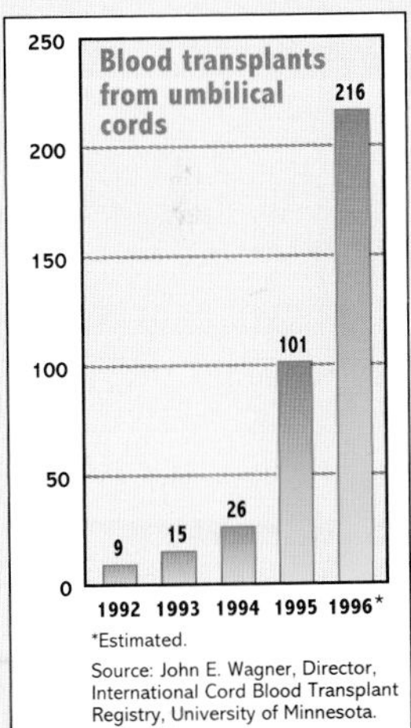

*Estimated.

Source: John E. Wagner, Director, International Cord Blood Transplant Registry, University of Minnesota.

Growing stem cells in the lab. German scientists reported in August 1995 that they had successfully grown *stem cells* in the laboratory from a small amount of patients' blood. Stem cells, which are present in very small numbers in the blood and bone marrow, give rise to all the different types of cells in blood. Patients on high doses of drug or radiation therapy for illnesses such as cancer must be given stem cells to replace those the therapy destroys. However, medical technicians have had to process large amounts of blood from such patients over several days to be able to collect an adequate number of stem cells. For some patients, adequate numbers cannot be obtained in this way.

The German researchers, at the Albert-Ludwigs University Medical Center in Freiburg, reported that they withdrew from 3.4 to 6.8 ounces (100 to 200 milliliters) of blood from six cancer patients who had undergone high-dose chemotherapy. The researchers collected stem cells from the blood and placed the cells in a medium that contained the patients' own *plasma* (the liquid component of blood) and factors that encouraged cell growth. The cells were allowed to grow and multiply for 12 days, then were transplanted to the patients. Five patients had normal recovery of blood cell counts. The sixth patient died of organ failure.

The researchers said their method may allow high-dose chemotherapy to be repeated since stem cells could be replenished. Also, the small amount of blood needed for the procedure may lower the risk of cancer cells being included with the stem cells. • G. David Roodman

In WORLD BOOK, see BLOOD.

Bone Disorders

- Lifestyle and bone mass
- Effects of exercise, calcium intake
- Sodium fluoride tablets
- Recovering from a hip fracture

Hip and spine fractures are frequent among older women with *osteoporosis* (bone thinning). An important indicator of bone strength is a measurement called bone mineral density (BMD). As BMD decreases, the chance of a hip or spine fracture increases. Investigators at several institutions in the United States reported studies in 1995 and 1996 indicating ways to maintain high BMD and avoid osteoporosis. Swedish researchers reported on the factors that help people recover from fractures.

Lifestyle and bone mass. In January 1996, several teams of investigators reported the results of a joint study on lifestyle factors that might increase BMD to prevent or minimize the effects of osteoporosis. The study, begun in the late 1980's, included 7,963 women aged 65 or older.

The researchers found that body weight is correlated with BMD. Women whose body weight was in the normal range tended to have stronger bone structure, while those who were excessively thin often had weak bones. Other factors found to be associated with stronger bone structure were the use of estrogen therapy after menopause, physical activity, and dietary calcium supplements.

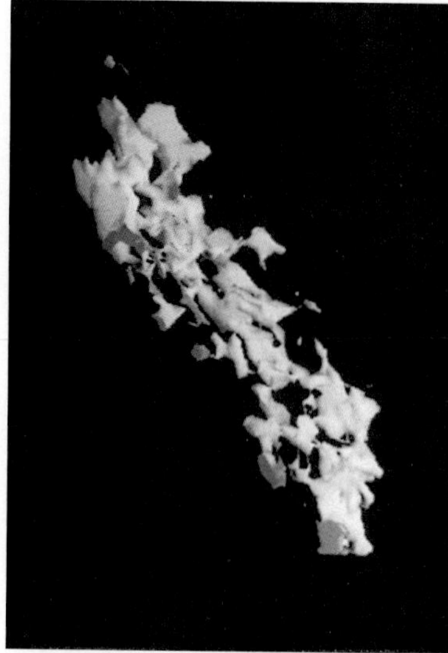

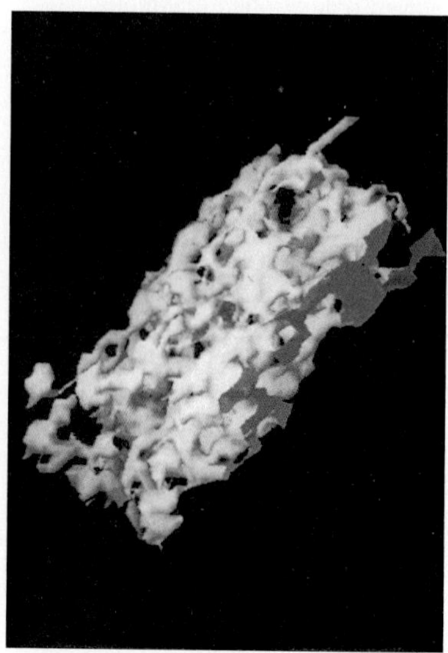

Building new bone

Images of an elderly woman's spine before, *right,* and after, *far right,* the woman was treated with a combination of slow-release sodium tablets and calcium citrate supplements reveal that the spine's bone mass increased dramatically. This study, reported in September 1995 by researchers at the University of Texas Southwestern Medical School in Dallas, marked the first time that a treatment was shown to rebuild lost spinal bone.

The investigators concluded that to avoid osteoporosis, women should maintain a normal body weight and take part in physical activity on a regular basis. Estrogen therapy and calcium supplements could offer an added degree of protection for women who are at higher risk of osteoporosis, including women with a family history of the disorder.

Effects of exercise, calcium intake. A lifetime of weight-bearing exercise, such as walking or jogging, is highly beneficial for maintaining strong bones in women, according to researchers in Seattle and in Portland, Oregon. In early 1996, the scientists reported the results of a study investigating what effect weight-bearing exercise and calcium intake have on BMD.

The study included 25 elderly women and their daughters. The researchers also found that mothers who took calcium supplements were less at risk for osteoporosis than mothers who did not take supplements. Surprisingly, however, the investigators were unable to find a link between milk drinking and BMD.

Sodium fluoride tablets. A new slow-release sodium fluoride tablet taken in conjunction with calcium citrate supplements can lessen the risk of spinal fractures and build bone in elderly women with severe osteoporosis. That finding, the first to show that lost spinal bone can be replaced, was reported in September 1996 by scientists at the University of Texas Southwestern Medical Center in Dallas. Their report came at the end of a four-year study of 110 women.

The researchers reported that the fluoride-calcium therapy increased spinal bone density by more than 4 percent a year. In addition, the new bone appeared to be just as strong as regular bone. Patients receiving the treatment had 70 percent fewer spinal fractures than patients who did not receive the therapy.

The scientists cautioned, however, that the sodium fluoride tablets must be taken in conjunction with calcium citrate supplements. Fluoride alone would produce abnormal and structurally weak bone, they said.

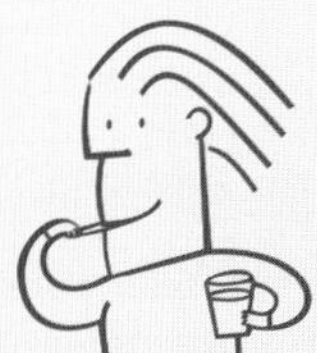

While you are sleeping

Old and damaged bone is broken down and removed in a normal process called resorption. Resorption occurs in conjunction with the production of new bone and goes on round the clock. However, researchers at Semmelweis University Medical School in Hungary and from several other institutions showed in 1995 that this process operates on a biological clock with the fastest bone loss occurring at around 3 a.m.

The investigators studied 15 healthy men and women. Blood samples from those individuals revealed that the resorption rate from 11 p.m. to 7 a.m. was 11 percent higher than during daytime hours.

Abnormalities in this rhythm may play a role in the development of *osteoporosis* (bone thinning) and other bone disorders. The research may be important in finding the best time to administer drugs that influence bone growth.

The research findings also indicate that a calcium-rich snack, such as a serving of milk, may be beneficial late at night.

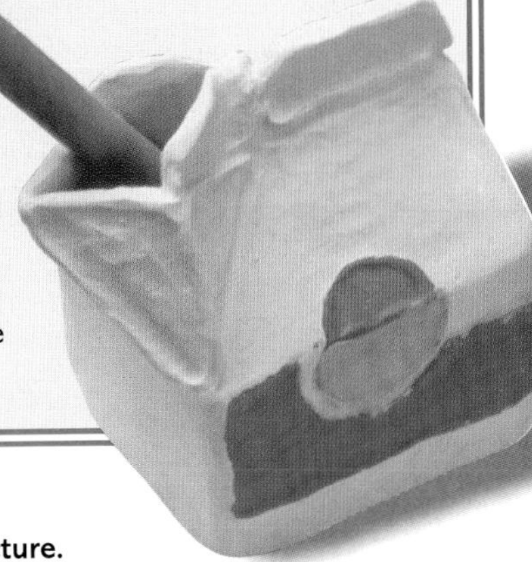

Recovering from a hip fracture. Fracture of the hip in elderly people is a serious injury from which many patients do not fully recover and some eventually die. Factors that can improve the chances of recovery were reported in January 1996 by investigators at Huddinge University Hospital in Huddinge, Sweden. The scientists found that good physical and mental health and an ability to perform the activities of daily living were the factors that best predicted a person's capacity for getting over a hip fracture and returning to an independent life. • John J. Gartland

In the section On the Medical Frontier, see ACTIVE LIVES WITH ARTIFICIAL JOINTS. In WORLD BOOK, see BONE; OSTEOPOROSIS.

Books of Health and Medicine

The following books on health and medicine topics were written for the general public. All were published in 1995 and 1996.

Breast cancer. *Breakthrough: The Race to Find the Breast Cancer Gene* by Kevin Davies and Michael White. The authors chronicle the roles of scientists in this fast-paced story combining history, medicine, science, politics, and human nature. (John Wiley & Sons, 1996. 310 pp. $24.95.)

Caregiving. *Caring for Yourself While Caring for Your Aging Parents: How to Help, How to Survive* by Claire Berman. Writing from her own perspective and that of other caregivers, Berman provides guidance for making important decisions about elderly parents—whether to invite parents to live with one or to place them in a nursing home. (Henry Holt, 1996. 255 pp. $22.50.)

Ways You Can Help: Creative, Practical Suggestions for Family and Friends of Patients and Caregivers by Margaret Cooke with Elizabeth Putnam. The authors recommend do's and don'ts for helping patients and providing emotional support for sick children and their healthy siblings. (Warner Books, 1996. 143 pp. $9.99.)

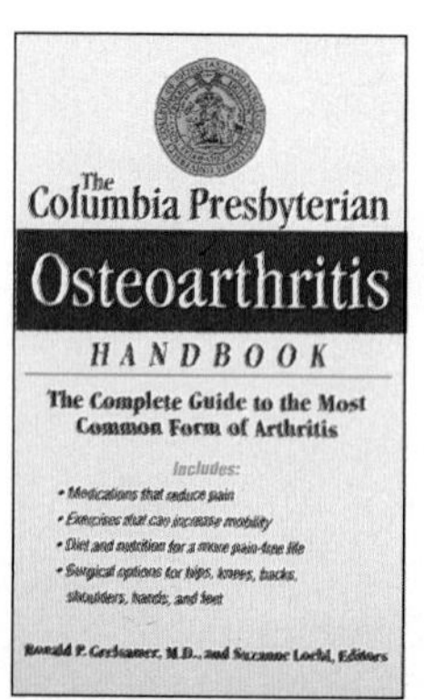

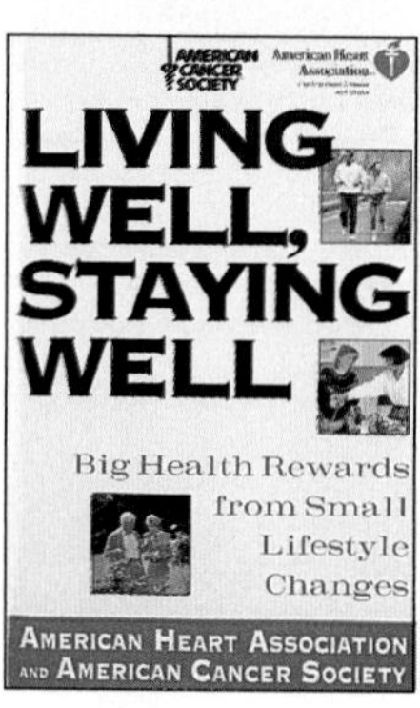

Chronic fatigue syndrome. *Osler's Web: Inside the Labyrinth of the Chronic Fatigue Syndrome Epidemic* by Hillary Johnson. This carefully researched history of chronic fatigue syndrome covers personalities, politics, scientific investigations, and the failure of the research establishment to take the syndrome seriously. (Crown, 1996. 720 pp. $30.)

Drugs. *People's Guide to Deadly Drug Interactions: How to Protect Yourself from Life Threatening Drug-Drug, Drug-Food, Drug-Vitamin Combinations* by Joe Graedon and Teresa Graedon. The authors—a pharmacologist and a medical anthropologist—organize over-the-counter and prescription drug information into easy-to-use charts, which address hazards posed by chemical interactions to drug users—particularly children, women, and older adults. (St. Martin's Press, 1995. 434 pp. $25.95.)

Essays. *Suspended Animation: Six Essays on the Preservation of Bodily Parts* by F. Gonzalez-Crussi. A pathologist elegantly expresses reverence for life and death in a book that was named one of 1995's best by *The New York Times Book Review.* (Harcourt Brace, 1995. 151 pp. $16.)

First-aid. *First Aid Pocket Guide* by the National Safety Council and Alton Thyerson. The guide offers clear, step-by-step instructions for dealing with medical emergencies, such as allergic reactions, snake bites, stings, heart attacks, strokes, wounds, fractures, sprains, frostbite, hypothermia, choking, burns, head and spinal cord injuries, and poisoning. (Jones & Bartlett, 1995. 115 pp. $7.95.)

General reference. *The American Heritage Stedman's Medical Dictionary.* This dictionary includes clear, accurate definitions of more than 45,000 medical terms and includes biographical entries, weights and measures, and an index. (Houghton Mifflin, 1995. 923 pp. $24.95.)

Health-care systems. *The System: The American Way of Politics at the Breaking Point* by Haynes Johnson and David S. Broder. Two Pulitzer Prize-winning journalists explore President Bill Clinton's attempt to reform health care, the media's role in the failure of that effort, and why reform failed when most Americans supported the idea. (Little, Brown & Co., 1996. 668 pp. $25.95.)

Tomorrow's Hospital: A Look to the Twenty-First Century by Eli Ginzberg. The author brings six decades of experience to this overview of trends in hospital care. He explores future troubles for hospitals, scenarios for better management, and hospital/physician realignments. (Yale University Press, 1996. 165 pp. $25.)

Heart. *Texas Heart Institute Heart Owner's Handbook: Live Longer and Feel Better.* This handbook guides the reader in developing a personal heart profile. Also discussed are habits for maintaining a healthy heart and ways to control stress, diabetes, hypertension, and cholesterol. (John Wiley & Sons, 1996. 396 pp. $16.95.)

Information on-line. *Health Online: The Complete Guide to Finding Information Through Your Computer* by Tom Ferguson. A reference guide to medical information on the Internet prepared by a senior associate at the Center for Clinical Computing at Harvard Medical School. (Addison-Wesley, 1996. 308 pp. $17.)

Infomedicine: A Consumer's Guide to the Latest Medical Research by Fred D. Baldwin and Suzanne McInerney. The authors provide guidance on how to choose the best treatment for various medical conditions and to find needed professionals, organizations, and self-help groups. (Little, Brown & Co. 1996. 283 pp. $14.95.)

Memoirs. *The Case of the Frozen Addicts* by J. William Langston and Jon Palfreman. Langston, a physician, discovered that his patient and five other addicts admitted to San Francisco-area emergency rooms in the 1980's had used the same tainted synthetic heroin, and it had destroyed an area of their brains essential for normal movement. This discovery eventually led to a treatment for Parkinson's disease. (Pantheon, 1995. 309 pp. $25.)

Emergency: True Stories from the Nation's ERs compiled by Mark Brown. This emergency-room physician and lawyer has compiled a collection of fascinating stories about emergency medicine. (Random House, 1996. 221 pp. $21.)

On the Ledge: A Doctor's Stories from the Inner City by Neil S. Skolnik. A physician relates gripping stories of his experiences providing health care for the urban poor, including the political and social issues involved. (Faber & Faber, 1996. 157 pp. $19.95.)

Nutrition. *Doctor, What Should I Eat? Nutrition Prescriptions for Ailments in Which Diet Can Really Make a Difference* by Isadore Rosenfeld. A physician offers specific diet prescriptions for many health problems in a readable, straightforward format. (Warner Books, 1996. 425 pp. $13.99.)

Osteoarthritis. *The Columbia-Presbyterian Osteoarthritis Handbook: The Complete Guide to the Most Common Form of Arthritis* edited by Ronald P. Grelsamer and Suzanne Loebl. This guide covers treatments, exercise, nutrition, physical therapy, and surgery for a disease affecting over 16 million people. (Macmillan, 1996. 279 pp. $24.95.)

Prostate. *Prostate Disease: A Massachusetts General Hospital Book* by W. Scott McDougal with P. J. Skerrett. McDougal, a professor of surgery at Harvard, has written a comprehensive guide to prostate disease—its causes, diagnosis, and treatment. (Times Books, 1996. 355 pp. $14.)

Wellness. *Living Well, Staying Well: Big Health Rewards from Small Lifestyle Changes* by the staffs of the American Heart Association and the American Cancer Society. This book guides the reader in the creation of a personal health-maintenance program aimed at preventing cancer and heart disease. (Crown, 1996. 316 pp. $25.)

Women's health. *Dr. Nancy Snyderman's Guide to Good Health: What Every Forty-Plus Woman Should Know About Her Changing Body* by Nancy Snyderman and Margaret Blackstone. The book covers pregnancy, child birth, sexuality, gynecological issues, menopause, cancer, chronic and progressive conditions, and aging. (Wm. Morrow & Co., 1996. 474 pp. $25.)

The Harvard Guide to Women's Health by Karen Carlson, Stephanie Eisenstat, and Terra Ziporyn. Authoritative, balanced A to Z entries guide the reader through such areas as how common disorders affect women differently than men. (Harvard University Press, 1996. 718 pp. $24.95.)

A New Prescription for Women's Health: Getting the Best Medical Care in a Man's World by Bernardine Healy. A former National Institutes of Health director offers advice on nutrition, sexually transmitted diseases, reproductive life, menopause, cancer, depression, anxiety, heart disease, stroke, osteoporosis, and Alzheimer's disease. (Viking Penguin, 1996. 560 pp. $12.95.)

• Margaret E. Moore

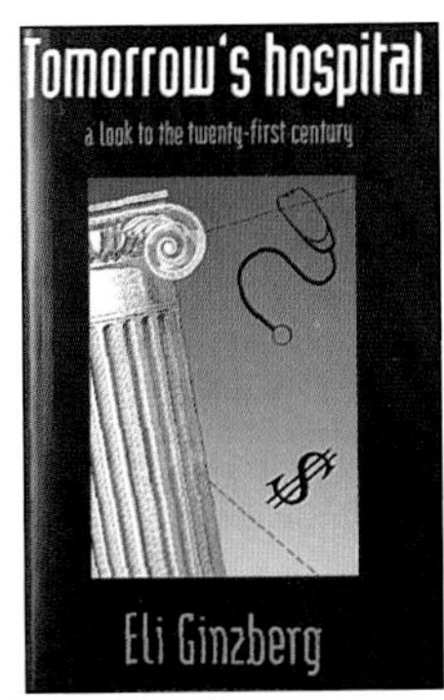

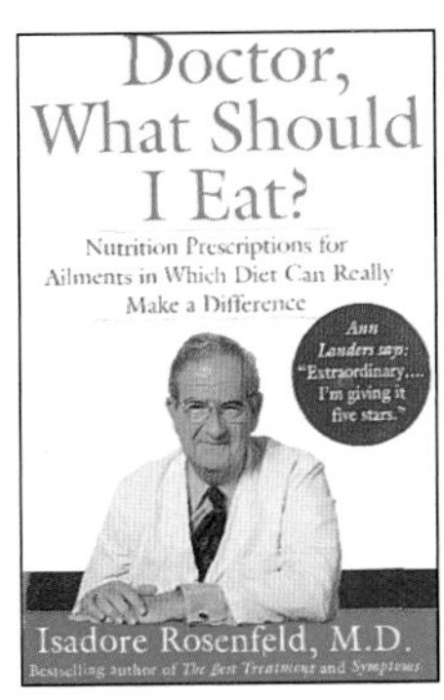

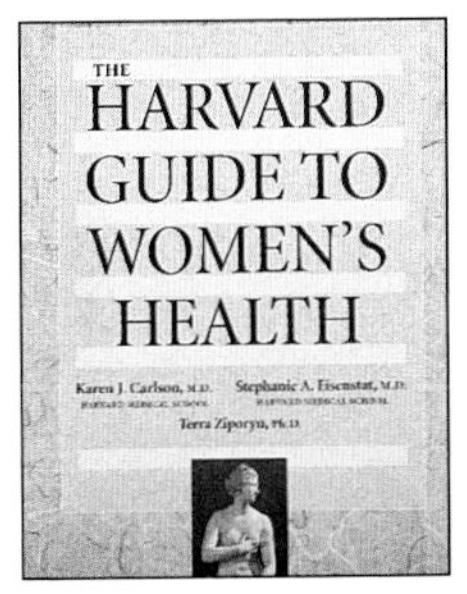

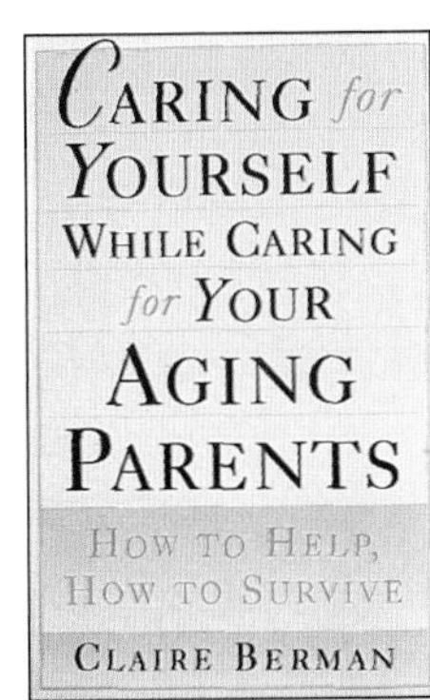

Brain and Nervous System

- Major advance in regenerating spinal cords
- New insight into prions
- Eating disorders
- Alzheimer's disease genes found

The first experimental evidence showing that function can be restored to a severed spinal cord was reported in July 1996 by researchers in Sweden. Although they did their work with rats, neuroscientists were hopeful that the results would be applicable to the human spinal cord.

The spinal cord and the brain constitute the *central nervous system* (CNS). The CNS can do many wonderful things, but one thing it cannot do very well is heal itself. There are a number of reasons for this. One of the most important is that certain cells in the CNS, such as *neurons* (nerve cells) and *oligodendrocytes* (cells that make myelin, the fatty insulation around nerve fibers) are unable to multiply. In addition, myelin contains proteins that prevent the regrowth of nerve-cell fibers.

As a result of these conditions, when the spinal cord is injured, the damage becomes permanent, and patients are usually unable to regain much of their previous functioning. In recent years, drugs had brightened this picture somewhat by making it possible, with speedy treatment, to limit spinal cord damage. But doctors wanted to do much more—to actually regenerate lost nerve connections.

The nature of the peripheral nervous system—the nerves outside the CNS—offered that possibility. These nerves can be cut and reattached and even have sections replaced with pieces of other nerves. More importantly, research had shown that nerve fibers called axons from CNS nerves will grow through peripheral nerves.

The researchers, at the Karolinska Institute in Stockholm, Sweden, severed the lower spinal cord of adult rats, making them unable to move their hind legs. They then took pieces of peripheral nerves and laid them in the gap between the ends of the severed cords. They cemented the nerve pieces in place with a protein "glue" that promoted axon growth and blocked the growth-inhibiting effects of the myelin proteins.

The investigators waited and watched, testing the animals repeatedly for their ability to use their back legs. Gradually, over a period of weeks and months, the rats began to recover. Although they never returned to normal, the animals could move their legs and even bear weight on them. A group of "control" rats with severed spinal cords that did not receive the nerve grafts did not recover any function in their legs.

The scientists made a microscopic examination of the spinal cords of the rats that received the grafts. They found that axons from nerve cells above and below the cut ends of each severed spinal cord had made their way through the graft and reconnected to nerve cells on the other side. Some fibers even connected as far away as the brain.

Many obstacles remained to be overcome in regenerating damaged spinal cords. For one thing, most human spinal cord injuries produce not clean surgical cuts but rather crushing and tearing wounds that can make the regrowth and reconnection of axons more difficult. Nonetheless, an essay in the journal *Science,* where the research report was published, hailed the results of the Swedish study as "a major milestone" and said it provided "a strong basis for hope" that damage to the human spinal cord can be reversed.

New insight into prions. Prions, abnormal proteins associated with a variety of degenerative brain diseases of human beings and animals, have been a subject of controversy since their discovery in the 1980's. In April 1996, teams of researchers in Switzerland and the United Kingdom reported that mice lacking the normal form of the prion protein suffer sleep disturbances.

Prions have been found in the central nervous system of humans with several degenerative brain diseases. One of these diseases, familial fatal insomnia, is a rare and mystifying illness in which people are unable to sleep. The association of prions with this disorder provided the starting point for the research conducted by the British and Swiss scientists.

Their findings indicated that the normal version of the protein has an important role in maintaining normal biological rhythms, including sleep and wakefulness. And it added to mounting evidence that the absence of the normal protein, rather than the presence of the abnormal protein, is what leads to disease. The normal form of the prion protein is present on the surfaces of neurons in both humans and animals. Neuroscientists, however, have been unable to determine the function of this naturally occurring protein.

The European researchers produced a group of mice in which the gene for the normal prion protein was inactivated. The altered mice looked and behaved normally, indicating that the function of the prion protein had been taken over by other proteins.

The investigators compared a group of these altered mice with a group of normal mice. They *entrained* (accustomed) both groups to a strict 12-hour cycle of alternating light and darkness. Because mice are nocturnal—that is, they sleep during the day and are active at night—the activities of all the animals increased dramatically in the dark.

The scientists then placed both groups of mice into 24-hour darkness and recorded their activities. Initially, all the mice maintained their previous cycle of activity—12 hours of sleep followed by 12 hours of activity. After a while, however, the mice whose bodies were producing the normal

Exercises for Parkinson's patients

Exercise can help Parkinson's disease patients maintain their mobility, balance, and coordination. But many Parkinson's disease patients become inactive, even when symptoms are still mild. These exercises are from a brochure, *Exercises for the Parkinson Patient,* available by writing the Parkinson's Disease Foundation, William Black Medical Research Building, Columbia University Medical Center, 650 West 168th Street, New York, NY 10032.

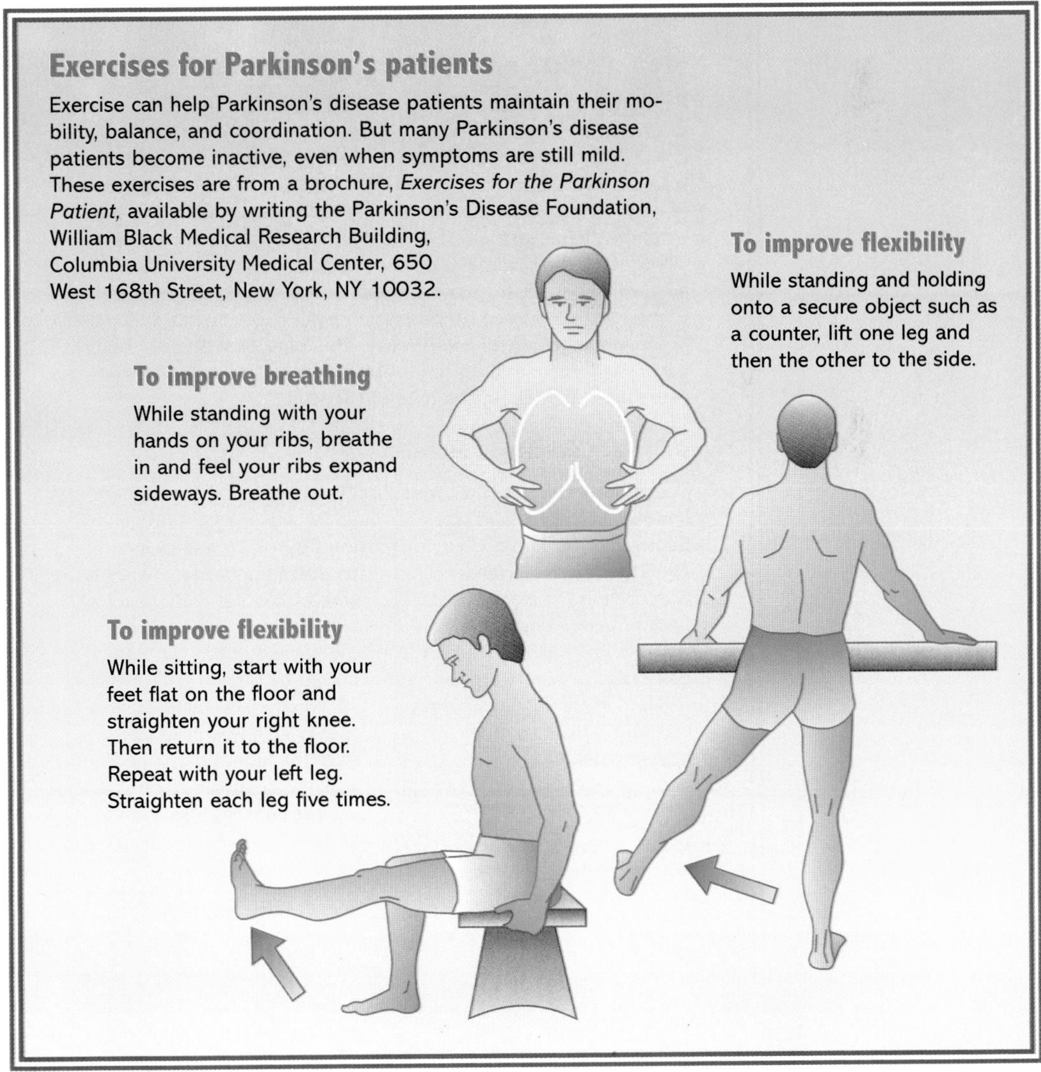

To improve breathing

While standing with your hands on your ribs, breathe in and feel your ribs expand sideways. Breathe out.

To improve flexibility

While standing and holding onto a secure object such as a counter, lift one leg and then the other to the side.

To improve flexibility

While sitting, start with your feet flat on the floor and straighten your right knee. Then return it to the floor. Repeat with your left leg. Straighten each leg five times.

protein gradually shortened their wake-rest cycles from 24 hours to between 22 and 23 hours.

In contrast, no such changes were observed in the genetically altered mice. Moreover, those animals were unable to have a deep or uninterrupted sleep after being kept awake for extended periods.

Although the researchers' findings were important, much remained to be learned about prions. Neuroscientists still did not know how the normal prion protein carries out its evident role in regulating sleep and other basic biological cycles. Nor could they explain how a lack of the normal protein in the body may lead to disease.

Eating disorders, both overeating and the avoidance of food, are major health problems. In April 1996, researchers at institutions in Paris and London reported findings that could lead to effective treatments for these medical conditions.

Hunger or a feeling of fullness are regulated by a number of different factors, including the interactions of certain groups of neurons in the brain. These cells communicate with one another by releasing a *neurotransmitter* (chemical messenger) called cholecystokinin (CCK).

CCK acts by binding to molecules called receptors on the surfaces of other neurons. There are two kinds of

Idea density and Alzheimer's disease

Researchers reported in February 1996 that it might be possible to predict who will develop Alzheimer's disease years before its onset. They based this conclusion on autobiographies written by 93 nuns just before they took their vows. By studying the density of ideas and the complexity of sentence construction in the nuns' writings, the researchers found they could predict who would develop Alzheimer's with 90 percent accuracy. The researchers, most of whom are from the University of Kentucky, also found that education offered no protection against the mental deterioration characteristic of the disease. The nuns were all born before 1917, and nearly a third had been diagnosed as suffering from Alzheimer's disease at the time of the study.

Which nun developed Alzheimer's?

"I was born in Eau Claire, Wis., on May 24, 1913, and was baptized in St. James Church. My father, Mr. L.M. Hallacher, was born in the city of Ross, County Cork, Ireland, and is now a sheet metal worker in Eau Claire ... .There are ten children in the family six boys and four girls. Two of the boys are dead."

This nun was diagnosed with Alzheimer's after her death. Sources: *New York Times, Journal of the American Medical Association.*

"The happiest day of my life so far was my First Communion Day which was in June nineteen hundred and twenty when I was but eight years of age, and four years later in the same month I was confirmed by Bishop D. D. McGavick. In nineteen hundred and twenty-six I was graduated from the eighth grade and now my great desire of entering the convent was soon to be gratified."

The names and places in the writing samples have been changed.

CCK receptors, CCK_A and CCK_B. The binding of CCK to A receptors results in a feeling of fullness. Binding of CCK to B receptors produces feelings of anxiety.

Because of these powerful biological effects, scientists have tried for years to regulate the activity of CCK. Such efforts have not been successful because CCK is also found in other parts of the body, where it has important functions, including controlling the emptying of the stomach. Drugs that regulate CCK in the brain were found to also affect its actions outside of the brain, producing unacceptable side-effects. But the new findings may lead to better ways of regulating CCK.

The investigators found an *enzyme* (a substance that speeds up biochemical reactions) that appears to be of major importance in breaking down CCK. This enzyme, called tripeptidyl peptidase II (TPPII) is present in the brain as well as in other organs, such as the liver and kidney. Because TPPII is so effective at rapidly deactivating CCK, the scientists reasoned that if the enzyme could be blocked, the concentrations of CCK would be raised and its effects amplified. With this in mind, and with a knowledge of the enzyme's structure and function, the scientists synthesized an inhibitor of TPPII.

When they administered the inhibitor to mice and rats, the actions of CCK, especially actions related to the CCK_A receptors, were greatly increased. As a result, the animals ate significantly less food.

This research promises to yield a new understanding of eating disorders as well as of mental illnesses associated with anxiety. The ability to regulate CCK in the brain could lead to new methods of treatment for these common, and often incurable, conditions.

Alzheimer's genes found. One of the most feared of illnesses is Alzheimer's disease, a devastating disorder in which brain cells degenerate and die, causing memory problems and, eventually, a complete loss of mental functions. The cause of the disease is not known but genetic factors are believed to play a role in many cases, particularly in familial, or early-onset, Alzheimer's. In August 1995, two teams of researchers in the United States announced that they had found a gene that causes perhaps 20 percent of all cases of familial Alzheimer's. That finding came soon after a group of Canadian scientists had reported finding a similar gene that is apparently responsible for nearly all of the other 80 percent of familial Alzheimer's.

Although about three-fourths of Alzheimer's patients are over 65 years of age, the other one-fourth suffer from the familial form of the disease, which usually strikes people in their 40's or 50's. This early-onset form of the disorder runs in families and has a very strong genetic component. The recently announced discoveries brought to three the number of genes known to be involved in early-onset Alzheimer's.

The American researchers, at Massachusetts General Hospital in Boston and the University of Washington in Seattle, studied a large group of families called the Volga Germans. These people are descended from a colony of ethnic Germans who lived in Russia's Volga Valley in the 1700's and 1800's. In a small number of these families, there is a high rate of early-onset Alzheimer's disease.

The scientists found that Alzheimer's victims among the Volga Germans had a *mutated* (changed) gene on chromosome 1. (Human cells contain 23 pairs of chromosomes. A chromosome number designates both members of a pair.) They called the newly discovered gene STM2.

An analysis of STM2 showed that it is amazingly similar to the gene, called S182, discovered earlier in the year by the Canadian researchers. Both genes appear to make a long, thin protein that is present in cell membranes. The functions of the similar yet different proteins produced by the two genes remained to be learned in late 1996, but clearly they must play an important role in the development of familial Alzheimer's.

• **Gary Birnbaum**

See also MENTAL HEALTH. In the section A HEALTHY FAMILY, see REMEMBERING NOT TO FORGET. In WORLD BOOK, see BRAIN; NERVOUS SYSTEM.

Cancer

- PET scan studies
- Advances in drug therapy
- Growth factors and chemotherapy
- Monoclonal antibodies

Lung cancer remained the leading cause of cancer deaths for both men and women in the United States in 1996. Although the lung cancer rate had begun to drop among men—reflecting a decline in smoking rates—the lung cancer rate among women was still rising, reflecting the fact that women took up the habit in large numbers more recently than men.

Positron emission tomography (PET) can accurately distinguish between cancerous tumors and *benign* (harmless) growths in the lung, researchers at Vanderbilt University in Nashville, Tennessee, reported in April 1996. PET represents a new technique of diagnostic imaging in cancer medicine. It can detect not only the presence of cancer but also the growth rate of cancerous tumors and the spread of the disease. Other imaging techniques, such as computerized tomography (CT) and magnetic resonance imaging (MRI), do not provide as much information.

PET scan studies make use of drugs known as radiopharmaceuticals that are labeled with radioactive molecules. These drugs travel through the patient's body and are absorbed by tumor cells. A machine called a scanner detects the radiation they emit.

A commonly used radiopharmaceutical, fluorodeoxy-glucose (FDG), is a form of sugar that incorporates a molecule of radioactive fluorine. Tumors absorb and *metabolize* (break down) FDG more avidly than normal tissue does. By detecting the radiation released by FDG, a PET scan can locate a tumor, define its boundaries, and spot any spread of the disease. The PET scanner then constructs a three-dimensional picture by putting together data collected from multiple cross-sectional images of body tissue.

The Vanderbilt study included 48 patients with suspicious growths in their lungs, some with a history of lung cancer. Laboratory tests and follow-ups determined whether these growths were indeed malignant. The FDG-PET scans accurately distinguished between benign and cancerous growths 88 percent of the time. The scans did produce six false positives (in six cases where the scans indicated a malignancy, the growth was actually benign) but they correctly predicted every actual malignancy.

Improvements in the ability to make early and accurate diagnoses of lung cancer through FDG-PET scans could make it possible for many patients with benign growths to avoid surgery. In patients who have already undergone surgery for lung cancer, FDG-PET scanning shows promise in distinguishing scar tissue and other changes in lung tissue following surgery from remaining cancerous tissue or a recurrence of the disease.

Cancer researchers continued to study possible applications for PET scanning in 1996. The National Cancer Institute (NCI) in February announced funding for a five-year study of the accuracy of PET scanning in detecting the spread of breast cancer to nearby lymph nodes. If the technique proves reliable, it could replace the current practice of surgically re-

STATISTICS

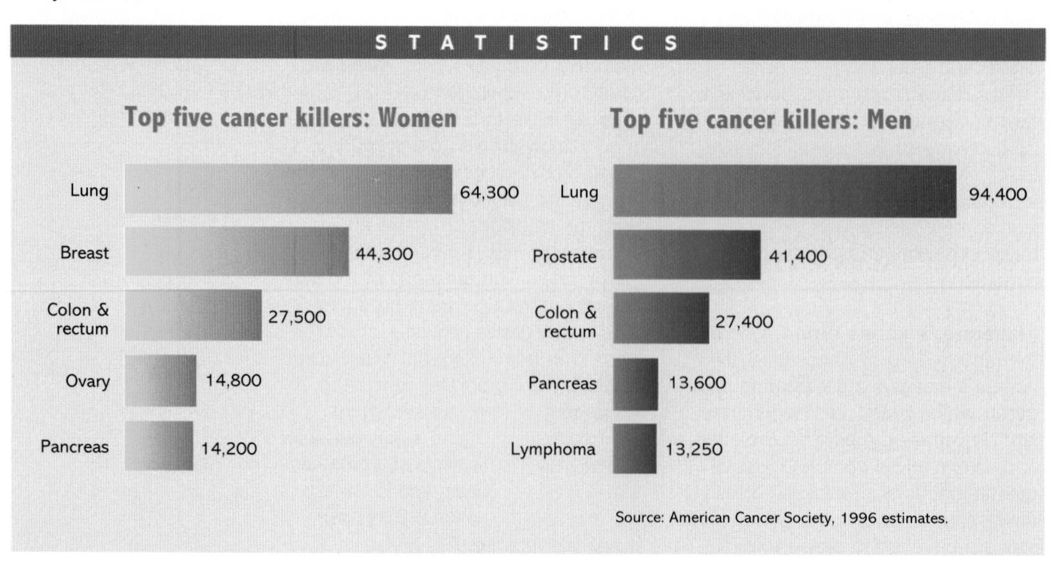

Source: American Cancer Society, 1996 estimates.

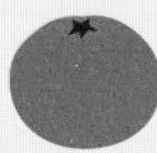

Tomatoes and prostate cancer

Could a plate of spaghetti with a rich tomato sauce or a slice of pizza smothered in tomatoes lower the risk of prostate cancer? That's what researchers at the Harvard School of Public Health found. In a six-year study involving about 48,000 male health professionals, the Harvard researchers found that men who ate four servings of foods rich in tomatoes every week lowered their risk of developing prostate cancer by 20 percent. Those eating 10 servings a week nearly halved their risk. The researchers theorized that the effect might result from a substance in tomatoes called lycopene, which is a close relative of the antioxidant beta-carotene.

moving the lymph nodes from breast cancer patients to determine whether cancer cells had spread to them. Researchers had already determined that FDG-PET scanning can dependably distinguish between normal and malignant tissue in diagnosing breast cancer. PET scanning may also help physicians evaluate how well a patient is responding to anticancer drugs. In a patient who is responding well to the drugs, a scan should show a reduced uptake of FDG, indicating that the tumor is shrinking.

FDG-PET scanning may prove useful in determining the extent of colorectal cancer prior to surgery and in detecting recurrences of tumors. In addition, it may enable physicians to distinguish between slowly growing and aggressive tumors in the brain. Such information should help physicians predict a patient's prognosis.

Advances in drug therapy. A number of studies were underway in 1996 to determine whether chemotherapy—treatment with anticancer drugs—prior to surgery for removal of a cancerous tumor could improve the outcome for patients with certain cancers. Researchers were also using chemotherapy to reduce the size of large, inoperable tumors sufficiently for surgeons to remove them.

People who have colon cancer, breast cancer, or melanoma—a potentially deadly form of skin cancer—and whose cancer has *metastasized* (spread) to lymph nodes in the region of the tumor have had a poor prognosis. In the past, only about a third of them survived for 5 to 10 years after diagnosis. This outcome remained true even when surgery successfully removed all visible signs of their tumor as well as the lymph nodes invaded by cancer cells.

One reason for the poor prognosis in most patients with lymph-node involvement has been that surgery leaves behind microscopic remnants of the disease. Another reason is that some cancer cells may already have spread to other sites in the body by the time of surgery. Over time, these cells multiply and spread throughout the body, eventually leading to death.

Adjuvant therapy (chemotherapy or immunotherapy with an immune-system protein called interferon for 4 to 12 months following surgery) has improved this prognosis in patients with colon cancer, breast cancer, or melanoma and regional lymph-node involvement. Chemotherapy drugs are chosen for their ability to produce partial or complete responses in patients. In melanoma, the drug used for adjuvant therapy is interferon.

Because such drugs proved at least partially effective in patients with advanced, detectable cancers, cancer specialists theorized that they should be even more effective for patients with microscopic, undetectable disease. This proved to be the case. Adjuvant therapy has reduced the incidence of tumor recurrence by about one-third in breast cancer patients, colon cancer patients, and melanoma patients with regional lymph-node involvement. It has also raised their long-term survival rates.

Encouraged by these results, cancer physicians and surgeons in 1996 had begun to study the use of neoadjuvant therapy—that is, drug treatment given before surgery. Trials were underway on the benefits of neoadjuvant therapy for certain types of lung cancer. And a large multicenter study to evaluate the drug paclitaxel (marketed as Taxol) in treating breast cancer was to begin in late 1996.

Growth factors and chemotherapy. A major side effect of most cancer chemotherapy has been a reduction in the number of blood-producing cells in the bone marrow. Research underway in 1996 indicated that certain hormones could stimulate production of blood cells and prevent some of the blood-related side effects of chemotherapy.

The body's cells increase in number when individual cells *replicate* (reproduce) their DNA (genetic material) and then divide into two new daughter cells. Each new daughter cell contains a full copy of the original cell's DNA. Cancer cells replicate their DNA and divide more rapidly than do normal cells. Most anticancer drugs act by interfering with a cell's ability to replicate its DNA and divide. These drugs seek out cancer cells because cancer cells are dividing at a rapid rate. But the drugs also kill a number of normal cells that are dividing at a relatively fast rate. Among these are blood-producing cells known as stem cells in bone marrow. Stem cells eventually develop into red blood cells, white blood cells, or platelets.

A reduction in oxygen-carrying red blood cells results in anemia; a reduction in infection-fighting white blood cells results in a condition called leucopenia; and a reduction in platelets, which bring about clotting, results in thrombocytopenia. Patients with anemia typically feel fatigued; patients with leucopenia are susceptible to infection; and patients with thrombocytopenia may bleed without clotting.

These disorders can complicate the treatment of cancer patients by limiting both the amount of an anticancer drug that can be given and the frequency with which that drug is given. And yet large dosages of a cancer drug administered frequently may be necessary to properly control a cancer patient's disease.

Since 1990 researchers have developed purified forms of new biological products that can help cancer patients recover more rapidly from anemia, leucopenia, and thrombocytopenia. These products are hormones called growth factors, which the body produces naturally and which stimulate the bone marrow to produce blood cells.

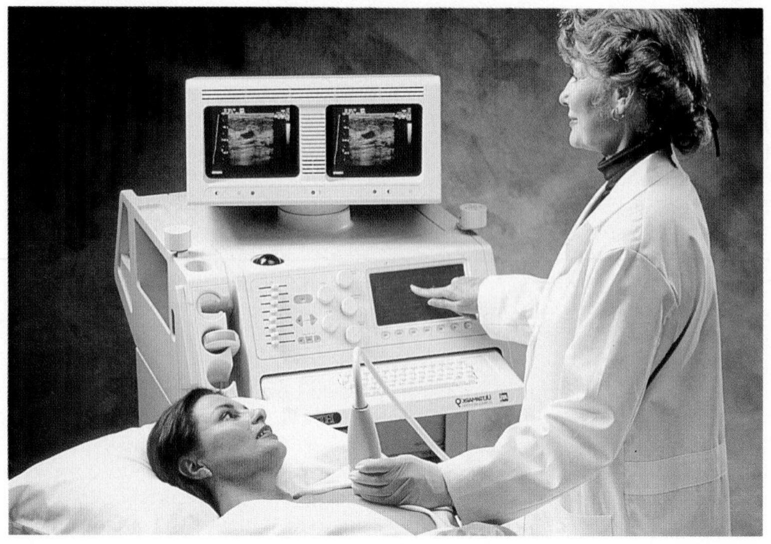

Ultrasound imaging for diagnosing breast lumps
Many women who find lumps in their breasts will be able to avoid a surgical *biopsy* (removal of tissue), currently the standard diagnostic procedure for breast cancer. In April 1996, the U.S. Food and Drug Administration approved a powerful new form of painless imaging by *ultrasound* (high-frequency sound waves) that can identify a noncancerous lump.

The growth factors are administered by an injection beneath the skin—in many cases, by the patients themselves. They have made it possible to give high dosages of cancer drugs to cancer patients at more frequent intervals, resulting in an improved quality of life and, for some patients, a stronger response to anticancer drugs and a longer life.

Monoclonal antibodies showed new promise for cancer diagnosis and treatment in 1995 and 1996. Antibodies are the body's disease-fighting proteins. The body produces them when immune-system cells recognize proteins known as antigens on the surface of such invaders as bacteria, viruses, and cancer cells.

Scientists produce monoclonal antibodies by first isolating an antibody-producing cell from an animal that has been exposed to a specific antigen, such as an antigen on a cancer cell. The antibody-producing cell is then fused with a cancer cell. Normal cells are programmed to die after dividing a certain number of times, but cancer cells escape this death sentence and can multiply forever.

The fused cell, called a hybridoma, grows in a laboratory culture or in the abdomen of an experimental animal. The hybridoma churns out huge quantities of the selected cancer antibody. The antibodies are called monoclonal because they all derive from the descendants, or clones, of the original hybridoma, and they react specifically with the antigen to which the animal was originally exposed.

Monoclonal antibodies can be used in cancer medicine alone or coupled with a radioactive molecule. For example, specialists now treat colon cancer patients with radioactive iodine bound to monoclonal antibodies that seek out and attach themselves to colon cancer cells. These antibodies are injected into colon cancer patients in whom a recurrence of the disease is suspected. After the antibodies bind to the antigens on the cancer cells, special cameras detect the release of radiation from the iodine. This information can help a surgeon decide how and whether to operate on patients suspected of having a recurrence of colon cancer.

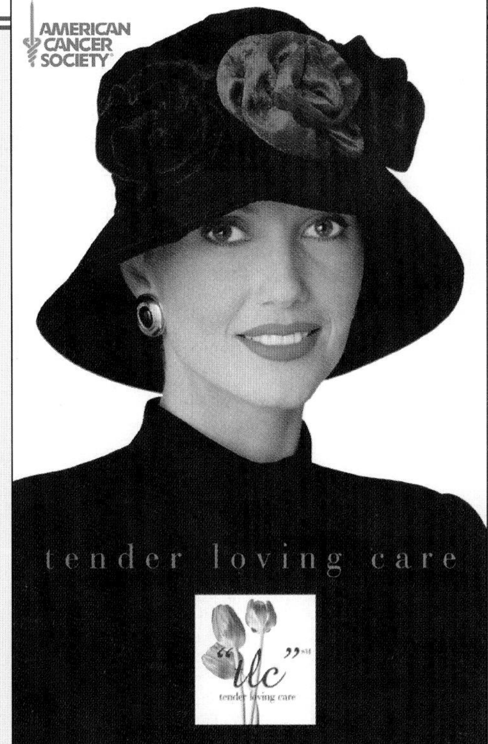

Fashionable alternatives

Tender Loving Care is a catalog that helps women who are undergoing treatment for breast cancer find stylish headgear, hairpieces, and mastectomy brassieres. The catalog is published by the American Cancer Society and available free of charge by telephoning 800/850-9445 or by writing TLC, Hanover, PA 17333-0080.

In April 1996, researchers from the University of California at Los Angeles reported success in treating breast cancer patients with monoclonal antibodies and the anticancer drug cisplatin. Together, the treatments pack a bigger punch than either one alone. The drug damages the cancer cell's genes, and the antibody prevents the cell from repairing the damage. As a result, the cell dies. The 36 women in the study had advanced breast cancer that had not responded to other therapies. Nine of them showed significant improvement. Further studies of treatments that combine anticancer drugs with monoclonal antibodies were planned.

• Jules E. Harris

In World Book, see Cancer.

Child Development

- Mother-child bonding and child care
- Children's grades and family size
- Sugar and hyperactivity
- Genes and hyperactivity
- Race and intelligence
- Early educational programs
- TV recommendations

The anxieties of working mothers were eased somewhat by research showing that placing an infant in a day-care center or with a baby sitter does not necessarily harm the emotional bonds between mother and child. The study, sponsored by the National Institute of Child Health and Development (a part of the National Institutes of Health in Bethesda, Maryland) was the largest, most comprehensive examination to date of how child development is influenced by day care. It involved 1,300 families at 10 sites in the United States.

Researchers began the study in 1991, when the infants were 1 month old or younger and planned to continue the study until the children reached the age of 7 years. In the phase of the study reported in 1996, researchers observed children, parents, and child-care providers when the infants were 15 months old.

The researchers studied infants from diverse economic, geographic, and ethnic backgrounds. The children were looked after at day-care centers and in several other settings, including at home by fathers or nonrelatives and at grandparents' homes. The investigators concluded that if an infant had good child care, was not moved frequently from one child-care setting to another, and had a mother who was sensitive and responsive during the time they spent together, the feeling of trust that the infant had toward its mother was not affected by being in day care.

These findings, however, applied only to infants who were in child care for 10 hours or less a week. Children of working mothers are often in child care from 40 to 50 hours a week.

The new research ran counter to a study reported in 1986 by child development specialist Jay Belsky of Pennsylvania State University, which suggested that infants in day care were more likely to have insecure maternal relationships and future problems. Belsky's study focused on children who spent more than 20 hours a week in day care.

Children's grades and family size. Youngsters with many siblings are more likely to bring home poor report cards and score lower on standardized tests than those who grow up in smaller households. That was the conclusion of a study at Ohio State University in Columbus, published in October 1995. However, the study also found that there are steps parents can take to counter this effect.

The study examined data collected by the National Center for Education Statistics on more than 24,000 eighth-graders from across the country. Researchers found that parents in families with four or more children had less time, attention, and encour-

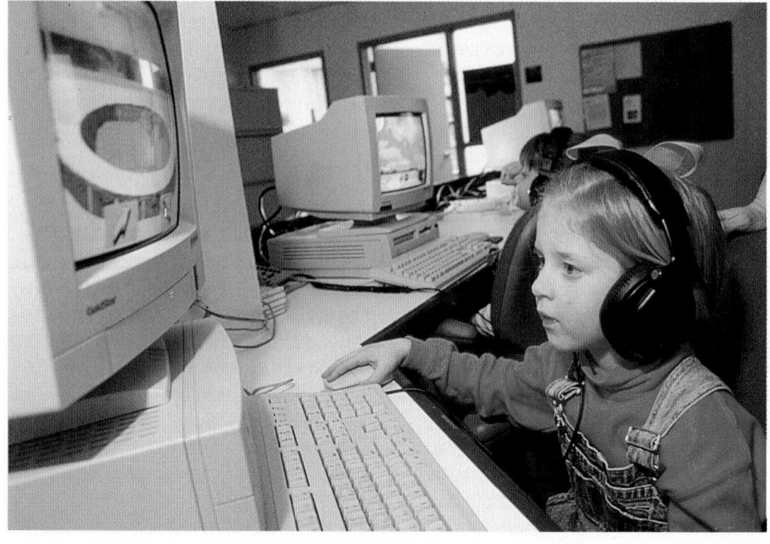

Building language skills
Video games with computer-generated speech can help many children with severe language problems. The games slow down consonant sounds, enabling youngsters to hear differences that they cannot discern in normal speech. The games were developed by physicians in New Jersey and California. The doctors reported in 1996 that after a month of therapy with this technique, children gained one to two years' worth of language ability and were better able to understand speech.

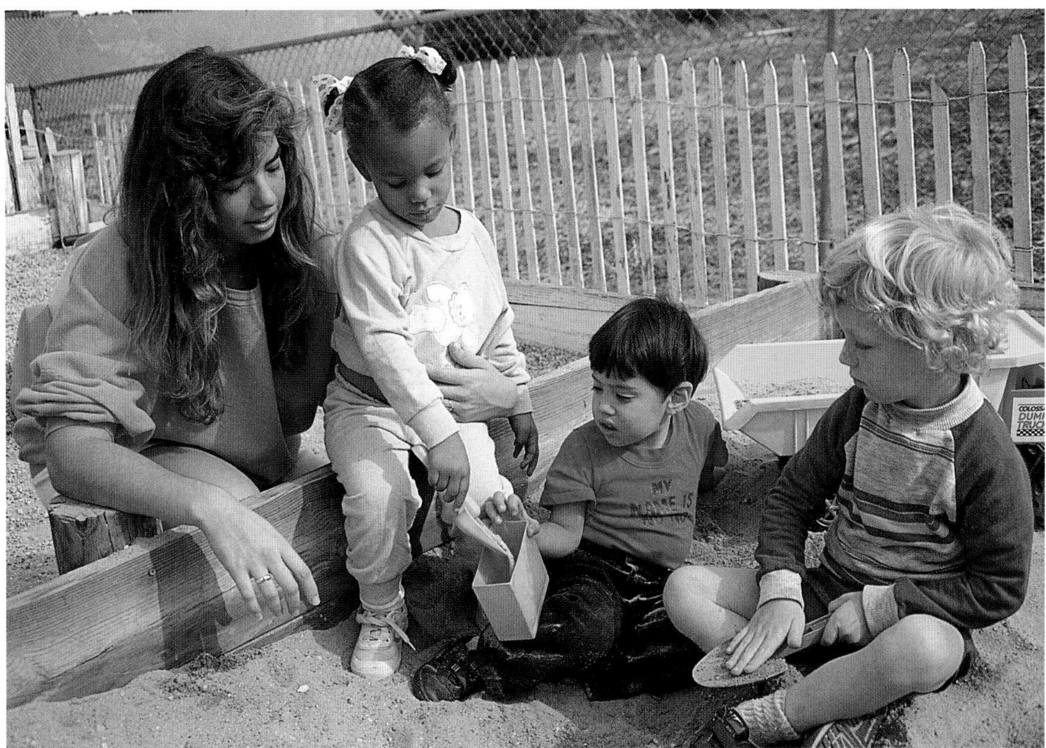

agement to give to each child, as well as fewer financial resources per child. As family size grew, the study reported, parents talked less to each child about school and had lower educational expectations for their children. Large families were also less likely to own a computer or to have educational materials, such as dictionaries and encyclopedias, available at home, and parents tended to save less money for their children's college tuition.

But the researchers also noted that when parents made the time to talk to the eighth-graders about school, became acquainted with their children's friends, and had high expectations for their children's academic success, family size did not have a negative impact on a child's success in school.

Sugar and hyperactivity. Investigators at the Vanderbilt University Child Development Center in Nashville, Tennessee, took another step in 1995 toward shattering the theory that sugar can cause attention deficit hyperactivity disorder (ADHD). Their report, published in November, concluded that sugar had no influence upon the behavior or intellectual performance of most children.

For years, many researchers theorized that the wild behavior of hyperactive children occurred in response to an intake of sweets, though studies did not always support that contention. According to the theory, after children eat sugar, their blood-sugar levels dive, causing *reactive hypoglycemia* (a condition in which a low level of sugar in the blood leads to nervousness and increased physical activity). This pattern is what some parents call a "sugar high."

In an attempt to settle the issue, Vanderbilt researchers reported in 1994 that two studies of children showed that high levels of sugar did not cause hyperactive behavior. In the 1995 study, the Vanderbilt researchers reevaluated the findings from these 2 studies and from 21 other studies conducted from 1982 to 1994 on the effects of sugar on children. Data on more than 500 youngsters, most under the age of 15, were analyzed. Some of the children were considered normal, while others

Day care and mother-child bonding

Day care does not harm the bond between a working mother and her child, as long as the mother is sensitive and responsive to the child when they are together. That was the conclusion of a study funded by the National Institute of Child Health and Development and reported in April 1996. The study examined 15-month-old children who were in day care 10 hours a week or less in 10 child-care sites throughout the United States.

were categorized as hyperactive, as being "sugar reactors," or as having problems with delinquency.

The Vanderbilt investigators acknowledged that some of the studies they examined did show a relationship between sugar intake and ADHD. However, because of the way those studies were structured, the researchers said it was difficult to tell whether sugar intake caused the ADHD, or whether hyperactive behavior led children to consume sugar.

The Vanderbilt team also pointed out that parents' own expectations of their child's activity level sometimes influenced how they thought their youngster behaved. At birthday parties, for example, children may have behaved wildly because of a high excitement level, not because of the sweets they ate. Still, the researchers said they could not eliminate the possibility that sugar might have an effect on some children.

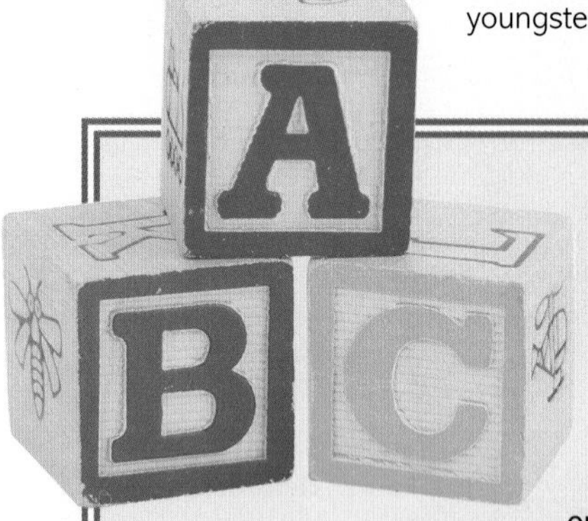

Fine-tuning motor skills

Children develop an amazing variety of motor skills in the earliest years of life. But they do not all develop them at exactly the same age or in exactly the same order. To help parents understand what a normal progression of development is, experts have averaged what many children do and the ages at which they do them to obtain the age-related milestones listed below. Since no child is "average," experts say that you should not expect your child's skills to match the chart perfectly. However, if you see that your child is seriously lagging in any area, you may want to share your concerns with your child's doctor.

Children's motor skills from birth to 3

Ages	Skills
0-12 months	**Sits without support, crawls, pulls self to standing and stands unaided, walks with aid, rolls ball, picks things up with thumb and one finger.**
12-24 months	**Walks alone, pulls and pushes toys, walks up and down stairs (hand-held), builds tower of three small blocks, throws ball.**
24–36 months	**Runs forward, kicks ball, jumps (two feet together), uses one hand consistently, holds crayon with thumb and fingers, turns pages, strings large beads.**

Source: *Mainstreaming Preschoolers*, Head Start Bureau.

Genes and hyperactivity. In other research on hyperactivity, investigators at the University of California at Irvine and the University of Toronto in Canada reported in May 1996 that they had identified an abnormal gene involved in ADHD. Earlier studies had suggested that genetics plays a part in many cases of ADHD, but this was the first time that a particular gene had been found to be associated with the disorder. The researchers emphasized, however, that the gene does not trigger ADHD by itself. Other, as-yet-unidentified factors also contribute to hyperactivity, they said.

The scientists analyzed genes that carry the coded information for creating brain-cell *receptors* (molecular docking sites) for dopamine, an important brain chemical. They studied the genes of 39 children with ADHD and a comparable number of children who were not hyperactive. About half of the ADHD youngsters had a dopamine gene called D4 that contained a defect, a segment that was repeated seven times. While not every child with ADHD carried this defective gene, those who did had a more severe form of the condition.

The researchers said they hoped the discovery of the faulty gene would lead to an understanding of how the drug Ritalin, widely prescribed to treat ADHD, works in the brain and give clues for the development of other treatments. They also expressed hope that finding the gene would make it possible to devise a diagnostic test for ADHD.

Race and intelligence. Lower IQ (intelligence quotient) scores among black children (as compared with white children) are caused by poverty and fewer learning opportunities, not race. That was the conclusion of researchers at Northwestern University in Evanston, Illinois, and Columbia University in New York City, who reported their findings in April 1996.

The investigators evaluated almost 500 children at eight health-care sites in the United States and found that, at the age of 5, the black children scored an average of 15 points lower on IQ tests than the white children. But an analysis of other information about these youngsters, such as their family structure, economic level, the degree to which learning was encouraged in the home, and neighborhood conditions, led the researchers to conclude that poverty was responsible for 52 percent of the differences in IQ scores between the races. The home environment, including the amount of learning stimulation there, accounted for most of the remainder. Once these factors were taken into account, the difference in IQ's was just 3 points, which was deemed statistically insignificant.

Researchers recommended job-training programs as one means of elevating poor single mothers and their children out of a low economic status. They said literacy programs and community resource centers for children and parents can also be effective. Most important, however, according to the researchers, was that children receive adequate mental stimulation very early in life—preferably between birth and age 3—when brain growth is most rapid.

Early educational programs. Another study also pointed out how important early educational opportunities are for children growing up in poverty. Researchers at the University of North Carolina at Chapel Hill and the University of Alabama at Birmingham reported in February 1996 that children experience improvements in intellectual development and academic performance if they are exposed to educational programs at an early age.

The study followed 110 black children from low-income families from their first six months of life through their teen-age years and into their 20's. Half of the children were initially placed in a year-round, full-day preschool program as infants, while the other half were placed in regular day-care or home-care programs. When the children entered kindergarten at the age of 5, they were redivided into two groups. One group took part in a three-year-long enrichment program that supplemented their elementary school education, while the other group did not.

The children were tested at 18 months and at yearly intervals thereafter until the age of 5. They were also tested at ages 8, 12, and 15. At every age, the children in the enriched programs scored higher on IQ tests and showed greater achievement in reading and mathematics than the children in the unenriched programs. They were also less likely to have to repeat a grade or to be placed in special-education programs. This advantage persisted until at least age 15.

The study showed that the children who received the most benefit over the long term were those who had been placed in the enrichment program in infancy. Children whose enrichment began at age 5 did not experience the same long-lasting benefits. The study added support to the argument that early education programs have significant and lasting value for very young children.

TV recommendations. In October 1995, the American Academy of Pediatrics (a professional society of children's physicians) issued a statement, making recommendations related to TV viewing. According to the academy, parents should limit the time their children watch TV to one to two hours a day, because television's influence on children increases the more they watch it. To take the place of time spent in front of the television, activities such as reading, athletics, and hobbies should be incorporated into children's lives. Parents should watch TV with their children, helping them to interpret what they see. Finally, parents should be aware of the negative impact of TV violence upon children, and pediatricians should urge that sexuality be depicted in a responsible manner.

In 1984, the academy had cautioned parents that television viewing may promote violent or aggressive behavior. In 1993, the academy noted that the average child in the United States watched 21 to 23 hours of television a week. • Richard Trubo

In World Book, see Child.

Dentistry

- Nonsurgical treatment for gum disease
- Newly discovered jaw muscle
- Estrogen and tooth loss

Many people with severe *periodontal* (gum) disease may be able to avoid tooth extraction or surgery, according to study results announced by the National Institute of Dental Research (NIDR) in May 1996. By administering antibiotics, researchers reduced the number of tooth extractions and gum surgeries by 88 percent.

The study, funded by NIDR—an agency of the National Institutes of Health in Bethesda, Maryland—was conducted at the University of Michigan and University of Detroit/Mercy schools of dentistry. Researchers examined 90 patients with advanced periodontal disease, a condition in which the gums and other tissues around the teeth become severely infected. The infection destroys the bones holding teeth in their sockets. The researchers determined that if the patients were being treated conventionally, 783 of their teeth would require extraction or surgery on the gums around the tooth.

All participants in the study first underwent scaling and planing, a traditional treatment in which the pockets of inflammation around teeth are cleared away. Researchers then gave patients oral doses of antibiotics that combat gum-disease bacteria. Finally, they placed films containing an antibiotic directly into infected areas around each tooth.

By the end of the study, only 93 teeth—12 percent—still needed extraction or surgery. The antibiotic treatment reduced the need for gum surgery by 93 percent, sparing 595 teeth, and the need for extraction by 81 percent, sparing 95 teeth. Seventy-three patients—81 percent of all who participated in the study—avoided surgery or extractions altogether.

Researchers found that the benefits of nonsurgical treatment lasted at least one year. They planned to follow the patients for five to eight years to learn the long-term benefits of nonsurgical treatment.

Newly discovered jaw muscle. The discovery of a new muscle involved in chewing and other movements of the jaw was reported in February 1996 by researchers at the University of Maryland School of Dentistry in Baltimore. Experts said discoveries of new anatomical structures are extremely rare because the human body has been so thoroughly studied.

Gary D. Hack, an assistant professor of dentistry, and Gwendolyn F. Dunn, an orthodontist, detected the muscle in studies on *cadavers* (corpses) by using an unusual angle in performing an autopsy of the head. They verified its existence in living people by using magnetic resonance imaging (MRI), a medical technique that uses powerful magnets to view tissues inside the body. The muscle,

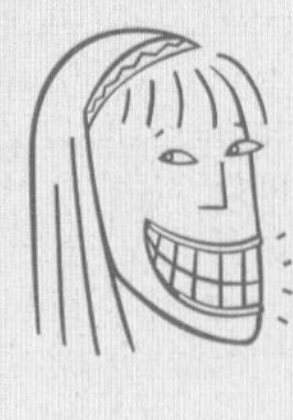

Too much of a good thing

Children under the age of 6 should use no more than a pea-sized amount of toothpaste daily, according to a study reported in December 1995 by researchers at the University of Connecticut. The researchers followed the health habits of 916 children through questionnaires and oral exams during the first eight years of life. They found that children who used too much toothpaste were at risk of fluorosis, a spotting or staining of the teeth.

Young children tend to swallow toothpaste instead of spitting it out, according to the researchers. If the body absorbs too much fluoride, the child can develop fluorosis. The authors of the study also recommended that parents supervise children while they brush to make sure they spit out the toothpaste.

Source: American Dental Association.

What to do in a dental emergency

If you have a tooth knocked out, a dentist can often save the tooth and replace it in the mouth. But dental injuries require immediate attention—within 30 minutes, the American Dental Association (ADA) advises. In an October 1995 address to the ADA, dentist Joe H. Camp recommended the following steps before reaching the dentist's office:

- Put the tooth back in the socket if possible.
- Put the tooth in a glass of milk to keep it moist if it cannot be put back in the socket.
- Place the tooth against the inside of the person's cheek if neither of the first two steps is possible. The important thing is to keep the tooth moist.
- Put the tooth in a glass of water as a last resort.

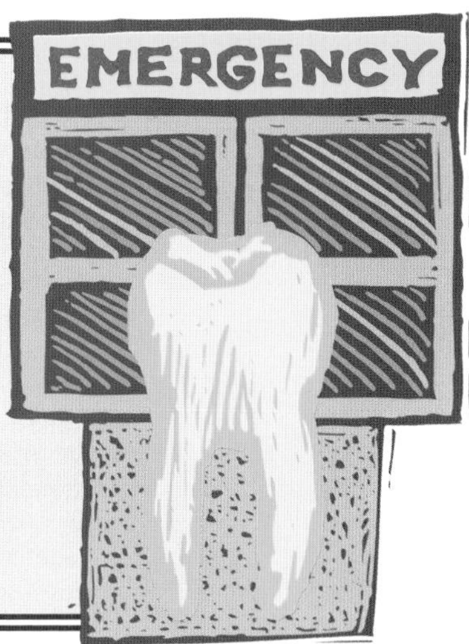

which the doctors named the sphenomandibularis muscle, extends from a bony outgrowth behind the eye socket to the lower jaw on both sides of the head. It is about 1½ inches (3.8 centimeters) long and ¾ of an inch (1.9 centimeters) wide.

The doctors said they suspected that further research might show the newly found muscle to be the source of certain hard-to-treat headaches. Some people complain that they get a headache behind their eyes when they are chewing.

Estrogen and tooth loss. Women taking the female hormone estrogen after *menopause* (the time in life when menstrual periods cease) may lower the risk of tooth loss, researchers at Harvard University in Cambridge, Massachusetts, reported in March 1996. Estrogen helps prevent bone weakening and other problems associated with menopause.

In a study of 42,000 postmenopausal nurses, the researchers found that women who took estrogen were 38 percent less likely to lose their teeth. Estrogen may protect against tooth loss by strengthening the jaw bone, the investigators said.

• Michael Woods

In the section A Healthy Family, see HEALTHY GUMS. In WORLD BOOK, see DENTISTRY.

Diabetes

- New oral drug approved
- Drug combination
- Gene linked to diabetes
- Islet cell transplants
- Bypass surgery
- Vitamin E and diabetes
- Preventing foot amputations

The Food and Drug Administration (FDA) in September 1995 approved the oral drug acarbose (sold as Precose) for people with Type II (noninsulin-dependent) diabetes. Acarbose slows down the digestion of carbohydrates, which the body turns into a simple sugar called glucose. In people with Type II diabetes, glucose can build up in the blood, sometimes leading to serious problems, such as coma, because the hormone insulin is not properly used. Insulin enables glucose to enter the body's cells, where it is converted to energy.

Acarbose can be administered in combination with metformin, another oral drug approved in 1994, or with drugs called sulfonylureas, for years the only oral drug for Type II diabetes approved for use in the United States. Metformin helps the body use insulin more efficiently. Sulfonylureas stimulate the production of insulin.

Drug combination. Diabetes patients taking a combination of metformin and a sulfonylurea called glyburide fared better than patients taking just one drug, according to a multicenter study of metformin reported in August 1995. In the study, 632 patients received one of three treatments: metformin alone, glyburide alone, or a combination of the two medications for 29 weeks. The group taking both drugs had the lowest glucose levels of all.

Gene linked to diabetes. Investigators at the Johns Hopkins University School of Medicine in Baltimore reported in August 1995 that a *mutated* (changed) gene, called the beta-3-adrenergic receptor gene, is linked to the early onset of Type II diabetes and that the same gene is associated with obesity. The gene directs fat cells to make a protein that increases the rate at which food is turned into energy. The scientists said a defective gene might slow this rate.

The researchers studied Pima Indians in Arizona, who have a high rate of diabetes—about half develop diabetes by age 40—and obesity. The scientists found that those who inherited the mutated gene did indeed burn fewer calories and became diabetic even earlier than average—by age 36. Those with the mutated gene gained weight particularly in the chest and abdomen, the so-called apple pattern, which past research had shown to be a high risk factor for diabetes and heart disease.

The scientists said that diet and exercise were still important to control Type II diabetes. But if further studies confirm their finding, genetic tests might make it possible to identify people prone to the disease, and treatment could begin early.

Islet cell transplants. In research involving mice reported in October 1995, investigators at the University of Massachusetts Medical Center in Worcester successfully transplanted insulin-producing cells called islet cells from healthy donor mice to mice with diabetes. Islet cells are made by the pancreas. However, instead of giving *antirejection drugs* (drugs to prevent the immune system from rejecting the transplant) to the recipient mice, the scientists gave them injections of white blood cells from the donor mice and *antibodies* (disease-fighting molecules) called CD40L. The two injections trained the immune systems of the recipient mice to accept the transplanted cells.

As a result, 37 of the 40 mice in the study demonstrated no evidence of rejection, and the transplanted cells subsequently produced insulin, thus halting the mice's diabetes. The scientists said the success of their procedure suggests that a similar means might someday be developed to cure diabetes in people.

Bypass surgery. Patients with diabetes who need treatment for blocked arteries in the heart survive better after bypass surgery than patients who undergo angioplasty. This was the finding of a major international study reported in September 1995 by the National Institutes of Health in Bethesda, Maryland. In angioplasty, an instrument with a tiny balloon on the end is threaded into a blocked artery. The balloon is inflated,

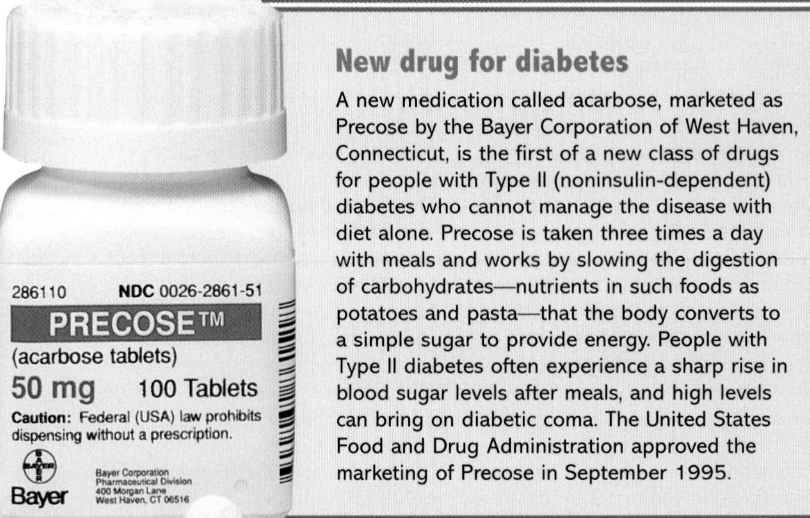

New drug for diabetes

A new medication called acarbose, marketed as Precose by the Bayer Corporation of West Haven, Connecticut, is the first of a new class of drugs for people with Type II (noninsulin-dependent) diabetes who cannot manage the disease with diet alone. Precose is taken three times a day with meals and works by slowing the digestion of carbohydrates—nutrients in such foods as potatoes and pasta—that the body converts to a simple sugar to provide energy. People with Type II diabetes often experience a sharp rise in blood sugar levels after meals, and high levels can bring on diabetic coma. The United States Food and Drug Administration approved the marketing of Precose in September 1995.

STATISTICS

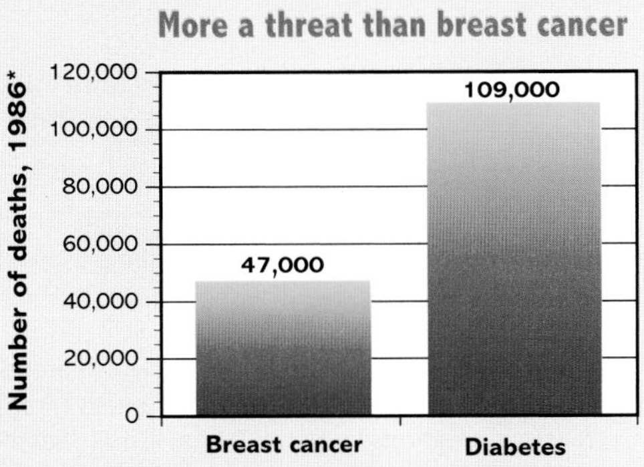

More a threat than breast cancer

Number of deaths, 1986*

	Number of deaths
Breast cancer	47,000
Diabetes	109,000

* Latest available figures from national surveys.
Source: Centers for Disease Control and Prevention.

Although women fear breast cancer more, diabetes poses a greater threat to their health, the Centers for Disease Control and Prevention reported in September 1995. Heart disease and all cancers combined are the top two killers of American women. After that, diabetes takes a disproportionately high toll among African American, Asian, Hispanic, and Native American women. It is the third-leading cause of death for African American and Hispanic women, the fourth-leading cause of death for Native American women (accidents rank third), and the fifth-leading cause of death for Asian women (accidents and pneumonia rank third and fourth, respectively).

flattening the blockage against the arterial wall, restoring blood flow. In the more invasive bypass surgery, veins taken from elsewhere in the patient's body are attached above and below a blockage, enabling blood to bypass the obstruction.

All 353 patients in the study had significant blockages in two or more coronary arteries and were randomly assigned to receive angioplasty or bypass surgery at 18 hospitals in the United States and Canada. Over a five-year period, 35 percent of the angioplasty group died, compared with 19 percent among those who had bypass surgery.

Diabetes is a major risk factor for coronary heart disease. Doctors had often chosen angioplasty over coronary bypass surgery because of the belief that bypass operations might increase the chances of infections and other diabetic complications. But the new study prompted U.S. health officials to issue a clinical alert to physicians, recommending bypass surgery for people already on diabetes drugs and with at least two blocked arteries.

Vitamin E and diabetes. A study by researchers at the University of Kuopio in Finland, published in October 1995, examined the role of vitamin E in protecting against Type II diabetes. The researchers said vitamin E may help prevent diabetes and may reduce the risk of complications in people who have the disease.

Until the study, little was known about the relationship between diabetes and vitamin E, a nutrient called an antioxidant. Scientists believe antioxidants may prevent certain types of cell damage by blocking the effects of *free radicals,* unstable molecules created when oxygen combines with food molecules to produce energy.

The Finnish researchers studied 944 nondiabetic men aged 42 to 60 for four years. All had low blood levels of vitamin E, and 60 percent had daily intakes of the vitamin below 10 milligrams, the recommended daily allowance for adult males. During the study period, 45 participants were diagnosed as having Type II diabetes. They had the lowest blood level of the vitamin. The scientists called for more studies in other population groups.

Preventing foot amputations. In November 1995, U.S. health officials launched a campaign for doctors to annually screen the feet of people with diabetes using a simple device. A bristle is pressed against 10 key spots on the foot to test for a loss of sensation caused by nerve damage and circulatory problems associated with diabetes. People with the disease face a risk of foot amputation 27 times greater than that of the general population. • **Richard Trubo**

In the section On the Medical Frontier, see LASER SURGERY COMES INTO FOCUS. In WORLD BOOK, see DIABETES.

Digestive System

- Antibodies for Crohn's disease
- Other antibody research
- Fish oil for Crohn's disease

Progress in treating the symptoms of Crohn's disease was reported by several research groups at the annual meeting of the American Gastroenterological Association held in San Francisco in May 1996.

Crohn's disease involves chronic inflammation of the gastrointestinal tract—in most cases, the *ileum* (lower half of the small intestine) or *colon* (part of the large intestine). Symptoms include abdominal pain, fever, diarrhea, rectal bleeding, and weight loss. The cause of the disease is unknown, and there is no cure. Treatment usually includes drugs called corticosteroids that reduce inflammation and keep symptoms under control. But these drugs have serious side effects, which make prolonged usage inadvisable.

Research on the development of inflammatory diseases—both those resulting from specific infections and those, like Crohn's disease, of unknown origin—has focused on immune system responses that help spread or control inflammation. These responses involve proteins in the blood called cytokines, which can stimulate or suppress inflammation. Researchers have found substantial amounts of one cytokine, called tumor necrosis factor alpha (TNF alpha), in the tissues and stools of patients with Crohn's disease.

Antibodies for Crohn's disease. The studies reported in May 1996 built on a 1995 study by researchers in the Netherlands. In the earlier study, the Dutch researchers selected 10 patients who had not responded to the standard drug treatment for Crohn's disease. Each of the patients received a single injection of an *antibody* (immune system protein) against TNF alpha. The antibody, cA2, was genetically engineered from human and mouse cells and was specifically designed to target TNF alpha and block its action.

Of the 10 patients, 1 required surgery and left the study. But in 8 of the 9 remaining patients, the disease entered remission—that is, symptoms markedly decreased.

The severity of symptoms was measured on a scale known as the Crohn's disease activity index (CDAI). At the beginning of the study, the patients had an average index of 257. (Physicians consider a drop in the index of at least 70 points to constitute a clinical response, and they consider the disease to be in remission when the patient's CDAI falls below 150.) Two weeks after the injection, the average CDAI of the patients in the study had dropped to 114, and after eight weeks, to 60. The researchers noted no harmful side effects from the treatment in any of the patients.

Other antibody research. Further progress toward an antibody treatment was reflected in several reports at the May 1996 meeting. Researchers from the University of Alabama reported on their study of the most effective dosage of cA2. They found that a dose as high as 20 milligrams per kilogram (mg/kg) of the patient's body weight effectively lowered the CDAI without provoking any adverse reaction from the body's immune system. The Dutch study had administered a dosage of 10 mg/kg. The Alabama team reported that after 12 weeks, 65 percent of patients receiving dosages of 5, 10, and 20 mg/kg had responded with a drop of at least 70 points in CDAI, and 40 percent were in remission.

A research team from Belgium reported on a study in which patients with Crohn's disease and patients with ulcerative colitis received either cA2 or a *placebo* (substance with no active ingredients). Ulcerative colitis is an inflammatory disease similar to Crohn's disease that affects the colon and rectum. Although researchers believe that TNF alpha is involved in the development of ulcerative colitis, these patients did not respond to the antibody treatment, whereas the Crohn's disease patients did.

A team from the United Kingdom reported at the May meeting on tests of another antibody against TNF alpha called CDP-571. The researchers engineered this antibody to reduce the immune system response to it. In so doing, they hoped to enable people with Crohn's disease to receive repeated doses.

Of the 30 patients in the study, 20

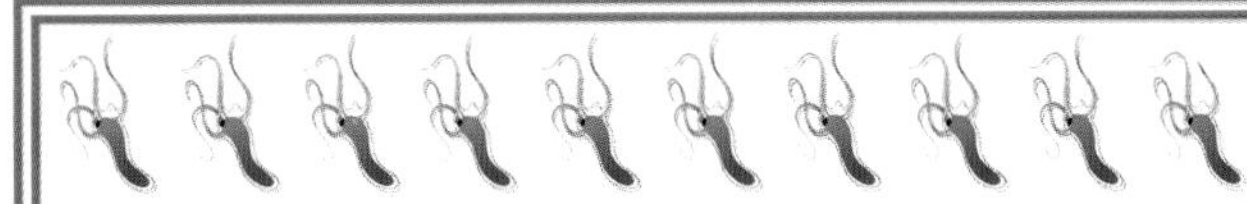

Changing the treatment of ulcers

The standard treatments for digestive tract ulcers have only relieved the symptoms. But in April 1996, the Food and Drug Administration (FDA) approved a combination of two medications that can also provide a cure.

One of the drugs is the antibiotic clarithromycin, sold as Biaxin, and the other is omeprazole, an antacid sold as Prilosec. In a study in Great Britain, this drug combination cured 83 percent of ulcer patients who received it. The therapy also reduced the chances of an ulcer's recurring.

For years, medical experts believed that ulcers resulted from stress and from habits such as smoking and consuming caffeine, which increased the production of stomach acid. The acid, in turn, irritated the lining of the stomach or small intestine, producing the sores known as ulcers. Treatment included changes in lifestyle, antacid drugs to alleviate pain, and changes in diet. But in 1984, an Australian researcher found a bacterium, *Helicobacter pylori,* in the stomachs of people with ulcers. He concluded that the bacteria caused the ulcers and that antibiotics could kill the bacteria.

This discovery has changed the treatment of ulcers only gradually. The FDA backed the combination therapy for ulcers to increase awareness of it in the medical community.

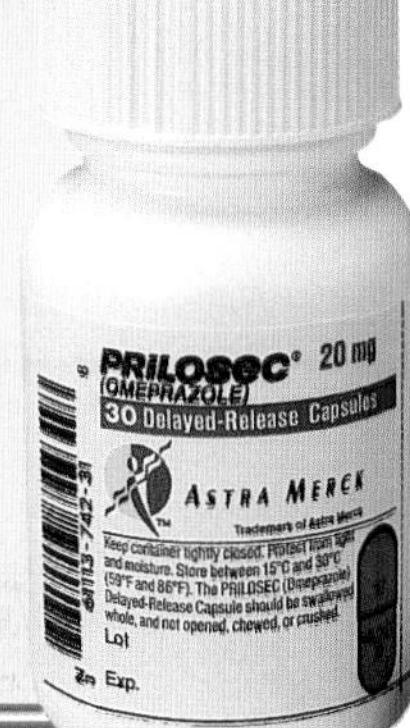

received CDP-571 and 10 received a placebo. In the treatment group, the average CDAI fell from 263 at the beginning of the study to 167 after two weeks. The placebo group also began with a CDAI of 263 but had a CDAI of 247 after two weeks. Benefits from the treatment lasted as long as eight weeks in some patients. Researchers found that the patients' immune systems did not mount a response to counteract the treatment.

These studies demonstrated the great potential for a Crohn's disease therapy that aims at suppressing the activity of TNF alpha. While antibodies against TNF alpha show great promise, researchers still must overcome the problem of administering repeated dosages without stimulating an immune system response that either diminishes the treatment's effectiveness or produces severe side effects. Hope remains strong of developing a drug that specifically blocks TNF alpha.

Fish oil for Crohn's disease. Fish-oil capsules with a new time-release coating can keep Crohn's disease in remission with few side effects. This finding was reported by a team at the University of Bologna in Italy in June 1996.

Physicians have prescribed fish-oil capsules in treating other inflammatory diseases, including ulcerative colitis and rheumatoid arthritis. However, many patients are unwilling to follow through with the treatment because of the unpleasant taste and the side effects of the fish oil. The side effects include diarrhea and a fishy smell.

The capsules used in the Italian study were coated with a resin that was capable of resisting the action of stomach acid for 30 minutes and of disintegrating within 60 minutes. This delay allowed the capsules to reach the small intestine before releasing the fish oil, thereby reducing the unpleasant side effects.

The 78 patients in the study had been in remission for at least three weeks but less than two years when the study began, and they had a CDAI of less than 150. They were, however, at high risk for a relapse of the disease. (The risk of relapse is 75 percent greater for people whose disease has been in remission less than two years than for those in remission longer than two years.) Over the course of a year, 39 patients received nine fish-oil capsules daily, and the other 39 received nine placebos. At the end of the year, 59 percent of the treated patients remained in remission, compared with only 26 percent of the placebo group.

The coated capsule had few side effects, and most of the patients were willing to complete the treatment. Only 10 percent of the patients taking the fish-oil capsules discontinued the treatment as a result of diarrhea.

• James L. Franklin

In the section A HEALTHY FAMILY, see HEARTBURN: TAKING AIM AT FIRE. In WORLD BOOK, see DIGESTIVE SYSTEM; ILEITIS.

Drugs

- AIDS drugs
- Fast track for cancer drugs
- New osteoporosis drug
- The first ALS drug
- A second drug for MS
- New drug for diabetes
- New antiobesity drug

Although there was still no drug in 1996 that would cure AIDS, significant progress was made in the development of new drugs that would prolong the survival of infected patients and reduce complications and the occurrence of other infections. In late 1995 and early 1996, the U.S. Food and Drug Administration (FDA) approved three new drugs for use in the treatment of patients infected with HIV, the virus that causes AIDS: saquinavir, ritonavir, and indinavir. With each of these drugs, the FDA set a new record for the speed with which it reviewed and approved a drug. FDA approval of indinavir came just 42 days after the company submitted a new-drug application.

All three new drugs are antiviral agents that work by inhibiting the action of HIV protease, a substance that is critical for the *replication* (reproduction) of HIV. They were expected to enhance the effectiveness of *combination therapies*—the use of two or more drugs at the same time—to combat HIV infection. Physicians use combination therapies to treat most HIV-infected patients because they provide a greater action against the virus and may also reduce the ability of the virus to develop resistance to the individual drugs.

The availability of three new anti-HIV drugs gave physicians the opportunity to combine them with older AIDS-fighting drugs, such as zidovudine (also known as AZT). These combinations interfere with two phases of the HIV replication cycle. Doctors had already been using various combinations of these drugs, and an increasing number of studies had reported that the drugs significantly reduce both the amount of HIV in the blood and the death rate from AIDS.

The approval of three new drugs represented an important advance in the effective management of HIV infection. But doctors cautioned that they must be used with care. For example, there is an extensive list of other drugs that people taking ritonavir must not use because of the risk of a harmful drug interaction.

Fast track for cancer drugs. The FDA announced new initiatives in March 1996 aimed at accelerating the approval of promising new cancer therapies and improving patient access to them. Prior to these changes, the approval process for new drugs typically took about 12 months. Experts hoped that the changes would cut approval times by 50 percent. Drugs to help fight the AIDS virus had already been receiving this kind of accelerated approval.

The steps taken by the FDA included shortening approval times for cancer treatments by recognizing that tumor shrinkage is often an early indi-

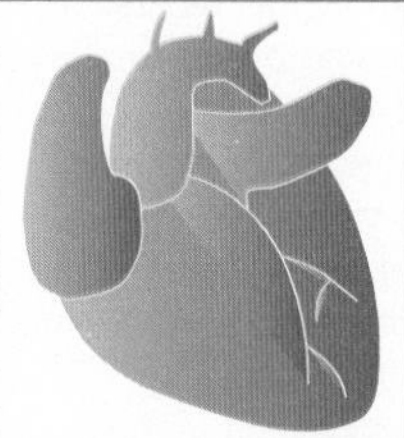

Controversy over CCB's

In February 1996, the U.S. Food and Drug Administration (FDA) moved to revise the labeling included with immediate-release nifedipine formulations to indicate that this version of the drug should not be used to treat certain cardiovascular diseases. Nifedipine is a calcium channel blocker (CCB)—a drug that blocks calcium *ions* (electrically charged atoms) from entering the cells of the heart and blood vessels. This action decreases the strength of muscular contractions and, therefore, lowers blood pressure. The FDA's action came amid a controversy over data that suggested that CCB's may increase the risk of heart attack. Many health experts disputed this conclusion because the data did not result from controlled clinical trials. The FDA concluded that the the data did not provide sufficient evidence to link CCB's with heart attacks. Other CCB's, as well as sustained-release formulations of nifedipine, were not affected by the FDA's action.

Immediate-release nifedipine formulations (sold as Adalat or Procardia, and in generic form) act quickly and are rapidly eliminated from the body. For this reason, they must be taken three or four times a day. The problem may be that the drug takes effect too abruptly, causing a rapid drop in blood pressure. Repeated doses several times a day may strain the heart. Sustained-release formulations of nifedipine (including Adalat CC and Procardia XL) work more slowly and so are only taken once a day.

Physicians in the United States may legally prescribe drugs for off-label uses, and many drugs have been used to treat conditions for which they were not specifically approved. Immediate-release nifedipine formulations have often been prescribed to treat hypertension. The FDA advised patients taking short-acting nifedipine formulations to continue following their doctor's instructions.

Drugs and vision

Don't believe your eyes? Check your medicine cabinet. A number of commonly prescribed drugs can also have an effect on your eyes. The drugs listed here include some of those most often associated with vision and other eye problems.

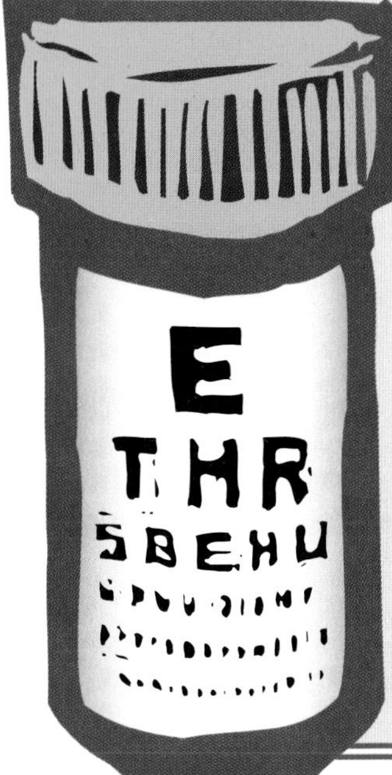

Drug Category	Eye Problem	Action
Antibiotics (Tetracycline, in particular)	• In rare cases, long-term use may cause blurred vision.	Sometimes the medication may need to be changed or even discontinued.
Anticoagulants (Coumadin, aspirin)	• May cause red spots on the surface of the eye.	None necessary. Spots do not affect vision and go away after medication is discontinued.
Antihistamines (Some over the counter and some prescription)	• Can cause eye dryness • Can cause changes in pupil size, which can lead to glaucoma.	Use "artificial tears" as needed. People at risk for glaucoma should use only with a doctor's approval.
Arthritis Drugs (Chloroquine, and Plaqueril; both also used for malaria)	• The drug can accumulate in the retina, leading to permanent loss of vision.	Eye exams are needed every 6 to 12 months.
Bladder/Stomach Antispasmodics (Ditropan, Donnatal, Levsin)	• Can cause blurred vision.	May need to lower dosage or discontinue use.
Heart Disease Drugs		
• Digoxin (for heart arrhythmias)	• High doses can cause blurred or "yellow-tinged" vision	Reduce dosage with approval of both prescribing physician and ophthalmologist.
• Cordarone (for heart arrhythmias)	• Can cause pigment deposits in the cornea.	Consult both prescribing physician and ophthalmologist.
• Diuretics (for hypertension)	• Can cause eye dryness	Use "artificial tears" as needed.
Steroids (including over-the-counter creams; avoid getting near the eyes)	• Can cause cataracts (clouding of the lens). • Can cause changes in pupil size, which can lead to glaucoma.	In rare cases, surgery may be required. Get an eye exam six weeks after starting medication, then others at the doctor's recommendation.

cator of a treatment's effectiveness. The agency also sought to make it easier for pharmaceutical companies to market promising cancer therapies that have been approved by other countries. Under the new guidelines, companies would be allowed to make such drugs available to patients in the United States before the drugs receive FDA approval.

In addition, a number of new drugs were approved in 1995 and 1996 for the management of various types of cancer. Among the most important were docetaxel and gemcitabine, both of which received approval from the FDA in May 1996. Docetaxel (sold under the brand name Taxotere) is used to treat advanced cases of breast cancer that have not responded to standard therapies. Gemcitabine (marketed as Gemzar) is prescribed for the treatment of cancer of the pancreas.

New osteoporosis drug. The FDA in September 1995 approved the marketing of alendronate sodium as the first nonhormonal treatment for postmenopausal *osteoporosis* (decreased bone density). The drug is sold under the brand name Fosamax.

Osteoporosis is a progressive disease that causes a person's bones to become more prone to fracture. It affects more than 25 million Americans, about 80 percent of them women. It occurs most commonly in women who have reached menopause. After menopause, a woman's body almost completely stops producing the female sex hormone estrogen. Research has shown that the reduced level of estrogen in a woman's body after menopause causes the rate of new bone formation to decrease. In women with postmenopausal osteoporosis, the rate of natural bone loss significantly exceeds the rate of new bone formation.

Prior to the approval of alendronate sodium, treatment options for postmenopausal osteoporosis were limited to estrogen replacement therapy, using such drugs as Premarin, and treatment with a naturally occurring hormone, calcitonin (sold as Miacalcin). However, some women do not tolerate estrogen treatment well. And many women were reluctant to use calcitonin, which until recently, when a nasal spray version was approved, was available only in an injectable form.

In the first five years after menopause, women may lose as much as 25 percent of their bone mass, increasing the possibility of fractures, height loss, curvature of the spine, restricted movement, and disability. Alendronate sodium helps increase bone strength because it slows down the natural destruction of bone tissue, thereby causing new bone formation to exceed bone loss.

However, alendronate sodium may cause irritation of the stomach and esophagus. In some patients, this irritation can be severe. For the drug to be used effectively and safely, patients must follow specific guidelines regarding its use. Because food, beverages, and other medications can significantly reduce its effectiveness, the drug should be taken with just a glass of plain water at least 30 minutes before the first food, beverage, or medication of the day. To help the drug reach the stomach and to reduce the risk of adverse effects to the esophagus, people should avoid lying down for at least 30 minutes after taking the drug.

The first ALS drug. In late 1995, the FDA approved the marketing of riluzole, the first drug shown to prolong the survival of people with amyotrophic lateral sclerosis (ALS), a disease that causes the progressive destruction of nerve cells, leading to increasing muscular weakness and then paralysis. ALS is often called Lou Gehrig's disease for the famous baseball player who died of it in 1941. It is usually fatal within five years after diagnosis. Approximately 30,000 people in the United States have ALS. Riluzole represented the first—and only—advance in the treatment of ALS since Lou Gehrig's death.

In clinical studies with about 1,000 ALS patients worldwide, riluzole prolonged survival an average of about three months. Although the effectiveness of riluzole proved to be limited, it represented a breakthrough in the treatment of ALS and offered the hope that more effective drugs could be developed in the future.

A second drug for MS. The drug interferon beta-1a (sold as Avonex) in May 1996 received FDA approval as the second drug to treat people with multiple sclerosis (MS). MS is a disease of the nervous system that causes tremors, paralysis, speech disorders, and other symptoms.

MS affects about 300,000 people in the United States. About half have the relapsing form, characterized by *relapses* (recurrent attacks) followed by *remissions* (periods of complete or incomplete recovery).

In 1993, interferon beta-1b (sold as Betaseron) was introduced as the first drug to be effective in reducing the frequency of relapses. However, the new drug is the first treatment shown also to slow the progression of the disease and the accumulation of physical disability.

Interferon beta-1a shares many of the properties of its predecessor but there are also several other differences between the two drugs. For example, the new drug is administered by *intramuscular* (into a muscle) injection once a week, whereas interferon beta-1b is administered by *subcutaneous* (between the skin and underlying muscle) injection every other day.

New drug for diabetes. In September 1995, the FDA approved the drug acarbose for use in the United States as a treatment for diabetes. Acarbose, sold under the brand name

Precose, works in conjunction with diets intended to lower blood *glucose* (sugar) concentrations. The drug delays the digestion of carbohydrates in food, resulting in a smaller rise in blood glucose concentrations after meals.

For the drug to be most effective, physicians said, it should be taken at the start of each main meal. One disadvantage of using the drug is that the undigested carbohydrates cause gastrointestinal side effects, such as flatulence, diarrhea, and abdominal pain, in most patients during the first few weeks of therapy. These effects diminish in most patients as treatment is continued.

New antiobesity drug. In April 1996, the FDA approved dexfenfluramine hydrochloride for use in controlling obesity. It was the first new antiobesity drug approved in more than 20 years. While other drugs used to suppress the appetite are recommended only for short-term use, the new drug (sold as Redux) was approved for longer-term use to help maintain weight loss. But the effectiveness and safety of the new drug when used for more than a year were not known. • Daniel A. Hussar

See also WEIGHT CONTROL. In the section A Healthy Family, see HORMONE REPLACEMENT THERAPY. In WORLD BOOK, see DRUG.

Ear and Hearing

- Broader use recommended for cochlear implants
- Pacifiers and child ear infections
- Flu vaccine fights ear infections
- Bigger ears with age

Cochlear implants have proved so effective as a treatment for some deaf people that a panel convened by the National Institutes of Health in Bethesda, Maryland, recommended in a December 1995 report that use of these electronic devices be expanded. By that time, more than 12,000 people worldwide with profound hearing loss had received cochlear implants. The panel recommended that people who have severe hearing impairment but retain some residual hearing be considered for the implants as well.

The panel noted that the devices improve communication abilities for the vast majority of recipients, particularly when used in combination with lip-reading. The greatest success was noted in children who had learned to speak prior to their hearing loss and who received an implant before the age of 6. Adult implant recipients who became deaf after learning to speak experienced an increased ability to read lips. Many implant recipients reported being able to hear and appreciate music and to recognize sounds around them.

The rate of complications associated with cochlear implantation, including failure of the device to function once implanted, had declined to

The big bang—dangers of toy noise

Toys that make noise may annoy parents, but they create a more serious threat to the child. Noise levels above 100 decibels (db) can permanently damage a child's hearing, according to the American Academy of Pediatrics (AAP). A pop gun, for example, registers at 122 db when held next to the ear. Even toys that measure lower than 100 db can create problems if the noise is repeated frequently.

Toy manufacturers have set limits for themselves on how much noise a toy can make, but the decibels are measured at 25 centimeters (about a child's arm length) from the source. Since children frequently hold noise-making toys up to their ears, a "safe" toy can still cause problems.

The AAP suggests testing the noise level of a toy at the store by holding it up to your ear. If it hurts your ear, it is definitely too loud for a child's more sensitive hearing. Other common-sense advice: If you can hear a toy from another room in the house, it is too loud.

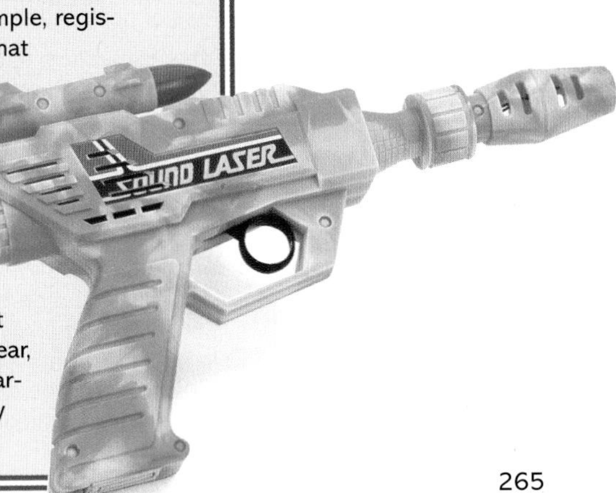

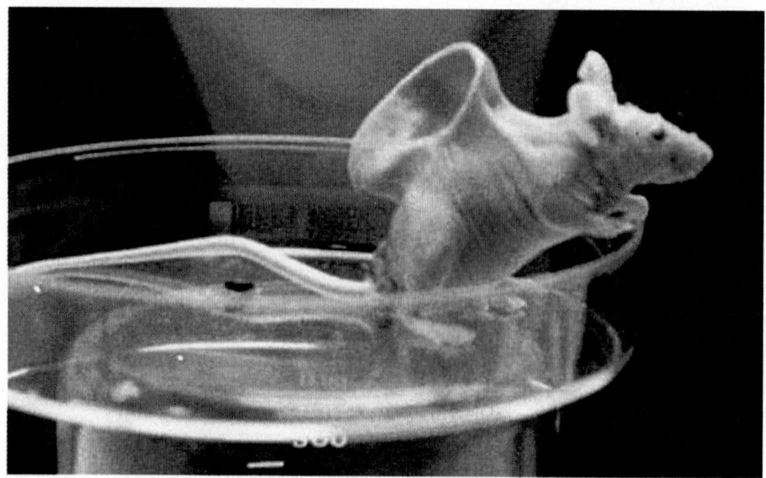

Mouse grows human ear
A human ear develops on the back of a mouse in an experiment reported in October 1995 by researchers at the University of Massachusetts. The mouse was bred to have no immune system so its body would not reject the ear, made from a biodegradable material "seeded" with human cartilage cells. The doctors hoped to develop a way for patients to grow their own replacement organs and other body parts from samples of their body tissues.

about 5 percent of cases in 1995. This compared favorably with other implanted devices, such as heart pacemakers, for which the complication rate was 10 percent.

Pacifiers and child ear infections. Investigators at the University of Oulu in Finland reported in November 1995 that children in day-care centers who sucked on pacifiers had a greater likelihood of developing *acute otitis media* (a middle-ear infection) than children who did not use pacifiers. Their conclusion was based on an evaluation of 845 children, 45 percent of whom had one or more ear infections during a 15-month period.

Children between ages 2 and 3 were found to be at the greatest risk of developing ear infections if they used a pacifier. Overall, the Finnish investigators concluded that pacifier use was responsible for 25 percent of the ear infections in children under 3 years old.

The researchers speculated that repeated sucking on pacifiers increases the production of saliva, a medium of transmission of the germs responsible for ear infections. They recommended restricting pacifier use to an infant's first 10 months of life, when ear infections are less prevalent and a baby's sucking urge is strongest.

Flu vaccine fights ear infections. A flu shot could be a defense for children against middle-ear infections. That was the conclusion of a study of infants and toddlers reported in October 1995 by doctors at Duke University in Durham, North Carolina.

The researchers evaluated 186 children between the ages of 6 and 30 months who attended eight day-care centers. Half of the children were vaccinated against influenza; the other half were not. The incidence of ear infections among the children was tracked from mid-November through mid-March, a period which includes the flu season.

During the flu season, the youngsters who received the vaccines had a 31 percent lower incidence of acute otitis media than the unvaccinated children. The researchers advised considering the use of influenza vaccines in children aged 6 months and older who attend day care.

Bigger ears with age. A group of physicians in England in December 1995 confirmed a commonly held belief: People's ears do get larger as they age. The doctors measured the ears of 206 patients aged 30 to 93 in the course of routine medical examinations. They found that ears grow an average of .009 inch (.22 millimeter) in a year—the equivalent of almost ½ inch over a 50-year period. The doctors could not offer an explanation as to why ears continue to grow as people age, when other parts of the body do not.

• Richard Trubo

In World Book, see Deafness; Ear.

Environmental Health

- Hormone disrupters
- Pesticides and immunity
- Lead and behavior
- Fine pollutants in the air
- Arsenic and cancer
- Cooking gas and asthma

The publication of the controversial book *Our Stolen Future* in March 1996 drew attention to research about chemicals in the environment. The authors compiled their findings from research suggesting that synthetic chemicals interfere with the function of hormones that control reproduction, the immune system, and mental and behavioral development.

These synthetic chemicals, called hormone disrupters, take the place of natural hormones in human cells and cause abnormal cellular reactions. For example, hormone disrupters are believed to interfere with the function of the male hormone testosterone. They may have caused an almost 50 percent drop in human male sperm counts since the mid-1940's.

Hormone disrupters belong to a group of chemicals called persistent organic pollutants (POP's), which do not degrade or dissolve in water, are carried around the world through the air and water, and are transmitted through the food chain. POP's include several pesticides and chlorine-containing compounds called polychlorinated biphenyls (PCB's) and dioxins.

Another report, released in May 1996 by investigators at several government agencies and universities in North America and Europe, warned that hormone disrupters can affect the development of the brain before birth and in the early years of life. Effects can range from almost imperceptible learning disabilities and behavioral problems to attention deficit disorder and severe mental retardation.

The researchers said that by mimicking the action of naturally occurring thyroid hormones, the chemicals interfere with the body's hormonal system, which plays a major role in guiding the development of the brain. The chemicals are so common that they are present in virtually every nursing mother's breast milk.

The scientists conceded that the results of the study are controversial since they based their conclusions on the evidence of several studies rather than any specific experiment. They said, however, that the evidence warrants more research to assess the potential risks of hormone disrupters.

Pesticides and immunity. Pesticides may reduce the body's ability to fight off diseases by impairing the immune system. That was the conclusion of a report released in March 1996 by the World Resources Institute, a research and advisory organization based in Washington, D.C. Examining studies on animals and humans from around the world, the authors concluded that pesticides are a major threat to health, particularly in developing countries where poor sanitation and nutrition already create risks of contracting infectious diseases.

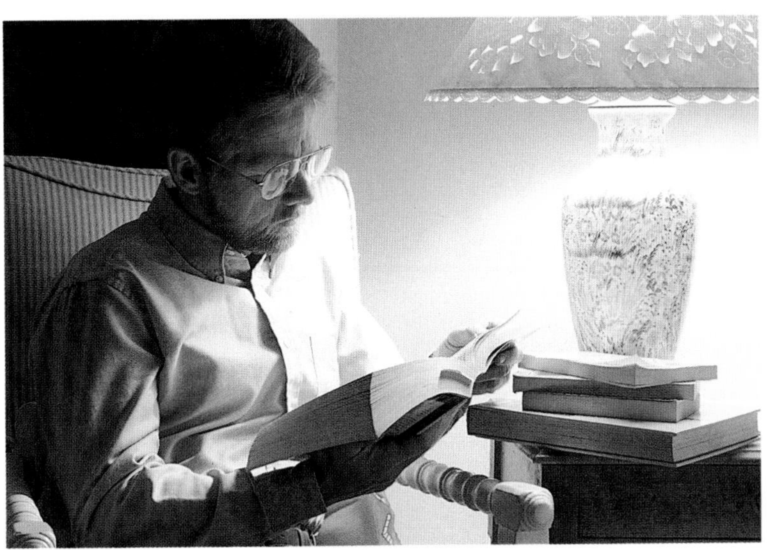

Reading yourself awake

A 1996 study at Boston's Brigham and Women's Hospital found that indoor lighting after sunset can reset your internal clock, which controls your sleep-wake cycle, alertness, body temperature, and metabolism. The internal time shift, similar to jet lag, can be as much as four to five hours. To counter the effect, the researchers recommended going to bed at the same time every day, getting eight hours of sleep, and reducing exposure to light before bedtime.

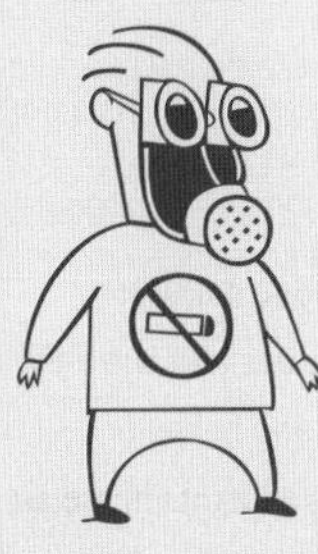

Clearing the air

Dust, pollen, animal dander, and soot are common indoor air particles that can irritate people with allergies and asthma. Air-cleaning devices can help reduce the amount of airborne particles and make breathing a little easier. They can also reduce the irritation from secondhand smoke, though experts say the devices will not minimize the more serious health risks of smoke, such as lung cancer. The following guidelines can help you select the right air-cleaning device for your home.

Device	What they do	Advantages	Disadvantages
Electrostatic precipitators	An electric field charges particles, which are trapped on metal plates.	Produce a steady flow of air and are energy-efficient.	The plate must be washed every one or two months. Improper maintenance can produce ozone, an eye and lung irritant.
Charged-media devices	Operate like electrostatic precipitators except that they trap particles with a replaceable filter.	Effective and energy-efficient if new filters are installed regularly.	The efficiency of these devices decreases with use. Filters need to be changed every two to three months.
Ion generators	Produce negatively charged gas molecules that cling to particles, weighing them down and causing them to drop from the air.	Energy-efficient and inexpensive to maintain.	Some models deposit dust on household surfaces, and some cannot trap large particles. They can also produce ozone.
HEPA filters	High-efficiency particulate air (HEPA) filters are mechanical filters that remove nearly all dust, pollen, and other airborne particles.	HEPA filters are available in several styles and in a wide price range.	Less energy-efficient than other filtration devices. The filters need to be replaced as often as every three months.

Source: *Indoor Air Quality Product & Service Guide*, Cutter Information Corporation.

One study was conducted in Kishinev, Moldova (a country between Ukraine and Romania), where pesticide use was 20 times the world average from the 1960's through the 1980's. Researchers found that Moldovan children had suffered abnormally high rates of acute respiratory diseases, skin diseases, ear infections, tuberculosis, and tooth decay. Adults had also suffered from high rates of infectious diseases.

Lead and behavior. Researchers at the University of Pittsburgh School of Medicine reported in February 1996 that exposure to lead in the environment can lead to antisocial behavior and delinquency.

The study evaluated 301 boys, aged 7 to 11, from Pittsburgh's inner city. The scientists estimated the boys' lifetime exposure to lead with a technique called X-ray fluorescence, which measures lead accumulated in bone. Boys whose bones contained above-normal amounts of lead were evaluated by teachers, parents, and themselves as being more aggressive and more prone to delinquent behavior. Such behaviors included bullying, vandalism, starting fires, theft, and fighting and were independent of social and economic factors.

Fine pollutants in the air. Fine airborne particles may cause as many as 64,000 heart- and lung-related deaths a year in the United States, the Natural Resources Defense Council (NRDC) reported in May 1996. The NRDC, an environmental organization in Washington, D.C., based that estimate on previous studies of the health effects of air pollution.

Environmental Protection Agency standards regulate the emission of particles as small as 10 microns in diameter, about a tenth the diameter of a human hair. But the NRDC claimed that particles as small as 2.5 microns cause the greatest health problems. The NRDC said that tougher standards controlling the emission of fine particles from vehicles and smokestacks could save as many as 56,000 lives per year.

Arsenic and cancer. A 1996 study in Argentina confirmed highly controversial findings in Taiwan indicating that high levels of arsenic in the water supply are associated with bladder cancer. Critics of the Taiwan study had speculated that the increased risk of cancer could be attributed to other causes—genetic susceptibility to the disease, malnutrition, or other pollutants in the water.

The results of the new study were of interest to American health officials because bladder cancer is among the nine most common forms of cancer in the United States, and several areas have water supplies containing high levels of naturally occurring arsenic.

The Argentina study was conducted by researchers from the University of California at Berkeley. They studied residents of Cordoba, a province in central Argentina, where the water contains high concentrations of arsenic but few other pollutants, the population is not known to be highly susceptible to the cancer, and there is a low incidence of malnutrition. The bladder cancer rate in Cordoba, however, is double the national average in Argentina—strong evidence that arsenic plays a major role in producing the disease.

Cooking gas and asthma. Epidemiologists from St. Thomas's Hospital in London reported in February 1996 that women who use gas stoves for cooking are at least twice as likely as those who use electric stoves to develop wheezing, shortness of breath, and other symptoms of asthma.

In a study of 659 women and 500 men, only the women showed the effects of gas appliances, presumably because they spent more time than men in the kitchen. Smokers were no more likely to develop the symptoms than nonsmokers. But when symptoms did occur, they were more severe among the smokers.

The researchers estimated that switching to electric appliances could cut the asthmatic symptoms among women by as much as 48 percent.

• Thomas H. Maugh II

In WORLD BOOK, see ENVIRONMENTAL POLLUTION.

Exercise and Fitness

- Reducing hypertension with aerobic exercise
- Exercise and heart attack risk
- Rating exercise machines
- Exercise to prevent weight gain

Regular aerobic exercise reduces severe *hypertension* (high blood pressure) and *left ventricular hypertrophy* (increased muscle thickness in the lower-left chamber of the heart). That finding was reported in November 1995 by researchers from the Veterans Affairs Medical Center and Georgetown University Medical Center, both in Washington, D.C.

The risk of heart attack and stroke is particularly high among African American men, who have a higher rate of severe hypertension than men in other racial groups. The researchers recruited 46 African American men ages 35 to 76 with severe hypertension and randomly divided them into two groups. One group received drug therapy and performed exercise training, while the other group received drug therapy alone. Men in the exercise group participated in moderately intense exercise—stationary cycling on exercise bicycles—at 60 to 80 percent of their maximum heart rate. They exercised three times per week for either 16 weeks or 32 weeks.

The researchers found that among the men who participated in the exercise training program, *diastolic* (when the heart relaxes after a contraction) blood pressure decreased after 16 weeks of training, whereas it slightly increased in those who did not exercise. Diastolic blood pressure remained lower after 32 weeks of exercise. The researchers also noted that the need for antihypertensive medication was reduced among the men who exercised. Thickness of the left-side heart muscle was also reduced. The findings suggested that efforts to control severe hypertension among African American men should include both medication and regular exercise of moderate intensity.

Exercise and heart attack risk. Participation in physical activities reduces the risk of a nonfatal heart attack among postmenopausal women, according to a study reported in November 1995 by researchers at the University of Washington in Seattle.

The researchers studied 268 women who had suffered a heart attack between 1986 and 1991 and 925 women who had not had a heart attack. All the women in the study belonged to a large health maintenance organization (HMO). Participation in physical activity was assessed from a telephone interview. The women were asked if they had participated in 26 leisure-time activities in the previous month, including walking for exercise, running, biking, aerobics, dancing, or mowing the lawn.

The researchers took into account other factors that might be related to both the level of physical activity and the risk of a heart attack, including prior heart disease, diabetes, smoking, body weight, blood pressure, family history, alcohol consumption, and education. Higher levels of energy expended in leisure-time physical activities were associated with a reduced risk of nonfatal heart attacks. Similar associations were observed for energy expended in nonstrenuous physical activity such as walking. The study found that modest leisure-time energy expenditure, equivalent to 30 to 45 minutes of walking three times a week, reduced the risk of a nonfatal heart attack by 50 percent.

Rating exercise machines. The treadmill is the best indoor exercise machine for maximizing energy expenditure in order to control weight, according to a study reported in May 1996 by researchers at the Medical College of Wisconsin and the Veterans Affairs Medical Center in Milwaukee. The study compared the energy and aerobic demands of six popular exercise machines.

The researchers studied eight men and five women who were in good health. Over a four-week period, the subjects were trained to use six indoor exercise machines—a cross-country skiing machine, an exercise bicycle, a rowing machine, a stair stepper, a treadmill, and an Airdyne, an exercise bicycle that combines arm motions with pedaling. The researchers then measured the amount of energy the men and women expended when using the machines.

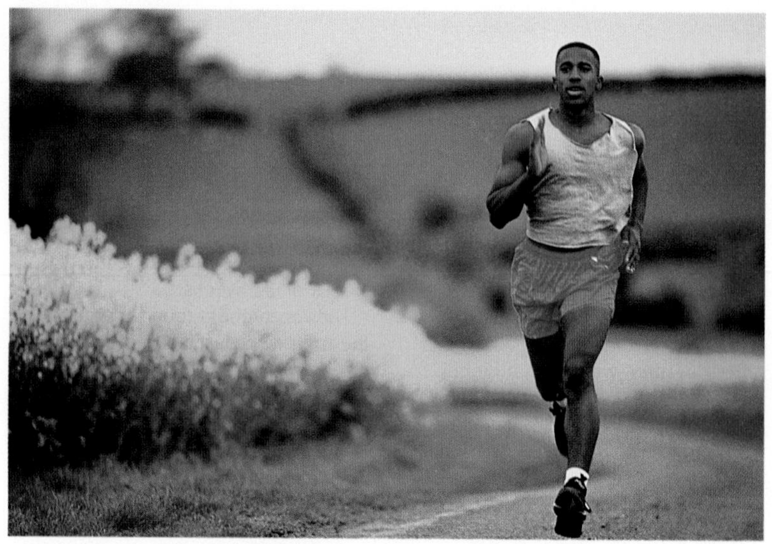

Help for hypertension

Regular aerobic exercise can reduce severe *hypertension* (high blood pressure), according to a November 1995 report. A study of African American men with severe hypertension found that those who exercised three times a week at 60 to 80 percent of their maximum heart rate had lower blood pressure after 16 weeks than those who did not exercise. The men who exercised also needed less medication to treat their hypertension.

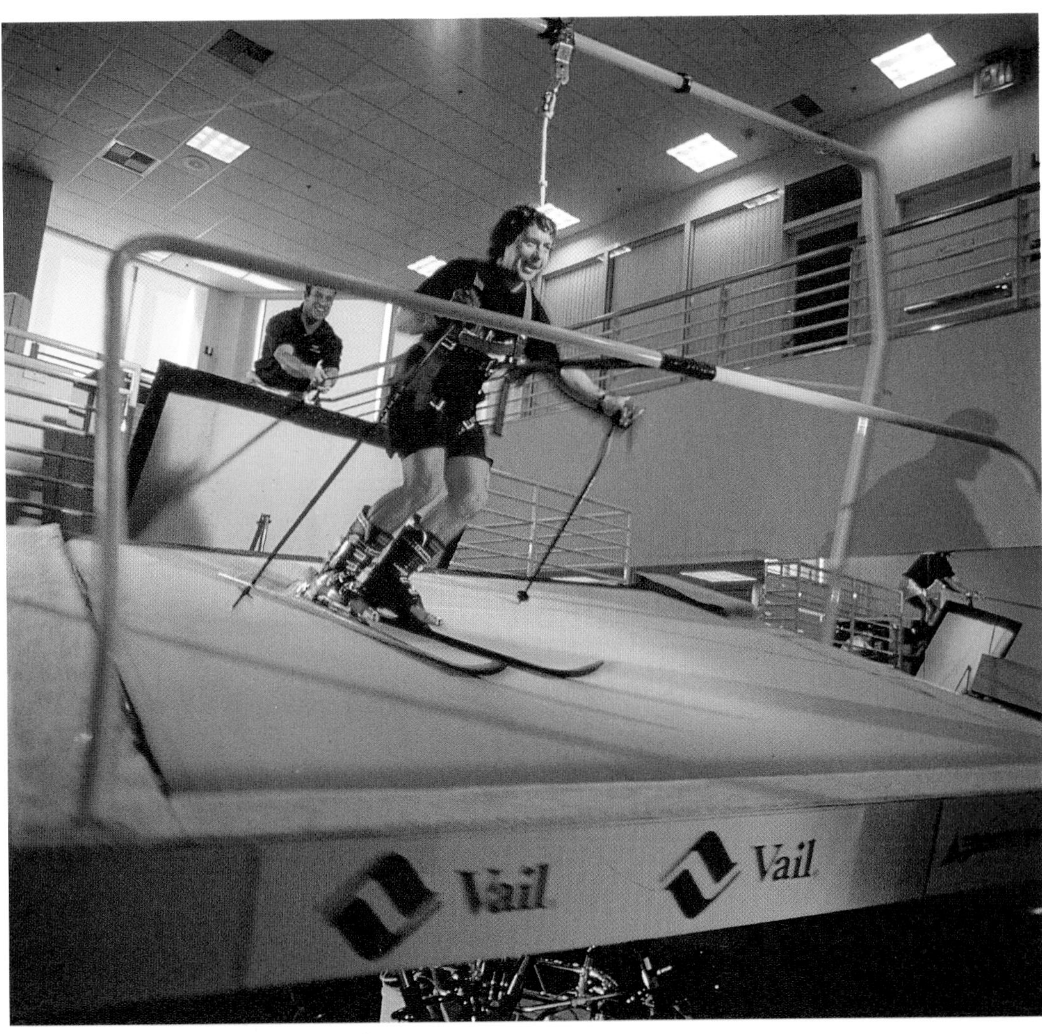

Subjects exercised on each machine for 15 minutes—5 minutes at each of three levels of exertion (fairly light, somewhat hard, and hard).

Walking on the treadmill was associated with the highest expenditure of energy. The cross-country skiing simulator, rowing machine, and stair stepper required less expenditure of energy than the treadmill, and the Airdyne machine and exercise bicycle required the least. Subjects' heart rates also varied depending on which machine they were using. The treadmill and stair stepper produced the greatest elevations of heart rate.

Exercise to prevent weight gain. Since maintaining a steady weight involves a balance between food intake and energy expenditure, it has long been recognized that exercise plays a role in weight control. A study reported in January 1996 by researchers at the Harvard University School of Public Health in Boston suggested that physical activity plays a more important role in preventing weight gain than in promoting weight loss.

The investigators studied nearly 18,000 nonobese male health professionals ranging in age from 41 to 78 who were free of cardiovascular disease, cancer, and other major illnesses. Each man completed a questionnaire in 1988 detailing how many hours he spent each week participating in various activities, including hiking, running, bicycling, swimming, tennis, heavy outdoor work, and

Virtual exercise

If you want to go skiing but there's no mountain nearby, try a skiing simulator. Health clubs in 1996 were increasingly offering exercise machines that simulate the movements, challenges, and sensations of various sports and outdoor activities. Machines have been developed to simulate swimming, windsurfing, kayaking, and in-line skating.

Exercises for back pain

If you're experiencing back pain, two simple exercises may help. You may try lying on your back and pulling your knees up to your chest, *right, top.* Another exercise is to lie on your stomach and prop yourself up on your elbows, *right, bottom.* Holding your body in these positions for five minutes every hour may help relieve the pain. People suffering from back pain should talk to their doctors to find out more information and to learn if these techniques are right for them.

Source: *American Family Physician.*

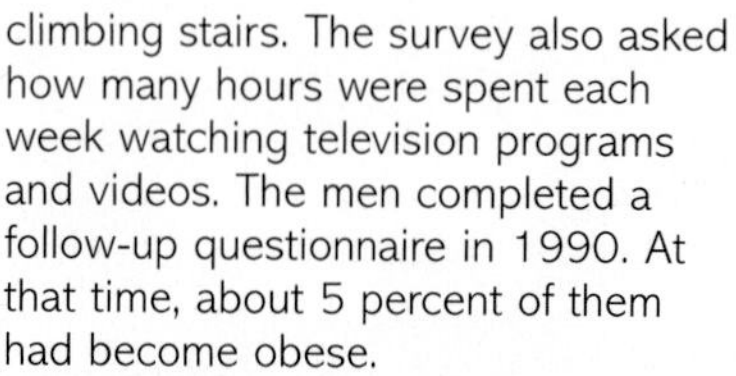

climbing stairs. The survey also asked how many hours were spent each week watching television programs and videos. The men completed a follow-up questionnaire in 1990. At that time, about 5 percent of them had become obese.

The researchers took into account factors that might influence activity levels and weight, such as age and cigarette smoking. They found that high levels of physical activity and less time spent in front of the television were associated independently with a reduced risk of becoming overweight over the two-year period. Engaging in light to moderately intense activities, such as brisk walking, jogging, and swimming, for at least 30 minutes daily, was associated with a 20 percent reduction in the risk of becoming overweight.

Given the increasing prevalence of obesity among middle-aged men in the United States and the health consequences of obesity, including high blood pressure, diabetes, and cardiovascular disease, the researchers recommended that people increase their level of physical activity and reduce the time they spend in sedentary pursuits.

• David S. Siscovick

In the section On the Medical Frontier, see NEW WEAPONS IN THE WAR AGAINST WEIGHT. In WORLD BOOK, see PHYSICAL FITNESS.

Eye and Vision

- The retina's 24-hour clock
- Medicare proposals for cataracts
- Antibiotics after cataract surgery
- Conquering river blindness
- Lasers for glaucoma
- Eye drug implant approved

The eye has its own biological clock unrelated to how the brain regulates such daily rhythms as the cycle of sleeping and wakefulness, researchers reported in April 1996. Neurobiologists Gianluca Tosini and Michael Menaker at the University of Virginia in Charlottesville reached that conclusion after studying the *retinas* of hamsters.

The retina makes up the innermost layer of the back wall of the eyeball. Light-sensitive cells in the retina absorb light rays and change them into electrical signals that are transmitted to the brain, which interprets them as images. The researchers reported that their study showed that the retina apparently regulates a 24-hour cycle in the eye of all mammals, including human beings. The researchers found that hamster retinas produce melatonin, a hormone made in the brain that is responsible for sleep and wakefulness.

The scientists removed the retinas of hamsters and kept them in laboratory dishes for several days. The retinas produced melatonin in quantities that over a 24-hour cycle peaked at night and decreased during the day.

Scientists believe that melatonin produced by the retina regulates the renewal of light-sensitive structures in the eye called rods and cones. Around dawn, melatonin renews the tips of the rods, which detect shades of gray and are needed for night vi-

Don't wear contact lenses overnight

No contact lens, including disposable soft lenses, should be worn overnight, according to ophthalmologist H. Dwight Cavanagh of the University of Texas Southwestern Medical Center at Dallas. Recent studies show that people who wear extended-wear lenses overnight have a 10 to 15 times greater risk of cornea infections than daily wear users. Wearing lenses while asleep prevents adequate amounts of oxygen from reaching the surface of the cornea. Such low-oxygen conditions are perfect for bacteria to thrive, and a bacterial infection of the eye carries the risk of permanent damage to vision. In 1996, clinical trials were underway on new lenses that allow the transmission of much higher levels of oxygen than any on the market.

sion. At about sundown, the retina renews the tips of the cones, which are used for color vision.

The discovery may further the understanding of eye diseases such as *retinitis pigmentosa,* in which the rods degenerate. Such disorders may be caused by faulty retinal clocks that do not produce melatonin at the proper times. Other researchers said the finding raises questions about the possible risk to eyes of taking melatonin supplements.

Medicare proposals for cataracts. The Health Care Financing Administration (HCFA) in October 1995 proposed new rules to limit Medicare coverage for surgery to remove *cataracts* (the clouding of the lens of the eye). Under the proposal, Medicare would pay only when eye surgeons could show that removal of a cataract was the only appropriate treatment. The HCFA is an agency of the United States Department of Health and Human Services that funds Medicare, the federal health insurance program for Americans 65 years or older or who are disabled.

Cataracts occur in 50 percent of people age 65 to 75 and 70 percent of those over age 75. Removal of a cataract and implantation of an artificial lens can improve vision and the ability to live independently.

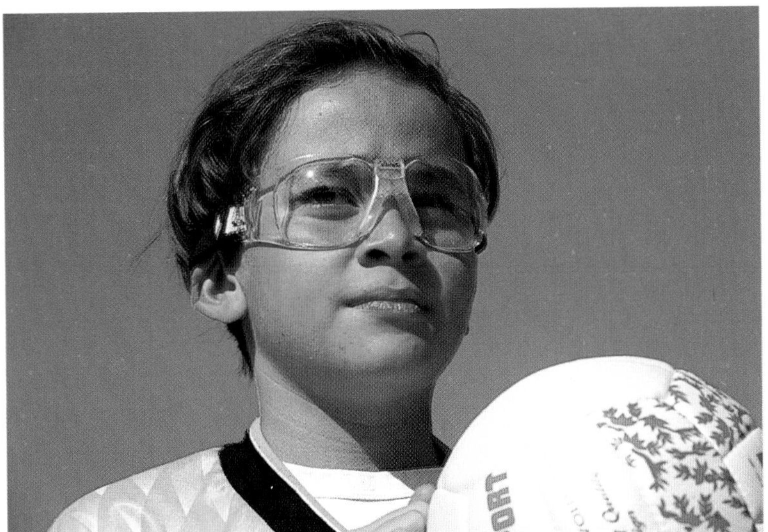

Preventing eye injuries when playing sports

Youngsters who wear goggles to play soccer greatly reduce their risk for injuring their eyes during a game. Eye experts say that more than 100,000 sports-related eye injuries occur in the United States every year, but as many as 90 percent of them could be prevented with goggles or other protective devices.

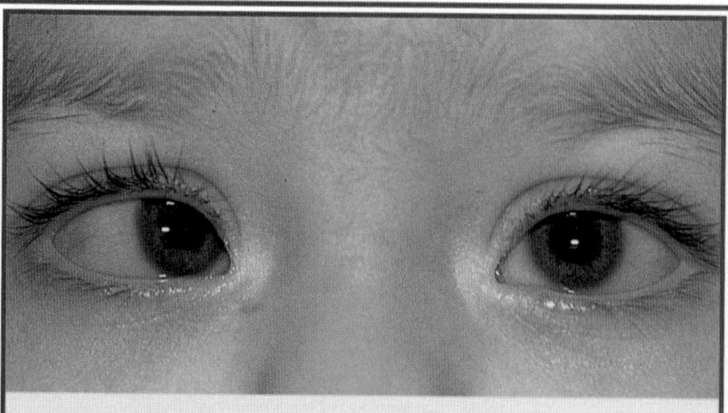

New way to treat "lazy eye"

Short-term treatment with a drug called levodopa in combination with patching improves the vision of older children with amblyopia, commonly called lazy eye because muscles of the eye are unable to control movement. That finding was reported at the annual meeting of the Research to Prevent Blindness (RPB) organization held in Orlando, Florida, in October 1995. According to ophthalmologist Lawrence E. Leguire of Ohio State University in Columbus, when amblyopia is diagnosed by about age 5, the traditional treatment of patching the good eye to force the child to use the lazy eye usually restores vision and the ability of the two eyes to work together. But a child diagnosed with amblyopia at age 8 or 9 is considered beyond the critical period for that treatment to succeed. Leguire and his colleagues studied 76 amblyopic children with an average age of 9. He found that daily doses of levodopa for seven weeks resulted in a 37 percent improvement in vision that was still evident six weeks after treatment ended. Children receiving levodopa and wearing a patch part of the day experienced greater improvement than those who just took levodopa.

If the rules are implemented, the HCFA would not pay for surgery if an individual could function normally or if vision could be corrected with eyeglasses. The action followed a 1993 government study indicating that Medicare spent $204 million in 1991 on unnecessary cataract surgery.

Antibiotics after cataract surgery. About 5,400 of the 1.35 million Americans who undergo cataract and lens-implant surgery annually develop a bacterial eye infection called endophthalmitis. The National Eye Institute (NEI) in September 1995 issued a clinical alert to more than 15,500 ophthalmologists warning that such patients need antibiotics injected directly into the eye rather than the traditional treatment of injections into a vein. The NEI is an agency of the National Institutes of Health in Bethesda, Maryland.

The NEI warning was based on the results of a study of 420 patients at 27 medical centers that compared the two drug delivery modes. Patients treated with direct injection were less likely to have complications or need a second surgical procedure known as a *vitrectomy,* in which the clear, jelly-like material that fills the eyeball behind the lens is removed.

Conquering river blindness. The World Health Organization (WHO) and other groups in December 1995 announced the start of a program intended to totally eliminate river blindness (onchocerciasis) in Africa within 12 years. WHO is an agency of the United Nations based in Geneva, Switzerland. River blindness infects about 17.6 million people in Africa. The disease is caused by a parasitic worm that is spread by tiny black flies, which breed in swiftly moving river water. The parasite's larvae bore through the skin, causing intense itching and disfiguring sores. Blindness occurs when the larvae reach and damage the eyes.

The new $124-million effort is based on a WHO program that since 1974 has virtually eliminated river blindness in 11 countries in West Africa. The program includes intensive spraying to control black flies and treatment with the drug invermectin, which kills newly hatched larvae in the body. Treatment costs only 70 cents per person per year.

Lasers for glaucoma. Laser therapy is as effective as eye drops in treating newly diagnosed patients with glaucoma. Also, patients treated with lasers experienced gradual improvement in vision. These were the findings, reported in December 1995, of a seven-year study conducted at U.S. medical centers nationwide.

The most common form of glaucoma, open-angle glaucoma, affects an estimated 3 million Americans. The disease occurs when the *aqueous humor* (the fluid that nourishes the cornea and the lens of the eye) does not drain properly. Accumulated fluid increases pressure inside the eye. If not treated, glaucoma can damage the optic nerve and cause blindness.

Treatment with daily eye drops reduces pressure in the eye. Laser therapy burns scores of tiny holes in tissue at the front of the eye to improve drainage. But uncertainty about the safety and effectiveness of laser therapy led physicians to reserve its use for patients who could not be treated with drugs.

Eye drug implant approved. The U.S. Food and Drug Administration (FDA) in March 1996 approved the Vitrasert Implant, the first device to provide a continuous dose of a drug to the eye. Vitrasert is used to treat a virus-caused form of *retinitis* (inflammation of the retina) in AIDS patients.

The implant, a small capsule, is inserted into the eye in a brief outpatient operation. The capsule releases the drug ganciclovir over an 8-month period. Ganciclovir combats cytomegalovirus, a microorganism that infects 15 to 40 percent of AIDS patients. The infection can spread throughout the eye, causing blindness. • Michael Woods

In the section Medical and Safety Alerts, see GLAUCOMA WATCH. In the section On the Medical Frontier, see LASER SURGERY COMES INTO FOCUS. In WORLD BOOK, see EYE.

Genetic Medicine

- Genetic link to skin cancer
- Genes and aging
- Genetic susceptibility to diabetes

In June 1996, researchers identified a gene linked to basal cell carcinoma, a skin cancer that is the most common form of cancer in humans. The finding was reported by two separate international teams of geneticists—one headed by Allen Bale of Yale University, the other by Matthew Scott of Stanford University.

Basal cell carcinoma, which affects approximately 750,000 people a year in the United States, is most likely to develop in people who are middle-aged or older and who have pale skin, which is especially sensitive to the damaging effects of the sun's ultraviolet rays. The cancerous growths appear most often on the face. Although this cancer can be treated with radiation or surgery, the identification of the suspect gene may lead to less drastic forms of treatment.

All cancers, which are characterized by uncontrolled cell division, are essentially genetic disorders. Normally, certain genes, called tumor-suppressor genes, regulate the division of cells, a necessary process that produces new cells in the body. Tumor-suppressor genes act as brakes on the development of cancer. If these genes are *mutated* (changed), however, the brakes are released and tumors may develop.

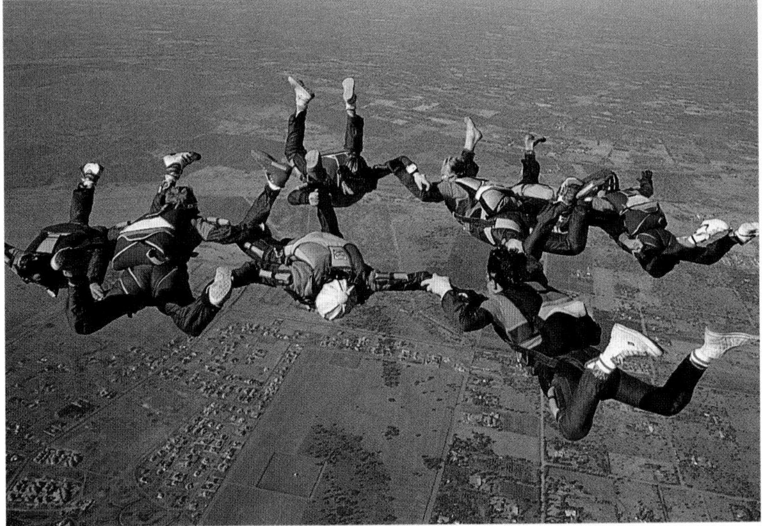

Genes for jumping

A gene may make some people more inclined to seek thrills, researchers in Jerusalem and at the National Institutes of Health in Bethesda, Maryland, reported in January 1996. The researchers found a variation of a gene that instructs brain cells to make larger receptors for dopamine, a chemical that transmits messages in the brain and is linked to novelty seeking. The study added to a controversial debate among specialists about the validity of associating genes with complex human behaviors.

The gene identified by the Yale and Stanford teams, called *patched,* probably acts as a tumor-suppressor gene. Both research groups came to that conclusion about *patched* and its role in basal cell carcinoma in a roundabout manner. Although neither group had set out to learn the causes of basal cell carcinoma, their research added to a growing body of evidence that genes linked to cancer are also involved in regulating the normal cell cycle and in the growth and development of the human body.

In 1989, researchers first identified *patched* in the fruit fly, long the workhorse of genetic research. In 1994, the Stanford team detected the same gene in mice and later in humans. When they noted that the mutations of *patched* in fruit flies led to developmental problems, they suspected that flaws in the human version of *patched* may cause similar problems. Their search for the gene's location led them to the region of a *chromosome* known to be the location of the gene linked to a developmental disorder called basal cell nevus syndrome or Gorlin's syndrome. (Chromosomes are tiny structures in the cell nucleus that carry the genes.)

Gorlin's syndrome, which occurs in about 1 in 100,000 people, is an inherited disorder. Those who have this syndrome have developmental abnormalities such as fused ribs and facial deformities, and they are highly susceptible to basal cell carcinoma. The Stanford researchers found mutated *patched* genes in the blood cells of patients with Gorlin's disease.

The Yale team started from the opposite direction; they set out to find the gene that causes Gorlin's syndrome. They found a gene resembling the fruit fly *patched* gene and noted similarities between the developmental problems associated with Gorlin's and developmental problems in fruit flies with a mutated *patched* gene.

Both teams identified mutated *patched* in the cells of people with the syndrome and in the basal cell carcinoma cells from people who had the cancer but not the syndrome. The researchers concluded that people who have Gorlin's syndrome inherit a mutated copy of *patched,* while people who develop the cancer alone inherit two normal copies of the gene. Years of exposure to the sun, however, damage one copy of the gene in a skin cell, giving rise to cancer. Because the cancerous skin cells are easy to reach, the scientists said, it might be possible to treat them effectively with drugs that reverse the effects of the mutated *patched.*

Genes and aging. An American-Japanese collaboration led in April 1996 to the discovery of a gene associated with Werner syndrome (WS), a rare disorder that accelerates the aging process. The teams of ge-

Gene test for embryos

A test developed in London in 1989 and available at several U.S. institutions in 1996 enables human embryos produced by laboratory fertilization of egg cells to be screened for a variety of genetic disorders. The test is used for couples who carry a known disease gene and want to be sure they are not passing it on. A delicate instrument is used to remove two cells from an embryo for testing, *right.* If the embryo is found to carry the defect, it is not implanted in the woman's womb.

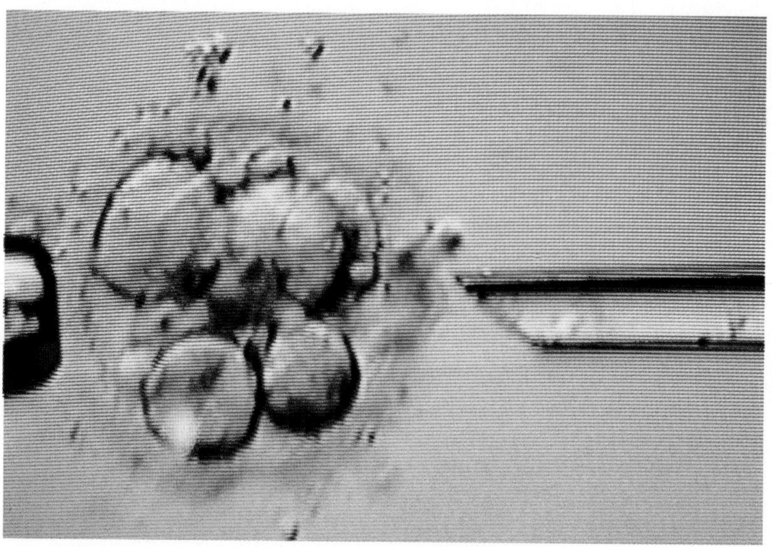

neticists led by Gerard Schellenberg of Seattle's Veterans Affairs Puget Sound Health System and Tetsuro Miki of Osaka University Medical School announced the breakthrough.

Individuals with WS often have gray hair and wrinkled skin in their 20's and develop disorders such as cataracts, cancer, and heart disease, problems usually associated with people more than twice that age. Most affected persons die before age 50. WS is a *recessive* disorder. That is, it occurs only when a person inherits two copies of the abnormal gene, one from each parent. Fewer than 200 cases of the syndrome had been reported worldwide as of 1996. Biologists believed, however, that the study of this rare phenomenon might contribute to a better understanding of the normal aging process.

After pooling tissue samples from families afflicted with WS, Schellenberg's and Miki's teams began the search in a particular region of chromosome 8, the location that a team at Tokyo Metropolitan Otsuka Hospital had identified in 1992 as the most likely place to find the suspect gene. They found the gene after studying over 650,000 *bases* of DNA (deoxyribonucleic acid, the molecule genes are made of).

Bases are four of the chemical subunits of DNA. Pairs of these bases create rung-like structures on a strand of DNA, which looks like a twisted ladder. Every gene has its own particular sequence of these bases, and each sequence provides a blue-print for one of the many proteins produced in the cell. If the sequence of bases in a gene is altered by a mutation, the gene produces a different—and most likely faulty—protein.

Schellenberg theorized that the WS gene provides the blueprint for the production of a protein known as a helicase, which helps unwind DNA from its *helical* (twisted) structure. DNA must be unwound to expose its bases to other proteins that carry out various biological processes. Any disruption of helicase could interfere with other important cellular functions, including the normal process of aging. Because WS is often accompanied by cancer, biologists speculated that the WS gene, like the gene associated with basal cell carcinoma, might interfere with genetically controlled processes that regulate cell division.

The discoveries of the WS gene and the gene involved in basal cell carcinoma furthered scientists' understanding of the role of genes in normal growth and development. Schellenberg's team noted that its work "provides evidence that at least some components of 'normal' aging and disease susceptibility in late life may be related to aberrations in DNA metabolism." The group cautioned, however, that the WS gene is just one small piece in the very complicated puzzle of the aging process.

Genetic susceptibility to diabetes. The search for genes associated with non-insulin-dependent diabetes mellitus (NIDDM) was narrowed in June 1996 to a stretch of genetic material on chromosome 2. A team of geneticists led by Graeme Bell at the University of Chicago reported the discovery.

NIDDM, also called Type II, is a form of diabetes affecting 10 to 20 percent of the population older than 45 and a major cause of illness and death in developed countries. As of 1996, it ranked as the fourth-leading cause of death in the United States and was responsible for an estimated $85.7 billion in annual medical costs.

Diabetes is a complex set of disorders associated with faulty processing of glucose, a simple sugar that is the primary source of energy for the body's cells. The disorders are related to the function of insulin, a hormone produced by the pancreas. The pancreas releases insulin when blood-sugar levels are high, usually after a meal. Insulin helps to move glucose from the blood into cells, and when the level of glucose in the blood drops, the pancreas stops releasing insulin.

The juvenile form of diabetes (onset before age 20) results from an insufficiency of insulin, and daily insulin injections are required to control it. In NIDDM, however, there is usually enough insulin in the blood, but for unknown reasons it does not do its job correctly. Most cases of NIDDM can be controlled by careful regulation of the diet. If uncontrolled, however, NIDDM can cause serious problems and premature death.

Although the causes of NIDDM are unclear, scientists have long suspected a genetic contribution. The disorder clusters in families, and when one identical twin has the disease, the other often has it also.

NIDDM is especially common among certain Native American populations and among people who share Native American ancestry, including Mexican Americans. Bell's team studied 408 Mexican Americans living in Starr County, Texas, where the death rate from NIDDM is unusually high.

Bell's group used a study method that focused on pairs of *siblings* (brothers and sisters) with NIDDM. After studying the DNA of 330 affected pairs of siblings, the scientists identified a *genetic marker* (a DNA sequence that is frequently present in people with the disorder) on chromosome 2 that suggested a genetic link to the disease. They did not isolate the disease-causing gene itself, but they significantly narrowed the search for it. The researchers stated that the next step would be to investigate this region of chromosome 2 to identify the gene or genes involved in NIDDM. Analysis of those genes might provide some clues to the underlying genetic basis of NIDDM.

• Joseph D. McInerney

In WORLD BOOK, see CANCER; CELL; GENETICS.

Glands and Hormones

- Growth hormone for the heart
- Treating goiter without surgery
- Testosterone skin patch

Growth hormone (GH) has been used for many years to promote growth in children whose bodies produce too little of the hormone on their own. Now, with the availability of *recombinant* (genetically engineered) GH, the spectrum of applications for GH therapy is widening. In March 1996, researchers at the University Federico II in Naples, Italy, reported on the use of recombinant GH to treat a type of heart disease called dilated cardiomyopathy.

Dilated cardiomyopathy is a disorder in which the left *ventricle* (lower chamber of the heart) becomes enlarged. This creates an additional load on the heart, which must then pump a larger volume of blood with each beat. Usually, the walls of the ventricle grow thicker to compensate for the increased workload. However, this growth does not occur in some people, and the heart then begins to fail. A heart transplant has been the only long-term solution for this condition.

In an earlier study, researchers had reported that a hormonelike substance called IGF-I appeared to be responsible for stimulating the growth of heart muscle and improving heart function in an experimental model. GH promotes growth in part by triggering the production of IGF-I by the body. The Italian doctors decided that growth hormone therapy could be effective in treating dilated cardiomyopathy in human beings.

The researchers studied seven people with dilated cardiomyopathy and impaired heart function. The patients received injections of GH every other day for three months. After the test period, the researchers found that the walls of the patients' left ventricles had significantly increased in thickness. The subjects' hearts grew stronger and the individuals became increasingly able to perform vigorous exercise. Three months after the treatment ended, however, the patients showed some reversal of those improvements.

The investigators concluded that although their results seemed promising, the study was only preliminary. Larger, more formalized trials conducted for longer periods of time were necessary, they said.

Treating goiter without surgery. Treatment with radioactive iodine has for many years been an accepted form of treatment for people with *hyperthyroidism* (excessive activity of the thyroid gland). People with hyperthyroidism typically also develop an enlarged thyroid gland, a condition known as a *goiter.* But many people who develop a goiter do not necessarily become hyperthyroid. In January 1996, researchers in Denmark reported on their analysis of data compiled from other studies that evaluated the effectiveness of I-131, a radioactive form of iodine, in treating people who had an enlarged thyroid gland but were not hyperthyroid.

The thyroid gland is located in the neck near the larynx and upper windpipe. It secretes thyroxine, a substance that helps regulate the body's metabolism and growth. In some cases, an enlarged thyroid gland can cause compression of a person's windpipe or esophagus, creating breathing or swallowing difficulties. Severe compression is usually treated by *thyroidectomy* (surgical removal of the thyroid gland), but surgery may not be an acceptable option for some patients. In recent years, medical researchers have administered I-131 to reduce the size of an enlarged thyroid gland in place of traditional surgery.

The Danish researchers examined data from eight studies that were conducted at various institutions between 1964 and 1995 comprising 1,219 patients. Reduction in goiter size was determined with several imaging techniques. The extent of reduction varied among the institutions from 39 to 99 percent. Some studies reported that thyroid volume was reduced by 40 percent after one year of I-131 therapy and 55 percent after two years. Patients who had suffered from compression of the esophagus or windpipe reported that they experienced substantial relief from their symptoms after treatment.

The study concluded that treatment with I-131 is an acceptable therapy for an enlarged thyroid gland that is not associated with hyperthyroidism. As such, the researchers stated, it can be used more widely in those patients who want to avoid the potential complications of anesthesia and surgery or who have medical conditions that prevent them from tolerating surgery.

Testosterone skin patch. Androderm, a skin patch representing a new treatment option for men whose bodies produce abnormally low levels of testosterone, received approval from the Food and Drug Administration in October 1995. Estimates are that between 4 million and 5 million men in the United States are testosterone deficient—a condition known as *hypogonadism.*

Testosterone is a naturally occurring hormone that triggers the development of male physical characteristics, such as a deep voice, increased muscle strength, and facial hair, beginning at puberty. Low levels of testosterone in men can be responsible for conditions that include sexual dysfunction, fatigue, and even osteoporosis and muscle atrophy.

Although the new treatment was considered safe, a number of doctors expressed concern over prescribing the patch for men who have had prostate cancer or those at high risk for cancer of the testicles. In addition, most subjects who used the patch in clinical trials reported some degree of skin irritation. • Andre J. Van Herle

In the section A Healthy Family, see Hormone Replacement Therapy. In World Book, see Gland; Hormone.

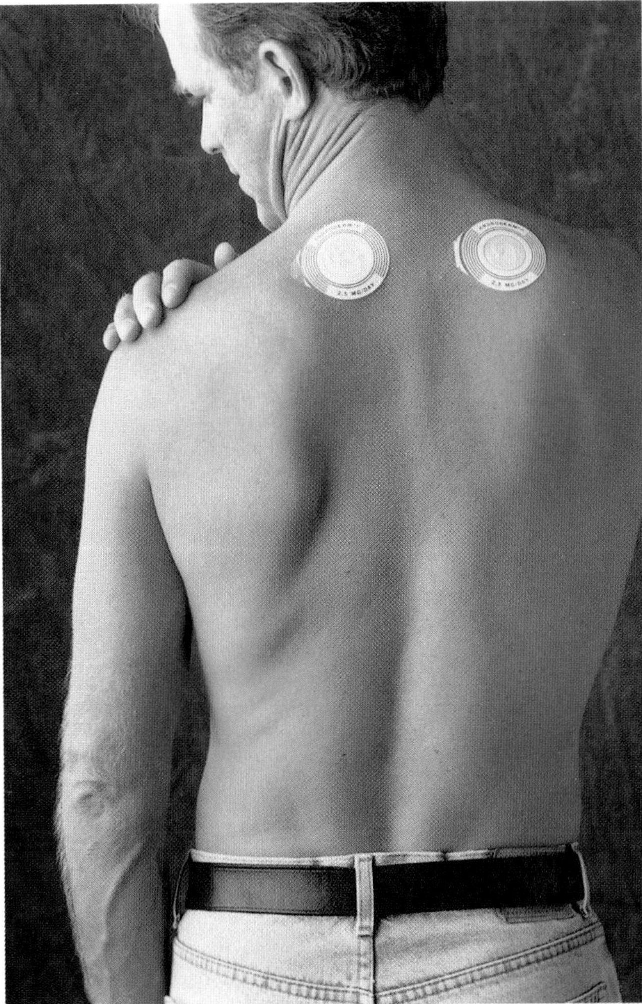

New testosterone patch

Androderm, a skin patch that releases the male hormone testosterone, was approved for use in October 1995 by the U.S. Food and Drug Administration. It was designed to be used by men whose bodies produce very low levels of the hormone. The body absorbs testosterone from the patch at a rate similar to the rate of normal testosterone production. Androderm was the first testosterone patch that could be worn on areas of the body other than the genitals.

Health Care Issues

- Medicare and medical savings accounts
- Medicaid debate continues
- Health insurance reform
- Managed-care backlash
- State health-care legislation
- Number of uninsured grows

The United States Congress in 1996 continued to struggle with the issue of controlling costs in the enormously popular Medicare program for the elderly. In September 1995, Republican leaders of the House of Representatives had unveiled a plan to rein in Medicare costs. The plan included broader use of *managed care* (enrollment in organized health plans), repeal of a reduction in the premiums paid by senior citizens, and a controversial concept called medical savings accounts (MSA's). The Republican Senate proposal, released later the same month, was similar but included more limited use of MSA's.

An MSA is a special type of savings account into which an individual can put nontaxable money to be used for the payment of routine health-care services. The individual then buys a health insurance policy that can be used for expenses over a set fee—for example, $10,000. If the MSA funds are not used for health care in a given year, they can be used later for non-health-care purposes.

Republican leaders argued that MSA's would increase consumer choice and cost consciousness. Democrats, especially President Bill Clinton, opposed them on the grounds that healthy, upper-income people would opt out of the current Medicare system and use MSA's instead. As a result, only the sickest and poorest people would be left in traditional Medicare. The program's costs would then escalate because healthy people's premiums, which would have helped defray the cost of sicker people's care, would no longer be available. Clinton said he would veto any health-care bill that included MSA's.

Meanwhile, on June 5, 1996, Medicare trustees reported that the part of the Medicare fund that covers hospital expenses would be $28.9 billion in debt by 2001 if no effective reforms were enacted.

Medicaid debate continues. Republicans in 1995 and 1996 supported a block-grant approach to Medicaid, in which federal funds would be provided in lump sums to the states. The states would then administer the program, which pays for health care for low-income people, with wide latitude in terms of coverage, services, and criteria for eligibility. Democrats opposed the plan, claiming that millions of people would be unfairly removed from Medicaid rolls.

On Feb. 6, 1996, the National Governors' Association (NGA) proposed a Medicaid plan that guaranteed access to care for pregnant women, children, the low-income elderly, and anyone the states deem disabled. Spending was to be controlled, and states were to have broad flexibility in deciding what benefits they would

Women are spending less time in the hospital after giving birth, and some health insurance plans provide coverage for only 24 hours of maternity stay. Growing opposition to this trend led the U.S. Senate in April 1996 to approve a bill requiring health plans to cover hospital stays of at least 48 hours. President Bill Clinton urged Congress to pass the bill, but it was still pending in August. Over half the states had already enacted laws requiring plans to pay for 48 hours of maternity stay.

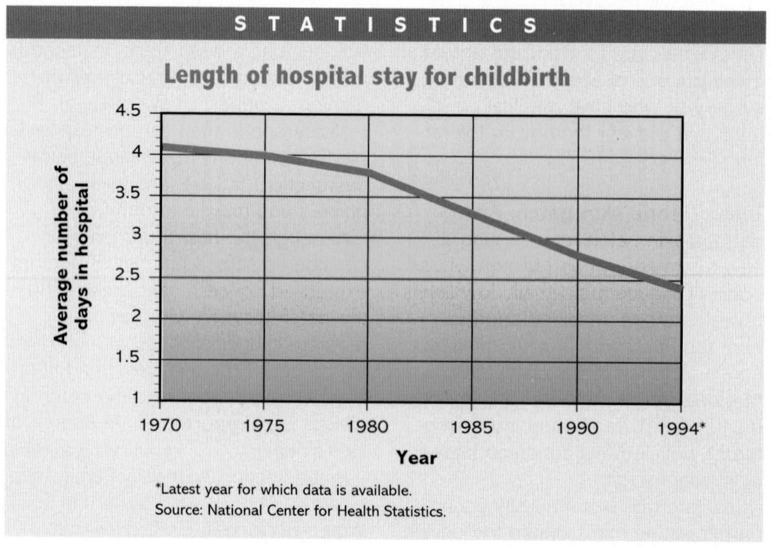

*Latest year for which data is available.
Source: National Center for Health Statistics.

provide. The plan, however, excluded coverage of children over the age of 12 and included little guidance on how the states could define disability.

Both Republicans and Democrats were cautiously supportive of the NGA plan, though the Republicans preferred block grants and the Democrats wanted more federal oversight. The plan was discussed a great deal but was not adopted as legislation.

On May 22, 1996, Republicans in the House and Senate introduced legislation to repeal the existing Medicaid law, tie Medicaid funding to welfare reform, provide states with block grants, and reduce overall program spending by $72 billion. Although the plan's supporters claimed that it was in keeping with the NGA proposal, opposition by Democratic governors made passage unlikely. House Minority Leader Richard Gephardt (D., Mo.) said that the plan would be vetoed by the president. An amended version of a similar but less radical bill passed the Senate on June 26, 1996; its fate was also uncertain.

Health insurance reform. A version of the health insurance reform bill first introduced in 1995 by Senators Edward Kennedy (D., Mass.) and Nancy Kassebaum (R., Kans.) was approved in 1996, after much negotiation. *Portability*—being able to retain eligibility for insurance when changing jobs or insurers—was the centerpiece of the Kennedy-Kassebaum bill.

The bill also required employers who offer insurance to provide coverage to all employees regardless of their health status and required insurers to offer coverage to any member of an employee group of two or more. In addition, the bill prevented insurers from requiring a person with a known health condition to undergo more than one waiting period before becoming eligible for coverage.

The Kennedy-Kassebaum bill was popular at first, but partisan forces soon altered it. Some Republicans sought to add provisions for the purchase of MSA's to the Senate bill. That proposal was defeated, but MSA's were added to the House bill.

An amendment cosponsored by Senators Pete Domenici (R., N.M.) and Paul Wellstone (D., Minn.) required insurers to provide *parity* (equal coverage) for mental health services, putting them on the same basis as other types of health care. Although this provision was already in place in some states, it was controversial because of the potentially high costs involved and because the benefits of many mental health services are difficult to measure.

On March 28, 1996, the House passed its version of the Kennedy-Kassebaum bill, including MSA's and other provisions opposed by President Clinton. On April 23, the Senate unanimously passed the bill, including the mental health parity amendment.

Reconciliation of the two sides was problematic. Although House Speaker Newt Gingrich (R., Ga.) had said that

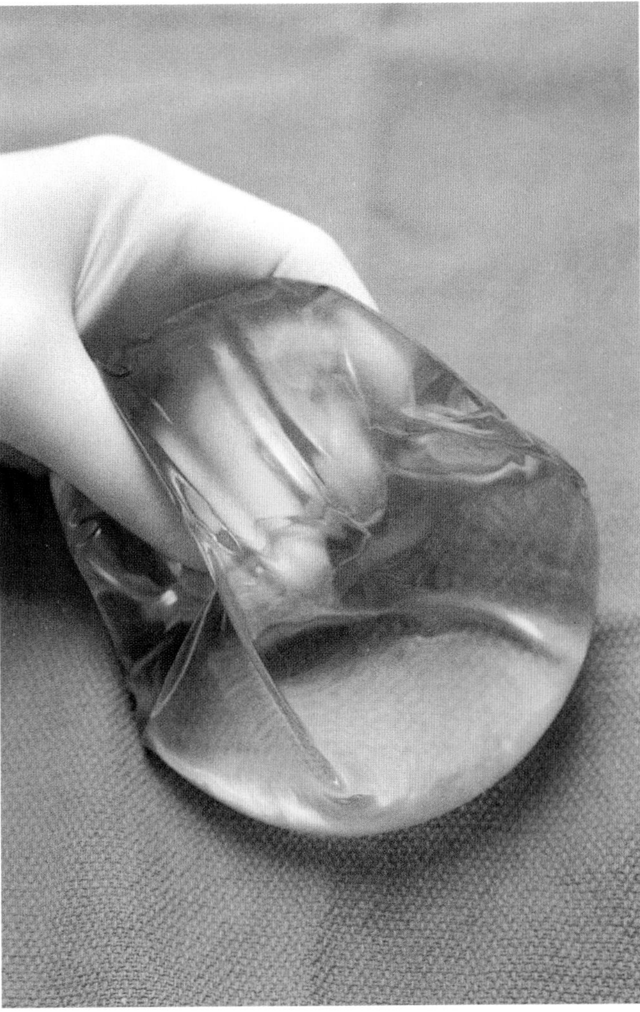

Breast implant debate
Women with silicone breast implants have a slightly increased risk of developing immune-system illnesses, according to a February 1996 report by researchers at Harvard Medical School in Boston. The researchers evaluated the health of over 10,000 female medical professionals with implants. Although implant manufacturers put a positive spin on the study, noting that it did not suggest a major risk, many physicians remained convinced that silicone breast implants can cause illness.

he would not allow the MSA provision to prevent passage of an insurance bill, he seemed determined to retain it. Senate Majority Leader Robert Dole (R., Kans.) (who resigned from the Senate in June 1996 to run for president) also supported MSA's.

On June 27, 1996, Republicans offered a compromise that called for allowing the introduction of MSA's, with limited participation, over four years as a demonstration. The House and Senate met on July 26 and worked out a bill that allowed some self-employed people and small groups to experiment with MSA's. The bill did not include a mental health parity provision and did not help people without health insurance. The House approved the bill on August 1, and the Senate passed it the next day. President Clinton signed the measure into law on August 21.

Managed-care backlash. Growth in managed care continued at a quick pace in 1995 and 1996. According to InterStudy, a research group in Minnesota, most enrollees belonged to for-profit plans. Profit, along with limitations on what physicians participating in these plans can tell patients, fed a growing backlash against managed care.

With many plans being bought and sold, corporate profits hit record levels. The California Medical Association reported in February 1996 that many for-profit health plans spent less than 80 percent of their revenue on patient care.

Also in February 1996, a much-quoted study by consultant Graef S. Crystal found that the heads of many for-profit HMO's had annual incomes over $2 million. In June 1996, the media revealed that Leonard Abramson, the president of for-profit U.S. Healthcare, would receive almost $1-billion in compensation as a result of the sale of his plan to Aetna Life & Casualty. Criticism of these large sums was keen—HMO's were accused of skimping on care and denying access to services in order to maximize profits. Opponents of managed-care excesses ranged from liberals to conservatives and from consumer groups to the American Medical Association, which historically has opposed most managed-care arrangements.

The media also reported HMO "horror stories": patients denied useful treatment, new mothers forced to leave the hospital too soon after giving birth, and plans refusing to pay for promising experimental treatments. In addition, many physicians were forced to sign agreements known as gag clauses. In some cases, a gag clause simply prohibited physicians from saying negative things about the plan or disclosing confidential information. In others, physicians were forbidden to discuss their financial incentives or alternative treatments with patients. Critics declared this last form of agreement to be unethical and a threat to the patient-physician relationship.

U.S. Representatives Greg Ganske (R., Iowa), who is a surgeon, and Edward Markey (D., Mass.) in February 1996 introduced the Patient Right to Know Act, which would ban health-plan agreements that forbid physicians to discuss treatment options or health-plan rules with patients. The bill quickly drew 100 cosponsors in a rare show of bipartisanship.

Hearings on the bill were held on May 30, 1996, and a House subcommittee approved a compromise version in late June. This bill did not include penalties on health plans that restrict or prohibit communications between health-care providers and their patients—a provision that was included in the original bill. Further hearings were held in July.

In the face of the growing firestorm, the American Association of Health Plans, the lobby to which most managed-care plans belong, issued a statement in May 1996. The association pledged support of the right of patients to have access to affordable, comprehensive care, a choice of provider within their health plans, and information about health plans and how they work. But a massive drop in the stock prices of several HMO's in July left observers wondering what the plans would do to recover.

State health-care legislation. Many states were pressured by medical societies in 1995 and 1996 to pass legislation that would broaden both

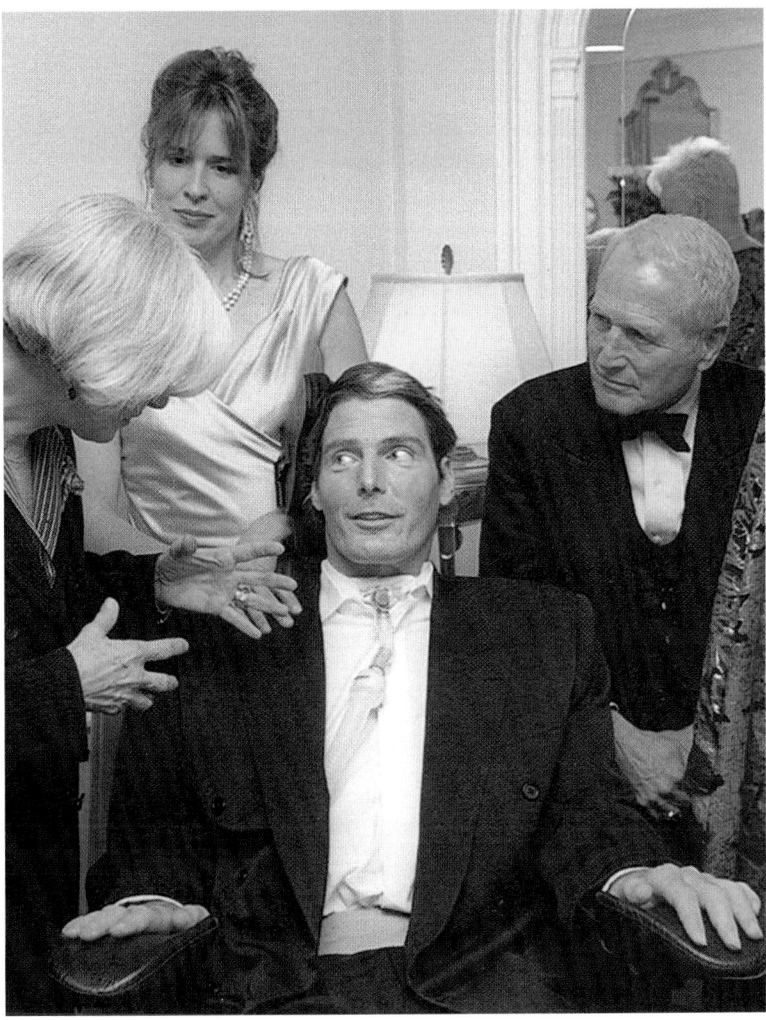

Celebrity spokesman
Actor Christopher Reeve, paralyzed as a result of a horseback-riding accident in May 1995, meets with fellow actors Joanne Woodward and Paul Newman before speaking at a benefit in New York City for the American Paralysis Association. Reeve's wife, Dana, stands behind him. The event, held in November 1995, raised funds for the association's research program.

patients' and physicians' rights in dealing with health plans. These proposals were usually known as patient protection acts.

According to the American Association of Health Plans, as of April 1996, 24 states required plans to contract with any health-care provider willing to abide by the plan's rules; 10 required plans to allow members to receive care from nonplan providers, with some or all of the cost paid by the plan; 14 required allowing patients direct access to specialist physicians without gaining permission from their primary-care physician first; 6 addressed plan responsibility to pay for emergency services for members; and 4 had passed patient protection acts of some type. Most states also required HMO's and other health plans to provide some kind of appeals process for enrollees to handle grievances. Initiatives and referenda concerning health plans were expected to appear on some state election ballots in November 1996.

Nonetheless, most health plans continued to be subject not to insurance law, but rather to less stringent corporate law, thus allowing the potential for lax regulation. Health-policy analysts expected that enthusiasm for managed care would grow among employers and others who provide health insurance—especially in light of the many estimates of significant cost savings over traditional insurance. But the fight over health-plan practices showed no sign of abating.

Number of uninsured grows. The core problem that led to calls for health-care reform in the first place—the number of Americans lacking health insurance—grew more severe in 1995 and 1996. In June 1996, the Census Bureau reported that 66.6 million people—about 27 percent of the population of the United States—had no health insurance coverage for at least one month of a 28-month period beginning in 1992.

Those most likely to be uninsured were young adults aged 18 to 24 and members of minority groups. Among Latin Americans, 49 percent lacked coverage for at least a month during the study period; among African Americans, 36 percent. The rate for whites was 23 percent.

Using Census Bureau data, the Employee Benefit Research Institute reported in April 1996 that 61.2 million Americans under the age of 65 were uninsured in March 1995—the highest figure ever reported.

Although some questioned the figures, it seemed obvious that shrinking private coverage, more employees being forced to pay for coverage that was once largely subsidized by employers, and limits on Medicaid eligibility were making it difficult for many Americans to receive adequate health insurance coverage. • **Emily Friedman**

See also Medical Ethics.

Heart and Blood Vessels

- Cholesterol and heart disease
- Fiber and heart disease
- Cholesterol drugs
- No risk seen from coffee
- Hormone therapy for cholesterol
- Earlobe creases

The health consequences of high cholesterol levels in the bloodstream continued to receive a large amount of attention in 1995 and 1996. Too much cholesterol can contribute to the build-up of fatty deposits in the coronary arteries—the arteries that supply the heart with blood. High cholesterol can result from inherited genetic characteristics or from a diet that includes excessive amounts of fat and cholesterol. Despite the efforts of health professionals to educate people about these risks, however, coronary heart disease remained the most common cause of heart-related deaths in the United States and other industrialized countries.

Research in the 1980's showed that a significant number of Americans had too much fat and cholesterol in their diet. In response, the federal government initiated an extensive public-health effort aimed at lowering cholesterol. A major part of this effort was the creation of the National Cholesterol Education Program (NCEP), a coalition of 38 health organizations coordinated by the National Heart, Lung and Blood Institute.

The NCEP published an extensive report detailing guidelines intended to control cholesterol. Some of the NCEP's recommendations, however, became a point of controversy among medical experts. For example, the NCEP recommended that people age 20 and older get regular blood cholesterol tests. The study also advised that these tests should measure not only total cholesterol, but HDL levels as well.

Cholesterol travels in the bloodstream attached to protein molecules called *lipoproteins.* Most cholesterol is carried by low-density lipoproteins (LDL's), but some is carried by high-density lipoproteins (HDL's). LDL's are known as "bad" cholesterol because they deposit cholesterol in cells, which can promote the development of fatty deposits in the arteries. HDL's, on the other hand, are called "good" cholesterol because they carry cholesterol to the liver, where it is broken down. Studies have shown that higher levels of HDL's are associated with reduced heart disease risk.

The American College of Physicians published a statement in March 1996 arguing that measuring only total cholesterol was sufficient to monitor heart disease risk, and that cholesterol screening was necessary only in middle-aged adults. This strategy, they said, would target the group whose risk is highest and for whom the chances for benefit are greatest. On the other hand, several organizations, the American Heart Association in particular, supported the NCEP recommendation. These experts argued that testing only middle-aged adults would deny people in other age groups the opportunity to gain the health benefits of maintaining low blood cholesterol.

Researchers at Montreal General

Hospital in Canada published a study in September 1995 evaluating the accuracy of cholesterol screening guidelines to estimate the risk of heart disease. The scientists studied 3,600 participants of a cholesterol study begun in the 1970's. They had followed the subjects for an average of 12 years to see how accurately they could predict whether coronary artery disease would develop.

The researchers evaluated the subjects using both cholesterol screening guidelines and other known risk factors for coronary artery disease, such as high blood pressure, diabetes, and smoking. The risk factor analysis correctly identified 70 percent of the individuals who developed coronary artery disease. By contrast, the accuracy rate of the NCEP guidelines was only 45 percent. The researchers concluded that future cholesterol screening guidelines should incorporate HDL cholesterol levels as well as other risk factors for coronary artery disease.

Fiber and heart disease. Eating more fiber to reduce cholesterol became a popular trend in the 1980's. But when studies showed that fiber alone did not significantly affect high blood cholesterol, its popularity faded. However, a study published in February 1996 by physicians and scientists at the Harvard School of Public Health in Boston brought fiber back into the headlines. The results of this study indicated that fiber in the diet helps reduce the risk of coronary artery disease.

In 1986, the researchers distributed a questionnaire to over 43,000 American male health professionals, asking about their dietary intake of fiber and foods known to be high in fiber. The researchers estimated each man's fruit, vegetable, and fiber intake from the questionnaire and compared it to the risk of developing coronary artery disease over a subsequent six-year follow-up. After controlling for other risk factors, the study showed that a high-fiber diet cut the risk of heart disease by 20 percent.

The three main food groups that contributed to this reduced risk were vegetables, fruit, and cereals. Cereal fiber was the most strongly associated with a reduced risk of coronary artery disease. The researchers concluded that their findings supported current dietary guidelines recommending that people increase their consumption of foods high in fiber.

Cholesterol drugs. Investigators in Scotland in November 1995 reported positive results of a study of the drug pavastatin, which is used to lower cholesterol. Pavastatin is a *reductase inhibitor,* a drug that lowers blood cholesterol levels by inhibiting the action of a substance in the liver which is necessary for the synthesis of

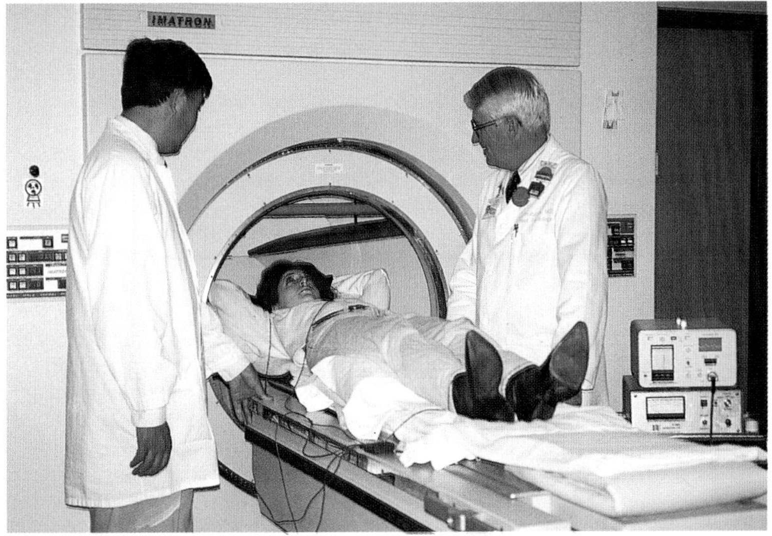

Ultrafast heart scans

New *CT* (computerized tomography) machines could help in the early detection of heart disease. They are able to take an X-ray image of a beating heart in just 0.1 second—so fast that the resulting image is not blurred from the movement of the heart. This means that doctors will be able to spot clues that indicate the build-up of fatty deposits in coronary arteries much sooner than with other diagnostic techniques, before the build-up has become severe.

cholesterol from dietary fat. These drugs reduce the level of LDL cholesterol, slow the progression of heart disease, and cut death rates in men with known coronary artery disease.

The Scottish study included more than 6,000 men aged 45 to 64 who had moderately high cholesterol levels but no family history of coronary artery disease. The men were randomly assigned to receive pavastatin or a *placebo* (inactive substance) and were followed for an average of five years. The data showed that pavastatin lowered LDL cholesterol by an average of 26 percent. In addition, the pavastatin group had a 30 percent lower incidence of heart disease than the placebo group and a 22 percent reduction in the risk of death from any cause. The investigators concluded that treatment with a reductase-inhibiting drug can significantly reduce the risk of heart attack or death from heart disease in men with moderately high blood cholesterol and no known heart disease.

Pavastatin is a costly method of treating high cholesterol, however, especially when viewed over the lifetime of an individual. The cost of a year's supply of the drug in 1996 was as much as $1,000.

No risk seen from coffee. Investigations of the possible role of coffee consumption in coronary artery disease continued in 1996. Earlier studies of this issue tended to show a slight increase in the risk of coronary artery disease in those with heaviest coffee consumption, but most of these studies were done only on men and were not controlled for other risk factors. In February 1996, physicians and scientists at the Harvard School of Public Health published the results of a comprehensive study of women coffee drinkers.

The study comprised more than 85,000 nurses aged 34 to 59, who were followed for 10 years. After adjusting for other risk factors for coronary artery disease, researchers found no association between drinking coffee and the risk of developing coronary artery disease. Nor did they find any heart risk associated with other sources of caffeine or from the consumption of decaffeinated coffee. The researchers also noted that previous studies had indicated that a person's sex makes no difference in terms of coffee consumption and heart disease risk.

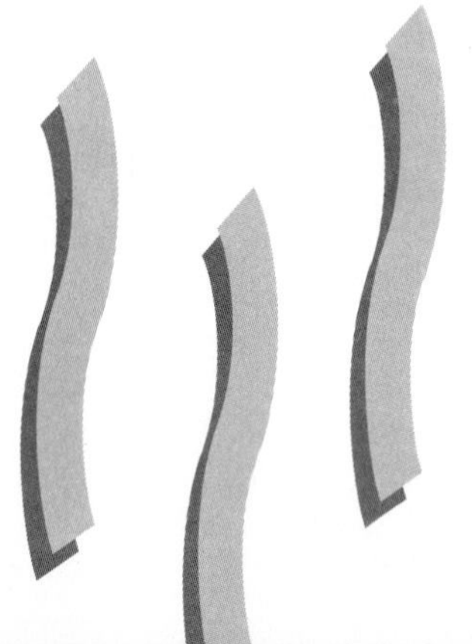

Coffee and heart disease

A study published in 1996 in the *Journal of the American Medical Association* found no link between coffee consumption and coronary heart disease among 85,000 American women. But that may not be the end of the story, because the study did show a link between drinking coffee and smoking. Of the women in the study, those who drank more coffee also were more likely to smoke—58 percent of women who drank six or more cups per day smoked; only 19 percent of those who drank less than a cup a month were smokers. Previous studies have conclusively linked smoking with heart disease.

Hormone therapy for cholesterol. Another important women's health issue in 1995 and 1996 was the continuing controversy over whether women should take female hormones after menopause. Researchers at several U.S. institutions published a study in January 1996 indicating that estrogen replacement has a positive effect on cholesterol levels in women.

In the study, 875 postmenopausal women taking four different hormone-

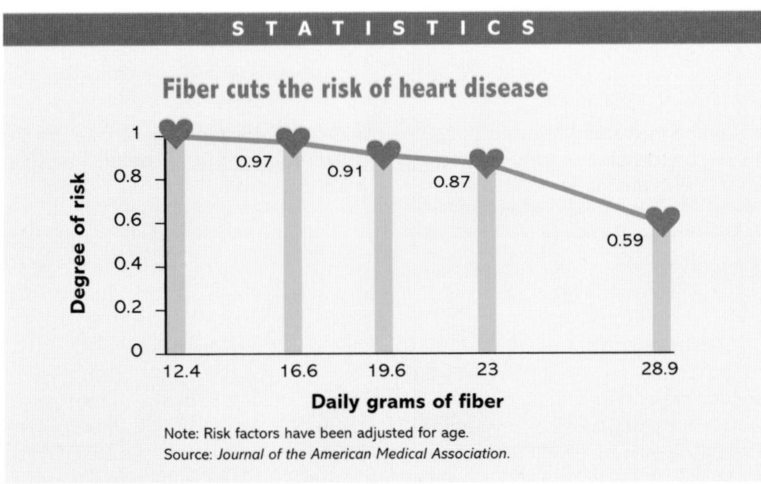

In a 1996 study, researchers in Boston reported a link between more fiber in the diet and a reduced risk of heart attack. Among men who consumed about 30 grams of fiber a day (about one cup of high-fiber bran cereal, for example) there were 41 percent fewer heart attacks. Men in the lowest-fiber group ate only about 12 grams of fiber per day. The researchers assigned this group the highest level of risk, represented by 1.

replacement treatments were followed for three years. The researchers found that estrogen replacement caused an increase in the levels of HDL cholesterol and also lowered the level of both LDL cholesterol and fibrinogen, a compound which contributes to the formation of blood clots. Other potential risk factors, such as blood pressure and blood-sugar levels, were not significantly affected by the hormones.

Although these results were encouraging and suggested that postmenopausal hormone-replacement therapy may reduce the risk of heart disease in older women, more study was needed. The length of the study was too short to determine whether the rate of heart disease among the women would also be reduced.

There was also continuing concern in 1996 that hormone-replacement therapy may increase the risk of certain types of cancer in women. However, many doctors said that postmenopausal women who were at risk for developing coronary artery disease (on the basis of family history, blood cholesterol levels, and other risk factors) might be well-advised to consider hormone-replacement therapy, because their chances of developing heart disease may be significantly greater than their cancer risk.

Earlobe creases are a reliable indication of whether an individual is likely to experience a heart attack or other heart problem, such as a blocked coronary artery. This finding was reported in February 1996 by researchers at Rush-Presbyterian-St. Luke's Medical Center in Chicago.

The physicians evaluated 264 patients who were admitted to the hospital in 1982 with suspected heart problems. At that time, the doctors noted whether or not the patients had a visible crease on one or both earlobes. The patients were followed for 10 years after being discharged from the hospital. After controlling for other factors that could contribute to heart problems, the researchers found that people who had a crease on one earlobe had a 33 percent greater incidence of heart problems than those with no ear creases; people with creases on both earlobes had a 77 percent higher incidence of such problems.

The researchers concluded that earlobe creases, which are caused by the hardening of small blood vessels in the lobes, are a more important predictor of heart disease than such traditional risk factors as smoking and a family history of heart disease. Furthermore, unlike traditional risk factors, earlobe creases do not rely on skilled observation or sophisticated testing to detect them. Health experts urged people with an earlobe crease to work hard to reduce the coronary risk factors within their control, such as by lowering their blood cholesterol levels, exercising more, and losing weight. • Michael H. Crawford

In World Book, see Heart.

Infectious Diseases

- Infectious diseases on the rebound
- Tuberculosis upsurge
- Mad cow disease
- Bacterial vaginosis
- Tick-borne microbe

The death rate from infectious diseases in the United States increased by 58 percent from 1980 to 1992, according to a study released in 1996 by the Centers for Disease Control and Prevention (CDC) in Atlanta, Georgia. Much of the increase resulted from the appearance of acquired immune deficiency syndrome (AIDS) in the 1980's and from the growth in the number of Americans aged 65 and over, who are susceptible to complications from pneumonia and influenza. But the CDC expressed most concern about the emergence of new antibiotic-resistant strains of bacteria.

Other reports also warned of a new health threat from infectious diseases, once thought to have been conquered by antibiotics and vaccines. The World Health Organization (WHO), an agency of the United Nations, reported in May 1996 that infectious diseases kill more than 17 million people throughout the world each year. Pneumonia, diarrheal diseases, and tuberculosis, which alone account for over 10 million deaths, all have strains that are resistant to common antibiotics. WHO also said that at least 30 new infectious diseases have emerged in the last 20 years and now threaten hundreds of millions of people.

A 1996 study at Ohio State University found that the bacterium *Streptococcus pneumoniae* became increasingly resistant to penicillin and other common antibiotics from 1991 to 1994. The bacterium causes about 500,000 cases of pneumonia each year in the United States. Researchers said the increased resistance resulted in part from the overuse of antibiotics. Some bacteria develop resistance after repeated exposure to an antibiotic, and these bacteria thrive as their competition dies off.

Tuberculosis upsurge. In March 1996, WHO reported that about 3 million people died from tuberculosis (TB) in 1995, more than in any previous year. During the worst stages of the last TB epidemic, which occurred around 1900, an estimated 2.1 million people died worldwide each year.

WHO warned that TB would take an even greater toll unless immediate action was taken. TB experts at WHO urged governments to adopt a strategy called directly observed treatment, short-course (DOTS). This strategy places responsibility for ensuring adequate treatment on health care workers, rather than on patients. The workers watch patients swallow their medication to be sure they take it.

Monitoring patients in this way ensures that they take the full course of the antibiotic, thus reducing the chances that some bacteria survive and multiply. WHO said DOTS could

Mad cow disease

Mad cow disease, which swept through the British cattle industry beginning in the mid-1980's, was linked with a rare and fatal human brain disorder by a report released by the British government in March 1996. The infection in cattle had been traced to feed supplements containing remains of sheep infected with a related disease. The March report concluded that people might have contracted the brain disorder, Creutzfeldt-Jakob disease (CJD), by eating beef from infected cattle. By July, 15 deaths had been attributed to CJD.

cure almost 95 percent of TB patients around the world at a cost of less than $11 per patient.

Mad cow disease. British scientists reported in March 1996 that bovine spongiform encephalopathy (BSE), popularly known as mad cow disease, provided the "most likely explanation" for a new strain of Creutzfeldt-Jakob disease (CJD), a rare and fatal disorder that destroys human brain cells. By July, British officials had attributed 15 deaths to the new strain of CJD.

Symptoms of CJD include memory loss, personality changes, and a decline in coordination and other motor skills. The brain, when dissected after death, appears spongy.

The scientists concluded that people might have contracted the disorder by eating beef from cattle infected with BSE. If so, it would mean that the disease could be transmitted from one species to another. The report caused other countries in Europe to ban imports of British beef.

An epidemic of mad cow disease began among British cattle in 1986. It was traced to the use of protein supplements made from the ground-up remains of sheep infected with a related disease called scrapie. Farmers in Britain had stopped using the supplements, but the disease has an extremely long incubation period—from 10 to 40 years. The long incubation period has made research on the disease difficult.

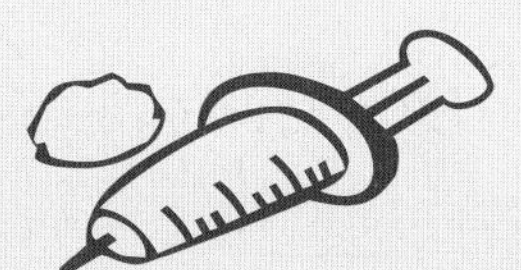

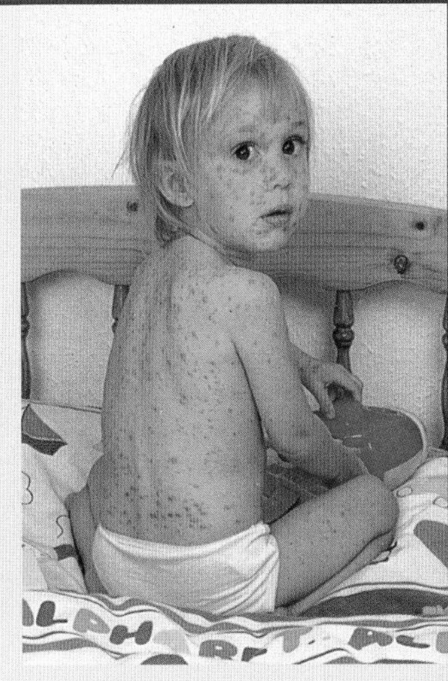

Chickenpox: To vaccinate or not?

In 1995, a vaccine against chickenpox became available and was strongly endorsed by the Centers for Disease Control and Prevention and the American Academy of Pediatrics (AAP). An estimated 4 million Americans, most of them children, get chickenpox each year. Some 5,000 to 10,000 of them are hospitalized, and about 100 die.

For most people, having chickenpox is as common a part of childhood as getting the first haircut. Most cases are mild, and getting the disease almost always guarantees lifetime immunity.

The AAP recommends the vaccine for children from 12 months through 18 years who have never had chickenpox. The vaccine affords protection to adults as well. Some physicians, however, hesitate to recommend the vaccine because of the cost—about $60—and uncertainties about how long it confers immunity. Should immunity wear off after 10 or 15 years, it could leave people vulnerable to the disease as adults, when chickenpox can be far more dangerous. So far, researchers have found that immunity lasts at least 6 to 10 years.

Bacterial vaginosis. A combination of two antibiotics may provide a cure for bacterial vaginosis, an infection believed to contribute to preterm, low-birth-weight deliveries, according to research at the University of Alabama in 1995. Bacterial vaginosis affects as many as 22 percent of pregnant women. But many of them do not know they are infected. The most common symptoms of infection are vaginal irritation and discharge.

Of the 258 women in the study with bacterial vaginosis, those taking a combination of two antibiotics—metronidazole and erythromycin—had a premature delivery rate of 31 percent. This compared with a rate of 49 percent among infected women not receiving the antibiotic treatment.

Another study reported in December found that women with bacterial vaginosis were 40 percent more likely to give birth to premature, low-birth-weight babies. The researchers were not sure how the infection triggers premature birth. But they suspected that the bacteria invade the amniotic fluid, which surrounds and cushions the fetus, or the sacklike membrane that encloses the fetus. The study was led by researchers at the University of Pittsburgh.

Infants with a birth weight of 5 pounds, 8 ounces (2.5 kilograms) or less are 40 times more likely than infants of normal weight to die in the first month of life. They also have a higher risk for mental retardation, blindness, and learning disabilities.

Epidemic in West Africa
An outbreak of bacterial meningitis in West Africa in 1996 claimed more than 10,000 lives. The disease, which spreads easily through sneezing and personal contact, causes inflammation of the lining of the brain and spinal cord. Although a vaccine exists and the disease can be cured with antibiotics, many cases were not treated soon enough. Also, the widespread outbreak depleted medical resources quickly.

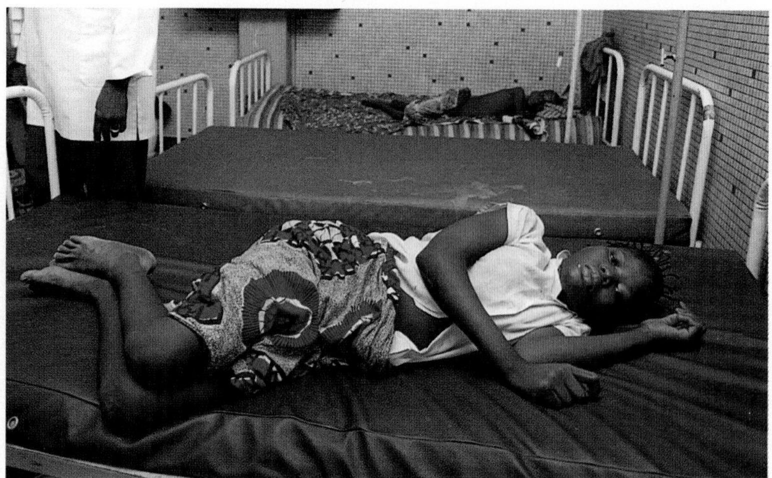

Tick-borne microbe. In January 1996, researchers at the University of Minnesota announced the isolation of the microbe that causes human granulocytic ehrlichiosis (HGE). This newly recognized and sometimes fatal disease is transmitted to human beings by ticks.

Symptoms of HGE include fever, chills, headaches, muscle aches, nausea, and vomiting. Severe cases can lead to kidney or respiratory failure. HGE can be treated with the antibiotics tetracycline and doxycycline.

The disease was first described in 1994 in patients in Minnesota and Wisconsin. It caused wide public concern as additional cases occurred in New York, California, Maryland, and Massachusetts. Experts believe HGE is transmitted by deer ticks, which also transmit Lyme disease. Some believe dog ticks also can transmit HGE. Patients can be infected with two or more tick-borne diseases at the same time, making diagnosis and treatment difficult.

Researchers said that isolation of the HGE bacterium would permit the development of better ways of diagnosing and treating HGE. It would also allow studies that explain exactly how the bacteria cause disease and how they are transmitted to human beings. • Michael Woods

In World Book, see Bacteria; Virus.

Kidney

- Fighting kidney rejection
- Preventing kidney failure
- Clue to a serious kidney disease

Rejection, the process by which the body's immune system attacks a transplanted organ, remained the main obstacle to successful organ transplantation in 1996. Mycophenolate mofetil (MMF), a drug to prevent kidney rejection, gained approval in 1995. It was just the second such drug to be aproved since 1983. However, several new antirejection drugs were under development and were expected to receive approval.

A study seeking new ways to prevent kidney rejection was published in April 1996 by an international team of scientists. In the study, 503 kidney patients were randomly divided into three groups, each of which received standard antirejection therapy with the drugs cyclosporine A and prednisone. One group was also given the antirejection drug azathioprine, while the other two received either 2 or 3 grams of MMF.

The patients treated with MMF experienced about 50 percent fewer rejection episodes. Moreover, those episodes were less severe and required less intensive treatment than those seen in the other group. The effect of the 2-gram dose of MMF was not as dramatic as the 3-gram dose, but patients in the 3-gram group developed more complications. The researchers concluded that MMF still appeared to be a valuable new tool in the prevention of kidney transplant rejection.

Preventing kidney failure. The effectiveness of the drug benazepril in treating various kidney diseases was being studied in 1995 and 1996 by a team of researchers in Italy, France, and Germany. The team published their results in April 1996.

Benazepril belongs to a class of drugs known as *ACE inhibitors*. These drugs block the production of *angiotensin II,* a hormone that produces a variety of effects in the body, including raising blood pressure and promoting cell growth. These effects are known to further harm already damaged kidneys. Researchers conducting studies with animals have also found that ACE inhibitors prevent diseased kidneys from further injury. Others have found that benazepril slowed the onset of kidney failure in people with diabetes.

The new study comprised 583 people with a variety of kidney diseases, each of whom had only 30 to 60 percent of normal kidney function (10 percent function is considered kidney failure). One group received benazepril, and the other received a *placebo* (inactive substance). Each group was monitored for up to three years. In the benazepril group, only 10 percent experienced a worsening of their condition, compared to 20 percent in the placebo group. The protective effect was especially pronounced in people with better kidney function at the outset and in those with higher levels of protein in their urine—a sign that the filtering system of a kidney may be damaged. However, patients with polycystic kidney disease, the most common form of inherited kidney disease, did not appear to benefit from benazepril.

Which drinks can prevent kidney stones?

About 12 percent of people in the United States develop a kidney stone during their lifetime. Kidney stones are a painful condition caused when minerals (mostly calcium) accumulate in the urinary tract, forming a "stone" that becomes too large to pass from the body easily. Drinking plenty of fluids has long been known to help prevent the formation of kidney stones. But a study by researchers at the Harvard School of Public Health in Boston, published in February 1996, indicated that certain beverages can lower the risk of kidney stones more dramatically than others. The study, which surveyed 45,000 men over a 6-year period, found that those who drank at least 8 ounces (236 ml) of water a day cut their risk of kidney stones by 4 percent. The same amount of other beverages yielded even better results. Wine drinkers for example, had a 39-percent lower incidence of kidney stones. However, the news was not all good: The study found that drinking apple or grapefruit juice actually increased the risk of kidney stones by an average of 36 percent.

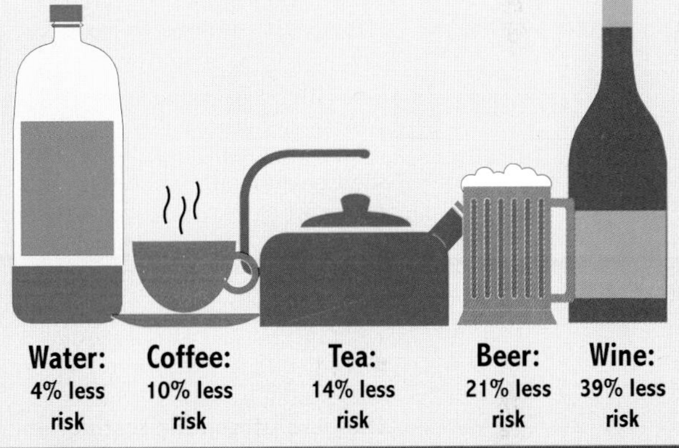

Water: 4% less risk
Coffee: 10% less risk
Tea: 14% less risk
Beer: 21% less risk
Wine: 39% less risk

Clue to a serious kidney disease. Researchers at a number of U.S. medical centers reported in April 1996 that they had found a clue to the cause of *focal segmental glomerulosclerosis* (FSGS). FSGS is a condition that affects the *glomeruli*—collections of tiny capillaries that are part of the filtering system of the kidney. Most patients with FSGS eventually experience kidney failure, and the condition redevelops in a transplanted kidney 40 percent of the time.

The researchers tested blood from healthy people and from people with FSGS or other kidney disorders. They used glomeruli taken from rats to determine that something in the blood was causing the glomeruli to become more permeable to protein—a characteristic of FSGS. They also analyzed the blood of patients with FSGS who had undergone *plasmapheresis*—a technique in which a patient's *plasma* (blood without the red blood cells) is removed and replaced with plasma from a donor. After plasmapheresis, previously positive tests for FSGS became negative, but the plasma that was removed remained positive. Therefore, the researchers concluded that FSGS is strongly linked to an unknown substance circulating in blood.

• Jeffrey R. Thompson

In World Book, see Kidney.

Medical Ethics

- Physician-assisted suicide
- Dangers of genetic testing
- HIV testing of pregnant women
- Infant organ donors

A Michigan jury in May 1996 acquitted retired physician Jack Kevorkian of criminal conduct in helping two women who were chronically but not terminally ill commit suicide in 1991. The acquittal was Kevorkian's fifth in two years. He argued that his intention was to end the suffering of the women, and that meant ending their lives. Kevorkian had assisted in over 30 suicides by mid-1996.

Two important rulings on physician-assisted suicide were issued in 1996. In March, the United States Court of Appeals for the 9th Circuit, in San Francisco, declared unconstitutional a Washington state law prohibiting physician-assisted suicide. The court held that the freedom of a mentally competent, terminally ill person to choose suicide is similar to a woman's right to choose abortion.

In April 1996, the 2nd U.S. Circuit Court of Appeals in New York City ruled that New York state's law banning physician-assisted suicide violated the "equal protection" clause of the Constitution. Under that clause, the court said, people can ask for assistance in suicide as long as the state allows people to hasten death by refusing medical treatment. Both federal court decisions were appealed to the U.S. Supreme Court.

Dangers of genetic testing. The results of a survey on genetic testing were reported in October 1995 at the annual meeting of the American Society of Human Genetics. The survey found that some laboratories offering the testing were bypassing regulatory controls and failing to inform physicians and patients of the experimental nature of many genetic tests.

Genetic testing expanded in 1995 and 1996 as a result of the federally funded Human Genome Project. The project, begun in 1990, is a large-scale effort aimed at mapping the entire human genetic profile—some 100,000 genes. As researchers began to identify genetic *mutations* (defects) linked to various diseases, serious questions emerged. Should people be encouraged to be tested for these genes? If so, what should be done with the information, which suggests susceptibility to various illnesses but cannot predict when—or often, if—they will occur? How can the commercialization of genetic testing be controlled? How can people with genetic flaws be protected from being discriminated against in certain situations, such as when seeking employment or applying for insurance?

An example of the genetic testing dilemma is the test for two newly discovered genes called BRCA1 and BRCA2, which sometimes contain mutations linked with hereditary breast cancer. Heredity accounts for less than 10 percent of all breast

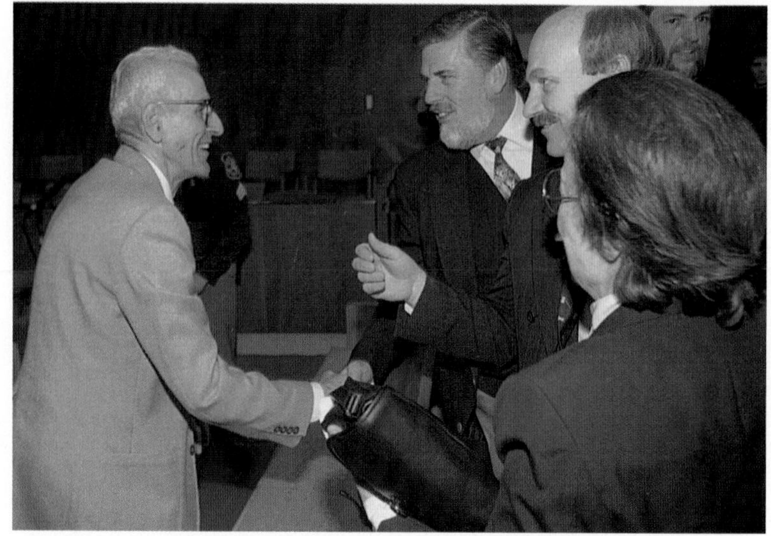

Kevorkian acquitted

Retired physician Jack Kevorkian receives congratulations in May 1996 after a Michigan jury acquitted him of criminal conduct in helping two chronically ill women commit suicide in 1991. Kevorkian's participation in more than 30 suicides has made him the focal point of legal battles and heated debates over the right of an individual to choose suicide and the right of physicians to assist patients in ending their lives.

cancer cases, but women who have a gene mutation and a family history of breast cancer are at increased risk for the disease. However, undergoing testing for the mutated genes offers little benefit. If a woman is found to have one of the flawed genes, there are no treatments that can guarantee to keep her from developing breast cancer. While most specialists urged women to be cautious about genetic testing, a commercial company planned to offer more widespread testing by the end of 1996.

Even when there is a clear benefit to testing and initiating treatment, many people are reluctant to be tested or to have their children tested, in part because they fear discrimination. Several bills introduced in Congress aimed at prohibiting insurance companies from discriminating on the basis of genetic information. But insurers claimed that, as businesses, they had the right to use risk-related information to set premiums and to deny coverage to some individuals.

HIV testing of pregnant women. In May 1996, the U.S. Congress reached a compromise in the debate about screening pregnant women and newborns for HIV, the virus that causes AIDS. Amendments to the Ryan White CARE Act of 1996, which funds much community-based care for people with HIV infection or AIDS, authorized $10 million to assist states in implementing guidelines set up by the Centers for Disease Control and Prevention (CDC) in Atlanta, Georgia. These guidelines encourage voluntary counseling, HIV testing, and treatment with the drug zidovudine (AZT) for pregnant women with HIV to help reduce the risk of HIV transmission to their fetuses.

To continue to receive federal Ryan White funding, states would have to meet one of three provisions: show that nearly all pregnant women in the state are agreeing to be counseled and tested, that new cases of transmission from mother to fetus have been reduced by 50 percent, or that the state has introduced a mandatory screening program for all newborns whose mothers have not had HIV testing. In June 1996, one such program was introduced in New York.

Infant organ donors. In December 1995, the American Medical Association (AMA) changed its opinion on the use of anencephalic newborns as organ donors. Anencephalic infants are born without a brain or with only a partial brain stem. The babies usually die within a few days or weeks.

The AMA's prior position, published in May 1995, was that it was ethically permissible, at the parents' request, to consider anencephalic newborns as organ donors. The AMA reversed that opinion. • Carol Levine

See also HEALTH CARE ISSUES.

Mental Health

- Managed care and mental health
- The ethics of managed care
- Variation in psychiatric treatment
- Early sign of Alzheimer's disease
- Eating disorders in decline

Since the mid-1980's, no aspect of psychiatric care—not biologic insights or new forms of treatment—has undergone greater change than the organization and financing of care. *Health Affairs,* a leading journal of health-care policy, devoted its fall 1995 issue to an evaluation of this transformation. In 1996, approximately 125 million Americans were covered by health plans that managed mental health care.

Managed care is a broad term used to describe an industry that arose to control health-care costs. Prior to managed care, insurance companies paid for medical services on a *fee-for-service* basis. Patients went to doctors when they were ill. Doctors treated them as they saw fit and sent the bill to the patient's insurance company. Typically, the insurer paid the bill without any questions. Because neither the doctor nor the patient had any reason to hold down costs, some analysts contended, this arrangement led to excess care and rising costs.

Managed-care organizations (MCO's), on the other hand, typically use various financial incentives to control costs. For example, most health maintenance organizations (HMO's) are paid a fixed fee for each person whose care they agree to cover, regardless of whether the individual stays healthy or requires large amounts of costly care. To control the costs of care, HMO's pay doctors a fixed salary, thereby removing the income incentives that typify a fee-for-service system. They also limit the use of costly diagnostic tests and referrals to health-care specialists.

Another form of managed care is *utilization review* (UR). Insurance companies hire UR firms to evaluate treatment decisions according to criteria based on the appropriateness and cost of treatment. Although the physician continues to send a bill to the patient's insurer, the doctor must get the UR firm's approval in advance before providing a particular treatment.

The ethics of managed care. The fall 1995 issue of *Health Affairs* featured a debate among leading ethicists and health-policy experts on ethical concerns arising from managed mental health care. The participants included Philip Boyle and Daniel Callahan, ethicists at The Hastings Center in Briarcliff Manor, New York, an organization that studies ethical issues in the sciences, and Mark Schlesinger of the Yale University School of Medicine.

Ethical issues in managed mental health care highlight many of the central issues in managed care throughout medicine. Advocates of managed care argued that it can lead to lower costs, more appropriate treatment, and greater access to care. MCO's hold down costs by limiting the use of services, through either financial incentives or criteria-based review. If the criteria are based on studies showing which treatments are most effective, then reviews could improve the appropriateness of care. Also, if cost savings are used to provide treatment to a greater proportion of the population, then access to care could improve.

Critics countered that MCO's may not adequately discriminate between necessary and unnecessary care. They noted that UR reviewers often lack sufficient experience to assess clinical cases and rarely evaluate patients firsthand. Review criteria may be inadequate to guide treatment decisions in complex cases. Also, research studies of treatment effectiveness often do not sufficiently address choices among alternative treatments or for specific types of patients. Critics also pointed out that cost savings may be consumed in administrative costs or taken as profit, rather than being used to expand access to care.

Some ethical concerns were specific to mental health care. To treat certain psychologically based problems, patients need a confidential relationship with the therapist. MCO's, however, often require a detailed review of the patient's history and illness. Many providers of mental health care believe this process disrupts the patient-therapist relationship and can be harmful to the treatment. Proponents of managed care suggest, on the other hand, that the MCO should be considered a part of this care-giving relationship and should protect patient confidentiality.

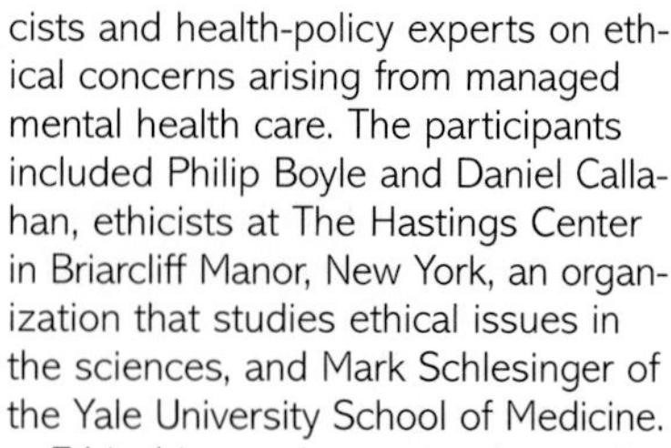

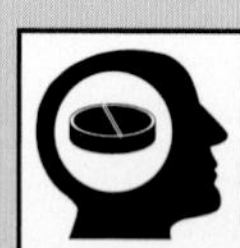

When cheaper may not be better

Health Maintenance Organizations (HMO's) decide what treatment for depression is most cost-effective and appropriate for the patients they enroll. Many mental-health specialists argue, however, that HMO's base decisions mostly on the cost rather than the quality of treatment. For example, many HMO's only approve older, less expensive generic antidepressants that have side effects much riskier than newer, more expensive drugs.

Drug	Wholesale price for typical daily dose for adult outpatient
Fewer side effects	(not available as generic)
Paxil	$1.90
Prozac	$2.24
Zoloft	$2.02
More side effects	(available as generic)
Amitriptyline	$0.21–$0.42
Desipramine	$0.22–$0.44
Imipramine	$0.09–$0.18

Source: *The Wall Street Journal*, Dec. 1, 1995.

Mental health specialists also argued that managed care can disrupt the continuity of care. MCO's often control costs by limiting patients to a selected group of clinicians. When an organization directs a patient to a new clinician, a previously established patient-therapist relationship can be disrupted.

Finally, ethicists were concerned that some MCO's provide less care or impose higher out-of-pocket expenses on patients with mental illnesses than those with physical aliments. This concern prompted Congress to address the issue. A health-care-reform bill passed in July 1996 originally would have guaranteed equitable coverage of mental health care, but that provision was dropped from the final version of the legislation. Nevertheless, President Bill Clinton signed the measure on August 21.

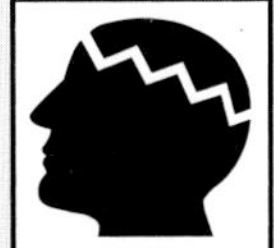

Diagnosing anxiety disorders

A little anxiety is a normal response to stress, change, and crises. A person may have an anxiety disorder, however, if he or she worries frequently and experiences physical symptoms, such as a rapid heart rate, shortness of breath, lightheadedness, insomnia, and diarrhea.

Anxiety disorders can be caused by the way a person responds to stress, but chemical imbalances, physical illnesses, and drugs can also cause the symptoms of anxiety. Most anxiety disorders can be managed by learning effective ways to express emotions, problem-solving skills, and relaxation techniques. Medications are sometimes prescribed as part of the treatment.

Physicians base a diagnosis partly on a series of questions, such as:

- Do your symptoms occur after a stressful event?
- Are there certain situations or settings that always make you feel anxious?
- Have you felt anxious over long periods of time even when you are not experiencing any problems?
- Do feelings of anxiety or the physical symptoms make you feel incapable of doing everyday activities?
- Do you do things or think about things repeatedly that do not make sense?
- Do you frequently have nightmares or thoughts about a painful time in your life?

Source: American Academy of Family Physicians.

Variation in psychiatric treatment. A July 1996 report concluded that research on geographical variations in psychiatric treatment are important to the future policy and financing of mental health care. Richard Hermann, a psychiatrist at McLean Hospital and Harvard Medical School, focused on a 1995 Harvard report about the use of *electroconvulsive therapy* (ECT), a treatment in which an electric current is sent through the brain to induce a seizure.

Many experimental studies had found ECT to be an effective treatment for severe depression, mania, and some forms of psychosis. With the use of anesthesia, monitoring, and drugs that cause muscle relaxation, ECT has been shown to be a relatively safe treatment as well. Between 30,000 and 100,000 Americans were treated annually with ECT in the mid-1990's.

The 1995 Harvard report, however, found the use of ECT to vary widely in different parts of the United States. In one-third of 317 cities studied, doctors reported that they did not use ECT. Among the cities reporting ECT use, rates of use varied more than five-fold. The availability of primary-care physicians, psychiatrists, and private psychiatric hospital beds in a city was strongly associated with the amount of ECT use. The study also showed that the more stringently states regulated the procedure, the less ECT was performed.

Studies of variation in medical practices have become influential in health-care policy, because the studies have found that the supply of clinicians and hospital beds influences both access to health-care services and the amount of treatment received. Furthermore, health-policy experts often associate a wide variation in treatment selection with a lack of consensus among clinicians about the effectiveness of treatments for a given condition.

To narrow variations in treatment, the federal government and medical organizations were developing practice guidelines to educate clinicians on the appropriate use of treatments. As cost-containment measures continued to be implemented, issues regarding access to treatments, appropriate use of treatments, and quality of clinical decision-making were expected to become more crucial.

Early sign of Alzheimer's disease. In a study of nuns who wrote autobiographical essays as young women, researchers found that poor linguistic ability early in life is a strong predictor of developing Alzheimer's disease in later years. Led by David Snowdon, a specialist in preventive medicine at the University of Kentucky, the researchers reported their findings in February 1996. Although it was felt that further studies would be needed, poor linguistic skills in early life may be an early expression of the disease.

Alzheimer's disease is a form of *dementia* (mental deterioration) most common among elderly people. The disease causes a progressive decline in memory, linguistic skills, and the ability to make judgments. Alzheimer's ultimately affects approximately one-third of all Americans and is the fourth most common cause of death among the elderly. Specialists had assumed that the changes in the brain structure associated with the illness begin late in life, but Snowdon's findings challenged that assumption.

Researchers from several medical centers studied 93 elderly nuns living in convents primarily in the Milwaukee area. Prior to taking their religious vows at an average age of 22, the women had written one-page autobiographies. To determine the women's early linguistic abilities, the researchers analyzed these essays using two measures: one assessing the complexity of the grammar, the other showing the density of ideas in their writing (the average number of ideas expressed for every 10 words).

The researchers then used several tests to determine the mental functioning of the women almost 60 years after writing the autobiographies. The investigators found that a low linguistic ability early in life increased the likelihood of developing Alzheimer's later in life.

Fourteen of the women subsequently died, and the investigators studied the structures of their brains. Five of these women's brains had *neurofibrillary tangles* (tangled fibers within nerve cells) and other malformations that indicate Alzheimer's. All five had written essays of low idea density in their youth. The other nine women, whose brains showed no signs of the disorder, had all written essays of high idea density.

The findings were indirectly supported by a 1995 study indicating that neurofibrillary tangles and other malformations associated with Alzheimer's may appear early in life and develop over many years.

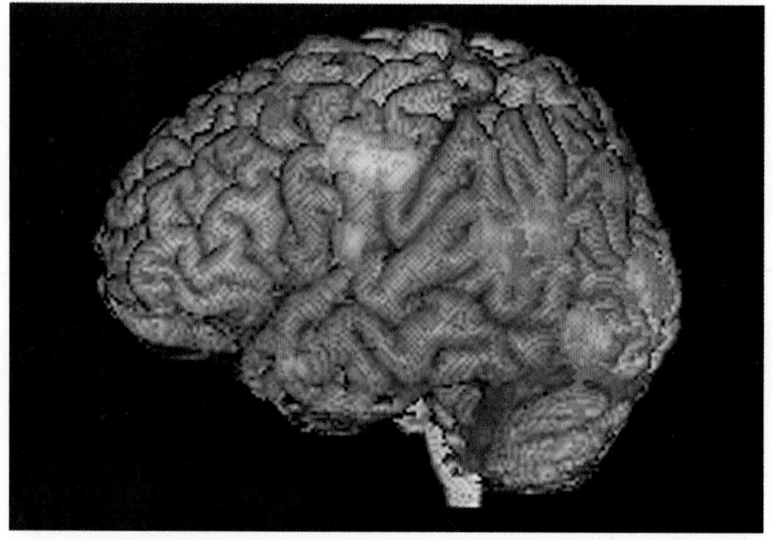

A map of schizophrenia

An image of the brain of a person with schizophrenia, made with a technique called positron emission tomography (PET), shows regions (bright patches) that were most active when the person was seeing hallucinations and hearing voices. The image, from the first study to use PET in this way, was released in November 1995 by researchers in London and at the Cornell Medical Center in New York City.

Eating disorders in decline. A reduction in problematic eating behaviors and distorted attitudes about body weight was shown in a comparison of two surveys of students conducted in 1982 and 1992 at a northeastern college. Researchers at Dartmouth College in Hanover, New Hampshire, reported their analysis of the surveys in November 1995.

Female students were on average five pounds heavier in 1992 than in 1982, while male students showed no significant change in average weight. Although less than 6 percent of women in either study were overweight, nearly one-half of the 1982 sample and one-third of the 1992 sample considered themselves overweight. The men's perceptions did not significantly differ from their actual weight.

The researchers found that the intensity of dieting, binge eating, vomiting, and the use of diet pills or *diuretic drugs* (which increase water loss) declined among women from 1982 to 1992. Although most symptoms of eating disorders declined, problematic attitudes persisted. More than 70 percent of female students in 1992 reported dissatisfaction with their body image and a desire to lose weight. • Richard C. Hermann

See also BRAIN AND NERVOUS SYSTEM. In WORLD BOOK, see MENTAL ILLNESS; ALZHEIMER'S DISEASE.

Nutrition and Food

- Beta-carotene studies
- Dietary fat and breast cancer
- Vitamin A and birth defects
- Soy and heart disease risk
- Chromium supplement safety

Some studies have suggested that the chemical compound beta-carotene may help prevent cancer and cardiovascular disease. But the safety and effectiveness of beta-carotene supplements were questioned in May 1996, when two major studies were reported. In the Physicians' Health Study, beta-carotene supplements were shown to have had no impact on the development of either cancer or heart disease. And researchers in the Beta-Carotene and Retinol Efficacy Trial (CARET) found that beta-carotene was not only ineffective in preventing cancer, but it may also have contributed to the development of lung cancer in smokers and individuals exposed to asbestos.

The CARET study examined over 18,000 men and women aged 50 to 69 who were current and former smokers and men aged 45 to 69 who had been exposed to asbestos. Half of the subjects took 30 milligrams (mg) of beta-carotene and 25,000 international units (IU) of retinol (vitamin A); the other half took a *placebo* (inactive substance). The investigation had been scheduled to continue until late 1997 but was discontinued in January 1996 because of the alarming results. Those taking beta-carotene and vitamin A had a 28

The egg redeemed?

A study reported in November 1995 concluded that many people on a low-fat diet can eat two eggs a day without doing any damage to their health.

Eggs have been targeted as a major source of cholesterol, blamed for clogging arteries and causing heart attacks. But it may be saturated fat, found in cheese and meats, that is the key cholesterol booster. Researchers at the University of Washington conducted a study of men and women with either high cholesterol alone or high cholesterol and elevated levels of *triglycerides* (fatty compounds) in their blood. Half of the participants ate two eggs a day for 12 weeks while the other half ate egg substitutes. Levels of LDL (harmful) cholesterol did not increase for people with high cholesterol alone. But the eggs raised the cholesterol of those who had high triglyceride levels. Health professionals suggested that people with high triglycerides should not eat eggs.

percent greater risk of getting lung cancer than the group taking a placebo; a 26 percent greater risk of developing *cardiovascular* (heart and blood vessels) disease; and a 17 percent greater overall risk of dying.

Some critics called the results a statistical fluke, noting that animal studies had not shown beta-carotene to be harmful. Perhaps what was harmful was that the study subjects took five times the recommended daily allowance of vitamin A.

The Physicians' Health Study involved over 22,000 male physicians from 40 to 84 years of age. For 12 years, half of them took 50 mg of beta-carotene every other day. Researchers suggested that the study may have found beta-carotene ineffective because smokers and asbestos-exposed workers, already at high risk for disease, would need to take the supplements earlier in life to see any benefits.

Most health professionals recommended that people get beta-carotene from fruits and vegetables in their diet. Further study is needed to identify the specific substance or substances in fruits and vegetables that protect against disease.

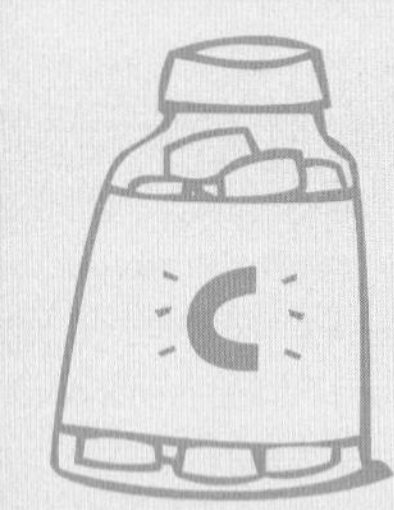

Getting your vitamin C

Researchers at the National Institutes of Health reported in April 1996 that the optimal daily amount of vitamin C is 200 milligrams. (The current Recommended Dietary Allowance is 60 milligrams.) Below are some of the best sources of vitamin C.

Food source	Serving	Amount of vitamin C (milligrams)
Guava	3 ounces, whole fruit	165.0
Sweet pepper	1 raw pepper	94.7
Orange	1 5-ounce navel	80.3
Grapefruit	1 cup sections with juice	79.1
Kiwi	1 medium fruit	74.5
Cranberry juice cocktail	6 ounces	67.3
Broccoli	½ cup, chopped, cooked	49.0
Brussels sprouts	½ cup, cooked	48.4
Papaya	½ cup cubes	43.2
Strawberries	½ cup, fresh	42.2
Potato, with skin	7 ounces, microwaved	30.5

Source: U.S. Department of Agriculture

Dietary fat and breast cancer. Scientists reported in February 1996 that they had found no relation between dietary fat and the risk of breast cancer. An international team of investigators found that even women who ate a very low-fat diet had no reduced risk of breast cancer.

Many other studies had found that high-fat diets do increase the risk of breast cancer. But these were animal studies, research comparing the diets of healthy women with those that already have breast cancer, and studies that look at different rates of the disease in different countries. For example, women in Japan and China have a low-fat diet and very low rates of breast cancer compared with the high breast cancer rates and high-fat diet of U.S. women. These studies had been criticized because they did not enroll enough women or look at a wide range of fat intakes.

The new study examined the data from seven studies that followed over 300,000 women in four countries: Canada, the Netherlands, Sweden, and the United States. The investigators said they could not rule out the possibility that eating a low-fat diet beginning in childhood could help prevent breast cancer. But for middle-aged and older women, they said, dietary changes to reduce fat consumption most likely will not reduce the risk of breast cancer.

Vitamin A and birth defects. A study reported in November 1995 found that pregnant women who took vitamin A supplements were more likely to give birth to babies with birth defects than those

Changing tastes

Americans have become more health conscious, an awareness that is reflected in the foods we choose. At right is a sample of how some familiar foods have increased or declined in popularity over the past 20 years.

Food	% Change
Broccoli	+520%
Yogurt	+438%
Low-fat milk	+180%
Turkey	+121%
Cheese	+121%
Whole milk	-60%
Sugar	-36%
Eggs	-25%
Butter	-22%
Beef	-21%

Source: Research Alert.

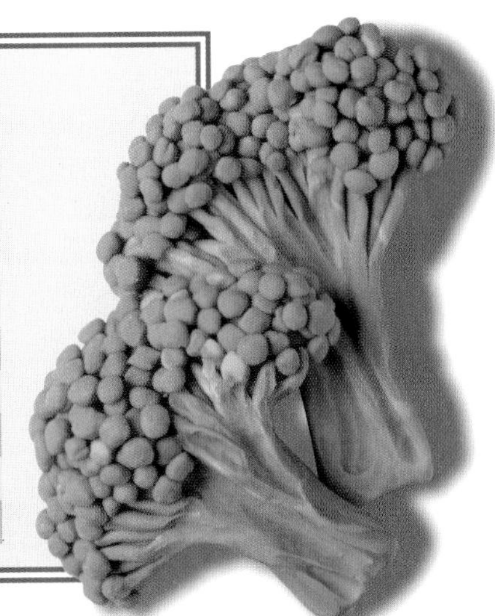

who did not take the supplements.

Researchers in Italy and at the Boston University School of Medicine reviewed data from studies of pregnant women who were being screened for birth defects. The women became part of the study between the 15th and 20th week of their pregnancy. They were asked about their diet, medications, and medical history and whether they were ill during the first three months of their pregnancy. They were also asked about vitamin A and multivitamin supplements—how much they took during the first three months of their pregnancy and when they started taking supplements. The women were followed up to check on the health of their newborn babies.

Of the 22,748 women in the study, 339 had babies with birth defects, including cleft palate and other deformities of the face, improper brain development, and heart defects. These defects were grouped together because they develop from the same group of cells in the embryo called the cranial-neural-crest (CRC).

The researchers found that the women who took more than 10,000 IU per day of vitamin A had almost five times the risk of having a baby with CRC defects compared with the women who took no more than the recommended daily amount, 5,000 IU. The investigators found that the worst time for a woman to be taking high doses of vitamin A is apparently from two weeks before to four weeks after conceiving.

Still, vitamin A—in appropriate amounts—is important for the growth and development of the embryo. This vitamin is found in liver, dairy foods, foods that are fortified and, of course, vitamin supplements. There does not seem to be a risk in taking the recommended amount of either vitamin A or beta-carotene, which the body converts to vitamin A.

Soy and heart disease risk. Soy protein, obtained from soybeans, may lower cholesterol, researchers at the University of Kentucky reported in August 1996. They analyzed 38 studies on soy and cholesterol and found that 84 percent of the studies showed that soy may lower cholesterol when it replaces animal protein in the diet.

The researchers found that blood-vessel-damaging LDL cholesterol—often called "bad" cholesterol—dropped by 13 percent and total cholesterol decreased by 9 percent in people who consumed 50 grams (almost 2 ounces) of soy protein daily.

Subjects with only slightly elevated cholesterol levels received little benefit from the added soy. But those with high cholesterol (259 to 333 milligrams/deciliter [mg/dl]) experienced a 7-percent reduction, and those with even higher levels (over 335 mg/dl) had a 20-percent decrease. The investigators found that 25 grams of soy protein a day lowered cholesterol by an average of 9 mg/dl, 50 grams

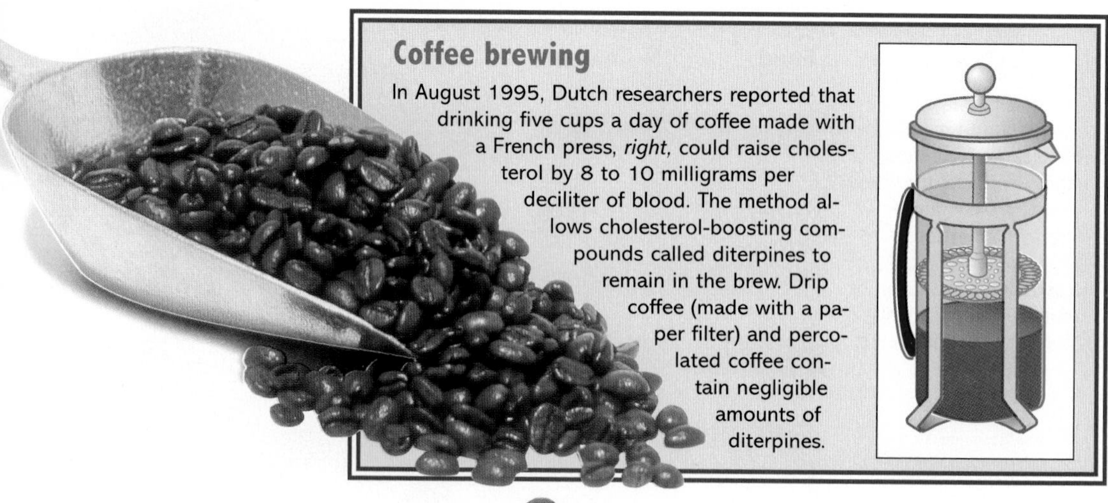

Coffee brewing

In August 1995, Dutch researchers reported that drinking five cups a day of coffee made with a French press, *right,* could raise cholesterol by 8 to 10 milligrams per deciliter of blood. The method allows cholesterol-boosting compounds called diterpines to remain in the brew. Drip coffee (made with a paper filter) and percolated coffee contain negligible amounts of diterpines.

caused a 17 mg/dl decline, and 75 grams reduced cholesterol by about 26 mg/dl.

The scientists were not sure what accounts for soy's effect on cholesterol. They said it may be the protein itself or substances called soy estrogens, chemically similar to the female hormone estrogen. Estrogen reduces the risk of heart disease in women by keeping LDL cholesterol low and beneficial HDL cholesterol ("good" cholesterol) high.

Soy protein can be added to the diet by eating such foods as soy milk, tofu, soy flour (added to a meat loaf or pancakes), or soyburgers. But experts caution that one cannot simply add soy to a poor diet and expect benefits. In most of the studies, soy protein replaced at least half of the animal protein. The reduction in saturated fat and cholesterol from meats and cheeses, for example, could account for the benefits.

Chromium supplement safety. The safety of chromium supplements was called into question by two groups of researchers in December 1995. Their findings caused many consumers to wonder if they should stop taking the mineral, which people use to reduce body fat, boost muscle bulk, and improve blood sugar control.

Investigators at Dartmouth College in Hanover, New Hampshire, and the George Washington University Medical Center in Washington, D.C., found that chromium picolinate, a form of the mineral found in many muscle-building supplements, may damage chromosomes, the cell structures that carry the genes. A substance that causes chromosome damage is considered likely to be cancer-causing.

Critics of the study, which was done with hamster cells, claimed that the dosages of chromium picolinate used were too high. But the researchers stated that chromium picolinate levels in the cells tested were about the amount that would be in the body of a person taking chromium picolinate supplements. Critics also said that a study in which chromium picolinate was injected into animal cells did not accurately reflect the effects of the substance on humans.

Because other forms of chromium did not damage the cells in the 1995 study, some investigators suggested that the results may have been due to the picolinate, a substance added to help the body absorb chromium.

Chromium is an essential trace element that helps the body metabolize blood sugar and plays a role in how the body processes fats and proteins. But nutritionists emphasize that there is no solid evidence that chromium will make anyone thinner or more muscular. And one of the study's authors pointed out that the long-term effects of chromium accumulation in the body are not well understood. Additional research is needed before chromium supplements are labeled as either toxic or safe. • Jeanine Barone

In World Book, see Nutrition.

A greater incidence of high blood pressure among African American women puts them at higher risk for developing certain complications in pregnancy. That finding was reported in April 1996 by researchers at the Morehouse School of Medicine in Atlanta, Georgia.

Some women have high blood pressure, or hypertension, before pregnancy; others develop it during pregnancy. If a woman has either of these forms of hypertension—called chronic and gestational, respectively—the fetus often does not grow properly or is born prematurely. Hypertension can also cause a woman to bleed from the uterus during pregnancy.

Using data from 1988 to 1992 from the National Center for Health Statistics in Hyattsville, Maryland, the investigators determined that the incidence of gestational hypertension did not vary much by race. But chronic hypertension was 2.5 times higher among African American women.

Compared with women who had normal blood pressure, women with hypertension—regardless of race—had almost twice as many preterm deliveries and about four times as many low-birth-weight babies. But African American women with hypertension experienced three times as many incidents of uterine bleeding as other women with that condition.

The researchers said the findings might explain much of the gap between African American women and other women in the United States in adverse birth outcomes—low birthweights, preterm deliveries, infant illnesses, and deaths.

Folic acid to prevent birth defects. In February 1996, the Food and Drug Administration (FDA) ordered food manufacturers to add *folic acid* (part of the vitamin B complex) to certain foods to help prevent *neural tube* defects in infants.

The neural tube is a structure in the fetus that develops into the baby's brain, spinal cord, and related tissues. With neural tube defects, these structures do not form properly. Two common forms of neural tube defects are *spina bifida* and *anencephaly.* With spina bifida, the spinal cord and vertabrae do not form normally, sometimes resulting in physical disabilities or other birth defects. Anencephaly occurs when the brain and head do not develop normally. Most infants with this condition are stillborn or die shortly after birth. Tests performed during pregnancy can detect these defects in a fetus.

As of July 1996, the exact cause of neural tube defects remained unknown, but earlier research indicated that women who consumed at least 0.4 milligram (mg) of folic acid per day lowered their chance of having an affected baby. In 1992, the Public

Pregnancy and Childbirth

- High-blood-pressure risks for pregnant African American women
- Folic acid to prevent birth defects
- Obesity and neural tube defects
- HIV tests for pregnant women

STATISTICS

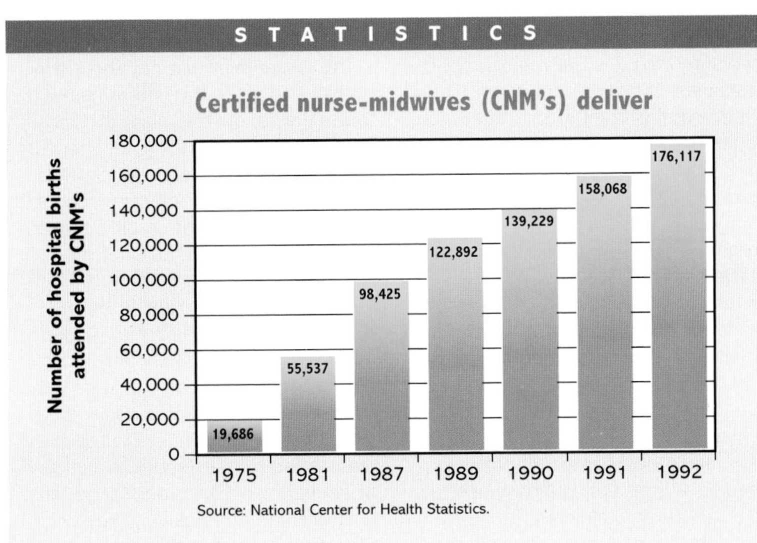

Source: National Center for Health Statistics.

Rise of low-tech births

The National Center for Health Statics, in Hyattsville, Maryland, reported in November 1995 that the number of hospital births attended by certified nurse-midwives increased by almost nine times from 1975 to 1992. A certified nurse-midwife is certified to care for normal, healthy pregnancies. The more natural, less high-tech care emphasizes support for women throughout pregancy. Hospitals with nurse-midwife deliveries offer backup from physicians to assist with any problems during delivery.

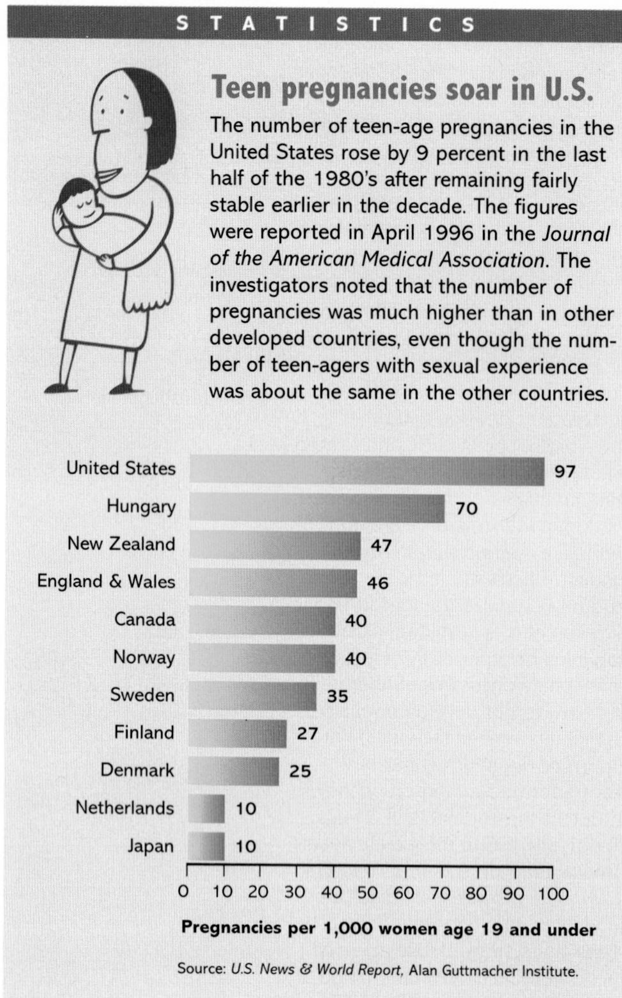

Health Service in Washington, D.C., recommended this daily allowance to all women of childbearing age. To be of benefit, this level of folic acid must be present in a woman's body in the early weeks of pregnancy when the fetus is first developing and the woman may not yet know that she is pregnant.

The FDA order, which was scheduled to go into effect Jan. 1, 1998, called for enriched bread, flour, and other grain products to be fortified with 0.43 to 1.4 mg of folic acid per pound of food. This level was designed to meet the recommended daily intake of 0.4 mg without exceeding 1 mg per day. Too much folic acid can mask vitamin B_{12} deficiencies, which can cause problems in older people. Other sources of folic acid include orange juice, leafy green vegetables, and dried beans.

Obesity and neural tube defects. Obese women have a higher risk of having a baby with a neural tube defect, according to two independent studies reported in April 1996. Both studies also noted that nutritional factors, such as taking recommended levels of folic acid, did not reduce the risk among heavier women.

Epidemiologist Martha Werler and her colleagues at the Boston University School of Public Health evaluated statistics from over 2,300 pregnancies from 1988 to 1994. They found the risk of having a baby with a neural tube defect was four times greater for a woman weighing over 240 pounds (110 kilograms) before pregnancy than for a woman weighing 110 to 130 pounds (50 to 59 kilograms). Although a daily intake of 0.4 mg of folic acid reduced the risk of neural tube defects by 40 percent among women weighing less than 155 pounds (70 kilograms), it did not offer any benefit among heavier women.

The second study, led by epidemiologist Gary Shaw of the California Birth Defects Monitoring Program in Emeryville, evaluated information from over 1,000 pregnancies. The investigators linked obesity with a twofold-increased risk of neural tube defects. The use of folic acid, the presence of diabetes, and other factors that could affect the nutrition of the mother had no effect on the risk.

The researchers did not know why obesity increases the risk of neural tube defects, but they said the link seems to be important since it occurs in at least one of every 1,000 pregnancies. The physicians concluded that lowering body weight before pregnancy could help prevent the defects.

HIV tests for pregnant women. Two medical groups recommended in August 1995 that all pregnant women receive—with their consent—counseling and testing for HIV, the virus that causes AIDS. The report was issued by the American Academy of Pediatrics in Elk Grove Village, Illinois, and the American College of Obstetricians and Gynecologists in Wash-

STATISTICS

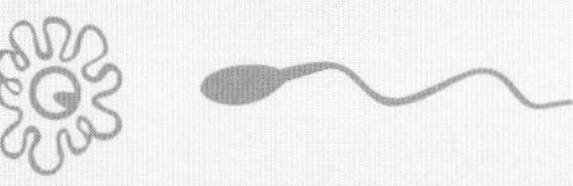

Misconceptions about conception

A report in December 1995 challenged beliefs about when women are most likely to conceive. According to former research and conventional wisdom, a woman's most fertile time lasts 2 to 13 days and ovulation occurs somewhere in the middle. But in a study of 212 women, researchers at the National Institute of Environmental Health Sciences found that the likelihood of conception is greatest on the day of ovulation and the two days preceding it. Fertility ceases, they concluded, when ovulation takes place.

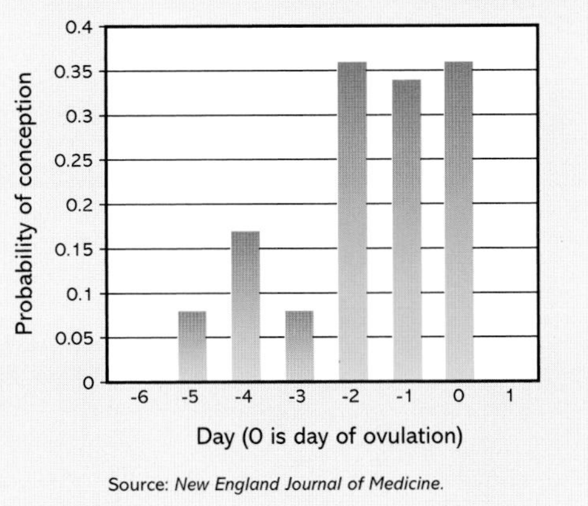

Source: *New England Journal of Medicine.*

ington, D.C., organizations representing the physicians who care for infants and their mothers. The report supported a July 1995 recommendation from the Centers for Disease Control and Prevention (CDC) in Atlanta.

According to the joint report, the HIV/AIDS epidemic had increased significantly among women and children. In September 1995, the CDC reported that approximately 6,530 HIV-infected women gave birth in the United States, and an estimated 1,630 of their babies were infected.

A mother can pass the virus to her baby during pregnancy, labor, or delivery. An estimated one-third of pregnant women infected with HIV pass the virus to their babies. Advances in prevention and treatment of HIV, however, have made early diagnosis important. A 1994 study showed that early treatment of pregnant women with the drug zidovudine (ZDV), also known as AZT, can lower the risk of passing the virus from mother to baby by about two-thirds. In addition, treatment of infants during the first months of life may help prolong their lives.

The joint report stressed the importance of having the mother's consent and providing counseling to ensure that her rights are protected and to make her aware of treatment options and resources. • Rebecca D. Rinehart

In WORLD BOOK, see PREGNANCY.

Respiratory System

- Smoking remains widespread
- Adult smoking can harm children
- Treating severely diseased lungs
- Treating respiratory failure
- Surgery for emphysema
- Antioxidants and lung cancer

Health experts in 1995 and 1996 continued to warn of the risks associated with cigarettes and other tobacco products, but many people still had not "kicked the habit." In the United States, sales of cigarettes and other tobacco products continued to be strong and even rose among some groups. Although progress continued in the development of new treatments for lung diseases, being a nonsmoker remained the simplest way to reduce the risk of developing *cardiopulmonary* (heart and lung) disease.

Adult smoking can harm children. In April 1996, physicians in Massachusetts published a comprehensive report on the effects of adult smoking on the health of children. The report combined the data collected by 119 smoking studies conducted since 1965. The study found that cigarette use among adults has a considerable negative impact on the health of children.

According to the study, approximately 300 children die each year of lung disease or in fires linked to adult smoking. In addition, the physicians found, cigarette smoke is associated with at least 354,000 doctor visits for middle-ear infections, 529,000 cases of asthma symptoms, and at least 1.3 million cases of coughing every year. In children under age 5, smoking by adults was associated with at least 260,000 cases of bronchitis and at least 115,000 cases of pneumonia.

The researchers said the results of the study emphasized that new regulations were needed to protect children from the health risks caused by exposure to second-hand smoke.

Treating severely diseased lungs. People with acute respiratory distress syndrome (ARDS), a severe failure of lung function, have a death rate of about 40 to 60 percent. In the mid-1990's, research into ways to manage these critically ill patients included finding new ways to restore lung function, halt the disease process, and protect the lung from further injury. In February 1996, researchers at the University of Michigan at Ann Arbor reported on their initial experience with one promising method, known as partial liquid ventilation. This procedure involved the use of *perfluorocarbon*, a fluid similar in some ways to blood, to help injured or diseased lungs do their job and perhaps also protect them from further damage.

Perfluorocarbon is a liquid that, like blood, absorbs oxygen and carbon dioxide. But it can carry greater amounts of these gases than blood. Partial liquid ventilation involves filling an injured lung with perfluorocarbon and then connecting the patient to a ventilator. The perfluorocarbon assists with gas exchange, opening collapsed *alveoli* (tiny air sacs in lung tissue) and helping to remove debris from the lung. The fluid is delivered into the lung in aerosol or drip form.

The researchers used partial liquid ventilation in 10 adults with ARDS. They found that the treatment contributed to an improvement in the exchange of oxygen and carbon dioxide, in lung function and physiology, and in survival rates compared with conventional treatments. However, the researchers stressed that the technique was experimental and required more extensive clinical evaluation.

Treating respiratory failure. In May 1996, researchers from the United States reported negative results in a nationwide clinical trial of another proposed treatment for ARDS. The physicians tested the benefit of artificial *surfactant* as a treatment for adults with lung failure. Surfactant is a substance secreted by lung cells that makes breathing easier by helping the lungs remain inflated.

Premature babies often develop infant respiratory distress syndrome (IRDS), a breathing problem associated with a shortage of surfactant in their underdeveloped lungs. Previous studies had shown that the survival rate of premature infants with IRDS improved if they were treated with artificial surfactant immediately after birth. The researchers suspected that surfactant treatment might produce a similar effect in adults.

The study consisted of 775 people who had ARDS caused by an infection. The patients were given artificial surfactant or a *placebo* (inactive substance) for five days. However, those receiving surfactant showed no improvement in pulmonary function, survival rate, length of hospital stay, or length of time spent on a ventilator.

Surgery for emphysema. An experimental surgical procedure for emphysema known as lung volume reduction surgery was being used at several medical centers in the United States in early 1996 and was producing significant improvements in many patients. The treatment involves removing diseased lung tissue, but doctors were uncertain how the procedure improves lung function. In April 1996, researchers at the University of Pittsburgh Medical Center and School of Medicine reported their findings on volume reduction surgery.

The study consisted of 20 people diagnosed with emphysema. Each patient's lung function and physiology were evaluated before and three months after surgery. After surgery, subjects showed several improvements, including increased airflow on lung function tests and less carbon dioxide in their arterial blood.

The researchers concluded that removing damaged lung tissue improves lung function by increasing the elasticity of the remaining lung tissue, which causes the lungs to return to a more normal capacity. However, they also emphasized that the treatment was still highly experimental and that further study was needed.

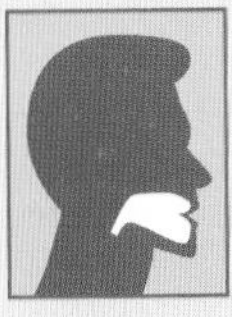

Some good old-fashioned hoarse sense

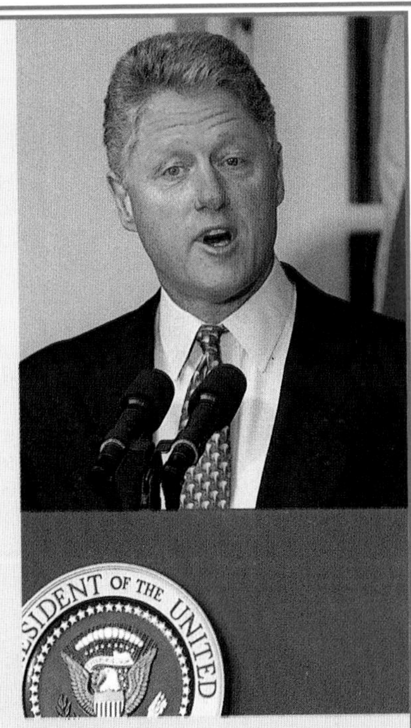

During his first campaign for the White House, Bill Clinton was forced to cancel speaking engagements or shorten speeches on a number of occasions to give his voice a break. By the end of the presidential campaign, he became literally speechless due to laryngitis.

Laryngitis is an inflammation of the *larynx* (voice box), which causes the voice to become hoarse or to disappear completely. Various conditions can irritate the throat and lead to laryngitis, including overuse of the voice, smoking, drinking, and colds and other infections of the respiratory tract. In President Clinton's case, nasal congestion and breathing difficulties caused by allergies make him susceptible to laryngitis.

The best and simplest way to treat laryngitis is to rest the voice and avoid smoking, alcohol, and caffeine. Using a humidifier and drinking water keeps the vocal chords moist and eases some of the discomfort and irritation. Treating the condition that contributes to the laryngitis, such as an infection or allergy, is also helpful. People who must speak frequently should consider seeking professional voice training.

Source: American Academy of Otolaryngology.

Antioxidants and lung cancer. The results of two clinical trials published in May 1996 cast doubt on the theory that antioxidants can reduce the risk of lung cancer. Antioxidants are chemical compounds that appear to protect cells from *oxidation,* a process in which the atoms of a substance lose electrons and become more reactive. Oxidation can damage cells and alter their genetic material, leading to cancer. Studies had indicated that people who eat a diet high in the antioxidant beta-carotene have a lower risk of lung cancer. Some yellow or green vegetables, such as carrots and spinach, are high in beta-carotene.

The first study reported no significant drop in the incidence of lung cancer development or death among 22,000 male physicians who were given beta-carotene or a placebo every other day for 11 to 14 years. The other study, which tested a combination of beta-carotene and vitamin A, also showed no benefit from antioxidant therapy. However, this trial was stopped 21 months early when researchers found a slightly higher risk of lung cancer and death—primarily from diseases of the heart and blood vessels—in the active treatment group. Both of these studies, however, tested beta-carotene in pill form only. The possible benefits of antioxidants received from food were not measured. (See also NUTRITION AND FOOD.)

• Robert A. Balk

In WORLD BOOK see Asthma; LUNG; RESPIRATION.

Safety

- Auto safety-rating labels
- Ford Motor recall
- Guidelines on workplace violence
- Children and bike helmets
- How safe are indoor playgrounds?
- Hazards of shopping carts
- Child restraints in airplanes

The National Research Council (NRC), an agency of the National Academy of Sciences in Washington, D.C., recommended in a March 1996 report that all new cars, vans, and light trucks carry a window safety label to help consumers compare safety features. At the time of the report, consumers were able to compare crash-test results for vehicles of similar size and weight, but not for vehicles of different styles and sizes, such as a midsized car and a sport-utility vehicle. The U.S. Congress requested the report, which was prepared by a group of highway safety experts.

The NRC said that the U.S. Department of Transportation should urge auto manufacturers to voluntarily display safety stickers by the year 2000. The stickers would include a crashworthiness score so that consumers could compare one vehicle to another and a list of crash-avoidance features, such as antilock brakes. Buyers would be able to get more detailed comparisons of vehicle safety from a brochure in the glove box and a book available in libraries or over the Internet, the global computer nework.

The NRC report said that more and more new buyers wanted autos with features that protect occupants, prevent accidents, and reduce insurance

Shopping cart danger
Children riding in supermarket shopping carts often suffer serious injury, doctors at Columbus (Ohio) Children's Hospital and the Ohio State University College of Medicine reported in February 1996. The doctors noted that the carts are designed with high seats and a narrow wheel base, giving the carts a high center of gravity and making them prone to tipping over. The physicians recommended that shopping carts be redesigned with a wider wheel base so that they would be less top-heavy.

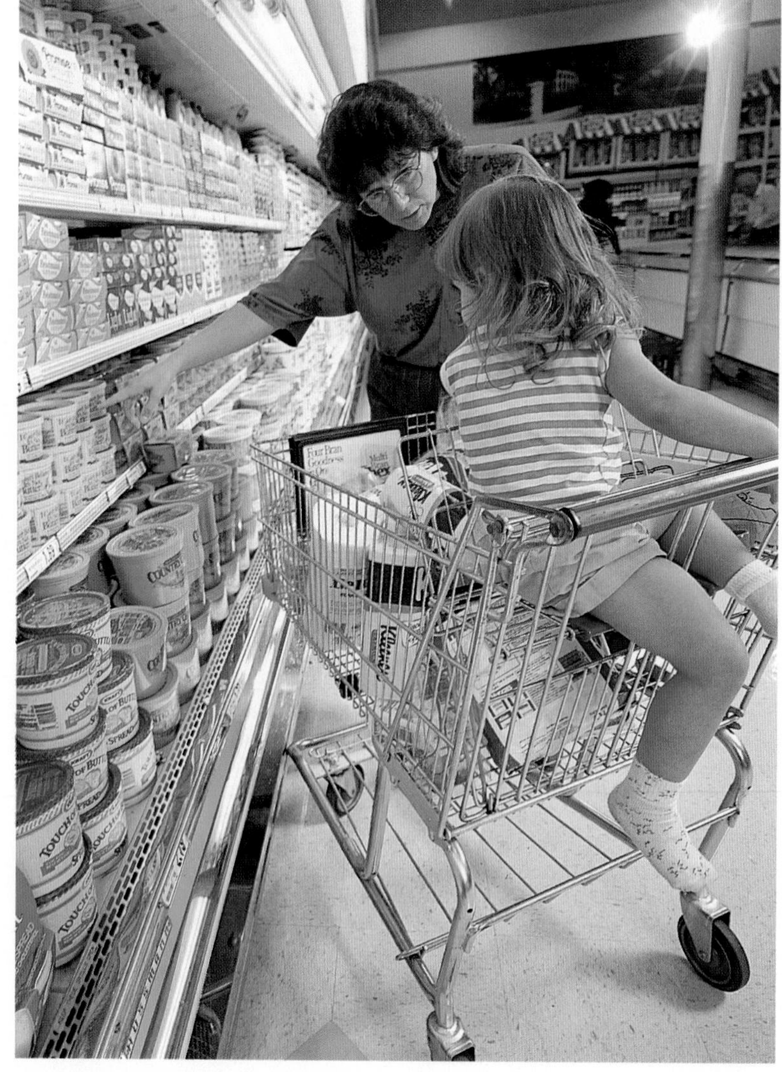

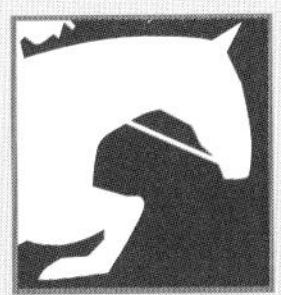

Riding into the sunset—safely

Horseback riding conjures up images of fox hunts and romantic rides at sunset, which make it easy to forget the dangers. One study found that more than 90,000 Americans were injured in riding accidents over a two-year period. The following precautions can make horseback riding a safer experience:

- Wear a hard hat. (They come in several traditional riding styles.)
- Take riding lessons if you are a beginner or have not ridden for years.
- Do not ride alone if you are a beginner.
- Wear a sturdy, smooth-soled shoe or boot with a heel that will not slip through a stirrup. (Athletic shoes are not appropriate.)
- Do not wear loose-fitting clothing or accessories.
- Wear riding gloves with a gripper surface.
- Do not mix alcohol and riding.

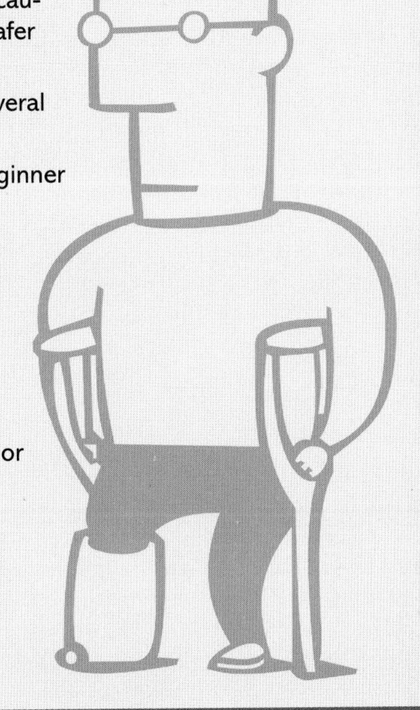

Source: *University of California at Berkeley Wellness Letter*, February 1996.

premiums. Though motor vehicle fatality rates had fallen by almost 70 percent since 1966, when the government first set safety standards, highway accidents remained a leading cause of accidental death in the mid-1990's, killing about 40,000 people annually and costing $140-billion in property damage, medical bills, and lost wages. Drivers and road conditions caused many accidents, the NRC experts noted. But in dangerous situations, design features such as vehicle stability sometimes helped avoid a crash.

Ford Motor recall. The Ford Motor Company in April 1996 recalled 8.7 million cars, trucks, minivans, and sport-utility vehicles to replace ignition switches that could cause fires. The recall—the largest ever by a single auto manufacturer—included almost all of Ford's 1988 to 1992 vehicles and some early 1993 models.

Ford said it had received reports that short circuits in the ignition switches caused at least 1,100 vehicles in the United States and 900 in Canada to catch fire. Some of the switches burst into flame after the vehicle was turned off, and some fires occurred in vehicles parked in home garages, destroying the homes.

The ignition switches were installed in about 26 million Ford vehicles built from 1984 to October 1992. But Ford said the danger involved only vehicles with switches produced after May 1987. A design change made the switches more likely to short circuit and catch fire.

Canada ordered a recall in November 1995 of 248,000 Ford vehicles with the defective switches. In the United States, Ford said it would notify owners of the vehicles by mail, so they could go to a dealer for free replacement of the switch. The following models were involved: 1988 EXP; 1988-89 Ford Crown Victoria, Mercury Grand Marquis, and Lincoln Town Car; 1988-90 Ford Escort; 1988-91 Ford Aerostar minivans, Bronco sport-utility vehicles, and F-series light trucks; 1988-92 and some 1993 Ford Mustangs, Ford Thunderbirds, Mercury Cougars, Ford Tempos, and Mercury Topazes.

Guidelines on workplace violence. The first federal guidelines on the prevention of workplace violence were issued in March 1996 by the Occupational Safety and Health Administration (OSHA), an agency of the U.S. Labor Department. The guidelines, which were not mandatory, focused on America's 8 million health-care and social-service workers, who accounted for 66 percent of the 1 million employees assaulted in 1994. OSHA planned similar guidelines for clerks and other retail sales workers, who faced the highest risk of being murdered at work.

OSHA recommended that hospitals, clinics, physicians, government agencies, and other employers assess security at their workplace. The guidelines said employers should then train employees to recognize and respond to early signs of violence in patients and visitors and adopt preventive measures. Such measures might include installing metal detectors, security cameras, "panic buttons" for employees who work alone, and wider counters that would form an effective barrier between employees and violent patients or visitors.

Children and bike helmets. The use of bicycle helmets by children under age 15 has increased greatly since the 1980's, the U.S. Consumer Product Safety Commission (CPSC), an independent agency of the federal government, reported in February 1996. The study, the first national survey of children's bike helmet use, reported that about 26 percent of American children who ride bikes owned or had use of a safety helmet in 1991. About 15 percent wore a helmet all or most of the time while bicycling.

The study included 399 children whose parents were part of a national telephone survey. Previous studies, conducted in individual U.S. cities in the middle and late 1980's, showed that only 2 to 3 percent of children were using bicycle helmets.

The CPSC study noted that helmet use was highest for children younger than 6 and lowest for children aged 12 to 14. The study also found that positive media coverage of helmets, state and local bike safety awareness programs, laws requiring helmet use, and the introduction of lighter, more attractive helmets contributed to the increased use of protective headgear.

The CPSC report also included the results of a CPSC survey of nationwide bicycle-accident statistics. The agency found that preventable deaths and injuries were still common among kids who did not wear helmets. About 300 children were killed and more than 400,000 went to hospital emergency rooms each year in the late 1980's because of bicycle injuries. Children aged 5 to 14 had the highest injury rate. Studies showed that helmets could have prevented most of the serious injuries, including 85 percent of the head injuries.

The CPSC said parents should be made aware of the seriousness of bike injuries and encouraged to have their children wear helmets every time they ride. Teen-agers needed special encouragement because they were the least likely to wear helmets. The CPSC also called for more community bike safety programs and programs to make helmets available to children from low-income households.

How safe are indoor playgrounds? In another study released in March 1996, the CPSC assured parents that properly supervised and maintained playgrounds made with Soft Contained Play Equipment (SCPE) were safe alternatives to traditional outdoor playgrounds. SCPE is playground equipment made primarily of plastic and enclosed so that children cannot

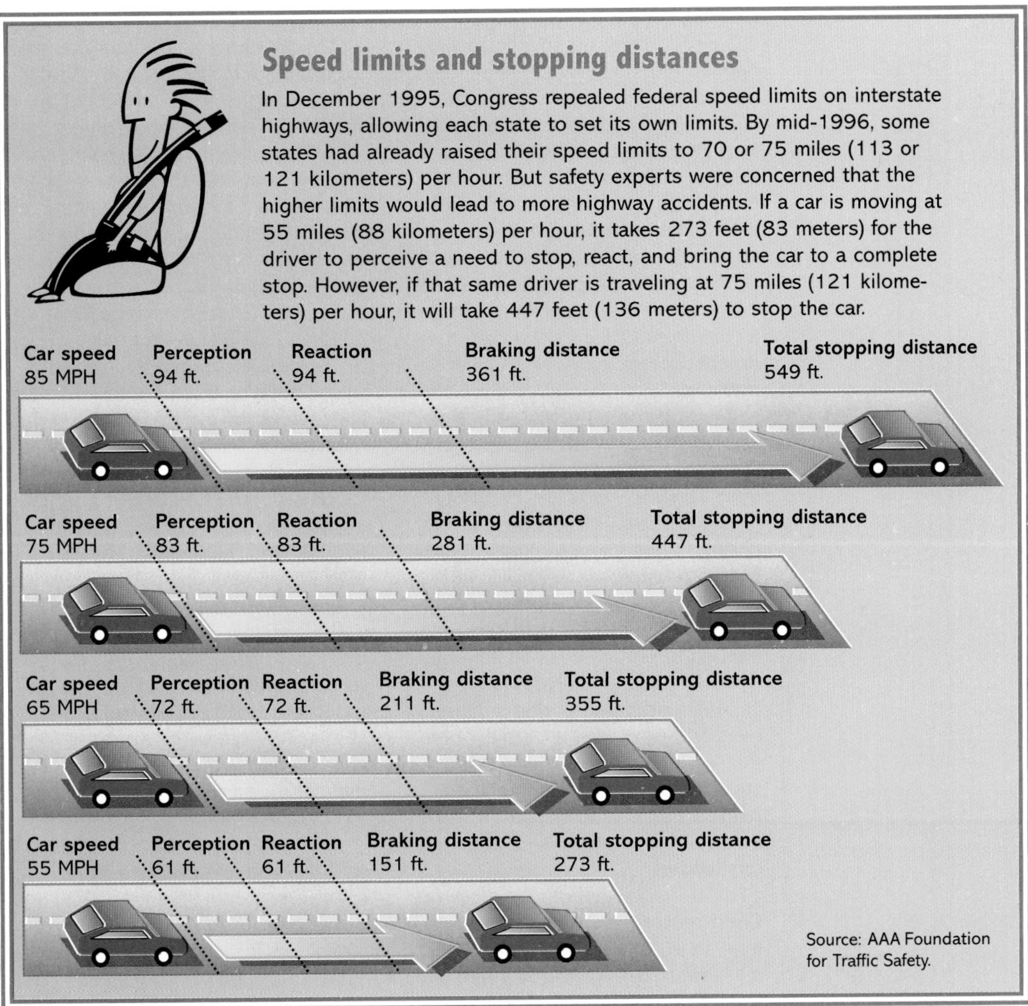

fall from it. SCPE was being used in the 1990's to make playgrounds of plastic tubes for children to crawl through, ball pools, climbing nets, slides, and padded floors. The playgrounds were built in pay-for-play chains, fast-food and family restaurants, shopping malls, and theme parks. Children, some less than 2 years old, teen-agers, and even adults used the equipment. Many parents became concerned about the safety of such playgrounds in 1995, after a 13-year-old boy buried himself in a pool of small plastic balls at the bottom of a slide and was killed by another child who landed on him after coming down the slide.

The CPSC study concluded that the playground equipment design, including its padded floors, actually minimized the risk of injuries that can result from falls. The CPSC noted, however, that adult supervision is critical to ensure proper use of the equipment and to prevent toddlers from getting in the way of older children. In addition, the agency emphasized the importance of proper maintenance of the equipment.

Hazards of shopping carts. Parents should stop the common practice of placing young children in shopping carts in supermarkets and other stores, researchers at Ohio State University in Columbus urged in February 1996. Their study of shopping cart injuries concluded that existing carts are too unstable for safe transport of kids during shopping trips.

Gary A. Smith, a pediatrician who headed the study, said that shopping carts should be redesigned with a wider wheel base or a lower center of gravity. Such features would reduce the tendency for carts to tip over, throwing children to the floor. Infant seats and safety belts do not reduce the risk of such injuries in young children, the researchers said. While safety belts and seats can keep a child from falling from a cart, they do not prevent injury when a cart overturns.

In another study reported in November 1995, Smith's group analyzed national injury data collected from 1990 to 1992 by the CPSC. They found that more than 25,000 children were seriously injured each year in accidents involving supermarket and department store shopping carts. All the injuries were serious enough to require hospital emergency-room treatment. Most involved children under age 5 who suffered head and neck injuries. Smith noted that while some stores had taken steps to alert parents about shopping cart safety, 80 percent of parents still left the child and cart unattended.

Child restraints in airplanes. In June 1996, the Federal Aviation Administration (FAA) issued a ban on the use of booster seats and harness- and vest-type child restraints on all U.S. air carriers. The ban was to go into effect in September 1996.

According to tests conducted by the FAA's Civil Aeromedical Institute (CAMI) in Oklahoma City, neither booster seats nor the harness- and vest-restraint systems adequately protect children during take-offs, landings, and while the airplane is moving on the ground. Based on the CAMI tests, the FAA recommended that children who weigh less than 20 pounds (9 kilograms) fly in a rear-facing child restraint approved by the National Highway Traffic Safety Administration (NHTSA); that children who weigh from 20 to 40 pounds (9 to 18 kilograms) fly in a forward-facing child restraint approved by the NHTSA; and that children weighing over 40 pounds use the standard lap belt attached to all airplane seats.

The National Transportation Safety Board, a federal agency that makes recommendations on airline safety, urged the FAA to make child restraints mandatory on airplanes for children under the age of 2. As of mid-1996, parents could still choose to hold their infants or toddlers on their laps during a flight. The FAA said that requiring parents to purchase a separate seat for a child under 2 in order to use the proper restraint would not be cost-effective.

• Michael Woods

In World Book, see Safety.

Sexually Transmitted Diseases

- Hope for a herpes vaccine?
- STD knowledge
- Hidden spread of genital herpes
- Acyclovir and genital herpes

Researchers in 1996 were exploring the possibility of a vaccine to protect against genital herpes. The search was conducted in the face of a growing herpes epidemic in the United States, inadequate public understanding of the prevalence of the disease, and the risk of transmission by people with no signs of infection. Large pharmaceutical firms continued to conduct clinical trials. If the trials prove successful, a vaccine might be available by the year 2000.

In the early stages of development were vaccines that might offer stronger protection against herpes infection. These included vaccines using genetic material from the virus, vaccines using live but weakened herpes viruses, and vaccines created from viruses that had been genetically engineered so they could not reproduce. Experts were hopeful, but many researchers remained concerned about how well such vaccines would work, how to decide who would receive a vaccine, and whether a vaccine could be widely administered.

STD knowledge. Although sexually transmitted diseases (STD's) are a significant health problem, most people in the United States and five European countries still know little about them, according to a survey reported in August 1995. Even though 30 percent of the people surveyed knew someone who had an STD, about 40 percent could not name an STD other than AIDS.

The survey was conducted by the Gallup Organization and commissioned by the American Social Health Association, a nonprofit organization dedicated to preventing STD's. It included 1,000 participants each from France, Italy, Spain, Sweden, the United Kingdom, and the United States.

The Gallup survey also asked respondents to estimate how many people in their country had genital herpes. Although official estimates for the countries in the survey ranged from 10 to 25 percent, most adults replied that only 1 percent or less of the population was infected with the virus. Many participants in the United States estimated that only 0.1 percent had herpes.

The survey found that most people did not learn about STD's from their health-care providers. Two-thirds of the teen-agers surveyed first learned about STD's in school, compared with 36 percent of the adults. The poll also showed that teens were more likely than adults to know that STD's were widespread, that some STD's other than AIDS were incurable, and that some STD's had no symptoms. More than half the respondents said their health-care provider spent no time discussing STD's with them.

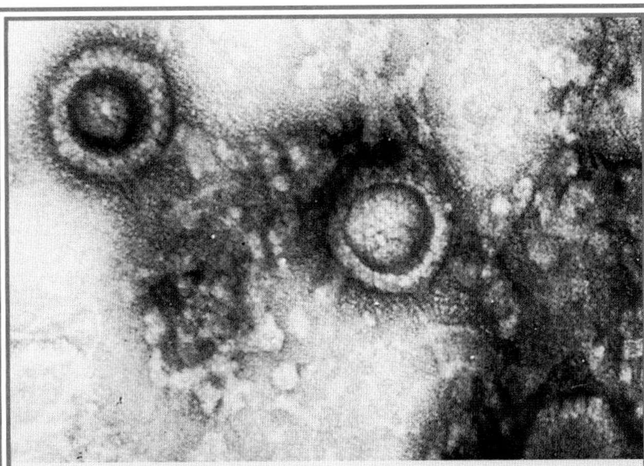

Living with a herpes infection

- A herpes outbreak usually begins 2 to 20 days after the initial infection and can last for several weeks.
- There is no cure for herpes. Although some people have no noticeable symptoms of the disease, the virus remains in the body. Most people with genital herpes experience five to eight outbreaks a year.
- Nonprescription pain relievers such as aspirin and ibuprofen can help ease the pain of an outbreak.
- The prescription drug acyclovir can reduce the duration and number of outbreaks, but it will not eliminate the virus. Acyclovir must be prescribed by a doctor.
- The National Herpes Hotline (sponsored by the American Social Health Association) offers assistance and information: (919) 361-8488 (Monday through Friday).

Sources: The National Herpes Hotline; *Herpes: A Complete Guide to Relief and Reassurance.*

Hidden spread of genital herpes. A theory that the herpes simplex virus (HSV) responsible for genital herpes is contagious even when a person has no symptoms of the disease received support from a study published in September 1995. Although physicians once thought HSV was contagious only when characteristic genital sores were present, researchers had suspected for more than a decade that the virus could be reactivated and transmitted without the presence of obvious symptoms—an occurrence known as *asymptomatic shedding.* But they did not know to what extent asymptomatic shedding occurred.

Over a period of 15 weeks, researchers at the University of Washington obtained daily samples of genital secretions from 110 women who were infected with HSV. The women also kept symptom diaries during the study period. On days when no observable *lesions* (sores) were present, researchers detected the live virus in the samples 2 percent of the time on average. Prior to the Washington study, some experts had estimated that up to 70 percent of people with herpes were infected by a partner who had no noticeable symptoms at the time of infection.

Acyclovir and genital herpes. Daily treatment with acyclovir—a drug designed to prevent the herpes virus from reproducing itself—greatly reduces the spread of herpes at times when no symptoms are present. This was the conclusion of another University of Washington study, which was published in January 1996.

In the study, women who had recently contracted genital herpes received daily treatment with acyclovir during half of a 15-week study period and a *placebo* (inactive substance) during the remaining half. Researchers found that acyclovir greatly reduced the number of days when the virus was active. Women receiving the placebo tested positive for the live virus on days when they had no lesions 5.8 percent of the time, compared with only 0.37 percent of the time for women on acyclovir—a reduction of 94 percent.

Researchers cautioned that they detected HSV by means of a *culture*—a test in which a virus grows in a substance—rather than through a more sensitive genetic test. Furthermore, because the study included only women, the researchers said additional studies were needed to examine the effects of acyclovir on asymptomatic shedding in men. Although the results indicate that acyclovir could become another tool for preventing the spread of genital herpes, the researchers stressed that using a condom at every sexual encounter was still the best defense.

• Peggy Clarke

In the section On the Medical Frontier, see SCIENCE VERSUS THE AIDS VIRUS. In WORLD BOOK, see AIDS; SEXUALLY TRANSMITTED DISEASE.

Skin

- Ulcer drug cures common warts
- New treatment for melanoma
- Pill treats fungal nail infections
- Creams help sun-damaged skin

Common warts can be eradicated with cimetidine, an oral drug which, under the trade name Tagamet, is used to treat gastrointestinal conditions such as ulcers. Researchers at the State University of New York at Brooklyn reported in June 1996 that they had successfully used cimetidine to treat warts in adults. Earlier tests had shown the effectiveness of cimetidine in treating children's warts.

Doctors had traditionally tried to remove warts—which are caused by a virus—at the skin surface by using *electrocautery* (a procedure in which an electrically heated wire is used to burn off the wart) or by applying liquid nitrogen or topical acids. None of these treatments is effective in all cases, and some are painful, especially if a patient has multiple warts.

The New York researchers gave 18 adults high doses of cimetidine three times a day for three months. By the end of the study, 67 percent of the patients were totally free of warts; 17 percent were partially free. Most of the patients who responded to the medication improved in six to eight weeks. After one year, the researchers reevaluated the patients who had improved and found that they were still free of warts. Cimetidine caused no adverse side effects, making it a safe and painless way to treat warts.

New treatment for melanoma. A significant breakthrough in the treatment of advanced melanoma, the most lethal form of skin cancer, was approved by the U.S. Food and Drug Administration (FDA) in December 1995. Researchers at 29 medical centers across the United States developed a treatment method using the drug interferon alpha-2b for patients who had been surgically treated for melanoma and were at high risk for developing a recurrence of the cancer. John M. Kirkwood, chief of medical *oncology* (cancer treatment) at the University of Pittsburgh, led the study.

Melanoma is a malignant tumor of the skin's pigment cells. According to the American Cancer Society, more than 38,000 people were expected to develop new cases of melanoma in 1996, and about 7,300 people would die of the disease.

Doctors at the 29 centers gave interferon alpha-2b—one of several kinds of interferon—to 287 patients for almost one year, both intravenously and by injection under the skin. Interferon is a naturally occurring protein produced by white blood cells that boosts the immune system. It was already being used to treat other cancers and hepatitis B, a liver disease caused by a virus.

The doctors found that interferon prolonged the time until the patient suffered a relapse of melanoma and lengthened the overall survival time by more than one year. While all patients experienced some side effects with interferon (usually of a flulike na-

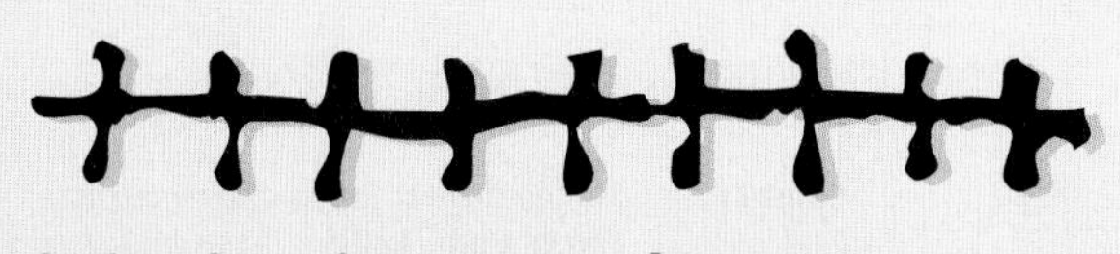

Caring for minor cuts and scrapes

Some wounds may seem minor but still require the attention of a physician. The American Academy of Family Physicians suggests that you call a doctor if any of the following conditions apply:

- The wound is jagged.
- The wound is on your face.
- The edges of the cut gape open.
- The cut becomes tender or inflamed.
- The cut drains a creamy, grayish fluid.
- You start to run a temperature over 100 °F (38 °C).
- The area around the wound feels numb.
- You can't move comfortably.
- Red streaks form near the wound.
- The wound is a deep cut or puncture wound, and you have not had a tetanus shot in the past five years.
- The cut bleeds in spurts, the blood soaks through the bandage, or the bleeding does not stop after 10 minutes of firm, direct pressure.

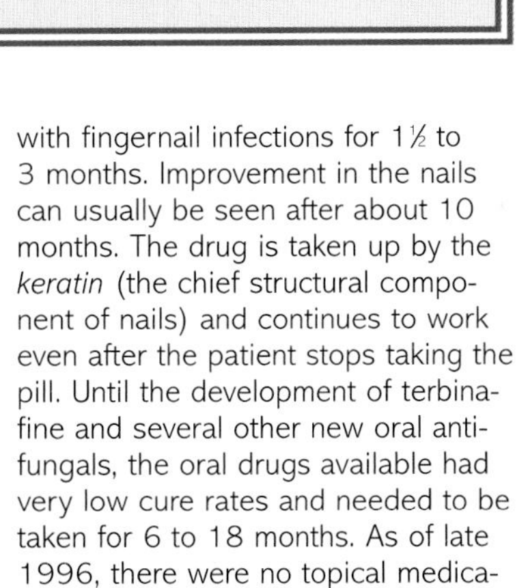

ture), it was the first agent to significantly benefit patients with advanced melanoma. Patients whose melanoma was recognized at an early stage—when the tumor was very shallow—had been successfully treated before, but no chemotherapy or radiation therapy had been effective once a melanoma *metastasized* (spread).

Pill treats fungal nail infections. An oral drug for treating fungal toenail and fingernail infections was approved for use by the FDA in May 1996. Terbinafine hydrochloride, whose trade name is Lamisil, had been available in pill form in 70 other countries for several years. In the United States, it had been used in a cream preparation. Fungal toenail and fingernail infections, in which nails become thick, discolored, misshapen, crumbly, and occasionally painful, affect about 10 million Americans.

Terbinafine is administered in doses of 250 milligrams once a day. Individuals with fungal toenail infections are treated for 3 to 6 months, and those with fingernail infections for 1½ to 3 months. Improvement in the nails can usually be seen after about 10 months. The drug is taken up by the *keratin* (the chief structural component of nails) and continues to work even after the patient stops taking the pill. Until the development of terbinafine and several other new oral antifungals, the oral drugs available had very low cure rates and needed to be taken for 6 to 18 months. As of late 1996, there were no topical medications that effectively cured fungal nail infections.

Terbinafine can safely be taken with many other commonly used medications, such as antihistamines, and, in most cases, causes only mild and temporary side effects. However, it is expensive: the average retail cost of one pill in 1996 was nearly $7, so a 12-week dose cost almost $600.

Creams help sun-damaged skin. Researchers at Massachusetts General Hospital in Boston reported in June 1996 that creams containing glycolic

UV index

The UV index is a forecast of the amount of ultraviolet radiation that will reach the earth's surface during the peak hour of sunlight. It is announced daily in many local weather reports. Find the UV index for a particular day in the left-hand column. The center column gives the general sunlight intensity corresponding to each value. The right-hand column gives the length of time you can safely stay in the sun.

UV index value	Sunlight intensity	Time until sunburn with unprotected exposure
0–2	Minimal	30 minutes for those who never tan/always burn; 120 for those who always tan/rarely burn.
3-4	Low	15 to 20 minutes for "always burns"; 75 to 90 minutes for "rarely burns."
5-6	Moderate	10 to 12 minutes for "always burns"; 50 to 60 minutes for "rarely burns."
7-9	High	7 to 8 minutes for "always burns"; 33 to 40 minutes for "rarely burns."
10-15	Very high	4 to 6 minutes for "always burns"; 20 to 30 minutes for "rarely burns."

Source: U.S. National Weather Service.

acid or lactic acid can help to decrease the signs of chronic sun damage to the skin. Glycolic and lactic acid are two of several alpha-hydroxy acids, which peel away dead skin. They are sold in cosmetic creams in varying concentrations.

The researchers divided the 67 participants in the study (women between 40 and 70 years of age) into two groups. One group applied a cream containing 8 percent glycolic acid to the face and forearms twice a day for 22 weeks; another group applied a cream containing 8 percent lactic acid; and a third group applied an acid-free cream. At the conclusion of the study, 70 percent of those using an acid-containing cream showed a modest improvement, while only 41 percent of the third group improved. The most significant improvements were a decrease in irregular pigmentation (brown spots), facial lines, and roughness. Only one patient experienced facial irritation, while several had facial redness. The researchers concluded that creams with 8 percent glycolic acid and 8 percent lactic acid are a safe over-the-counter preparation that can modestly improve the results of chronic sun damage.

• Kathryn E. Bowers

In the section A Healthy Family, see FEET: A USER'S MANUAL. In WORLD BOOK, see SKIN.

Smoking

- Youth smoking
- The tobacco war
- Ex-smoker wins lawsuit
- Organized medicine gets involved
- Smoking and childhood cancers
- Kicking the habit

President Bill Clinton in August 1996 announced new rules allowing the Food and Drug Administration (FDA) to regulate tobacco products. The new rules authorized the FDA to restrict tobacco advertising and sales in an effort to stop the sale and marketing of cigarettes to children. This new stance was triggered by an increase in teen-age smoking and mounting evidence that nicotine, a major component of tobacco, is a highly addictive drug.

According to a 1995 report from the Centers for Disease Control and Prevention in Atlanta, Georgia, the percentage of teen-agers who smoke had risen sharply since 1991. Smoking increased by 22 percent among eighth-graders between 1991 and 1994 and by 16 percent among tenth-graders. Such findings suggested the need for smoking-prevention programs that focus on youths as soon as they enter grade school.

Antitobacco activists and health officials in 1995 and 1996 became more vehement in accusing tobacco companies of targeting youths. While smoking among adults seemed to have steadily decreased over the previous few years, smoking among underage youths rose at an alarming rate. The FDA estimated that teens were spending about $1.26 billion on cigarettes each year.

Many medical experts contend that cigarette smoking is primarily a childhood addiction or disease and that most adults who smoke started in their youth and found later that they could not quit. In January 1996, the federal government issued rules governing how states should enforce a 1992 law that prohibits the sale of tobacco products to anyone under 18 years of age.

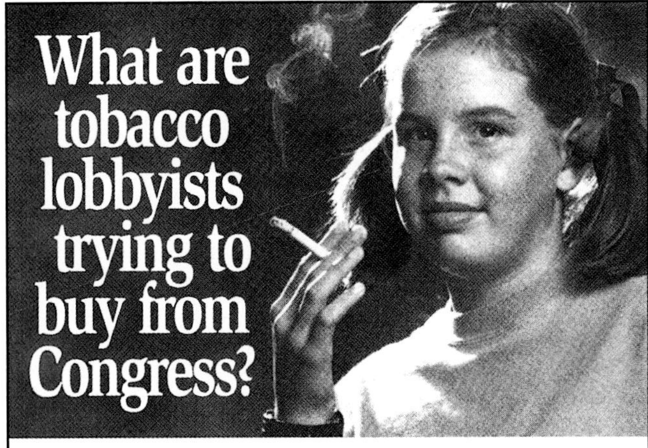

After decades of lying about addiction and disease, tobacco companies have launched a last-ditch scheme to continue marketing to kids: flood Congress with cash.

During the first half of 1995, tobacco industry contributions to political parties skyrocketed more than 400 percent. Tobacco companies gave more than $1.6 million ($1.5 million to Republicans), becoming the GOP's largest donor by far.

Why the sudden surge? President Clinton and Members of Congress from both parties are backing new limits on tobacco marketing to kids—limits that could save thousands of children from addiction, disease and death. Tobacco companies are desperately trying to buy opposition.

Voters want Congress to say no to the tobacco industry. More than 85 percent say Congress should support the administration's effort to protect children.

Write your Members of Congress today (U.S. Senate, Washington, DC 20510; U.S. House of Representatives, Washington, DC 20515). Tell them ***America's children aren't for sale.***

To learn more, call ***1-800-284-KIDS.***

This ad sponsored by the Congress of National Black Churches; American Academy of Family Physicians; Nationa Association of Elementary School Principals; Catholic Health Association; InterHealth/Protestant Health Alliance; National Association of County and City Health Officials; National Association of Evangelicals; American Public Health Association; General Board of Church and Society of the United Methodist Church; Secondhand Smoke Awareness Program, National Medical Association; and NETWORK: A National Catholic Social Justice Lobby.

CAMPAIGN for TOBACCO-FREE Kids

Attack on tobacco

The tobacco industry came under heavy attack in 1995 and 1996, particularly for its alleged targeting of young people in marketing cigarettes. President Bill Clinton in August 1996 authorized the Food and Drug Administration (FDA) to regulate tobacco products and set up a new program to stop the sale and marketing of cigarettes to children.

The tobacco war. The cigarette industry has stirred up controversy for decades, but tobacco companies bebecame much more aggressive in defending their rights in 1995, when the FDA began to consider recategorizing nicotine-containing tobacco products as drugs.

After Clinton's August 1996 announcement 1996, tobacco companies challenged the FDA's new powers in federal court. The business of selling cigarettes is extremely profitable, with expected sales of over $50 billion in 1996. Moreover, taxes on tobacco sales are an important source of revenue for governments throughout the world.

But states and individuals were increasingly filing lawsuits against tobacco companies to recover health expenditures for individuals who had suffered smoking-related illnesses and deaths. In May 1996, an important lawsuit against major U.S. tobacco companies and a tobacco lobbying group was dismissed by a federal appeals court in New Orleans, Louisiana. Three smokers and the husband of a smoker who died of lung cancer originally filed the suit in 1994. They had accused the tobacco industry of manipulating nicotine levels in cigarettes to keep smokers addicted and concealing knowledge of the dangers of smoking. The suit could have covered up to 50 million American smokers, but the court claimed that the case was too complex to manage.

Ex-smoker wins lawsuit. In August 1996, a jury in Jacksonville, Florida, awarded $750,000 to a man who developed lung cancer after more than 40 years of smoking. Grady Carter, who began smoking Lucky Strike cigarettes in 1947, sued the maker of the cigarettes, Brown & Williamson Tobacco Corporation, for $1.5 million. The jury found that the cigarette maker had been negligent in failing to inform the public about the danger of its product.

The verdict was only the second monetary award against a tobacco company in a liability case. The first was a $400,000 award won by a New Jersey family in 1988. That award was overturned on appeal.

Many observers believed that the outcome of the Florida case would open the door for future successful lawsuits against the tobacco industry. But Brown & Williamson expected to get the verdict overturned, and tobacco industry spokespersons called the jury's decision an aberration.

Organized medicine gets involved. In April 1996, the American Medical

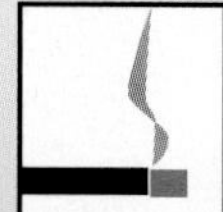

The smoker's "high"

Nicotine may not be the only reason why smoking is addictive, researchers at Brookhaven National Laboratory reported in February 1996. Using brain scans, the researchers found that smokers had 40 percent less than nonsmokers of a brain enzyme called monoamine oxidase B (MAO B). The function of MAO B is to break down dopamine, a brain chemical associated with feelings of pleasure. Less MAO B means more dopamine and increased pleasure.

Nerve cells communicate with one another by releasing chemicals such as dopamine. After release, some dopamine attaches to receptors on adjacent nerve cells, some is taken back up by the releasing cell, and some is broken down by the enzyme MAO B. An unidentified substance in tobacco smoke appears to deplete MAO B stores in the brain. As a result, more dopamine remains available to enhance the smoker's "high" that nicotine produces. Nicotine, scientists already knew, stimulates the release of dopamine.

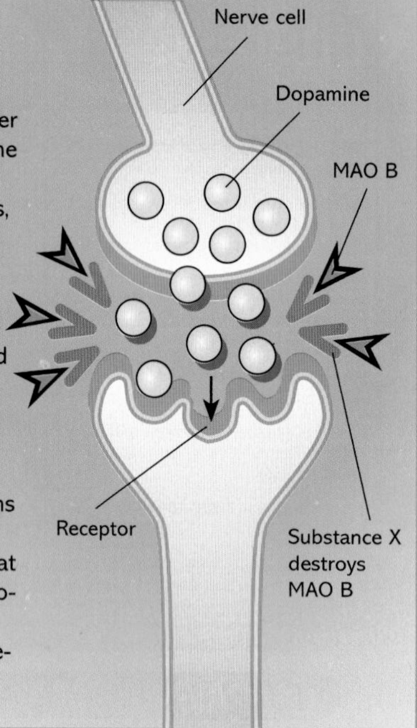

Association (AMA) called on individual and institutional investors to sell their holdings in 13 tobacco companies. In June, the AMA called for insurance companies and health maintenance organizations to do so as well.

The AMA also continued to support FDA involvement in regulating tobacco products, a vigorous physician campaign to help patients quit smoking, clear AMA positions emphasizing the addictive potential of nicotine, and attacks on tobacco advertising, particularly ads directed at youths.

Smoking and childhood cancers. *Carcinogens* (substances that can cause cancer) found in cigarette smoke can be transferred from a mother to her baby during pregnancy. That finding was reported in April 1996 by researchers at the University of Louisville School of Medicine in Kentucky.

The researchers obtained detailed smoking histories from over 400 pregnant women and took blood samples from both mother and baby after the women gave birth. They found that not only the smoking mothers, but also the nonsmoking mothers who spent several hours a day around smokers, had passed a significant amount of the toxic substances on to their babies. These compounds can cause damage to the genetic material in cells and may lead to childhood leukemia and cancers developing later in the babies, the researchers said.

Kicking the habit. In July 1996, the FDA approved the sale of two smoking-cessation aids without a prescription. Researchers and physicians have found that the nicotine *transdermal* patch (containing drugs that enter the body through the skin) and nicotine chewing gum are effective in helping patients stop smoking.

These two nicotine-replacement methods administer a controlled dose of nicotine that alleviates the difficulties associated with withdrawal from the drug. The dose is gradually lowered until the patient is no longer dependent on nicotine. In addition to helping eliminate addiction, nicotine-replacement therapy does not deliver the toxic contaminants found in cigarette smoke that are responsible for most of smoking's harmful effects.

Researchers also began exploring the potential of nicotine nasal sprays and inhalers as aids in smoking cessation. In March 1996, the FDA announced that it had approved the nasal sprays for sale, by prescription only. Nicotine nasal sprays work in much the same way as the nicotine patches or gum. But the FDA warned that smokers could become as dependent on a nasal spray as they are on cigarettes. The FDA advised that smokers should not use a nicotine spray for longer than six months.

• David C. Lewis

In WORLD BOOK, see SMOKING.

Stroke

- New treatment for stroke approved
- A second treatment for stroke
- Lower cholesterol prevents strokes

In June 1996, the Food and Drug Administration (FDA) approved *tissue plasminogen activator* (TPA), a clot-dissolving drug, for the treatment of *ischemic stroke,* a sudden loss of brain function caused by a blood clot.

Before the introduction of TPA, physicians could prescribe drugs to prevent strokes, but they had no medications with which to treat a stroke in progress. Often physicians could only wait for natural chemicals in the bloodstream to dissolve the clot, and then they assessed the damage to the brain.

The genetically engineered TPA is the same as the body's clot-dissolving chemicals, but the large dose restores blood flow sooner and, therefore, minimizes the damage to the brain. In December 1995, the National Institutes of Health in Bethesda, Maryland, reported that patients who received TPA were less likely to suffer disabilities from a stroke.

TPA does involve risks. Although it can treat ischemic stroke, it could worsen a stroke caused by a *cerebral hemorrhage* (bleeding from a blood vessel in the brain). Therefore, physicians must determine the cause of a stroke before administering TPA. Also, TPA can itself cause bleeding if the patient does not receive treatment within three hours of the onset of the stroke. Since timing is crucial, advocates of TPA began an effort to educate people about the early warning signs of stroke. Those signs include sudden weakness, loss of sensation on one side of the body, partial loss of vision, slurred speech, dizziness, mental confusion, and personality changes.

A second treatment for stroke. In December 1995, physicians at the Prince of Wales Hospital in Hong Kong reported successful results with a second treatment for stroke—*low-molecular-weight heparin.*

Low-molecular-weight heparin is an *anticoagulant* (also called a blood thinner), a chemical substance that inhibits the clotting of blood. Low-molecular-weight heparin has been used in conjunction with a high-molecular-weight form of the drug for the treatment of blood clots in the lower extremities.

Over a 10-day period, the 312 patients in the study received either low-molecular-weight heparin or a *placebo* (substance with no active ingredients) within 48 hours of the onset of a stroke. An analysis six months later showed fewer deaths and disabilities among the patients who received the low-molecular-weight heparin. While specialists stated the need for further research, the study offered hope for stroke victims who cannot be treated with TPA. As of July 1996, the FDA had not yet approved this treatment.

First treatment for stroke

In June 1996, the Food and Drug Administration approved *tissue plasminogen activator* (TPA) for the treatment of *ischemic stroke,* which is caused by a blood clot in the brain. A large dose of TPA breaks up the clot and restores the flow of blood, preventing further damage to the brain. Diagnosing the stroke quickly is important. If more than three hours have elapsed since the onset of the stroke, TPA can cause *hemorrhaging* (bleeding) in the brain. The effectiveness of this treatment depends on knowing the symptoms of a stroke and seeking immediate help.

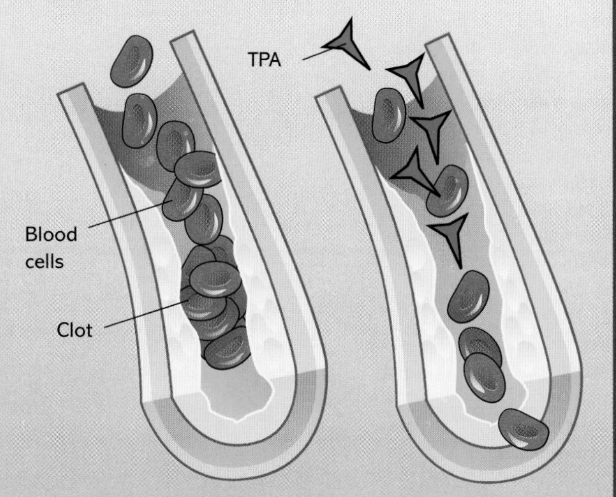

Lower cholesterol prevents strokes. In March 1996, researchers at the University of Southern California reported that lowering cholesterol can help prevent strokes.

As people age, cholesterol can contribute to the build-up of fatty deposits on the walls of the *carotid arteries,* causing them to thicken and harden. The carotid arteries are the major blood vessels supplying the brain with oxygen and nutrients. Blood clots can form in the hardened arteries and break loose, causing a stroke when they lodge in the brain.

The researchers studied the thickness of the carotid arteries in 188 patients, ranging in age from 37 to 67. The researchers divided the patients into two groups, one receiving a low-cholesterol diet and the drug lovastatin to lower cholesterol, and the other receiving the same diet with a placebo. Lovastatin treatment reversed the build-up of deposits in the carotid arteries. After four years of treatment, the deposits in the arteries of the drug-treated group were not as thick as the deposits in the other group's arteries. The investigators concluded that careful attention to cholesterol levels and aggressive treatment of individuals with high cholesterol could lead to a reduction in strokes. • James N. Davis

In WORLD BOOK, see STROKE.

Surgery

- Cancer risk associated with drug for chronic heartburn
- Treating breast cancer
- Cool operating rooms may be bad for patients

Many people suffer chronic attacks of heartburn, known medically as gastroesophageal reflux disease, and are put on long-term treatment with omeprazole, a drug that suppresses acid production in the stomach. But a study reported in April 1996 by investigators at the University of Gothenburg in Sweden and the Free University Hospital in Amsterdam, the Netherlands, found that some people treated with omeprazole are at increased risk for developing a condition that can lead to stomach cancer.

Doctors have long known that the suppression of stomach acid over long periods can pave the way for infection with *Helicobacter pylori.* An infection of *H. pylori* destroys the stomach's inner lining, a condition called atrophic gastritis, which increases the risk of developing stomach cancer.

The researchers studied patients in Sweden who underwent an operation to prevent stomach acid from backing up into the *esophagus,* the tube connecting the mouth and the stomach. In this procedure, called a fundoplication, part of the stomach is wrapped around the lower esophagus to increase pressure on a muscle that blocks the backward flow of acid.

The researchers compared the Swedish patients with patients in the

Troubling success

The success of organ transplants in the United States has created an increased demand for organs, but the number of donors has not increased proportionately. In 1994, surgeons in the United States performed more than 18,000 organ transplants, according to the United Network for Organ Sharing. Thousands of others met the criteria to qualify for a transplant, but some 3,000 died while waiting for an organ to become available.

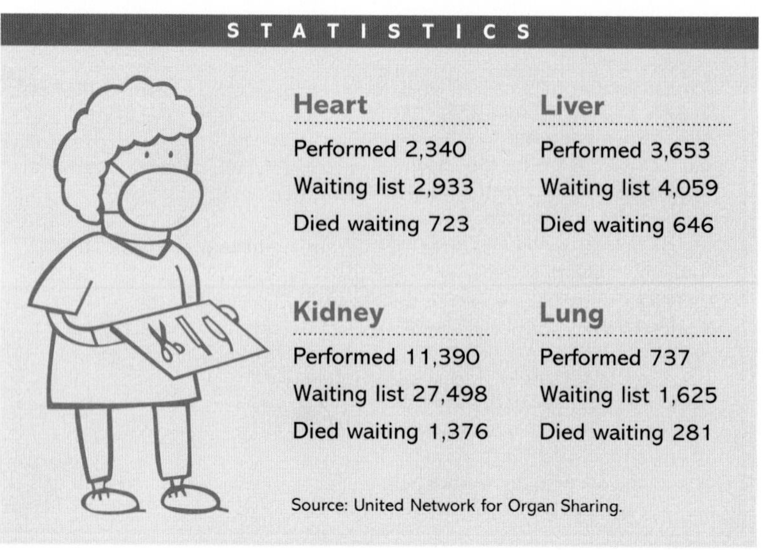

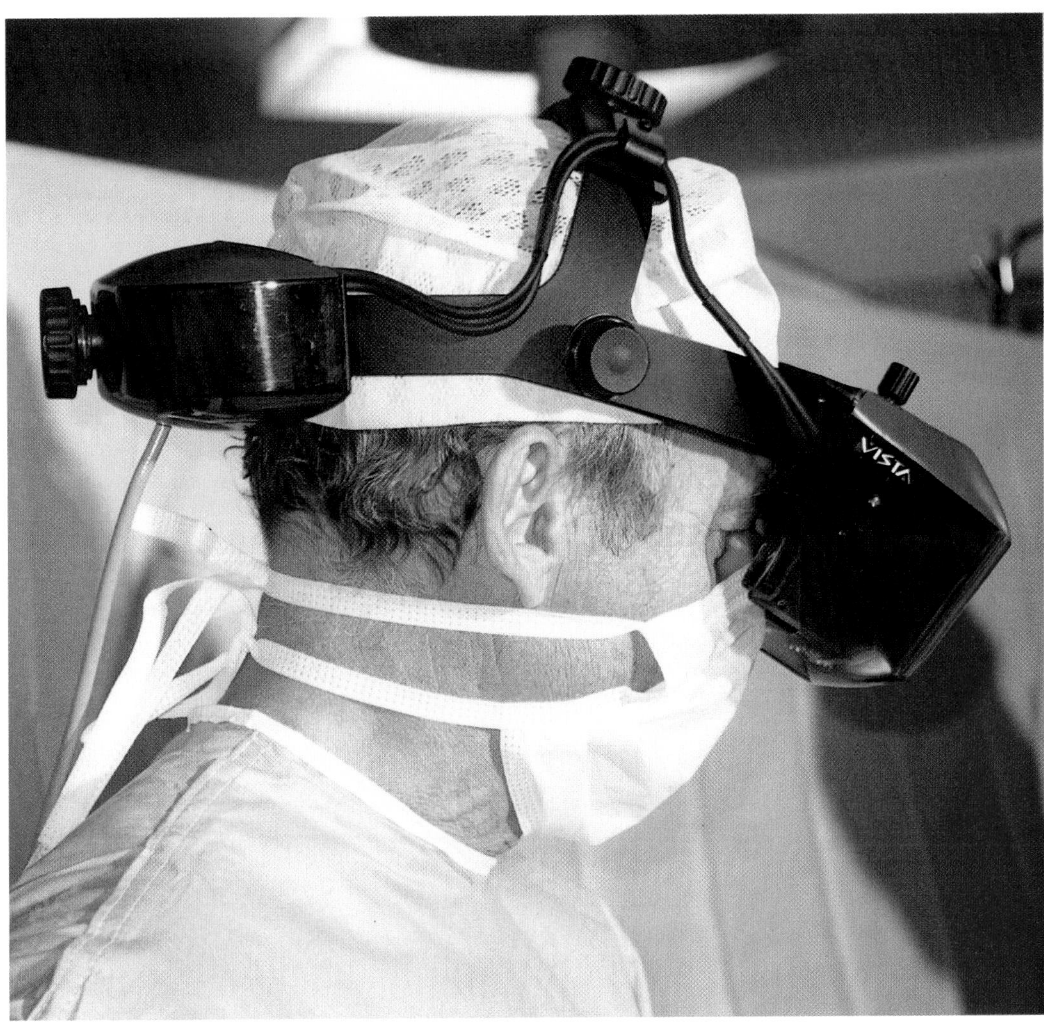

Heart surgery in 3D

A surgeon at the New England Medical Center in Boston performs an operation to replace heart valves assisted by a special visor developed by Vista Medical Technologies of Carlsbad, California, that enables him to view his work in three dimensions. Tiny screens in the visor, one for each eye, receive transmissions from a camera that processes two separate signals from optical fibers in an *endoscope,* a lighted, tubular device that is threaded through an artery to view interior organs.

Netherlands who were given daily doses of omeprazole, which blocks the activity of cells that produce acid in the stomach. The scientists followed both sets of patients from three to eight years in order to compare the long-term effects of the two treatments.

None of the 72 Swedish patients developed atrophic gastritis, even though 31 had been diagnosed as being infected with *H. pylori* before surgery. None of the 105 Dutch patients had atrophic gastritis at the beginning of the study. However, 18 of the 59 Dutch patients infected with *H. pylori* at the beginning of the study and 2 of the 46 patients who were not infected did develop gastritis.

The researchers concluded that patients with chronic heartburn and *H. pylori* infection who are treated with omeprazole are at increased risk for atrophic gastritis. They advised doctors to consider the long-term effects when choosing between surgery or drug treatment.

Treating breast cancer. Patients with early-stage invasive breast cancer are increasingly being treated with surgery followed by radiation, then *chemotherapy* (drugs that kill cancer cells). However, no research on the effectiveness of this treatment order had been reported until May 1996, when Boston researchers reported the results of their study of 244 patients with breast cancer that showed signs of spreading.

The treatment of breast cancer long focused on surgery to remove the tumor with all or part of the breast. When necessary, this was followed by radiation. In the mid-1970's, this approach was challenged by the fact that, despite the treatment, many cancers still spread and patient survival rates were poor. Therefore, doctors increasingly added chemotherapy to the treatment regimen for breast cancer patients.

In their study, the Boston scientists randomly assigned the 244 patients to receive a 12-week course of chemotherapy either before or after radiation therapy. The patients had all undergone surgery that removed the tumor with a small rim of normal tissue. The operations were performed between June 1984 and December 1992.

The researchers found that 38 percent of the patients in the radiation-first group had a recurrence of cancer. For the patients who received chemotherapy before radiation, 31 percent had a recurrence of cancer. Overall, 73 percent of the patients treated with radiation first were alive five years after surgery, compared with 81 percent of the patients treated with chemotherapy first.

The researchers concluded that early treatment with 12 weeks of chemotherapy followed by radiation controlled the spread of cancer better than radiation followed by chemotherapy. They said further study was needed to confirm their findings. They also said they had not studied the effects of taking tamoxifen, a drug commonly given to breast cancer patients in the 1990's, because too few patients in their study were taking it.

Cool operating rooms. The temperature in an operating room is often kept relatively low for the comfort of the surgical team, who work in gowns, gloves, and masks under hot lights. But for patients, this often leads to *hypothermia* (subnormal body temperature). A study reported in May 1996 found a link between surgical patients' hypothermia and delayed healing, as well as a possible predisposition to infections.

Researchers at the University of California at San Francisco and the University of Vienna in Austria enrolled 200 patients who were having major colon and rectal surgery at various Austrian hospitals. The patients were assigned at random either to receive measures to keep their body temperature near normal during surgery, such as with warm air or warm intravenous solutions, or to not receive such measures. In the patients who were not warmed, the average body temperature during surgery dropped to about 95 °F (35 °C). In the group receiving warming, the average body temperature held at about 98 °F (37 °C).

The researchers examined the patients' wounds throughout the postoperative period to see if body temperature during surgery had any impact on healing. Infections occurred in 18 of the 96 patients in the hypothermia group, and in only 6 of the 104 patients kept warm during surgery. The average length of stay in the hospital for the hypothermia group was 2.6 days longer than the average stay for the group that was kept warm.

Mild hypothermia is common in patients having major abdominal surgery. In addition to exposure to cold air in the operating room, anesthesia impairs the ability of the body to regulate heat and to distribute it throughout the body.

However, the California study suggested that maintaining normal body temperature during surgery might both improve surgical outcomes and lower the cost of care by making it possible to release patients sooner from the hospital. Moreover, measures to control the operating-room temperature or to keep a patient's body temperature near normal were relatively inexpensive. The scientists said more studies were needed to determine whether the findings for colon and rectal surgery would hold true for other kinds of abdominal surgery as well and to identify any adverse effects of patient warming.

• **Richard A. Prinz**

In the section A Healthy Family, see HEARTBURN: TAKING AIM AT FIRE. In the section On the Medical Frontier, see ACTIVE LIVES WITH ARTIFICIAL JOINTS; LASER SURGERY COMES INTO FOCUS. In WORLD BOOK, see SURGERY.

Urology

A six-month clinical study conducted in the United States concluded in April 1996 that an injection used to treat men with *impotence* (the inability to achieve an erection) is both safe and effective. The drug, prostaglandin E1 (alprostadil), was approved for general use by the Food and Drug Administration (FDA) in mid-1995. It is sold under the brand name Caverject. The study reported that the drug produced an erection 94 percent of the time, and that sexual intercourse was described as satisfactory by 87 percent of the men and 86 percent of their partners.

Impotence is a common problem in men, and it increases in frequency with age. Its causes can include hormonal imbalance, nerve damage, inadequate blood flow to the penis, and psychological causes. Alprostadil works by relaxing muscle tissue, which allows dilation of blood vessels in the penis, leading to an erection.

Treatment with alprostadil begins with a test injection in a physician's office. After the proper dosage is determined, patients are instructed how to perform penile injections and receive a prescription for the medication. The injection is generally effective in producing an erection within 5 to 20 minutes. Potential side effects associated with the use of penile injections of alprostadil include bruising and swelling, prolonged erections, pain, and scarring on the penis. However, physicians who tested the new therapy said that, when used correctly, it is generally safe and effective.

Significance of prostate tumors. In recent years, a new method of prostate cancer detection has increased both the number of men diagnosed with prostate cancer and the percentage of men whose tumors are detected early and are potentially curable. However, concern has been raised that some cancers detected by the new method—a blood test known as a PSA test—may not require treatment, because they are growing too slowly to cause significant symptoms during a patient's lifetime.

In a report published in January 1996, researchers at the Mayo Clinic in Rochester, Minnesota, and the University of Michigan analyzed prostate tumors surgically removed from 337 men. Using such factors as the time required for cancers to develop and the age and overall health of the subjects, the investigators tried to determine how many of the tumors would have remained harmless during the men's natural lifetime and therefore did not need to be removed. The study concluded that most of the tumors would most likely have caused symptoms and death if left untreated. However, reliable evidence of when screening and treatment are of bene-

Preventing cystitis

Cystitis is an inflammation of the bladder usually caused by a bacterial infection. The primary symptoms are a burning sensation during urination and a frequent urge to urinate. The bacteria usually enter through the *urethra,* the tube that carries urine from the bladder. Because their urethra is much shorter than men's, women are more likely to contract cystitis. In some women, cystitis becomes chronic. Physicians recommend several precautions to help prevent recurrences:

- Drinking plenty of fluids—one glass every hour—helps flush bacteria from the urinary tract. Cranberry juice can also help by making the bladder less hospitable to bacteria.
- Wiping from front to back can help women prevent intestinal bacteria from entering the urethra.
- Emptying the bladder immediately after sexual intercourse can help flush bacteria from the urethra.

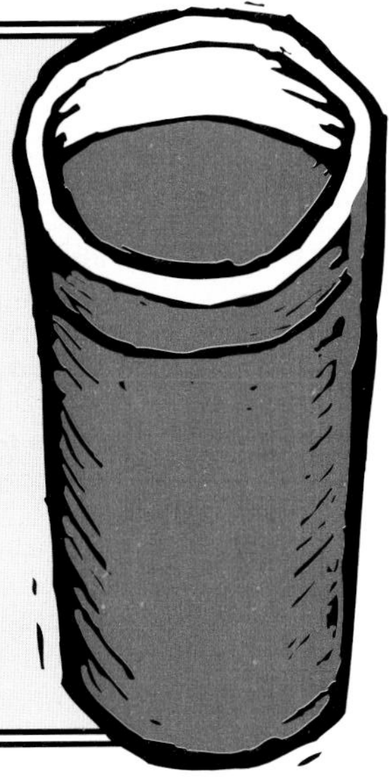

fit can come only from randomized clinical trials. Such trials were underway in the U.S. and Europe in 1996.

A new test for bladder cancer received FDA approval in late 1995. The procedure, called a BTA test, uses a urine sample to tell if cells in the lining of the urinary bladder have been damaged by BTA, a substance secreted by bladder tumors.

Most people with bladder cancer have tumors that can be removed using an *endoscope,* a thin, flexible tube with a tiny video camera on the end. A cutting tool can be threaded through the tube. The endoscope is inserted through the urethra into the bladder. However, tumors may reappear in many patients, making frequent follow-up procedures necessary. Most patients must undergo an endoscopic examination of the bladder every three months. The BTA test, however, requires only a urine sample. A test strip is inserted into the sample, and immediate color changes in the strip indicate the result.

Studies have indicated that the BTA test is up to 70 percent accurate, a rate much higher than other nonsurgical methods. However, visual inspection with an endoscope remains the most accurate means of diagnosing bladder cancer. • Glenn S. Gerber

In World Book, see Prostate gland.

Veterinary Medicine

- Mad cow disease in the United Kingdom (UK)
- Cat vaccines and cancer
- Wolf hybrids as pets

Veterinary medicine, human health, and food safety intertwined in a controversial issue on March 20, 1996, when a panel of British scientists claimed that 10 people in England who had a rare, fatal brain disease may have contracted the illness by eating contaminated beef. The cattle were afflicted with an unusual central nervous system disorder called bovine spongiform encephalopathy (BSE), commonly called mad cow disease because an infected animal stumbles in circles, appearing crazy.

Since 1986, over 160,000 cattle on 33,000 farms in Britain had been diagnosed with BSE, compared with fewer than 400 cattle in the rest of the world. British scientists said domestic herds became infected with BSE through feed supplements made from the tissue of sheep that had scrapie, a disease closely related to BSE. The UK banned the use of sheep by-products in cattle feed in 1988, and BSE declined. New cases occurred mainly in cattle born before the ban was fully implemented.

BSE and scrapie are caused by a poorly understood type of protein called a prion rather than by a bacterium or a virus. The diseases slowly create tiny holes in the nerve cells of the brain, causing mental deterioration and eventually death.

Like BSE and scrapie in animals, the human illness—Creutzfeldt-Jakob Disease (CJD)—also damages the brain by creating tiny holes in nerve cells. Under the microscope, brain tissue from people with CJD closely resembles that from cattle with BSE and sheep with scrapie. CJD usually strikes people in their 50's and 60's, but the average age of the 10 British people was 27 years.

The causal link between eating beef from cattle with BSE and CJD remained far from proven. Still, in June 1996, the UK agreed to a program to destroy about 120,000 cattle most at risk for BSE in an effort to convince the public that diseased beef would not reach world markets. The United States stopped importing British beef in 1989 to protect Americans from contaminated meat. The United States has had no documented cases of BSE.

Cat vaccines and cancer. Vaccines are designed to protect against disease, but in some cats vaccination gives rise to a deadly cancer. Since the late 1980's, an increasing number of cats have been diagnosed with sarcoma, a type of cancerous tumor that often leads to death. The tumor arises at the vaccination site several months to several years after a vaccination has been administered.

In most cases, vaccines against either the feline leukemia virus or the rabies virus are the culprits, according to a review of the literature on cancer and vaccines reported in January 1996. These vaccines contain high levels of viral *antigen* (a foreign

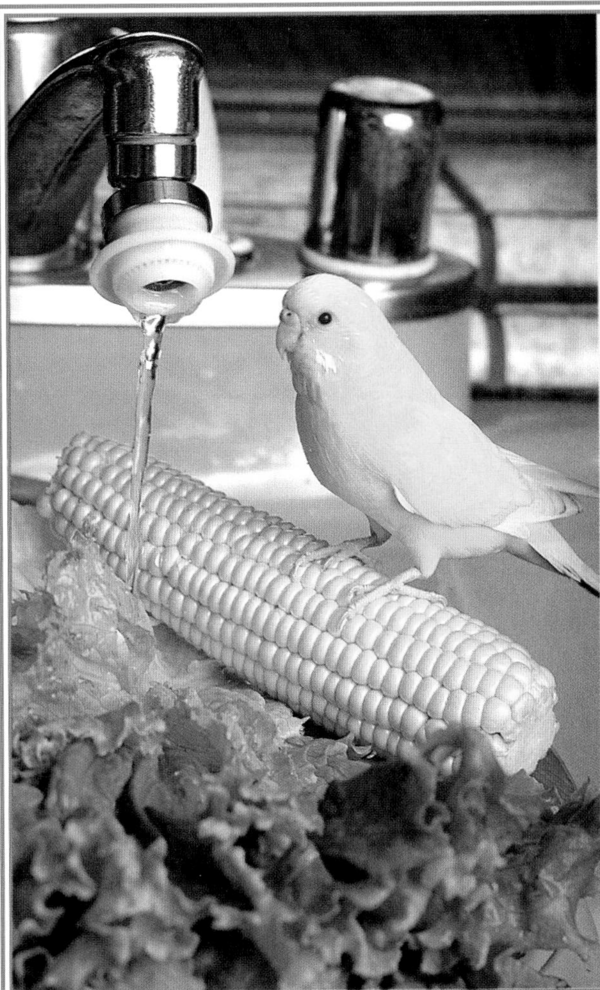

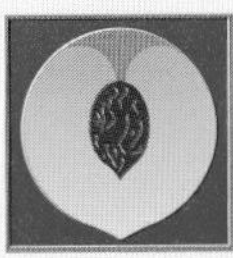

Pet birds need veggies

Beets, corn, kale, red peppers, and squash, cooked or raw, should be part of a pet bird's diet, according to the Association of Avian Veterinarians (AAV). Vegetables and fruits such as raisins, apples, pears, and melon should make up about 25 percent of a bird's diet. Pasta, beans, potatoes, and other starches, including seed—often the only food a pet bird gets—should constitute only about half its daily fare. The AVA says the rest of the diet for parakeets, cockatiels, parrots, and lovebirds—all hookbills—should be protein provided by cooked meat, poultry, fish, and eggs, or yogurt and cheese. Good nutrition can add years to a pet's life.

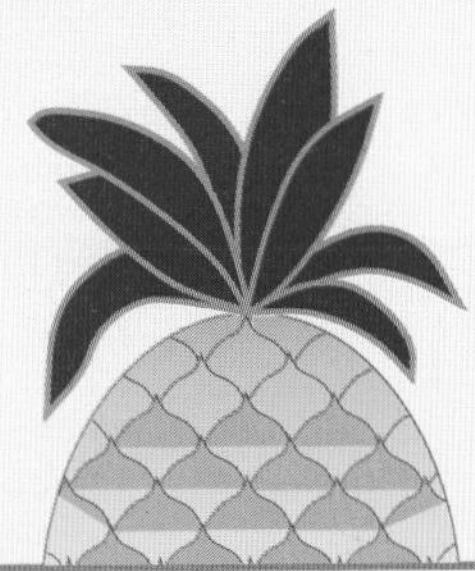

substance against which the body mounts an immune reaction) or a chemical that boosts the cat's immune response. Veterinary scientists theorized that the inflammation routinely occurring after a vaccination somehow induces normal cells to multiply out of control, forming a tumor.

Veterinarians estimated that approximately 1 in 5,000 to 10,000 vaccinated cats develops sarcoma. Still, they continued to recommend vaccination for the benefit of feline and public health because in many areas cats are at high risk of exposure to feline leukemia and rabies. Researchers advised that the vaccines be given at different body sites to minimize the risk of tumors.

Wolf hybrids as pets. In late 1995, the American Veterinary Medical Association (AVMA) came out strongly against keeping the hybrid offspring of wolves and dogs as pets. It said the selling of such animals should cease. The AVMA cited strong evidence of the aggressive, unpredictable behavior of dog-wolf hybrids and warned that the half-wild canines can inflict severe injuries on other animals and people. No rabies vaccine had been approved for hybrids. Some states had outlawed ownership of hybrids, potentially making it illegal for veterinarians to treat them. But the animals rose in popularity in 1995 and 1996. • Philip H. Kass

In World Book, see Veterinary medicine.

Weight Control

- Physical activity and overweight
- Fake fat gets FDA OK
- Researchers find leptin receptor
- New antiobesity drug

More than one-third of overweight adults in the United States are physically inactive during their leisure time. That was the finding reported by researchers at the Centers for Disease Control and Prevention (CDC) in Atlanta, Georgia, in March 1996. The researchers also noted that people who were trying to lose pounds or prevent weight gain were more active than those who were not trying to do either.

Many weight-loss experts define overweight by using a measurement called body mass index (BMI), which reflects body fat more accurately than a standard height and weight chart. BMI can be calculated by taking a person's weight (measured in kilograms) and dividing it by his or her height (measured in meters) squared. Men are considered overweight if their BMI is over 27.8, and women, if their BMI is over 27.3. In the United States, 28 percent of men and 27 percent of women were overweight in 1994, according to the CDC report.

The CDC researchers analyzed the results of a random telephone survey of 103,690 adults conducted in 1994 in all 50 U.S. states and Washington, D.C. More than 25,000 of the adults in the survey indicated that they were overweight. The researchers found that 37 percent of the overweight adults (33 percent of the men and 41 percent of the women) reported that they participated in no physical activity during their leisure time. The researchers also noted that older people and those who were the most overweight reported less physical activity than other respondents. In addition, the respondents with higher levels of education were more active than those with less education. This finding suggested to the researchers that awareness of the value of exercise may play a role in how likely a person is to be physically active.

The CDC and the American College of Sports Medicine recommend that adults engage in moderate to intense physical activity for 30 minutes on most, and preferably all, days of the week. This is especially important for people who are overweight, because they are at higher risk for developing heart disease, diabetes, and some cancers.

Fake fat gets FDA OK. The U.S. Food and Drug Administration (FDA) in January 1996 approved the use of olestra, a fat-based substitute for ordinary fat, in certain snack foods. Procter & Gamble, the developer of olestra, began test-marketing potato and tortilla chips made with the product in three cities in the United States in mid-1996.

Olestra, marketed under the name Olean, is composed of sucrose polyester, a substance made from sugar

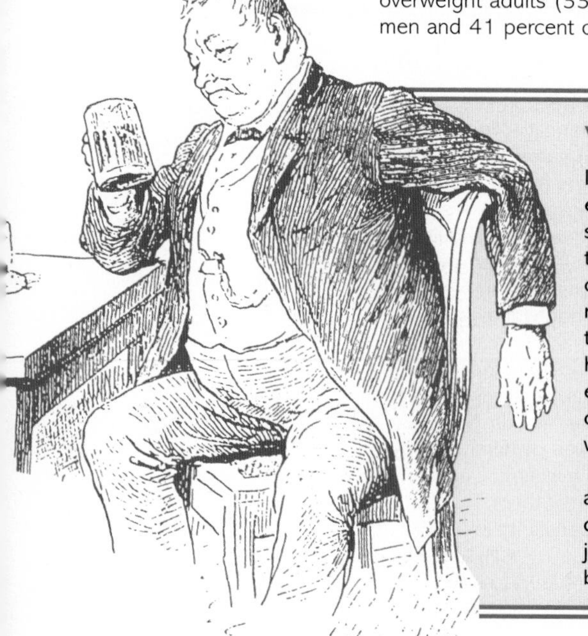

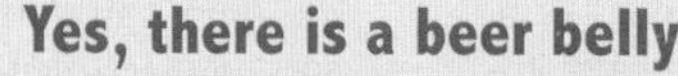

Yes, there is a beer belly

In case you thought the term *beer belly* offered a naive explanation for an oversized waistline, think again. A study of more than 12,000 American adults confirmed that people who drink at least six beers a week have, on average, a slightly greater waist-to-hip ratio than nondrinkers. (A high waist-to-hip ratio has been shown to increase a person's risk for high blood pressure, heart disease, stroke, and diabetes.) The study, reported in November 1995 by researchers at the University of North Carolina, also found that people who drink wine tend to have smaller waists than nondrinkers.

The results, however, were not an invitation to build a wine cellar. The study did not say that the drinks caused the differences in waistlines. The culprit may just as well have been the burgers and fries that the beers washed down.

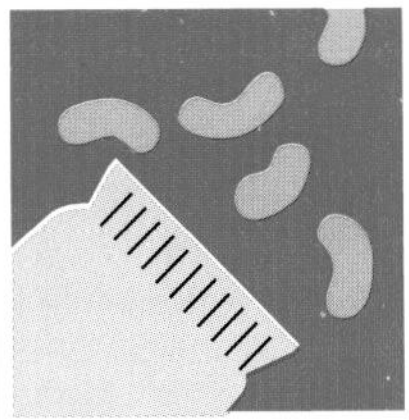

A dieter's dream?

In January 1996, the Food and Drug Administration (FDA) approved the use of olestra, a fat substitute, in snack foods such as potato chips. Some health experts and consumer groups, however, were not pleased with the action.

Olestra, marketed as Olean, tastes like fat and feels oily like fat, but it does not add calories to food because the body cannot absorb it. Olestra is intended to let people enjoy their favorite snack foods and still control their weight.

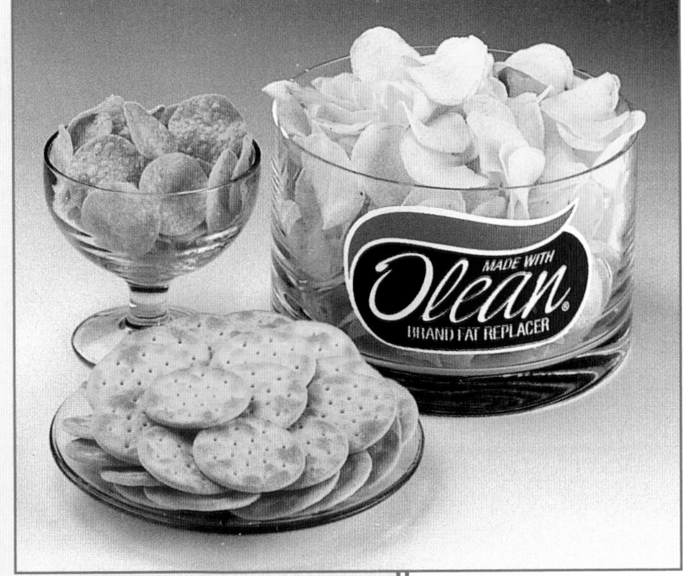

Olestra does have drawbacks. It can cause abdominal cramps and diarrhea, and it robs the body of the fat-soluble vitamins A, D, E, and K as well as carotenoids, a group of nutrients believed to protect against heart disease and cancer. The FDA requires olestra's manufacturer, Procter & Gamble, to add the four vitamins to snack foods made with olestra, but it does not require the addition of carotenoids.

Critics of the FDA action expressed concern about the lack of research on olestra's long-term safety. Some nutrition experts also disapproved of promoting fat-free snack foods with little nutritional value as a healthy choice for weight loss.

and vegetable oil. The vegetable oil contains extra molecular components called fatty acids, making it impossible for digestive enzymes to break down the oil. Thus, olestra passes through the body without being digested, and the body absorbs none of the calories or fat that it normally takes in from fatty foods.

Although many chip lovers said the fat-free chips taste like the real thing, olestra-based products were expected to cost up to twice as much as regular snacks. A bigger concern than price, however, was that some people experience gastrointestinal problems after eating products containing olestra. The Center for Science in the Public Interest, a Washington, D.C.-based consumer interest group, began a campaign to overturn the FDA approval, claiming that people eating olestra are "uninformed guinea pigs."

Because of the concern over safety, the FDA required that products containing olestra carry a warning label saying that they "may cause abdominal cramping and loose stools." The FDA also required that Procter & Gamble add vitamins A, D, E, and K to olestra, since olestra inhibits the absorption of these nutrients. Procter & Gamble agreed to conduct follow-up studies on the long-term effects of olestra, and the FDA planned to review the studies within 30 months of the approval date. To avoid side effects, nutritionists cautioned snackers to limit their chip consumption to an ounce (28 grams) or so at a time.

Researchers find leptin receptor. Three research groups reported the discovery of a *receptor* (molecular docking site) for the hormone leptin in February 1996. Leptin was found to be a key weight-control hormone in 1994, when molecular biologist Jeffrey Friedman of Rockefeller University in New York City and his coworkers first identified it in a genetically obese strain of mice. The Friedman group reported that the *ob* (for obese) strain of mice was deficient in leptin and, when given leptin, lost weight. Leptin is thought to serve as a fullness signal, telling the brain to block the feeling of hunger. Friedman's group found that humans also manufacture leptin, which led researchers to hope that increasing the body's supply of leptin might be a new way to lose weight.

But that hope was soon disappointed. Just days after Friedman's group reported its findings, biochemist Robert Considine of Thomas Jefferson University in Philadelphia and his colleagues reported that the concentration of leptin in fat tissue increases in proportion to increasing body weight in humans. Because obese people were found to have high leptin levels, a deficit of the hormone was obviously not responsible for their condition. In addition, Considine found that in seven obese people who lost weight, leptin levels continued to decline until they stopped losing weight, then increased as they maintained the lower weight. The researchers concluded that obesity in humans may result from a failure of cells in the brain to respond to leptin, rather than to a lack of leptin.

The search was on to identify the gene that produces the leptin receptor. An important breakthrough came from the study of a different type of genetically obese mice, called *db* for diabetic. This strain of mice, researchers had shown in the 1970's, has high leptin levels but apparently cannot process leptin's signal to stop eating. Thus, the researchers suspected that the *db* gene may be the one that encodes the leptin receptor.

Jeffrey Friedman's group at Rockefeller University, molecular biologist Rudolph Liebel's team at the same institution, and molecular biologist Louis Tartaglia's group at Millennium Pharmaceuticals Inc. in Cambridge, Massachusetts, all reported in February 1996 that the leptin receptor is the product of the *db* gene. They hoped that further studies on how the leptin receptor works may lead to the development of new weight-control drugs or other treatments.

New antiobesity drug. Dexfenfluramine, a new drug to fight obesity, received FDA approval in April 1996. Wyeth-Ayerst Laboratories, the developer of dexfenfluramine, sold the drug by prescription under the name Redux. Dexfenfluramine was the first antiobesity drug to receive FDA approval since 1974.

Dexfenfluramine works by increasing levels of a *neurotransmitter* (chemical that transmits nerve signals) called serotonin. Serotonin produces a feeling of fullness and satisfaction, thus limiting the amount that a person wants to eat. However, dexfenfluramine is not a miracle cure for obesity. In clinical studies the drug enabled about 60 percent of obese subjects to lose 10 percent of their body weight in a year's time, but that was just half the amount they needed to lose. Generally, diet and exercise result in a 10 percent weight loss over the course of a year in about 30 percent of obese individuals. In some people, the use of the drug resulted in no weight loss at all.

Some consumer groups and neurologists raised concern over the FDA approval of the new drug, citing the fact that long-term side effects were unknown. In addition, dexfenfluramine caused a potentially fatal heart and lung condition in a small number of laboratory animals. However, as some of the FDA committee members pointed out, in most cases the side effects of dexfenfluramine—sleep disruption, moodiness, and short-term memory lapses—were less severe than those of other drugs prescribed for weight control. Redux must be taken under a physician's supervision, with frequent blood tests to monitor its effects. • Ricki Lewis

In the section On the Medical Frontier, see NEW WEAPONS IN THE WAR AGAINST WEIGHT. In WORLD BOOK, see WEIGHT CONTROL.

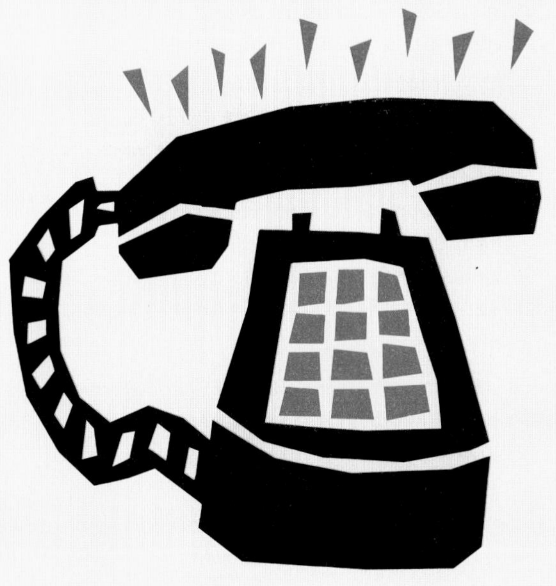

1997 Directory of health resources

A wealth of health information is available by telephone and through your home computer. Listed below are some useful phone numbers and on-line addresses. If you know of a toll-free service that is not listed here, you can call toll-free directory assistance at 800-555-1212.

AGING

☎ **National Institute on Aging Information Center** (800-222-2225) provides written information and referrals on various issues affecting aging or elderly people weekdays from 8:30 a.m. to 5 p.m. Eastern time. Hearing-impaired people can reach the institute by TDD at 800-222-4225.
Web site: http://www.aoa.dhhs.gov/aoa/resource.html

☎ **Older Women's League** (800-825-3695) provides written information, answers questions, and makes referrals to support groups and local chapters weekdays from 9 a.m. to 5 p.m. Eastern time.
E-mail: seidokid@aol

AIDS

☎ **HIV/AIDS Clinical Trials Information Service** (800-874-2572) answers questions and sends written materials on trials for drugs and experimental therapies weekdays from 9 a.m. to 7 p.m. Eastern time.
E-mail: actis@cdcnac.org
Web site: http://www.actis.org

☎ **HIV/AIDS Treatment Information Service** (800-448-0440) provides information on treatment options and treatment guidelines and refers callers to sources of additional information on these topics weekdays from 9 a.m. to 7 p.m. Eastern time.
E-mail: atis@cdcnac.org
Web site: http://www.hivatis.org

☎ **National AIDS Hot Line** (800-342-AIDS), operated by the Centers for Disease Control and Prevention, provides information and referrals 24 hours a day, 7 days a week. Spanish-language information is available at 800-344-7432, 7 days a week from 8 a.m. to 2 a.m. Eastern time. People who are hearing impaired can call 800-243-7889 weekdays from 10 a.m. to 10 p.m. Eastern time.
Web site: http://sunsite.unc.edu/ASHA/

☎ **Project Inform National HIV/AIDS Treatment Hot Line** (800-822-7422) answers questions about treatment of HIV and AIDS and provides referrals to local sources of assistance for HIV- and AIDS-related problems Monday through Saturday from 10 a.m. to 4 p.m. Pacific time.
Web site: http://www.projinf.org/

ALCOHOLISM AND DRUG ABUSE

☎ **Alcohol and Drug Help Line** (800-821-4357) provides referrals to local treatment centers nationwide 24 hours a day, 7 days a week.

☎ **American Council on Alcoholism** (800-527-5344) answers questions and provides written information and educational materials weekdays from 9 a.m. to 5 p.m. Eastern time. An answering service operates after regular hours.

☎ **National Cocaine Hot Line** (800-262-2463) provides referrals to local treatment centers 24 hours a day, 7 days a week.

☎ **National Council on Alcoholism and Drug Dependence, Inc.** (800-622-2255) provides referrals through voice mail to affiliates that offer counseling and answer questions.

☎ **Center for Substance Abuse Treatment** (800-662-HELP) sends written information, provides counseling, and refers callers to treatment centers and support groups weekdays from 9 a.m. to 3 a.m. and weekends from noon to 3 a.m. Eastern time.

ALZHEIMER'S DISEASE

☎ **Alzheimer's Association** (800-272-3900) provides written information and referrals to local chapters weekdays from 8:30 a.m. to 5 p.m. Central time.
Web site: http://www.alz.org/

☎ **Alzheimer's Disease Education and Referral Center** (800-438-4380) answers questions, provides written materials, makes referrals to research centers for diagnosis and treatment, provides information on state services for patients, publishes information on research, and provides an on-line database of information weekdays from 8:30 a.m. to 5 p.m. Eastern time.
Web site: http://www.alzheimers.org/adear

AMYOTROPHIC LATERAL SCLEROSIS (Lou Gehrig's disease)

☎ **Amyotrophic Lateral Sclerosis (ALS) Association, National Office** (800-782-4747) answers questions, supplies written information, and provides referrals to support groups and local chapters weekdays from 8 a.m. to 5 p.m. Pacific time.
Web site: http://www.alsa.org

ARTHRITIS

☎ **Arthritis Foundation** (800-283-7800) sends written information on treatment and local chapters to callers who leave their names and addresses on its answering machine. Callers also may listen to taped information.
Web site: http://www.arthritis.org

☎ **The American Lupus Society** (800-331-1802) sends written information to those who leave their names and addresses on its answering machine.

☎ **Lupus Foundation of America** (800-558-0121) provides written information to those who leave their names and addresses on its answering machine.

ASTHMA AND LUNG DISORDERS

☎ **Asthma and Allergy Foundation of America** (800-7-ASTHMA) provides free written information weekdays from 9 a.m. to 5 p.m. Eastern time.

☎ **Lungline** (800-222-LUNG) provides written information on respiratory and immunological problems and an opportunity to speak with registered nurses weekdays from 8 a.m. to 5 p.m. Mountain time.
Web site: http://www.hjc.org

ATTENTION-DEFICIT DISORDER

☎ **National Attention-Deficit Disorder Association** (800-487-2282) provides written information, including referrals to local support groups, to people who leave their names and addresses on its answering machine.

BLADDER DISORDERS

☎ **Bladder Health Council** (800-242-2383) operated by the American Foundation for Urologic Disease provides written materials on bladder cancer and urinary tract infections weekdays from 8:30 a.m. to 5:30 p.m. Eastern time. Callers can also obtain information on other urologic disorders, such as prostate disease, kidney disease, and sexual function.
Web site: http://www.access.digex.net~afud

BRAIN INJURY

☎ **Brain Injury Association Family Help Line** (formerly National Head Injury Foundation) (800-444-6443) answers questions, provides written information, and makes referrals to local resources weekdays from 9 a.m. to 5 p.m. Eastern time.

CANCER

☎ **Cancer Information Service** (800-4-CANCER) of the National Cancer Institute answers questions and provides written information and referrals to treatment centers, mammography facilities, and support groups weekdays from 9 a.m. to 4:30 p.m. local time. Hearing-impaired people can reach the service by TDD at 800-332-8615.
Web site: http://www.icic.nci.nih.gov

☎ **Cancer Response System (CRS)** (800-ACS-2345) of the American Cancer Society (ACS) provides written information and referrals to local ACS programs and resources weekdays from 9 a.m. to 5 p.m. local time.
Web site: http://www.cancer.org

☎ **Y-ME National Breast Cancer Organization** (800-221-2141) allows callers to speak to counselors who have survived breast cancer; offers a men's hot line staffed by male counselors; provides written information; and supplies wigs and prostheses to women who cannot afford them. The line operates 7 days a week, 24 hours a day. Spanish speakers may call 800-986-9505.
Web site: http://www.y-me.org

☎ **Prostate Cancer Support Network** (800-828-7866) sends written information and provides referrals to local support groups weekdays from 8:30 a.m. to 5:00 p.m. Eastern time.
Web site: http://www.access.digex.net~afud

CHILD ABUSE AND NEGLECT

☎ **American Human Association, Children's Division** (800-227-4645) answers questions and provides written information weekdays from 8:30 a.m. to 4:30 p.m. Mountain time.

☎ **Boys Town National Hotline** (800-448-3000) provides counseling to young people and adults and makes referrals to local counselors, shelters, and social services 24 hours a day, 7 days a week.

☎ **Childhelp/IOF Foresters National Child Abuse Hotline** (800-4 A CHILD) provides trained professional counselors for crisis intervention 24 hours a day, 7 days a week. Written information and referrals to local resources and agencies for assistance with issues related to child abuse, adult survivors of abuse, domestic violence, and parenting are also available. Hearing impaired people can reach the hot line at 800-2 A CHILD.

CHRONIC FATIGUE SYNDROME

☎ **Chronic Fatigue and Immune Dysfunction Syndrome Association of America** (800-442-3437) provides free information, including lists of local support groups, to callers who leave a message on their answering machine.

CROHN'S DISEASE AND COLITIS

☎ **Crohn's and Colitis Foundation of America,** Inc. (800-932-2423) provides written information and referrals to physicians and support groups weekdays from 9 a.m. to 5 p.m. Eastern time. Callers can speak to a counselor weekdays from 2:15 to 4 p.m. Eastern time.
E-mail: mhda37b@prodigy.com

CYSTIC FIBROSIS

☎ **Cystic Fibrosis Foundation** (800-FIGHT CF) provides written information and referrals to accredited cystic fibrosis care centers weekdays from 8:30 a.m. to 5:30 p.m. Eastern time.

DIABETES

☎ **American Diabetes Association** (800-ADA-DISC) answers questions and provides written information weekdays from 8:30 a.m. to 5 p.m. Eastern time.

☎ **Juvenile Diabetes Foundation International Hot Line** (800-223-1138) answers general questions and supplies written information weekdays from 9 a.m. to 5 p.m. Eastern time.
E-mail: info@jdfcure.com
Web site: http://www.jdfcure.com

DISABILITY AND REHABILITATION

☎ **National Rehabilitation Information Center** (800-346-2742) acts as a library on topics relating to disability and rehabilitation by searching databases and providing written information. The center also answers questions and provides referrals weekdays from 8 a.m. to 6 p.m. Eastern time.
Web site: http://www.naric.com/naric

DOWN SYNDROME

☎ **National Down Syndrome Society Hot Line** (800-221-4602) answers questions, supplies written information, and provides referrals to local parent-support groups weekdays from 9 a.m. to 5 p.m. Eastern time.
Web site: http://www.pcsltd.com/ndss/

DRINKING WATER

☎ **Safe Drinking Water Hot Line** (800-426-4791), operated under contract for the Environmental Protection Agency, answers questions and provides written information about federal regulation of public water weekdays from 9 a.m. to 5:30 p.m. Eastern time.

DYSLEXIA

☎ **The Orton Dyslexia Society** (800-222-3123) sends written information to callers who leave their names and addresses on its answering machine. Staff members answer questions at 410-296-0232 weekdays from 8:30 a.m. to 4:30 p.m. Eastern time.

ELDERLY

☎ **Eldercare Locator** (800-677-1116) answers questions, provides written information, and makes referrals to local support groups and sources of assistance for the elderly weekdays from 9 a.m. to 11 p.m. Eastern time.

EPILEPSY

☎ **Epilepsy Foundation of America** (800-EFA-1000) answers questions; provides information; and makes referrals to physicians, local support groups, and organizations that supply assistance with issues such as employment and legal matters weekdays from 9 a.m. to 5 p.m. Eastern time. If the line is busy, the foundation can be reached at 301-459-3700.
E-mail: postmaster@efa.org
Web site: http://www.efa.org

EYES AND VISION

☎ **American Council of the Blind** (800-424-8666) answers questions, makes referrals, and provides information on consumer items for blind people weekdays from 3 to 5:30 p.m. Eastern time. At all other times, an answering service provides updates on legislation affecting the blind.
Web site: http://www.acb.org

☎ **Guide Dog Foundation for the Blind, Inc.** (800-548-4337) provides guide dogs free of charge to qualified people who are legally blind. The toll-free line has information specialists who answer questions weekdays from 8 a.m. to 5:15 p.m. Eastern time. An answering service operates outside those hours.
E-mail: ebiegel@guidedog.org
Web site: http://www.guidedog.org

☎ **National Association for Parents of the Visually Impaired** (800-562-6265) answers questions and provides referrals to support groups weekdays from 9 a.m. to 5 p.m. Eastern time.

☎ **National Eye Care Project** (800-222-EYES) provides referrals to physicians who treat on a volunteer basis people 65 years and older who are unable to afford eye care. Callers also can request written materials on various subjects related to the eyes. The line operates weekdays from 8 a.m. to 4 p.m. Pacific time.

☎ **National Eye Research Foundation** (800-621-2258) answers questions, sends out written information, and provides referrals weekdays from 9 a.m. to 5 p.m. Central time.
E-mail: nerf1955@aol.com

☎ **Prevent Blindness America** (800-331-2020) answers general questions and provides written information on eye health and safety weekdays from 8 a.m. to 5 p.m. Central time.
E-mail: 74777.100@compuserve.com
Web site: http://www.prevent-blindness.org

FOOD AND NUTRITION

☎ **Consumer Nutrition Hot Line** (800-366-1655) of the American Dietetic Association's National Center for Nutrition and Dietetics provides registered dietitians who answer questions on food and nutrition and provides referrals to local dietitians weekdays from 9 a.m. to 4 p.m. Central time. Callers can listen to taped messages on food and nutrition from 8 a.m. to 8 p.m. Central time.
Web site: http://www/.eatright.org

☎ **Meat and Poultry Hot Line** (800-535-4555), operated by the United States Department of Agriculture, provides an opportunity to speak to a food safety specialist weekdays from 10 a.m. to 4 p.m. Eastern time. Callers can listen to recorded messages 24 hours a day.
Web site: http://www.usda.gov/agency/fsis/homepage.htm

☎ **Seafood Hot Line** (800-FDA-4010), operated by the United States Food and Drug Administration, provides written information and answers questions weekdays from noon to 4 p.m. Eastern time. Taped messages are provided 24 hours a day.
Web site: http://www.fda.gov/

FEET

☎ **Foot Care Information Center** (800-FOOT CARE), operated by the American Podiatric Medical Association, provides written materials and information on how to obtain local physician referrals to callers who leave their names and addresses on its voice mail.

GENERAL HEALTH AND SAFETY

☎ **Agency for Health Care Policy and Research** (800-358-9295), operated by the Public Health Service, provides written information on a variety of health-related topics weekdays from 9 a.m. to 5 p.m. Eastern time.
Web site: http://www.ahcpr.gov

☎ **Auto Safety Hot Line** (800-424-9393) provides taped information on recalls, crash-test results, tire quality, and other automotive safety topics 24 hours a day, 7 days a week. Callers can also obtain written information and report auto safety problems.
Web site: http://www.nhtsa.dot.gov/index.

☎ **Consumer Product Safety Commission Hot Line** (800-638-2772) provides taped information on product recalls, corrective actions, and other product safety questions 24 hours a day, 7 days a week. Callers also can file complaints about unsafe products.

☎ **Medic Alert Foundation** (800-825-3785) operates a worldwide medical information service. Members receive a pendant that alerts medical personnel to wearer's medical conditions, allergies, or medications. Members also are registered with a 24-hour emergency response center that transmits vital medical facts worldwide.
E-mail: info@medicalert.org

☎ **National Health Information Center** (800-336-4797) provides referrals to national health organizations and support groups weekdays from 1 p.m. to 5 p.m. Eastern time. Recorded messages about some organizations can be heard 24 hours a day.
E-mail: nhicinfo@health.org
Web site: http://nhic-nt.health.org

GENETIC DISEASES

☎ **Alliance of Genetic Support Groups** (800-336-GENE) provides callers with information on how to contact genetic services and national support groups for various genetic disorders weekdays from 9 a.m. to 5 p.m. Eastern time.
Web site: http://medhelp.org/www/agsg.htm
E-mail: alliance@capaccess.org

HEADACHE

☎ **National Headache Foundation** (800-843-2256) answers questions, supplies written information, provides referrals to support groups, and offers audiotapes, books and a videotape for sale weekdays from 9 a.m. to 5 p.m. Central time.
Web site: http://www.headaches.org

HEARING

☎ **American Speech-Language-Hearing Information Resource Center** (800-638-8255) provides information on speech, language, and hearing disorders as well as referrals weekdays from 8:30 a.m. to 5 p.m. Eastern time.
Web site: http://www.asha.org

☎ **Dial a Hearing Screening Test** (800-222-EARS) answers questions, sends written information, and makes referrals to local physicians, audiologists, and hearing-aid specialists weekdays from 9 a.m. to 5 p.m. Eastern time. The organization also puts callers in touch with regional centers that give free hearing screening tests over the phone.
E-mail: dabiddle@aol.com

☎ **Hearing Aid Help Line** (800-521-5247), operated by the International Hearing Society, answers questions, sends written information on hearing aids and hearing loss, and makes referrals to local hearing-aid specialists weekdays from 10 a.m. to 4 p.m. Eastern time.

☎ **Hearing HelpLine** (800-EAR-WELL) provides written information weekdays from 9 a.m. to 5 p.m. Eastern time.

HEART DISEASE

☎ **American Heart Association** (800-AHA-USA-1) provides written information on cholesterol and all aspects of heart disease as well as referrals to local chapters weekdays during local business hours.
Web site: http://www.amhrt.org

HEPATITIS

☎ **Hepatitis/Liver Disease Hotline** (800-223-HEPABC), operated by the American Liver Foundation, answers questions, provides written information, and makes referrals to physicians and local support groups weekdays from 9 a.m. to 5 p.m. Eastern time.
Web site: http://sadieo.ucsf.edu/alf/alffinal/homepagealt.html

HOSPICE CARE

☎ **National Hospice Organization** (800-658-8898) provides written information and answers general questions on hospice and makes referrals to local hospices weekdays from 8:30 a.m. to 5 p.m. Eastern time.
E-mail: drsnho@cais.com
Web site: http://www.nho.org

HUNTINGTON'S DISEASE

☎ **Huntington's Disease Society of America** (800-345-4372) provides written information to callers who leave their names and addresses on its answering machine 24 hours a day, 7 days a week.
Web site: http://neuro-www2.mgh.harvard.edu/hdsa/hdsamain.nclk

HYPERTENSION

☎ **National Heart, Lung, and Blood Institute's Information Line** (800-575-WELL) mails written information on high blood pressure and high blood cholesterol to callers who leave their names and addresses on its answering machine.

IMMUNIZATION

☎ **National Immunization Campaign** (800-525-6789) sends information to people who leave a message on their answering machine.

INCONTINENCE

☎ **The Simon Foundation for Continence** (800-237-4666) provides free written information and sample products 24 hours a day, 7 days a week.

KIDNEY DISEASE

☎ **American Association of Kidney Patients** (800-749-2257) provides free written information and makes referrals to local support groups weekdays from 8:30 a.m. to 5 p.m. Eastern time.
E-mail: AAKPNat@aol.com

☎ **National Kidney Foundation** (800-622-9010) answers questions and provides written information on various types of kidney disease, research, dialysis, transplants, and diet weekdays from 8:30 a.m. to 5:30 p.m. Eastern time.

LEAD POISONING

☎ **National Lead Information Hot Line** (800-LEAD-FYI) provides written information on preventing lead poisoning and referrals to agencies that can provide further information to callers who leave their addresses and phone numbers on its answering machine. People who are hearing impaired may call 800-526-5456.

LIVING WILLS

☎ **Choice in Dying** (800-989-9455) provides free legal, medical, and mental health counseling and crisis intervention weekdays from 9 a.m. to 5 p.m. Eastern time. For a small charge, callers can also obtain state-specific materials for preparing living wills and medical power of attorney documents.
E-mail: cid@choices.org
Web site: http://www.choices.org

MARFAN SYNDROME

☎ **National Marfan Foundation** (800-8-MAR-FAN) answers questions, sends written information, and makes referrals to local support groups weekdays from 8 a.m. to 3:30 p.m. Eastern time.
Web site: http://www.marfan.org

MENTAL ILLNESS

☎ **National Alliance for the Mentally Ill** (800-950-6264) provides written information and makes referrals to support groups to callers who leave their names and addresses on its answering machine. Callers may speak to an information specialist weekdays between 9 a.m. and 5 p.m. Eastern time.
E-mail: namiofc@aol.com
Web site: http://www.cais.com/vikings/nami/index.html

☎ **National Institute of Mental Health** (800-421-4211) sends written information on clinical depression to those who leave their names and addresses on its voice mail.

☎ **National Foundation for Depressive Illness** (800-248-4344) provides a recorded message describing the symptoms of depression and manic depression, and an address where further information is available.

☎ **National Mental Health Association** (800-969-6642) supplies written information on more than 200 mental health topics, makes referrals to local mental health providers, and provides a directory of local mental health associations to callers who leave their names and addresses on its voice mail.

☎ **Panic Disorder Information Line** (800-64-PANIC), operated by the National Institute of Mental Health, provides written information weekdays from 9 a.m. to 9 p.m. Eastern time.
Web site: http://www.nimh.nih.gov

MULTIPLE SCLEROSIS

☎ **Multiple Sclerosis Association of America** (800-833-4672; 800-LEARN MS) provides an opportunity to speak with peer counselors and health-care counselors weekdays between 9 a.m. and 6 p.m. Eastern time. Callers also can request written information and referrals to local support groups as well as obtain information on the association's equipment loan program, symptom-management research and therapies, and barrier-free construction assistance.

☎ **National Multiple Sclerosis Society** (800-FIGHT-MS) provides educational information about MS, counseling, family and social support, equipment assistance, clinical trials, and employment programs. Callers seeking local services are transferred automatically to their nearest chapters or can speak to trained national staff weekdays from 11 a.m. to 5 p.m. Eastern time.
E-mail: info@nmss.org
Web site: http://www.nmss.org

MYASTHENIA GRAVIS

☎ **Myasthenia Gravis Foundation of America, Inc.** (800-541-5454) answers questions and provides written information weekdays from 8:45 a.m. to 4:45 p.m. Central time.
E-mail: mgfa@aol.com
Web site: http://www.med.unc.edu/mgfa/

NEUROLOGICAL DISORDERS

☎ **National Institute of Neurological Disorders and Stroke** (800-352-9424) answers questions, provides written information, and makes referrals to local agencies weekdays from 8:30 a.m. to 5 p.m. Eastern time.
Web site: http://www.nih.gov/ninds/

ORGAN DONATION

☎ **United Network for Organ Sharing** (800-243-6667) sends organ donor cards and written information to callers who leave their names and addresses on its answering machine.

OSTEOPOROSIS

☎ **National Osteoporosis Foundation** (800-223-9994) provides written information 24 hours a day, 7 days a week.
Web site: http:www.nof.org

PARENTING AND CHILDBIRTH

☎ **La Leche League Help Line** (800-LA LECHE) answers questions and provides written information weekdays from 9 a.m. to 3 p.m. Central time.

☎ **Depression After Delivery Information Request Line** (800-944-4773) sends written information to callers who leave their names and addresses on its answering machine.

PARKINSON DISEASE

☎ **American Parkinson Disease Association, Inc.** (800-223-2732) sends written information, loans videotapes, and makes referrals to local referral centers weekdays from 9 a.m. to 5 p.m. Eastern time. Outside these hours, callers may leave a message on its answering machine.
E-mail: apda@admin.con2.com
Web site: http://neuro-chief-e.mgh.harvard.edu/parkinsonsweb/main/pdmain.html

☎ **National Parkinson Foundation Inc.** (800-327-4545; 800-433-7022 within Florida) answers questions and provides referrals weekdays from 8 a.m. to 5 p.m. Eastern time. An answering machine takes messages outside these hours.

PREMENSTRUAL SYNDROME

☎ **PMS Access** (800-222-4767) provides recorded information and sends written information to callers who leave their names and addresses on its answering machine.

RARE DISORDERS

☎ **Office of Orphan Products Development** (800-300-7469), operated by the United States Food and Drug Administration, sends written information and answers questions on the development of drugs and biological products to treat rare diseases weekdays from 8 a.m. to 5 p.m. Eastern time.

☎ **National Organization for Rare Disorders** (800-999-6673) collects and provides information on more than 1,000 rare disorders and refers victims of rare disorders to information networks weekdays from 9 a.m. to 5 p.m. Eastern time. NORD also makes referrals to other organizations, support groups, clearing houses, patient services, and registries pertaining to specific rare disorders. An answering machine operates outside regular hours.
E-mail: orphan@nord-rdb.com
Web site: http://www.nord-rdb.com/~orphan

REYE'S SYNDROME

☎ **National Reye's Syndrome Foundation** (800-233-7393) answers questions and provides written information weekdays from 8 a.m. to noon and 1 p.m. to 5 p.m. Eastern time.

SCLERODERMA

☎ **United Scleroderma Foundation** (800-722-HOPE) answers questions; provides written information; and makes referrals to physicians, local chapters, and support groups weekdays from 8 a.m. to 5 p.m. Pacific time.
Web site: http://www.scleroderma.com

SEXUALLY TRANSMITTED DISEASES

☎ **Centers for Disease Control National STD Hot Line** (800-227-8922) answers questions and provides written information and referrals weekdays from 8 a.m. to 11 p.m. Eastern time.
Web site: http://sunsite.unc.edu/ASHA/

SICKLE CELL ANEMIA

☎ **Sickle Cell Disease Association of America Inc.** (800-421-8453) answers general questions, provides educational materials, and makes referrals to physicians and local chapters weekdays from 8:30 a.m. to 5 p.m. Pacific time.

SPINA BIFIDA

☎ **Spina Bifida Information and Referral** (800-621-3141) sends written information 24 hours and day, 7 days a week to callers who leave their names and addresses on its answering machine.

SPINAL CORD INJURY OR DISORDER

☎ **National Spinal Cord Injury Association** (800-962-9629) answers questions, provides written information, makes referrals to facilities, and puts callers in touch with local chapters that know of support groups. The line operates weekdays from 10 a.m. to 2 p.m. Eastern time.
Web site: http://[to come-call]

☎ **National Spinal Cord Injury Hot Line** (800-526-3456) answers questions weekdays from 9 a.m. to 5 p.m. Eastern time. The hot line also makes referrals to peer support groups, rehabilitation centers, housing advice, and sources of other information to assist people who have suffered paralyzing spinal cord injuries.
E-mail: scihotline@aol.com
Web site: http://users.aol.com/scihotline

☎ **Spondylitis Association of America** (800-777-8189) sends written information to callers who leave their names and addresses on its answering machine, and returns the calls of those who leave a phone number. The association also operates an on-line chat room at firenze@aol.com
Web site: http://www.usa.net/welcome/saapage.html

STROKE

☎ **American Heart Association Stroke Connection** (800-553-6321) makes referrals to agencies and support groups and provides written information weekdays from 8:30 a.m. to 5 p.m. Central time. An answering service operates outside regular hours.
Web site: http://www.amhrt.org/stroke

☎ **National Stroke Association** (800-STROKES) answers questions and provides written information about stroke and stroke prevention Monday through Thursday from 8 a.m. to 4:30 p.m. and Friday from 8 a.m. to 4 p.m. Mountain time.
E-mail: info@stroke.org
Web site: http://www.stroke.org

STUTTERING

☎ **National Center for Stuttering** (800-221-2483) answers questions, offers suggestions for parents of children who have begun to stutter, makes referrals, and provides written information weekdays from 9:30 a.m. to 5:30 p.m. Eastern time.
Web site: http://www.stuttering.com

☎ **Stuttering Foundation of America** (800-992-9392) answers questions, provides written material, and supplies a list of specialists weekdays from 9 a.m. to 5 p.m. Eastern time.

SUDDEN INFANT DEATH SYNDROME

☎ **American SIDS Institute** (800-232-7437; 800-847-7437 within Georgia) provides the opportunity to talk with a doctor or social worker weekdays between 9 a.m. and 5 p.m. Eastern time. Also sends written information and makes referrals to local support groups. After regular hours, an answering service at the same number will page a doctor or social worker.
E-mail: prevent@sids.org
Web site: http://www.sids.org

☎ **SIDS Alliance** (800-221-7437) provides written information and referrals to support groups weekdays from 9 a.m. to 5 p.m. Eastern time. The alliance also allows SIDS families to speak to a counselor 24 hours a day.

THYROID DISORDERS

☎ **Thyroid Foundation of America** (800-832-8321) provides written information and referrals to physicians weekdays from 8:30 a.m. to 4 p.m. Eastern time.

TOURETTE SYNDROME

☎ **Tourette Syndrome Association** (800-237-0717) sends written information to callers who write to the address given on the answering machine. Callers can speak to an information specialist for referrals to physicians and local chapters by calling 718-224-2999 weekdays between 9 a.m. and 5 p.m. Eastern time.

VICTIMS OF VIOLENCE

☎ **National Victim Center** (800-FYI CALL) answers questions, sends written materials, and makes referrals to local support groups and organizations for victims of violence weekdays from 9 a.m. to 5:30 p.m. Eastern time.
E-mail: nvc@mail.nvc.org
Web site: http://www.nvc.org

INDEX

How to use the index

This index covers the contents of the 1995, 1996, and 1997 editions of *The World Book Health & Medical Annual.*

Each entry gives the last two digits of the edition year and the page number or numbers. For example, this entry means that information on stomach acid may be found on pages 98 through 105 of the 1997 edition.

When there are many references to a topic, they are grouped alphabetically by clue words under the main topic. For example, the clue words under the general reference for *stress* group the other references under several subtopics.

An entry in all capital letters indicates that there is a Health Updates article with that name in at least one of the three volumes covered by this index. References to the topic may also appear after the topic name.

An entry that only begins with a capital letter indicates that there are no Health Updates articles with that title but that information on this topic may be found in the edition and on the pages listed.

The "see" and "see also" cross-references indicate that references to the topic are listed under another entry in the index.

The indication (il.) after a page number means that the reference is to an illustration only.

A

D

E

F

G

H

N

O

P

Q

R

S

T

Acknowledgments

The publishers of *The World Book Health & Medical Annual* gratefully acknowledge the courtesy of the following artists, photographers, publishers, institutions, agencies, and corporations for the illustrations in this volume. Credits should read from top to bottom, left to right on their respective pages. All entries marked with an asterisk (*) denote illustrations created exclusively for *The World Book Health & Medical Annual*. All maps, charts, and diagrams were prepared by *The World Book Health & Medical Annual* staff unless otherwise noted.

2 Michael Rosenfeld, Tony Stone Images; Skjold, The Image Works
3 John Manders*; Ron Chapple, FPG
4 Eileen Mueller Neill*; Telegraph Colour Library from FPG; Charles Welleck*; Dan Osborn*
5 John Zielinski*; Remi Benali, Gamma/Liaison; Candela Laser Corporation; Bob Thomas, Tony Stone Images
10 Bob Schatz, Gamma/Liaison; Bill Nation, Sygma; Mark Richards, PhotoEdit; David Waldorf, FPG
11 Gary Buss, FPG; Erin Elders, *McClean's* Magazine
13 T. Orban, Sygma; Bob Schatz, Gamma/Liaison
16 Based upon Yerkes and Dodson's Law, *Journal of Comparative Neurology and Psychology*, 1908
18 Mark Richards, PhotoEdit
23 Erin Elders, *McClean's* Magazine
27 Gary Buss, FPG
28-29 Joe Rogers*
31 Bill Nation, Sygma
33 David Waldorf, FPG
36-37 Joe Rogers*
40 Eileen Mueller Neill*; Bill Goes*; Bill Goes*; Telegraph Colour Library from FPG
41 Charles Welleck*; Charles Welleck*; Ron Chapple, FPG
43-54 Eileen Mueller Neill*
56-57 Bill Goes*
59 Barbara Cousins*
60-62 Bill Goes*
70-71 Ron Chapple, FPG
73 Ciba Pharmaceuticals; Jeff Guerrant*; Jeff Guerrant*
75 Ron Chapple, FPG
76 L. Steinmark, Custom Medical
82 Telegraph Colour Library from FPG
88 Chuck Savage, The Stock Market
89 Dick Luria, FPG
91 Superstock
94 Ron Chapple, FPG
98 Bill Goes*
101 Barbara Cousins*
106 Bill Goes*
109-113 Charles Wellek*
116 Dan Osborn*
122 Custom Medical; John Zielinski*
123 John Zielinski*; Kathryn Adams*
124-136 John Zielinski*
140-146 Kathryn Adams*
148 Nathan Benn, Stock, Boston
150 Michael Newman, PhotoEdit
151 Mary Kate Denny, PhotoEdit
154 Custom Medical
156 Roger Phillips, Bausch & Lomb
157-158 Linda Kinnaman*
160 Custom Medical
164 John Manders*; Will & Deni McIntyre, Photo Researchers; Michael Rosenfeld, Tony Stone Images; John Manders*
165 Candela Laser Corporation; Kristin Mount*
166-170 John Manders*
171 Remi Benali, Gamma/Liaison
174 U.S. Department of Agriculture and U.S. Department of Health & Human Services
175 © 1978 George A. Bray; NYT Graphics
176 John Manders*
177 Reprinted with permission from *Eat For Life: The Food and Nutrition Board's Guide to Reducing Your Risk of Chronic Disease* © 1992 National Academy of Sciences; National Academy Press
181 Will & Deni McIntyre, Photo Researchers
182 Barbara Cousins*
185 Barbara Cousins*; Dan McCoy, Rainbow
186 Custom Medical; Custom Medical; David McDaniel, M.D., Laser Center of Virginia
187 David McDaniel, M.D., Laser Center of Virginia; Sherri L. Rowen, M.D.; Sherri L. Rowen, M.D.
188 Barbara Cousins*
190 Alexander Tsiaras/SS from Photo Researchers
191 Candela Laser Corporation
192 Fritz Hoffman, JB Pictures
194 NIBSC/SPL from Photo Researchers; Bobbeh, *Figaro* from Gamma/Liaison
197 Barbara Cousins*
201 Barbara Cousins*; Barbara Cousins*; Barbara Cousins*; Michael Rosenfeld, Tony Stone Images
203 Hank Morgan, Photo Researchers; Barbara Cousins*; Barbara Cousins*
206 Hank Morgan, Photo Researchers
208-212 Kristin Mount*

216 Alexander Tsiaras/SS from Photo Researchers; SIU from Photo Researchers; Wedgeworth, Custom Medical; Kristin Mount*
218-219 Kristin Mount*
220 L. Steinmark, Custom Medical
222 Peter Lamberti, Tony Stone Images; Bob Thomas, Tony Stone Images; David Silberswig, M.D., Cornell Medical Center; Myrleen Ferguson, PhotoEdit; Robert Pearcy, Animals Animals
223 Ralph Wetmore, Tony Stone Images
224 Skjold, The Image Works
226 Brian Palmer, *U.S. News & World Report*
227 AP/Wide World
233 Ralph Wetmore, Tony Stone Images
239 Ann States, SABA
240 Charles Y. C. Pak, University of Texas Southwestern Medical Center
242-243 Jeff Guerrant*
245 Barbara Cousins*
250 Advanced Technology Laboratories
252 Nina Berman, Sipa Press
253 Myrleen Ferguson, PhotoEdit
258 Bayer Corporation
266 AP/Wide World
267 Frank Pedrick, The Image Works
270 Bob Thomas, Tony Stone Images
271 John Carnett, © 1996 *Popular Science*
272 Barbara Cousins*
273 Tony Freeman, PhotoEdit
274 Biophoto/SS from Photo Researchers
275 Peter Lamberti, Tony Stone Images
276 Chien-Chi Chang, *The Baltimore Sun*
279 Theratech/Brown and Powers
281 Susan Van Etten, PhotoEdit
283 AP/Wide World
285 Mark S. Scott, Harbor-UCLA Research and Education Institute
289 Alex Bartel/SPL from Photo Researchers
290 Robert Grossman, NYT Pictures
292 AP/Wide World
294 David Silberswig, M.D., Cornell Medical Center
305 AP/Wide World
306 Robert Daemmrich, Tony Stone Images
309 Barbara Cousins*
311 Centers for Disease Control and Prevention
315 Campaign for Tobacco-Free Kids
316-317 Barbara Cousins*
319 Vista Medical Technologies
323 Robert Pearcy, Animals Animals
325 Procter & Gamble Company